D1250743

How Snakes Work

How Snakes Work

Structure, Function, and Behavior of
the World's Snakes

Harvey B. Lillywhite

OXFORD
UNIVERSITY PRESS

OXFORD
UNIVERSITY PRESS

Oxford University Press is a department of the University of Oxford.
It furthers the University's objective of excellence in research,
scholarship, and education by publishing worldwide.

Oxford   New York
Auckland   Cape Town   Dar es Salaam   Hong Kong   Karachi
Kuala Lumpur   Madrid   Melbourne   Mexico City   Nairobi
New Delhi   Shanghai   Taipei   Toronto

With offices in
Argentina   Austria   Brazil   Chile   Czech Republic   France   Greece
Guatemala   Hungary   Italy   Japan   Poland   Portugal   Singapore
South Korea   Switzerland   Thailand   Turkey   Ukraine   Vietnam

Oxford is a registered trade mark of Oxford University Press
in the UK and certain other countries.

Published in the United States of America by
Oxford University Press
198 Madison Avenue, New York, NY 10016

Library of Congress Cataloging-in-Publication Data
Lillywhite, Harvey B., 1943–
How snakes work : structure, function, and behavior of the world's snakes / Harvey B. Lillywhite.
    pages   cm
ISBN 978-0-19-538037-8 (alk. paper)
1. Snakes. I. Title.
QL666.O6L724   2014
597.96—dc23   2013019018

9 8 7 6 5 4 3 2 1

Printed in China
on acid-free paper

This book is dedicated to

Rodolfo Ruibal,

George Bartholomew, and

Kenneth Norris,

who inspired and mentored my passion

for discovery and science.

CONTENTS

FOREWORD

We share this beautiful planet with an astonishing array of different kinds of creatures, but few are as remarkable as snakes. Some people worship snakes, some are terrified of them, and some even keep them as pets. Despite a wide public interest in serpents, however, we still know very little about the day-to-day lives of most species—including really basic issues such as how they move around, find food or mates, or influence the ecosystems in which they occur.

Dedicated field biologists like Harvey Lillywhite are shedding new light on these questions. Over his long career, Harvey has pioneered many new insights into snake biology—not just in the laboratory, but also out in the field, where he can explore an animal's functioning in the conditions that it actually encounters. Harvey has worked on a very wide variety of snake species, in many parts of the world, and thus brings a truly broad perspective to this engaging book. Importantly, Harvey is one of the very few researchers to have focused on the physiology of snakes—that is, the ways that these mysterious animals deal with basic challenges such as finding, capturing, and digesting their food, maintaining their water balance, and regulating their body temperature. By embedding his research in the field biology of his study animals, Harvey has revealed the fascinating complexity and elegance of these much-misunderstood creatures.

This book brings together a lifetime of experience, to explain in easy-to-understand terms what snakes do, and how and why they do it. I am sure that this attractive volume not only will educate people about snakes, but also will inspire its readers and help them to understand why we need to conserve these amazing creatures for future generations.

—*Rick Shine, Sydney, January 2013*

PREFACE

Since childhood I have marveled at the sleek form, rich colors, and absolutely intriguing behaviors of snakes. Having no limbs, these reptiles possess incredible stealth, grace, and beauty. They exhibit a wonderful capacity for actions that amuse, startle, or evoke intense curiosity. Snakes live in a rich variety of habitats, from oceans to rocky hillsides, from subterranean spaces to open sand deserts. They have evolved colors and patterns that awaken the artist, and they have inspired mythical reverence and respect from many cultures. They persistently survive, and yet they are perhaps the most maligned group of vertebrates—misunderstood by far too many humans who carry out death sentences at every opportunity.

For many years I have planned to write a book about snakes, one that is intended to interest both the general reader and professionals. There are numerous books that have been written about snakes—gems of information as well as collections of great photographs. As more and more books appeared with snakes as their subjects, I had cause to ponder how I might make a meaningful contribution in the form of another "snake book." My professional training and much of my career as a scientist has been related to physiology and the subdiscipline that is generally known as "physiological ecology." My perspectives are quite broad, however, and much of what interests me as a research scientist involves interdisciplinary investigation and integrative studies of structure, function, and behavior—focused with questions related to the ecology and natural world of the animals that fascinate me. The majority of books that have been written about snakes provide relatively little in-depth coverage of these topics, and none to my knowledge focuses on physiology—or structure and function—as the principal subject of treatment. Thus, I decided to write this book, which specifically targets this "niche" of subject matter.

There are comparatively few persons with rigorous training in physiology who focus their research on snakes, and many of the persons with physiological training who do investigate snakes at one time or another may not have a background of knowledge that includes extensive firsthand field experience as well as a passionate appreciation for the natural history of this group of animals. Thus, I hope that in some manner I might bring a unique perspective to the subject matter, and to cover a range of topics in this book that will interest a wide group of readers. Snakes are wonderful animals, and they have become very popular in the pet trade as well as a high-priority attraction at zoological parks. As one begins to understand and appreciate their inner "workings," snakes become even more fascinating and evoke even greater emotional as well as intellectual response. My sincerest hope is that readers of this book will find enjoyment in discovering new knowledge, increased curiosity, and a greater respect for a group of animals that reflect an amazing amount of innovation and success in life's evolutionary game. Insofar as possible, I have attempted to illustrate the many fascinating features of snakes—sometimes related to complex or difficult concepts—using photographs instead of relying on dense and tedious text. I shall be extremely delighted if many persons enjoy reading this book as much as I have enjoyed producing it.

To assist readers with understanding the terminology that is used throughout the book, I have defined many useful and specialized terms in the glossary. I have avoided the use of equations or complicated graphs, but I have provided lists of additional readings that provide roads to further—often more technical—presentation of the subject matter. Such readings are listed at the end of each chapter, and they include articles by the authors who are mentioned specifically in the text.

ACKNOWLEDGMENTS

I owe a debt of gratitude to many persons who helped to make this book possible. First, I thank my parents, who allowed me to keep snakes at home when I was a very young boy. Reluctant at first, they encouraged me in very important ways as it became evident that my interest in snakes began to open many other doors in the world of science and learning. I am equally indebted to my wife Jamie, who has assisted me with patience, tolerance, and also encouragement for a meaningful project. My son and daughter, Steve and Shauna, have also been supportive in various important ways.

I am grateful to the many persons who have contributed to the illustrations, both photographs and drawings. These include Dan Dourson, Coleman Sheehy, Elliott Jacobson, Jason Bourque, Rom Whitaker, Laurie Vitt, Gowri Shankar, Richard Shine, Indraneil Das, John C. Murphy, Sara Murphy, Joseph Pfaller, Xavier Bonnet, Irene Arpayoglou, David and Tracy Barker, John Randall, Phil Nicodemo, Blair Hedges, Tony Crocetta, Ray Carson, Akira Mori, Ming-Chung Tu, Erik Frausing, Jesús Rivas, Dhiraj Bhaisare, Parag Dandge, Howie Choset, Thimappa, James Nifong, Lincoln Brower, Alejandro Solórzano, John Roberts, Lauren Dibben, Nicholas Millichamp, Arne Rasmussen, Amanda Ropp, Gavin Delacour, Nikolai L. Orlov, Stephen Beaupre, Guido Westhoff, Richard Sajdak, Shauna Lillywhite, Steven Lillywhite, Jake Socha, Tracy Langkilde, Mac Stone, Glenn J. Tattersall, William Montgomery, and Kanishka Ukuwela.

Numerous other persons were invaluable for contributing stimulating discussions, reviews of chapters, scientific clarification, and general support of the project. These include, but are not limited to, Coleman Sheehy III, Richard Shine, Harold Heatwole, Harry Greene, Phil Nicodemo, David Barker, Roger Seymour, Bruce Jayne, Natalia Ananjeva, François Brischoux, John C. Murphy, Michael Thompson, Paul Maderson, Michael Douglas, Bruce Means, Carl Franklin, Bruce Young, Xavier Bonnet, Matthew Edwards, Elliott Jacobson, Stephen Secor, Brad Moon, Max Nickerson, Sergio Gonzalez, Jennifer Van Deven, Joe Pfaller, Li-Wen Chang, and Lauren Dibben. There are numerous other persons—friends, associates, and students—who also deserve thanks, but who are too numerous too mention without error of missing one or two individuals.

Finally, I also express my appreciation to the editors and other production staff at Oxford University Press who encouraged me and provided professional assistance in the production of this book.

How Snakes Work

EVOLUTIONARY HISTORY AND CLASSIFICATION OF THE WORLD'S SNAKES

It has been truly said that we do not know a species until we know everything about it, its anatomy, its physiology, its development, its habits. The variations in structure in different families and genera, sometimes even in species that are placed in the same genus, have no doubt their interpretation in their varying modes of life, and the correlation of the two is a fascinating study. It is one that has been much neglected by the field naturalist. Here is a great field of research waiting for him, for it is upon the living creature that all our theories concerning the function of structure must finally be tested.

—*Malcolm A. Smith*, Reptilia and Amphibia, *vol. 3*, Serpentes *(1943), p. 2*

What Is a Snake?

If we think about snakes we might have seen, and also about other animals that look much like snakes in superficial resemblance, we begin to ponder what features there are that actually define a snake. If we focus carefully on some of the more obvious features of snakes, we can enumerate some important and potentially diagnostic characters. A *diagnostic character* is an attribute that is unique to a particular chosen taxon or group of related animals—in our case the snakes. Snakes are elongate in body form, they have no legs or arms, they are covered with scales and do not bear fur or feathers (fig. 1.1). All snakes possess a forked tongue, and they do not have external ear openings of any sort (fig. 1.2). Internally, it is important to notice that any snake we might examine has a bony and segmented vertebral column bearing ribs (fig. 1.3). All of these characteristics, however, are not diagnostic because they can be found in some other groups of animals as well.

Let us think about some other animals that we know appear superficially snakelike but are not what taxonomists or systematists call a snake. These might include eels, worms, legless lizards, and some elongate amphibians that are also without limbs. Many persons, including trained biologists, might mistake some of these animals for a snake in certain circumstances (fig. 1.4). Some species of eels, for example, resemble sea snakes in both size and color, and the distinctions are not clear when the animal is seen swimming at some distance. Upon closer inspection, of course, the eel is seen to possess gills, mouth, skin, and other features that allow us to recognize it as a fish and not a snake. Worms and limbless amphibians (caecilians) might appear very snakelike if we catch but a glimpse of one of these creatures as it slips away quickly in moist, low vegetation, or into soil beneath a log or rock that we might turn while looking for these animals. If one of these animals is in our hand, however, we note the creature—which might even be a slender and nearly legless salamander—has no scales, and its tongue is not forked. Similarly, a worm has neither scales nor a defined head with jaws, nor a vertebral column internally. So, what are the characters that determine with certainty that we have a snake and not one of these other animals?

If we explore further, we find there are other characters that are peculiar to snakes when compared with other vertebrates. The eyes of snakes appear always "open." This is because snakes have no eyelids, and the cornea is covered with a clear extension of the skin called a *spectacle* (also *brille* or *eyecap*) (fig. 1.5; also compare with fig. 1.2 and figs. 7.3, 7.4). The spectacle is fixed in place, transparent, and serves a protective function as do eyelids. This feature distinguishes snakes from many lizards, but some aquatic amphibians, cave salamanders, and some lizards also exhibit partial fusion of the skin with the eye to form a spectacle or similar structure. Thus, by itself, this feature is not explicitly diagnostic of snakes, although it is helpful in most cases.

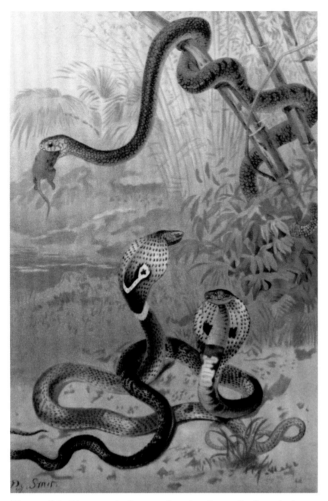

Figure 1.1. Photograph of a reproduced antique print from the late 19th century (1890–1899) featuring cobras and a rat snake eating a rodent. Original sources include Warne and Co. Ltd. (1895) and "Royal Natural History" by Richard Lydekker (1896).

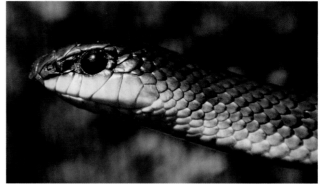

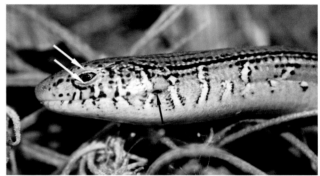

Figure 1.2. Comparison of the external characters on the head of a snake and a lizard. The **upper photo** is of a Herald Snake (*Crotaphopeltis hoamboeia*), which is an African colubrid. The **lower photo** features a legless Eastern Glass Lizard (*Ophisaurus ventralis*). Note that unlike the snake, the glass lizard has eyelids (white arrows) and an external ear opening (black arrow), whereas the only external opening on the head of the snake is the nostril that is visible near the snout. Photographs by the author.

Many snakes also possess a lightened and highly movable skull with jaws that are modified to engulf and swallow large prey items, although some groups of snakes such as blind snakes are exceptions. Many snakes also are venomous; but an even larger number of species are relatively harmless. Moreover, the Gila Monster lizard also can envenomate prey, and the saliva of varanid lizards is toxic. Thus, we need to look at still more characters.

Snakes are unlike other reptiles in that the skin undergoes synchronous shedding cycles in which the entire outer epidermis is sloughed from the body all at one time. The underlying cycle of epidermal renewal occurs also in other *lepidosaurs*—snakes, lizards, amphisbaenians, and tuatara—but the old generation of snake epidermis is typically shed as one sheet and at one time, instead of in pieces. Exceptions sometime occur in dehydrated, stressed, or older and larger snakes, which may shed patches of skin (see also discussion of blind snakes below). Normal whole-body

ecdysis (skin shedding), however, is one of the earliest phenomenological observations about snakes and is another distinct and ubiquitous characteristic of these reptiles (fig. 1.6). Some amphibians might also slough the epidermis all at once, but the shed skin does not consist of scales like that of snakes. Also, in snakes there is a vertical alternation of synthesized keratin proteins known as α and β during the renewal of epidermis in shedding cycles (see chapter 5). Only in snakes and in other lepidosaurs is this vertical alternation of keratins expressed throughout life over the entire body.

The more we examine features of snakes, the more we appreciate that a number of characteristics are shared with other vertebrates, whereas some characters are unique attributes of snakes. The shared attributes suggest relationships during evolutionary history, whereas the unique attributes evolved exclusively in the group in question and are said to be *derived*. All of these features have been useful in classifying snakes among living organisms in a manner that reflects their evolutionary history, and such a classification is reflected in a branching structure called a *phylogenetic tree*. Increasingly, molecular data related to genetic structure and

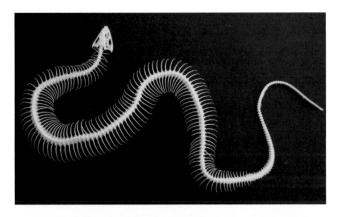

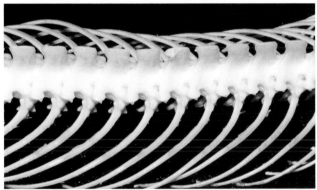

Figure 1.3. The **upper photo** features a fully articulated skeleton of a water snake (*Nerodia* spp.), photographed by Phil Nicodemo. The **lower photo** shows a segment of the vertebral column of a Florida Cottonmouth (*Agkistrodon piscivorus conanti*). Each pair of ribs articulate with processes on the vertebrae. See also fig. 3.2 for further details. Skeleton courtesy of the Florida Museum of Natural History, photographed by the author.

biochemical properties are used, sometimes in combination with the observable structures (or phenotype), to resolve details of the phylogeny. This subject will be elaborated in the next section of this chapter.

Back to the question: What is a snake? We can describe a snake using a list of characters that confer specificity when considered collectively. We may call this an informal description that has utility when one is inspecting a newly found animal and wants to decide whether or not it is a snake. The other way in which the question can be answered is by what I call a formal definition. In order to understand the more formal approach, we need first to consider the evolutionary history of snakes and their relationships with other vertebrates.

Evolutionary History of Snakes

There is great difficulty in determining the evolutionary history of snakes, including the origins and classification of currently living species. There are many reasons why this is so. The fossil record of snakes is quite scattered and scanty, and piecing together the origins of snakes is difficult without

a more complete record. Furthermore, many specimens are either poorly preserved or incomplete, and there are few researchers who study the material. When characteristics of snakes are considered—including fossil and living forms—human judgments and personalities sometime lead to disagreement when it comes to forming hard conclusions. With respect to living species, there are more characters to be considered than what is present in fossilized material, including internal organs, coloration, DNA, proteins, and other properties of tissues. But again, disagreements can emerge when different people examine different characters and attempt to construct an evolutionary tree. Indeed, the classification of living snakes has been fraught with disagreement and controversy. What follows is an assessment of our current state of knowledge concerning these subjects.

Fossils and Origins

Snakes are unquestionably *tetrapods*, which are four-limbed vertebrates including amphibians, reptiles (including birds), and mammals. Thus, snakes represent a specialized branch of vertebrates that descended from limbed ancestors. Representatives of some snake families possess vestiges of a pelvic girdle or posterior limbs, although in living snakes the pelvic girdle has lost direct contact with the vertebral column or is absent altogether. The vestigial elements that are present in living snakes are greatly reduced bones representing the femur and/or pelvis. In male specimens of boas and pythons these are associated with external protrusions of keratinized tissue called *spurs* (see chapter 9, fig. 9.21). There is no trace of forelimbs or an anterior limb girdle in either living or fossil snakes.

Most paleontologists believe that reptiles shared a common ancestor with a prominent group of extinct amphibians known as labyrinthodonts, named for a distinctive structure of teeth having complexly infolded enamel. These ancient tetrapods comprised a diverse group of animals that lived during the Paleozoic era more than 300 million years ago (fig. 1.7). It is not clear from which group of labyrinthodont amphibians the reptiles evolved, and there might well have been multiple origins from ancient amphibians that appeared to be developing reptilian characteristics. The oldest known fossils that are definitely recognized as reptiles are from small animals resembling lizards and classified as cotylosaurs, also called the "stem reptiles" (fig. 1.8). These ancient reptiles are believed to be ancestral to all the taxa of reptiles that are living on the earth today. The cotylosaurs appeared first during the late Carboniferous or early Permian period over 275 million years ago. Subsequently these early reptiles diversified and gave rise to lineages that produced turtles, dinosaurs, mammals, crocodilians, birds, tuatara, and the modern lizards and snakes (Squamata).

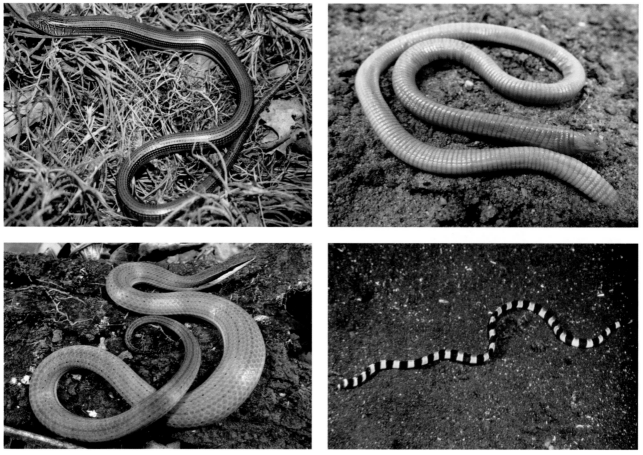

Figure 1.4. Some vertebrate animals that people might mistake for a snake. **Upper left:** An Eastern Glass Lizard (*Ophisaurus ventralis*) is a legless anguid lizard common in the eastern United States. Photograph by the author. **Upper right:** A Florida Worm Lizard (*Rhineura floridana*), which is an amphisbaenid squamate and not a true lizard. This is a subterranean species, characterized by having degenerated eyes, a blunt worm-like tail, and a rigid head that helps it burrow its way through soil. Photograph by the author. **Lower left:** Burton's Snake Lizard (*Lialis burtonis*) is a legless gekkonid lizard that lives in Australia. Photograph by the author. **Lower right:** A species of eel (*Myrichthys colubrinus*) that very closely resembles a banded sea snake that also lives in its habitat. This specimen was photographed in Bali, Indonesia, by John E. Randall, Bishop Museum, Hawaii.

The oldest fossil snakes come from the middle of the Cretaceous period roughly 70 to 95 million years ago. Fossil snakes are by no means abundant, and the historical record is incomplete, as is the case with many other vertebrates. Sometimes the fossil consists of only a few ribs or vertebrae, or other bones, and a proper interpretation can be quite challenging. For example, one of the earliest fossils thought to be a snake later proved to share some characters that also existed in Cretaceous lizards and is no longer regarded as a snake. The oldest unequivocal snakes have a snakelike vertebral column with evidence of limbs. A fossil snake named *Najash rionegrina*, recently discovered in Argentina's Rio Negro province, has a primitive pelvis and legs that were presumably functional outside the rib cage. It is purported to be the earliest limbed snake to be found in a terrestrial deposit. The skeletal structure of this snake appears to be closer to that of a quadrupedal ancestor than is that of previous fossils, but the closest ancestor remains unknown.

Because *Najash rionegrina* was found in a terrestrial deposit, it supports the hypothesis that snakes evolved on land. The idea that snakes evolved from terrestrial ancestors, eventually losing their limbs after they adopted habits of burrowing in soil, was popular for most of the 20th century and enjoys considerable support. The skull of snakes resembles that of lizards with respect to certain features, for example a moveable quadrate bone at the rear of the jaw and the absence of a quadratojugal bone at the rear of the skull. Snakes probably evolved during the Jurassic—perhaps 150 million years ago—however, there are currently no fossils dating back that far. During the early Cretaceous (about 120 million years ago) these early snakes radiated into a number of forms, including some that were aquatic and some that were terrestrial. Both terrestrial and aquatic species of snakes existed in the mid-Cretaceous (about 95 million years ago), and there is still debate about which type evolved first.

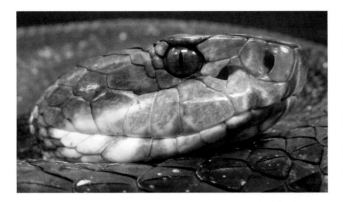

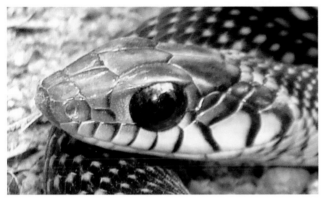

Figure 1.5. The eyes of snakes are covered with a spectacle or brille. The **upper photo** features the eye of a Florida Cottonmouth (*Agkistrodon piscivorus conanti*) photographed by the author. The facial pit, an infrared thermal imaging receptor, and the nostril are also easily seen. This snake is largely nocturnal and has a vertically elliptical pupil. The **lower photo features** the relatively large eye and round pupil of a Speckled Racer (*Drymobius margaritiferus*), a diurnally active forager. Note the complete absence of any sort of eyelid or covering at the edges of the pupil. Compare this photograph with that of the lizard that is featured in fig. 1.2. The racer was photographed in Belize by Dan Dourson.

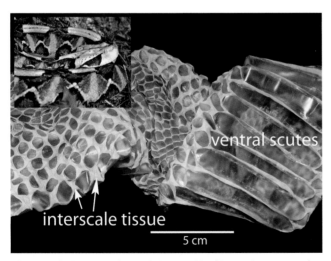

Figure 1.6. Shed skin from a Gaboon Adder (*Bitis gabonica*, inset) showing dorsal scales and ventral scutes separated by interscale tissue. The shed skin is epidermis from the entire body surface, intact and inside out as it "peels" from the snake and subsequently dries. Photographs by the author.

Some of the earliest fossil snakes are marine forms that have been unearthed in 95-million-year-old marine deposits in North Africa, the Middle East, and eastern Europe. One of these possesses a complete hind limb that extends beyond the body wall, but is certainly a snake. Thus, some scientists argue that snakes lost their limbs in the ocean instead of on land, the immediate ancestors being now-extinct marine lizards called *mosasaurs* (fig. 1.8). Fossils identified in marine environments are at least 8 million years older than are those from terrestrial deposits. The question of "Who came first?" may never be resolved with universal consensus. And, of course, both of these alternative evolutionary scenarios might have played out in ancient times roughly in parallel. If this was the case, the marine forms probably died out and the current lineages of snakes evolved from the terrestrial ancestors. DNA sequencing and other data suggest that the living lineages of snakes have a *monophyletic* origin, which means they all evolved from a single common ancestor or ancestral lineage.

Studies of fossil snakes and their comparisons with anatomical features of modern reptiles have led a number of scientists to suggest that snakes evolved from a family of lizards during the time when dinosaurs were prominent. Varanid lizards (monitor lizards or goannas) are very similar to snakes in the structure of the skull, sensory systems, and also other features. The Earless Monitor (*Lanthanotus borneensis*) of Borneo, Indonesia, has movable eyelids, but the lower lid bears a clear "window" resembling the snake's eyecap. As its name implies, the Earless Monitor lacks an external ear, just as in snakes, and also exhibits a number of snakelike features in the architecture of its skull. Based on such similarities, some scientists have theorized that ancient lizards related to monitors adopted a burrowing mode of life, tunneling through loose dirt or sand as do a number of lizard species today. In this manner, a number of features characteristic of snakes evolved, such as reduction and eventual loss of limbs and external ears, and the development of a spectacle to protect the eyes while moving through earth. The various descendants of these burrowing forms diversified and radiated into terrestrial habitats after emerging from a subterranean lifestyle to exploit a variety of terrestrial niches. Once the limbs were lost during the subterranean existence, they were not regained by "reversals" in the other environments. Rather, the limbless creatures we call snakes evolved many specializations and marvelous means of living without arms or legs.

It is interesting to note that numerous losses and reductions of limbs have occurred during vertebrate evolution, including many species of skinks and other reptiles beside snakes. The loss of limbs and elongation of the trunk of snakes is related to changes in the expression of genes called *Hox* genes. These genes are known to control development

Eon	Era	Period		Epoch	millions of years
Phanerozoic	Cenozoic	Quaternary		Holocene (recent)	− 0.01
				Pleistocene	− 1.8
		Tertiary	Neogene	Pliocene	− 5.2
				Miocene	− 23.8
			Paleogene	Oligocene	− 33.5
				Eocene	− 55.6
				Paleocene	− 65.0
	Mesozoic	Cretaceous			− 144
		Jurassic			− 206
		Triassic			− 251
	Paleozoic	Permian			− 290
		Carboniferous			− 354
		Devonian			− 409
		Silurian			− 439
		Ordovician			− 500
		Cambrian			− 543
	Proterozoic				− 2500

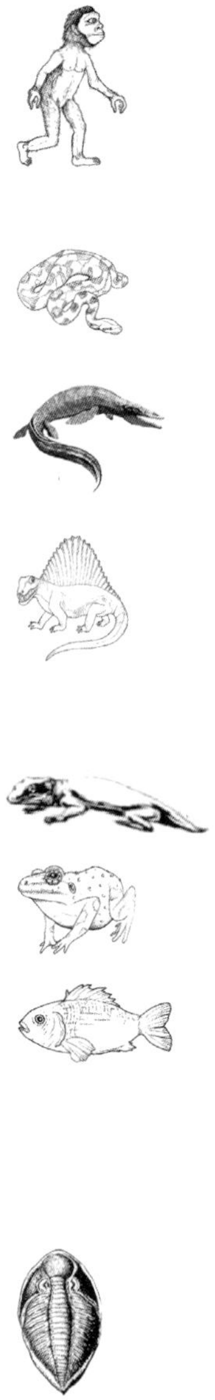

Figure 1.7. Geologic time scale with nomenclature for major units of time in millions of years before the present. The figure illustrates the major units of geological time related to definitive events of the Earth's history. The animal cartoons to the right of the table indicate approximate times of radiation and dominance, not the earliest points of origin. Cartoons by Dan Dourson.

by specifying embryonic cell division along the long axis of the body and determine limb development and specific boundaries of related morphological changes. Martin Cohn and Cheryll Tickle have shown that the patterns of Hox gene expression along the body axis in developing embryos of pythons accounts for the absence of forelimbs and the expansion of the thoracic axial skeleton. These authors also suggested that the failure of signaling pathways to activate the development of limbs might be related to changes in the expression of Hox genes during the early evolution of snakes.

The Concept of Phylogeny

Phylogeny refers to an evolutionary history of species, or a group of species, and is represented by a branching diagram. Such a diagram is called a dendrogram, cladogram, phenogram, or tree, depending on the methods used to construct the diagram and the information content it is intended to convey. For our purposes we will call such a diagram simply a *phylogeny* or *tree*. Scientists use many alternative methods, indeed incorporating even entire philosophies, for building a phylogenetic tree. The process involves reconstructing

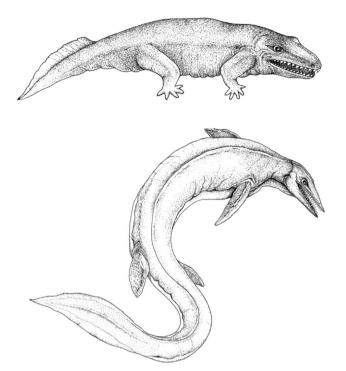

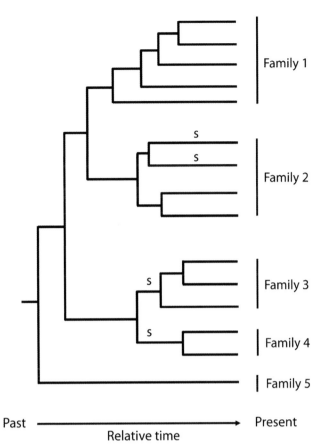

Past ————————————————→ Present

Relative time

Figure 1.9. Hypothetical phylogeny of several taxa of snakes, illustrating variation in topology and lengths of branches for different taxa. The scale of time is relative and arbitrary. Alternate scales (with more variable branch lengths) could be expressed in terms of genetic substitutions assuming availability of molecular data. Two examples of sister taxa are represented by pairs of the letter "s" above the two respective branches. Drawing by Coleman Sheehy III and the author.

Figure 1.8. The **upper drawing** illustrates a *cotylosaur*, representing one of the earliest families of reptiles. Cotylosaurs were small lizard-like reptiles that date from the late Carboniferous through the Permian (see fig. 1.7), and they have sometimes been called "stem reptiles" or "root reptiles" in reference to their basal position in reptilian phylogeny. The **lower drawing** depicts an extinct marine lizard known as a *mosasaur*. These reptiles were powerful swimmers and well adapted to living in the warm, shallow seas that were prevalent during the late Cretaceous period. Mosasaurs probably evolved from semiaquatic squamates and have a body shape that is similar to that of modern terrestrial monitor lizards (varanids), except for being longer and streamlined for swimming. Mosasaurs are considered to be close relatives to snakes, judged from analysis of the jaw and skull anatomy. Drawings by Dan Dourson.

evolutionary events, inferred from changes in *character states* (different forms of the same character) represented by different taxa or lineages. Various characters are used, usually depicting *phenotypic traits* such as anatomical features, or molecular data such as properties of proteins or DNA. Phenotypic traits are observable features that are expressed from the genetic makeup of an organism. Molecular data are increasingly being used to reconstruct evolutionary histories, and recent technological advances in genetics and genomics have greatly enriched the data base and helped to produce many new and sometimes radical changes in phylogenetic trees. This is true for many organisms, not just snakes.

A tree-shaped branching diagram conveys potentially two kinds of information: the tree *topology*, or sequential order in which the taxa branch from one another, and the lengths of the individual branches (fig. 1.9). Typically, the length of a branch on a tree is scaled as proportional to trait

changes, commonly expressed using molecular data as the number of mutations in a genetic sequence. Hence, species evolving at different rates will have unequal branch lengths. If such empirical data are not available, branch lengths may be represented in terms of relative time, or constructed from evolutionary models. The branching order is determined from phylogenetic methods that estimate or infer ancestral phenotypes from characters studied in living species. The methods are used to optimize character states at internal nodes (branching points) of the tree, which are hypothesized to represent speciation events. Comparison of trait values at ancestral and descendant nodes of the tree allow the history of phenotypic changes to be traced.

Species descend from each other in a hierarchical fashion—that is, a branching or treelike process of speciation. So character evolution is regarded as a process of historical transformation from a primitive to a derived state. *Primitive* or *ancestral* traits are characteristics that resemble ancestral or early conditions, whereas *derived* traits are those that have undergone change (phenotypic or molecular) from the ancestral condition in relatively recent time. Thus, character evolution is perceived as trait change on a tree.

Because species descend from common ancestors in a hierarchical fashion, closely related species tend to resemble each other more than they do distantly related species. Traits can be shared among species through common descent (called *homology*) or by independent origin (called *convergence* or *homoplasy*). Homologous characters are ones that are inherited from a shared common ancestor, whereas homoplastic characters are convergent because of similar functional pressures and natural selection. Thus, two species that are unrelated might resemble each other in some character simply because of similar selection pressures in similar kinds of environments. For example, two independent lineages of sea snakes both evolved a paddle-shaped tail that is used as an aid in swimming. These structures represent two independent origins of the same character (see fig. 3.8). Within each group, however, paddle-shaped tails are inherited through separate lineages; each can be traced to a common ancestor, and they are therefore homologous. The concept extends to other character states, including color and behavior (see below).

Many persons will assume that the value of phylogenetic trees is simply to provide a picture image of how snakes are related as part of understanding their evolutionary history. Indeed, this is the intention implicit in this conceptual overview and the more detailed discussion that follows in the next sections of this chapter. However, the reader should also appreciate that phylogenetic trees are being used in concert with evolutionary approaches using comparative data to study the evolution of various characters ranging from molecular and biochemical features to attributes of morphology, physiology, and behavior. Indeed, a richer understanding of how snakes or other organisms work is growing from an interdisciplinary approach to evolutionary questions using tools from both phylogenetics and comparative anatomy or physiology.

Classification and Phylogeny of the World's Snakes

Deciphering the evolutionary relationships among the world's snakes has been very challenging for scientists. Constructing a phylogeny can be time-consuming and expensive, and is subject to error, reinterpretation, and controversy. Certain groups of snakes, such as the speciose colubrids (Colubridae) have been especially problematical, and there remains disagreement and many questions about the details of relationships.

From a long-standing conventional viewpoint, snakes are classified in the class Reptilia (reptiles), which includes all the ectothermic animals with dry scaly skin. By this criterion, reptiles include the traditional divisions into tuataras, turtles, crocodilians, snakes, and lizards. In recent years, however, most taxonomists have begun to agree that natural groups, or *taxa*, should be monophyletic to include all the descendants of a particular ancestral form. By this convention, "reptiles" (or the class Reptilia) would include all birds because it is clear that birds and crocodilians are sister taxa (fig. 1.10). Thus, traditional members of the class "Reptilia" are often now referred to as "non-avian reptiles" to emphasize the close relationship between crocodilians and birds. For clarity and ease of understanding, however, we shall consider snakes as part of the traditional class Reptilia and refer to them simply as reptiles.

As part of the reptiles, snakes comprise a *clade* or monophyletic lineage within the order Squamata, which also includes lizards and amphisbaenians. The latter are essentially highly derived lizards. Amphisbaenians are elongate and generally limbless, and they are characterized by heavily ossified skulls that are modified for subterranean digging (fig. 1.4). All squamates are characterized by generally prominent and obvious scalation, and they share some other characteristics as well. The tuataras of New Zealand, which superficially

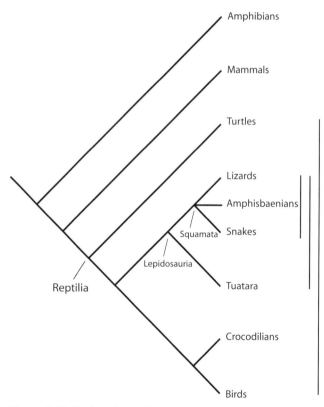

Figure 1.10. Phylogenic tree illustrating a schematic representation of the evolution of vertebrates. The vertical bars at the right-hand side of figure encompass clades that are identified to the left: Squamata, Lepidosauria, and Reptilia (in reverse hierarchical order). Drawing by Coleman M. Sheehy III and the author.

resemble lizards, belong to a separate and ancient order that is a sister taxon to the Squamata having a separate evolutionary history. Collectively, all snakes are classified as a suborder of Squamata, called Ophidia or Serpentes. Hence, when people speak or write about "ophidians" (or use this term as a descriptor), they are referring to snakes.

The following discussion is an attempt to summarize what is currently known about these relationships, with emphasis on broad patterns rather than details and hardened opinions about alternate classification schemes. Thus, one may well consider the relationships to be a work in progress. What is important is for the reader to acquire an appreciation for the diversity and marvelous adaptations that characterize snakes as a living and successful group of vertebrates. Some lineages contain only one or a few species, while others are extremely rich and include hundreds of species. There is evidence from the fossil record which indicates that some groups were more diverse in the past, so the present diversity has been impacted by past extinctions. Let's now explore the living diversity of snakes.

Scolecophidia: The Blind Snakes

The Scolecophidia, technically an infraorder or superfamily, represents one branch of a primary dichotomy of snakes. This is a monophyletic group of snakes consisting of three families: Leptotyphlopidae, known as thread snakes, worm snakes, or blind snakes; Typhlopidae, also called blind snakes; and Anomalepididae, also called blind snakes or dawn blind snakes. All of the snakes classified within these families—a little over 300 species—are considered to be evolved from a common ancestral form. This conclusion is inferred largely from possession of common characters unlike those of other snakes, including features of the skull, eyes, and soft anatomy. The collective vernacular name of blind snakes is derived from the eyes being reduced or vestigial—usually buried beneath the head scales—and in some species absent entirely or reduced to small patches of dark pigment (fig. 1.11).

Collectively, Scolecophidians resemble each other in having uniformly smooth scales encircling the body without enlargement of the ventral scales as in other snakes. The skin is smooth and shiny, adheres tightly around a cylindrical body, and sometimes separates into discrete multiple rings of sloughed epidermis during skin shedding. This feature is unlike other snakes in which the outer generation of epidermis is shed generally as one entire piece. Whereas the skin of snakes is generally without glands, some species of blind snakes possess numerous small glands in the skin covering the head.

Blind snakes generally have rounded or blunt heads as well as blunt tails, the latter often tipped with a harmless spine (fig. 1.11). Members of Typhlopidae and Leptotyphlopidae have a remnant pelvic girdle, but this is variably lacking in the Anomalepididae. Some leptotyphlopid species in Africa possess external spurs. The skulls are highly modified and quite peculiar in some species. Typically, the small, curved mouth is set well below the snout, somewhat like that of a shark, and some species have enlarged, shovel-like or sharpened snouts that presumably facilitate digging. The rostral scale is enlarged and sometimes covers much of the anterior head (fig. 1.11). The two lower jaws are attached anteriorly, a character state that is similar to most other vertebrates but unlike other snakes. Some worm snakes (Leptotyphlopidae) possess relatively large teeth on the lower jaws while lacking teeth on the upper jaws, whereas others (Typhlopidae) have teeth only on the upper jaws or on both upper and lower jaws (Anomalepididae). Little is known about the functional biology of worm snakes, but one recent study describes an unusual manner of feeding (see chapter 2).

Blind snakes are nonvenomous and harmless, although when aroused they often emit a strong and offensive odor related to secretions from well-developed musk glands located in the base of the tail. These secretions might assist aggregation behaviors in addition to defensive functions. Chemical stimuli as well as the sensory capacity for response are probably very important to these animals, which have weak or no vision and live in a world where vision is not very useful.

These snakes are typically small, and so they have been difficult to study. Some species are less than 2 mm wide in body girth and weigh less than a single gram. The group includes the world's smallest snake—*Leptotyphlops carlae*—discovered by Blair Hedges in June 2006 on the Caribbean island of Barbados. Fully grown adults of this species stretch less than 10 cm and can coil upon a coin the size of a US

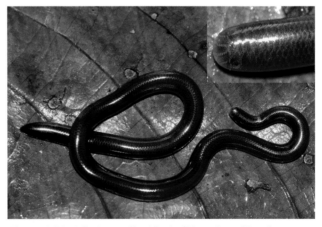

Figure 1.11. A Brahminy Blind Snake (*Rhamphotyphlops braminus*, Leptotyphlopidae), sometimes called Flowerpot Blind Snake, photographed in India by Indraneil Das. The head is shown in the inset. Note the enlarged rostral scale, rounded snout, smooth scales, degenerative eyes, and short blunt tail.

quarter (fig. 1.12). Larger species of blind snakes generally range in length up to about 40–41 cm, but several species measure more than 60 cm, and there are two unusual species of blind snakes reaching lengths approaching 80 cm. The body color of most species is generally brown, pink, or black. Because of their colors and long, thin appearance, some species of blind snakes are also called worm snakes or thread snakes.

Owing to their small size and tendencies to burrow, blind snakes are difficult to find. They feed on several life history stages of social insects. Many species prey on the larvae and pupae of ants or termites, so the probability of finding them increases greatly inside ant or termite nests. All species burrow, and most spend much of their time in deep, loose soil, only to be seen when found by flipping logs or rocks, or when crawling on the surface of the soil at night and especially after rainfall. They also emerge following

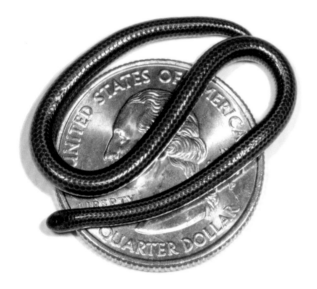

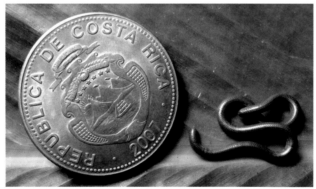

Figure 1.12. The **upper photo** shows the world's smallest species of snake, *Leptotyphlops carlae*, the Barbados Threadsnake. This diminutive species was discovered in 2006 on the Caribbean island of Barbados. The species is less than 10 cm (4 inches) in length. Photograph by S. Blair Hedges. The **lower photo** features a juvenile Black Threadsnake, *Leptopyphlops ater*, photographed by the author in Guanacaste, Costa Rica. The 50 colones coin in this photograph measures 2.7 cm in diameter and is 3 mm wider than the US quarter.

saturating rainfall that can flood their subterranean homes. The Flowerpot Blind Snake (*Ramphotyphlops braminus*, fig. 1.11) is so named because it is often transported from location to location in garden soil or plant debris. Although scolecophidians are characteristically fossorial, some species live among roots of tree ferns, while others crawl over vegetation at night and are occasionally found several meters above ground. Interestingly, blind snakes can sometimes be found in the nests of large birds, where they are apparently brought by the parents to feed the chicks, inadvertently or not. Blind snakes are found in the Americas, from southwestern United States southward to Uruguay and Argentina, and they also occur in parts of the Caribbean, Europe, Africa, southwestern Asia, and Australia.

Blind snakes reproduce by laying eggs, and the female Texas Blind Snake (*Leptotyphlops dulcis*) coils around her eggs and shivers like some pythons to elevate temperatures during egg incubation. This is an extraordinary feat considering the small size of these snakes! Equally fascinating, the Flowerpot Blind Snake is the only snake that is known to be *parthenogenetic*. This is a unisexual species in which eggs develop without being fertilized by sperm. Probably most blind snakes are *oviparous* and reproduce by laying eggs, but Diard's Blindsnake (*Typhlops diardii*) is possibly *viviparous* (live bearing) in some parts of Asia. Again, because of their secretive habits, much more remains to be learned about the reproduction, behavior, and ecology of this primitive group of snakes.

The systematics and ecology of blind snakes are very poorly known in comparison with other terrestrial vertebrates. They are the closest relatives of all other snakes (Alethinophidia). A recent molecular study of the Leptotyphlopidae suggests that living lineages diversified as early as the mid-Cretaceous (~ 100 Ma), influenced by the breakup of continents. The diversity of species appears to be much greater than is currently recognized, and new species are continually being discovered all over the world.

Alethinophidia: The "Modern Lineages"

This grouping of snakes is the second branch in the basal dichotomy of the world's snakes. These are so-called true snakes or advanced snakes and include all of the modern lineages except for the Scolecophidia. Within this large group of snakes there is a primary dichotomy between what some call Henophidia (formerly Booidea) and Xenophidia, or Caenophidia (formerly called Colubroidea). The former group, henophidians, include dwarf pipe snakes, pipe snakes, shieldtail snakes, sunbeam snakes, boas, and pythons. All of these are relatively basal lineages within the Alethinophidia. The remaining more advanced snakes, Caenophidia, include the well-known colubrids, elapids, and viperids; the lesser known homalopsids, lamprophiids, pareatids, and xenodermatids;

plus the acrochordids, which are sister to all the others. The position of the Acrochordidae is now fairly well accepted, and the sister caenophidians collectively comprise the Colubroidea in current terminology. We begin with a discussion of the more basal groups.

Henophidia: The Basal Lineages

Several taxa of basal lineages are collectively referred to by many herpetologists as "pipe snakes." So-called dwarf pipe snakes (family Anomochilidae) were once considered to be transitional between the blind snakes and the other alethinophidians, but this supposition is no longer supported by molecular studies (see below). There are three species of dwarf pipe snakes—also called "stump heads"—known from Indonesia and all belonging to a single genus, *Anomochilus* (fig. 1.13). We have very little knowledge about the natural history and functional biology of these animals. Historically, these snakes have long been associated with other pipe snakes, but they appear to be a sister taxon to other alethinophidians and thus have been placed in their own family.

The other pipe snakes include a single neotropical species (fig. 1.14) belonging to its own family, Aniliidae, and nine species of Asian pipe snakes belonging to the family Cylindrophiidae (fig. 1.15). Pipe snakes are small to medium-size snakes, ranging in length from roughly 0.5 to 1 m. They are generally somewhat stouter than blind snakes, possess smooth scales, rounded heads, and short, blunt tails. The head is no wider than the neck; the eyes are degenerate and diminutive. Pipe snakes are usually dark brown to black and may have colorful yellow or reddish bands, which can be pale and difficult to see. The neotropical Red Pipe Snake, *Anilius scytale*, is colorful, and to some—most importantly potential predators—it resembles a coral snake (fig. 1.14; see chapter 5).

Pipe snakes burrow in loose soil or vegetation, like blind snakes, and are strong diggers. They inhabit lowland forests near sources of water and can be common at rice paddies and other places that are disturbed by humans. Prey items are constricted and consist of elongated animals such as eels, lizards, and other snakes. Captive snakes also eat small mice and fish. Defensive behaviors include flattening the body and waving a curled tail to show its colorful underside while hiding the head beneath part of the body. When touched or attacked, pipe snakes emit a foul-smelling secretion from their postcloacal musk glands. These snakes are viviparous and give birth to living young.

The family Uropeltidae contains almost 50 species of small snakes (15–40 cm) called shield-tail snakes, inhabiting Sri Lanka and southern India. These snakes are highly specialized burrowers that are closely related to the pipe snakes, which they are sometimes called. The head is conical, more slender than the trunk, and often bears a distinct keel (fig. 1.15). The tail is blunt and in many species bears a single large scale that is roughened at the very end of the snake. The tail collects a plug of dirt or mud and protects the snake when it is inside a tunnel. The anterior body musculature is specialized structurally and biochemically for sustained burrowing. These muscles together with the vertebral column and viscera move relative to the skin and thus allow these snakes to use a portion of the body to anchor within a tunnel while the head and anterior body move forward. The head is then used to enlarge and compact the sides of the tunnel by moving from side to side, after which it anchors while the posterior body is dragged forward to find a new point of friction anchor. Most species of uropeltids are poorly known and unstudied, while others are quite common. These interesting snakes are thought to eat earthworms, and most or possibly all reproduce by giving birth to live young.

Two other small families are known as sunbeam snakes because of their highly iridescent scales. These are the Loxocemidae and Xenopeltidae. The Loxocemidae has a single species, the Mexican Burrowing Python (*Loxocemus bicolor*, fig. 1.16), which grows to a length of about 1 m, lives a secretive and burrowing lifestyle in forests, but emerges at night (often during heavy rains) to forage on small mammals and other reptiles. *Loxocemus* ranges along the Pacific coast of Mexico and Central America. This species is oviparous and oviposits small clutches of relatively large eggs. The Xenopeltidae includes two species of Asian sunbeam snakes in the genus *Xenopeltis* that grow to a length of just a little more than 1 m. They live in burrows or beneath logs or vegetation, and they prey on various small animals including other snakes. Like *Loxocemus*, these snakes lay eggs. Several studies place the families Loxocemidae and Xenopeltidae as sister taxa, and both of these taxa as sister to the pythons.

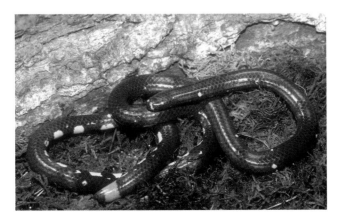

Figure 1.13. A recently described species of pipe snake, *Anomochilus monticola*, photographed in Borneo by Indraneil Das.

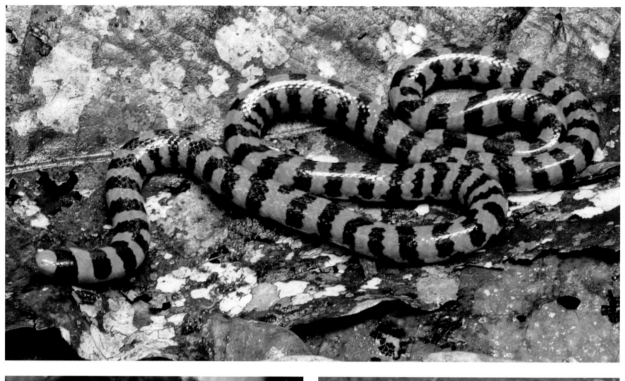

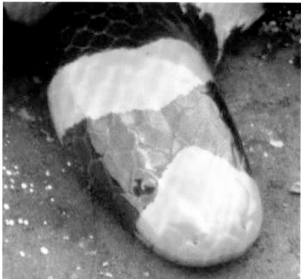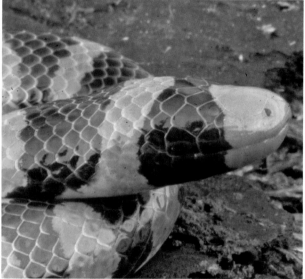

Figure 1.14. The **upper photo** features a beautiful Red Pipe Snake (*Anilius scytale*)—also called a False Coral Snake—photographed in the Mato Grosso, Brazil. This is the only species currently recognized in the monotypic family Aniliidae. It possesses a pair of cloacal spurs, presumably representing a vestigial pelvic girdle. The **lower photos** feature the head of *A. scytale*, which is somewhat flattened and shows diminutive eyes. This specimen is from Pará, Brazil. All photographs are courtesy of Laurie J. Vitt.

Boas and Pythons: Big Is Beautiful

The boas and pythons are snakes that are well known because of their popularity in movies, storybooks, and the current pet trade. They are simultaneously loathed and loved for being large, and clearly certain boas and pythons represent the world's largest snakes. The Reticulated Python (*Broghammerus reticulatus*; formerly *Python reticulatus*) of Southeast Asia is probably the world's longest living snake and grows to maximum length of about 10 m (although most specimens are no longer than 6 m) (fig. 1.17). South American anacondas are probably the world's heaviest snake, if the measure is relative mass. Wild Green Anacondas (*Eunectes murinus*) can grow to lengths of about 5 m and weigh up to 45 kg (fig. 1.18). There are reports of longer and heavier anacondas, but their validity is questionable. Since the early 1900s the Wildlife Conservation

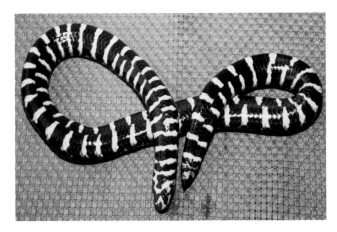

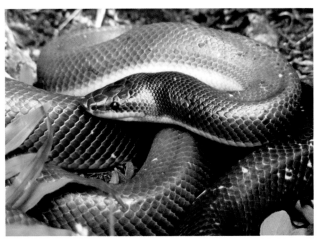

Figure 1.16. A Mexican Burrowing Python (*Loxocemus bicolor*) photographed by the author at Palo Verde Field Station, Guanacaste, Costa Rica. Note the smooth scales, stout body, and enlarged rostral scale.

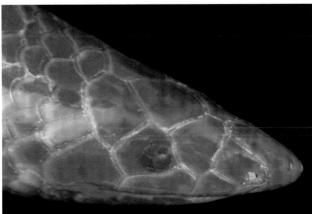

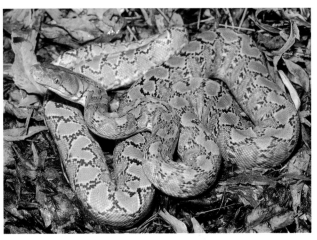

Figure 1.15. The **upper photo** shows the underside of a Red-tailed Pipe Snake (*Cylindrophis rufus*) photographed by the author in Thailand. This is a burrowing snake found throughout many parts of Southeast Asia. The scales are smooth and shiny. The tail is blunt and pointed with variable red coloration and is used defensively to deter predators. The **lower photo** features a head view of a shield-tailed snake (Blyth's Earth Snake, *Rhinophis blythii*). This is a burrowing snake, like other species of uropeltids, and it exhibits specializations for a fossorial life. The head and skull are primitive and inflexible, with a rigid jaw, pointed snout, and degenerative eyes that lie beneath a head shield lacking a spectacle. This is a preserved specimen from Sri Lanka photographed by John C. Murphy.

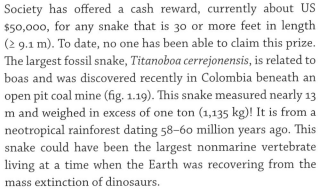

Figure 1.17. A recently described subspecies of Reticulated Python (*Broghammerus reticulatus jampeanus*) from Jampea Island in the Flores Sea. This is the first adult wild-caught specimen in captivity, measuring five feet in length. Photograph by David Barker.

Society has offered a cash reward, currently about US $50,000, for any snake that is 30 or more feet in length (≥ 9.1 m). To date, no one has been able to claim this prize. The largest fossil snake, *Titanoboa cerrejonensis*, is related to boas and was discovered recently in Colombia beneath an open pit coal mine (fig. 1.19). This snake measured nearly 13 m and weighed in excess of one ton (1,135 kg)! It is from a neotropical rainforest dating 58–60 million years ago. This snake could have been the largest nonmarine vertebrate living at a time when the Earth was recovering from the mass extinction of dinosaurs.

Boas and pythons are classified into three or four separate families depending on one's view of the classification scheme. These snakes were previously classified as a single family, but clearly they represent two to four independent lineages that diverged from ancestral snakes leading to the Caenophidia. The largest living snakes are boas and pythons that inhabit the tropics of South America and Southeast Asia. However, not all species of boas and pythons are large.

An assemblage of about 21 species of relatively small snakes called dwarf boas are contained in the family Tropidophiidae, distributed in Middle America (Central America including tropical Mexico and northern South America), Caribbean islands, and Malaysia. These snakes grow to a maximum length of about 1m, but most species are 30–50 cm and usually moderately slender with a somewhat enlarged head.

Another species of boa (*Casarea dussumieri*) is placed in the family Bolyeridae, confined to Round Island near

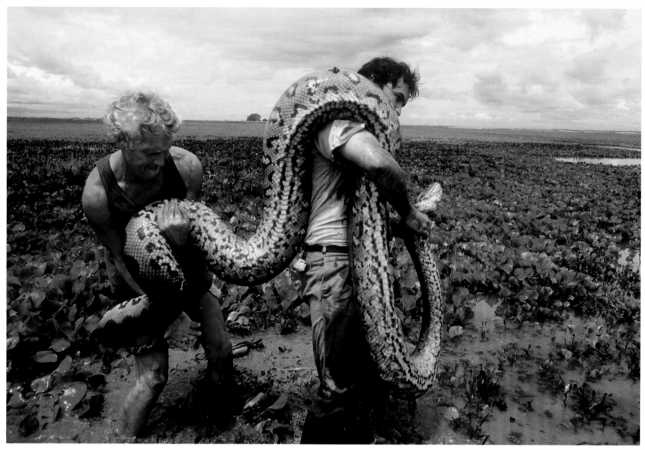

Figure 1.18. A Green Anaconda (*Eunectes murinus*) captured by Ed George and Jesús A. Rivas at El Frio, Apure, Venezuela. Photograph by Tony Crocetta.

Mauritius in the Indian Ocean and called the Round Island Boa or Split-jawed Boa. This species is unique among tetrapods in having divided maxillary bones with movable front and rear parts. A second species called *Bolyeria multocarinata* is thought to have gone extinct only recently within the past 30 years. Round Island Boas are oviparous and eat primarily skinks and geckos.

There are roughly 28 species of boas and sand boas in the family Boidae. Some 15 species of sand boas have been separated from the other boas for at least 50 million years, and some scientists place these in a separate family (Erycidae) or subfamily (Erycinae). These are semifossorial small to medium-sized snakes distributed across central and northern Africa, the Middle East, and parts of Eurasia, and also include rubber boas (*Charina* spp.) and Rosy Boa (*Lichanura trivirgata*) of western North America. The Old World sand boas (*Eryx* spp.) exhibit some marvelous adaptations for living in sandy habitats, including dorsally placed eyes and nostrils and a countersunk lower jaw (fig. 1.20). Other boas occur largely in neotropical forests, and many of these have infrared-sensitive pits commonly present on or between upper or lower labial scales. Among these species are the popular and well-known Boa Constrictor (*Boa constrictor*) (fig. 1.21) and the anaconda (*Eunectes* spp.), which is specialized for aquatic life (fig. 1.18). All boas are viviparous and collectively consume a variety of vertebrate prey.

There are roughly 27 species of pythons in the family Boidae. These are sometimes treated as a separate family (Pythonidae) and are distributed through central Africa through Southeast Asia, southern China, and the East Indies to Australia and Papua New Guinea. Most pythons have premaxillary teeth directly beneath the snout, and both boas and pythons have long, curved teeth for snaring prey that might include large mammals and birds. All pythons are oviparous, and some incubate their eggs by coiling about them and shivering the body muscles to produce heat. Pythons are diverse in size, color pattern, and habitat. Some species are arboreal or climb readily, and these are generally more slender than are terrestrial species (also true for boas). Snakes of the genus *Python* evolved as part of an Australasian radiation and include stout species such as the Ball Python (*P. regius*) and very long species such as the Burmese Python (*P. molurus*), African Rock Python (*P. sebae*), and Reticulated Python (*Broghammerus reticulatus*; = *Python*

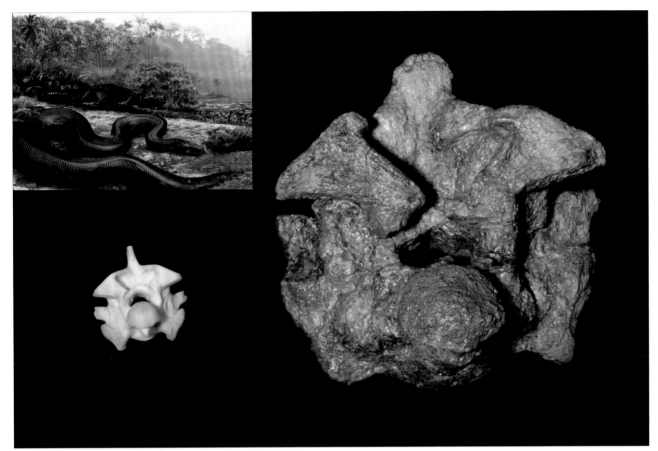

Figure 1.19. Vertebra of the world's largest fossil snake (*Titanoboa cerrejonensis*, **right**) shown side by side with the vertebra of a Green Anaconda (*Eunectes murinus*, **left**). The length of *Titanoboa* was 13 m (42 feet), and the snake was estimated to weigh as much as 1.3 tons—30 times the weight of an anaconda! The scientific name *Titanoboa cerrejonensis* means "titanic boa from Cerrejon," which is the region where the fossil was found. Photograph by Ray Carson, University of Florida Photography. The inset depicts what the snake might have looked like (drawn by Jason Bourque, Florida Museum of Natural History).

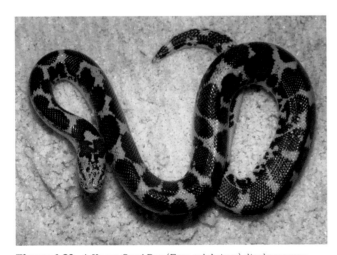

Figure 1.20. A Kenya Sand Boa (*Eryx colubrinus*) displays some prominent characteristics of semifossorial boas. These include a muscular body, dorsally placed and upward-looking eyes, a prominent rostral scale with countersunk lower jaw beneath, and a short, blunt or spine-like tail. This is a captive specimen owned by Phil Nicodemo and photographed by the author.

reticulatus of earlier nomenclature), which might exceed 10 m in total length. Some of the Australian species of pythons also grow to great lengths, with Scrub Pythons (*Morelia amethystina*) reaching lengths of around 8.5 m. Australian pythons of the Australian genus *Aspidites* comprises a *sister taxon* of all other living pythons. The Green Tree Python (*Morelia viridis*), common to New Guinea, is highly specialized for arboreal life, as is the neotropical Emerald Tree Boa (*Corallus caninus*) (fig. 1.22).

Caenophidia: Advanced Snakes

The Caenophidia is a monophyletic group of snakes, including what are generally regarded as the more advanced lineages of snakes (Colubroidea) and a sister group (Acrochordoidea) of odd snakes, the family Acrochordidae. The Colubroidea also is a monophyletic group and contains the families Colubridae, Elapidae, Homalopsidae, Lamprophiidae, Pareatidae, Viperidae, and Xenodermatidae. The colubrids contain the most

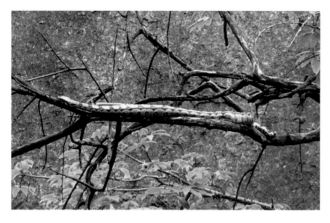

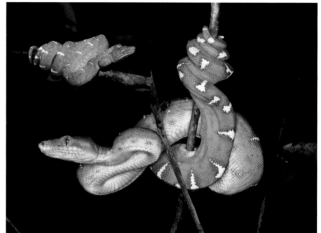

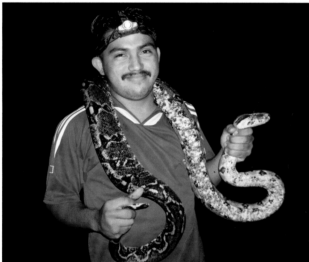

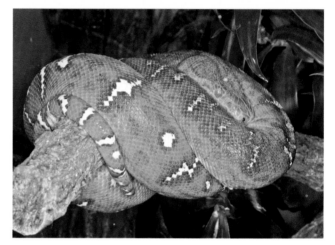

Figure 1.21. In the bush and in the hand. The **upper photo** captures a wild Boa Constrictor (*Boa constrictor*) resting on a tree branch against a steep rock face in Río de Janeiro, Brazil (photograph by Steven Lillywhite). The **lower photo** shows William Garcia holding a Boa Constrictor, soon after its capture in Belize (photograph by Dan Dourson).

Figure 1.22. Evolutionary convergence in the trees. The **upper photograph** shows a New World Emerald Tree Boa (*Corallus caninus*), and the **lower photograph** features an Old World Green Tree Python (*Morelia viridis*). Both snakes are highly arboreal and exhibit remarkable convergence in body form, behavior, and color. The inset at the top shows a juvenile Emerald Tree Boa, which often differs in color from the adult. The juveniles are typically yellow to orange. Both photographs are by Laurie J. Vitt.

species of any family of snakes. Caenophidia is characterized by several osteological and anatomical characters, and the close relationships among the inclusive groups are now strongly supported by molecular data.

File Snakes: The Bizarre and the Ugly

File snakes are among the more unusual snakes by almost any measure. They are indeed bizarre and fascinate almost all persons who might have the good fortune to see one. Three species belong to a single genus and collectively comprise the family Acrochordidae. The two larger species, *Acrochordus javanicus* and *A. arafurae*, are also called elephant trunk snakes, which inhabit freshwater streams or estuaries in tropical Asia and northern Australia, respectively (fig. 1.23). The third species of this family, *A. granulatus*, is smaller than the other two and is largely

marine (fig. 1.23). This snake inhabits mostly mangroves and shallow, coastal waters, but there are populations that also occur in freshwater streams, ponds, and lakes. All three species are entirely aquatic and rarely leave water except when they occasionally become stranded on tidal mud flats.

All of the file snakes possess small tuberculate scales terminating outwardly in small spines, creating a rough body surface that gave rise to the popular name (see chapter 5). The small, granular scales encircle the body, and there is very little enlargement of the mid-ventral scales. The tail is only slightly compressed, but the ventral skin protrudes to form a small ridge, and the body is flattened laterally when swimming. File snakes are capable swimmers, but they mostly crawl along the muddy bottoms of

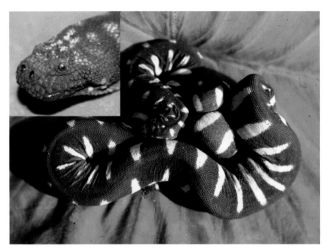

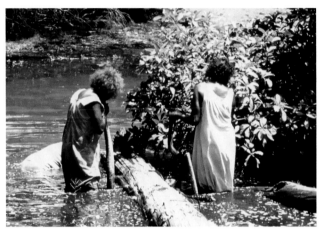

Figure 1.23. File snakes (Acrochordidae). The **upper photo** illustrates the smaller marine species, *Acrochordus granulatus*, photographed by the author in the Philippines. The inset illustrates the bead-like scales and the dorsally positioned eyes and nostrils. The **lower photo** features aboriginal women hunting the Australian species, *A. arafurae*, which they collect for food. The lower photograph is by Richard Shine.

streams, ponds, or mangroves. They are secretive and hide among roots of aquatic vegetation or in holes or burrows formed by other aquatic animals. The skin is loose and very flaccid, and the body of these snakes tends to collapse downward against a surface when they are taken out of water. They crawl slowly with seeming effort when outside of water, and the skin collapses in various directions with the body as the animal moves. The eyes are small and bead-like, while the nostrils are upturned with an internal valve that is an aquatic specialization (fig. 1.23). File snakes feed on fish and sometimes crustaceans, and they are capable of rapidly capturing prey by ensnaring it within a body coil. The snake does not constrict the prey, but the granular scales assist in holding the prey until the head locates the item and quickly swallows it. All file snakes are viviparous and reach high population densities in local waters.

Mole Vipers: Packing a Dangerous, Unusual Bite

About 60 species of snakes inhabiting sub-Saharan Africa and Arabian Peninsula are called mole vipers because of their burrowing habits. They do not look like typical vipers, but most possess a venom apparatus. Mole vipers were formerly classified as a family Atractaspididae, but the member species are now considered to be two colubroid subfamilies within the family Lamprophiidae. The subfamily Atractaspidinae contains about 23 species of snakes, most in the genus *Atractaspis* and known as stiletto snakes. The Aparallactinae is a sister subfamily containing about 50 species of small (less than 1 m), nocturnal, and usually secretive or burrowing snakes that are distributed throughout sub-Saharan Africa and the Middle East. Most of these snakes eat elongate vertebrates such as snakes, skinks, and caecilians, but species of *Aparallactus* eat centipedes almost exclusively. Some of these species bear resemblance to stiletto snakes (*Atractaspis*). The composition of these two sister taxa includes several lineages of snakes previously classified in the other colubroid families—Colubridae, Elapidae, and Viperidae. However, these are now shown to bear closer relationships among each other, warranting a separate classification, although the phylogeny of this group remains somewhat unclear. In the following discussion, we will consider both subfamilies together.

Mole vipers are small to medium-size snakes (up to 1 m), usually black or brown, but some species have stripes or bright bands of color. The head has a compact skull and small eyes, and it joins a cylindrical body with a short, pointed tail. The scales are smooth or keeled, and those on the head are relatively enlarged (fig. 1.24). Most species are oviparous, but one species is a live bearer (*Aparallactus jacksoni*) and the reproductive habits of several species are presently not known.

Most species of mole vipers have grooved rear fangs that are preceded by smaller solid teeth on the more anterior parts of the maxillary bone, resembling some colubrid species of snakes. Another species (*Aparallactus modestus*) lacks grooved teeth and is possibly nonvenomous. Yet other species have fixed front fangs resembling those of cobras and other elapid snakes. The stiletto snakes (*Atractaspis* spp.) possess movable front fangs resembling those of vipers, but these fangs are employed differently during prey capture. A distinctive feature of these snakes is a reduced maxilla that bears an enormous hollow or grooved fang (fig. 1.24). These are not true vipers, but like them, the maxilla has a complex articulation and can move to erect the fang. Because of the nature of the jaw movement and the large size of the fangs, the "erected" fangs protrude just a little from the jaw margin and are directed posteriorly. Striking and envenomating prey are accomplished by a lateral and posterior stabbing

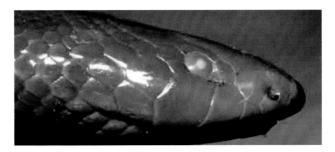

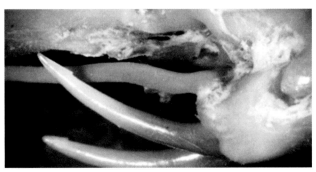

Figure 1.24. Head views of a Small-scaled Burrowing Asp (*Atractaspis microlepidota*), one of the "mole vipers" present in the middle part of Africa. The **upper photo** illustrates the flattened head with a blunt snout, adaptations for burrowing in soil. This species grows to lengths between 45 and 75 cm. The **lower photo** shows the fangs of this snake, which are relatively long and hollow—resembling fangs of viperid snakes but uniquely different. The fangs are situated such that the snake can approach its prey (say a rodent) inside a burrow and impale a single fang deep into the animal without completely opening its mouth. Little is known about this behavior, but the snake can use just one fang at a time. Photographs by John C. Murphy.

motion of the head, which is the reason for the name stiletto snake. The ability to bear the fangs without greatly opening the mouth is no doubt an advantage to these snakes when they forage within subterranean tunnels where they feed on small mammals (mostly rodents and shrews), nestling birds, and other reptiles.

The diversity of venoms and venom delivery systems in this group probably reflects adaptations to diverse diet specializations. Many eat elongate reptiles or other small vertebrates, some eat earthworms, and some like to eat centipedes. Most species of mole vipers present little danger and are too small to envenomate a person effectively. However, the venom glands of *Atractaspis* spp. are distinctive from elapids and viperids, containing unusual toxins that subdue prey and can be dangerous to humans. These snakes are well known and feared in parts of rural Africa where inquisitive children, snake catchers, and others are often bitten because the snakes cannot be picked up safely using one's hands. The stiletto snakes resemble other harmless species and often respond defensively by becoming immobile but suddenly striking with a slashing, backward movement. These snakes occupy

diverse habitats from forests to sandy semideserts. All of these snakes burrow and are generally secluded in soil or hiding beneath objects during the day. As with other burrowing snakes, movements above ground often occur at night, especially following rainstorms.

Other Lamprophiid African Snakes

The Lamprophiidae, of which the mole vipers are a part, also contains many other species representing a late Eocene radiation of nocturnal snakes endemic to the African continent. These include a widespread genus *Lamprophis*, many members of which are known as house snakes, water snakes (*Lycodonomorphus*), racer-like sand snakes, *Psammophis* spp., and other lesser known taxa. Aside from the mole vipers and stiletto snakes (Atractaspidinae and Aparallactinae), the family incorporates many of the more characteristic and widespread nonvenomous snake species of Africa. Altogether, there are more than 290 species of snakes represented within this family.

Vipers and Pit Vipers

Vipers and pit vipers (Viperinae and Crotalinae, respectively) are among the more spectacular, interesting, misunderstood, and maligned snakes. These are all venomous with prominent fangs and defensive behaviors that feature striking toward a threatening human or animal, as featured popularly on movie and television screens. These are reactive behaviors, however, and venomous snakes like all the others do not harbor aggressive tendencies toward humans. Many people believe they are aggressive, but their impressions that lead to such stories are misguided exaggerations, possibly with a few exceptions. Snakes are perceived as aggressive and "on the attack" only after they have been attacked or treated with aggression first. The toxins of venomous snakes evolved primarily in relation to prey capture, and defensive functions are usually secondary with few possible exceptions (e.g., spitting cobras; see chapter 2).

Collectively, vipers and pit vipers are members of the family Viperidae, which contains some 230 species. The typical vipers or adders of the Old World represent one major lineage of viperid snakes, and these are placed in the subfamily Viperinae. Member species of the family exhibit "typical" viper-like appearance with relatively short and bulky bodies, distinct and slightly triangular heads—often with enlarged cheeks to accommodate the venom glands—heavily keeled scales with small scale size adorning the head, and sometimes spectacular defensive behaviors. Most species feed on mammalian or avian (endothermic) prey and often swallow relatively large items potentially harmful to the snake. Other species, however, consume a variety of prey including insects (e.g., Orsini's Viper, *Vipera ursinii*), other reptiles, and carrion (especially Cottonmouths, *Agkistrodon piscivorus*). Most vipers, including viperine species, give birth to live young except members of the genus *Causus*, which lay eggs.

Vipers belonging to the genus *Vipera*, also called adders, comprise a diverse group of smaller species ranging across a variety of habitats and are, at northerly latitudes, active in cool weather with rather low body temperatures (fig. 1.25). There are about 20 species of Eurasian viperines that belong to the genus *Vipera*, and these include the only vipers that are familiar to many central and northern Europeans. *Vipera berus* is one of only two species of snakes to range into the Arctic Circle (the other is *Thamnophis sirtalis*).

Other groups or related lineages of vipers are distinctive in various interesting ways. Six species of African vipers belonging to the genus *Causus*, commonly called night adders, are distinctive in having smooth scales, large head plates,

round pupils, and dietary specialization for eating anurans (frogs or toads). Some have an upturned snout (fig. 1.26), perhaps of some value for digging loose earth or debris in search for toads, and two species have very elongate venom glands extending into the trunk beneath the skin. Another group of African vipers includes arboreal species known as bush vipers (genus *Atheris*). The more arboreal forms largely occupy the equatorial forests of central Africa, while others range further south (fig. 1.27).

Thirteen species of African vipers belonging to the genus *Bitis*, and many of these have exceptionally massive, stout bodies and are truly spectacular (fig. 1.28). Some of the better known species include the Gaboon Adder (*Bitis gabonica*), the Rhinoceros Adder (*B. nasicornis*), and the Puff Adder (*B. arietans*). These snakes move slowly but can strike

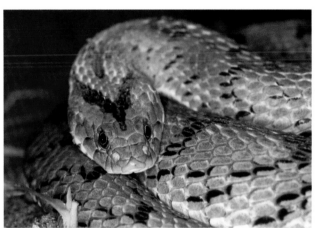

Figure 1.26. Spotted Night Adder (*Causus maculatus*), photographed in the Ivory Coast by Xavier Bonnet.

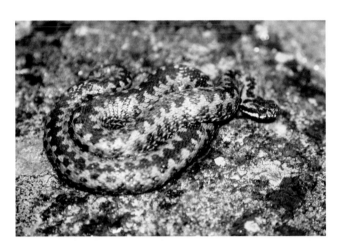

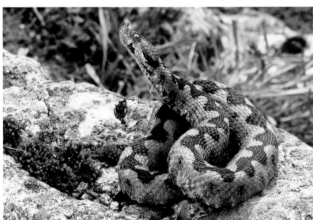

Figure 1.25. Two species of European viper. The **upper photo** features a common European Adder or Viper (*Vipera berus*) photographed by the author on an island off the coast of Sweden. This scene illustrates the camouflage value of the color pattern when seen against the rocks in the snake's habitat. The **lower photo** shows a Nose-horned Viper (*Vipera ammodytes*) photographed by Xavier Bonnet in its native habitat in Golem Grad, Macedonia.

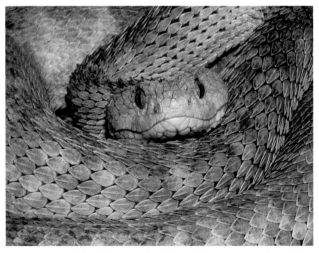

Figure 1.27. A female African Bush Viper (*Atheris squamigera*), also called Rough-scaled Bush Viper, found in western and central Africa, usually in low bushes. The coloration is variable, and females are usually larger than males. This is a captive specimen photographed by Elliott Jacobson.

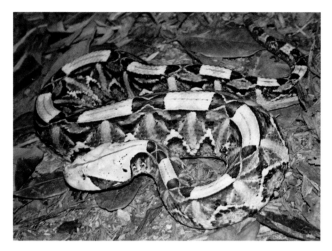

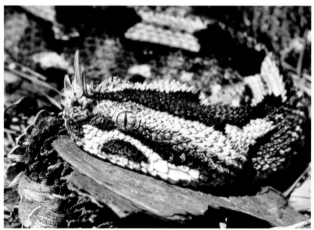

Figure 1.28. Two large and very heavy-bodied viperid snakes native to west-central Africa south of the Sahara, especially forested areas. The **upper photo** features a Gaboon Adder, *Bitis gabonica*—the world's heaviest viperid snake. This species also has the longest fangs and the highest yield of venom of any venomous species. The **lower photo** features a Rhinoceros Viper, *Bitis nasicornis*, which is stout with several prominent keratinized horns on its snout. Both species are largely ambush foragers and are very nicely camouflaged against backgrounds of dappled light and leaf litter. These are captive specimens photographed by the author.

extremely fast and with much force. They possess unusually long fangs—up to 4 cm in *B. gabonica*—and feed on generally large endothermic prey relative to their body size (see chapter 2). The color patterns are beautiful and provide effective camouflage. When disturbed or threatened, these snakes may emit a sharp, loud, and frightening hiss, which is sometimes repeated at regular or irregular intervals. The Puff Adder derives its name from this behavior.

Snakes widely known as pit vipers belong to the subfamily Crotalinae, which includes a diversity of species distributed in eastern Asia and the Western Hemisphere. The name is derived from the presence of paired facial pits, each located between the nostril and eye. The inner recess of the pit bears a thin, vascular, and densely innervated membrane that is sensitive to heat and infrared radiation. These pits function to detect warm prey and objects in the environment (see chapter 7).

Rattlesnakes are familiar pit vipers, represented by some 30 species of *Crotalus* and three species of *Sistrurus* collectively distributed from North to South America but with greatest diversity in the southern United States and Mexico (fig. 1.29). The tip of the tail bears a characteristic appendage (the "rattle") consisting of interlocking segments of rigid, dead tissue (keratin) derived from successive shedding of the outer skin. Individual segments are added to the rattle at its base during skin shedding (chapter 5). When a rattlesnake is disturbed or acts defensively, the tail is shaken rapidly and produces a loud sound (scaled to body size of the species) that resembles the sound of escaping steam. Specialized muscles in the tail of a rattlesnake vibrate the interlocking rattle segments which move against each other to produce the rattling sound. The rattle is characteristic of all species except for its secondary loss in two insular species, *Crotalus catalinensis* (Santa Catalina Island Rattlesnake) and *C. ruber lorenzoensis* (San Lorenzo Island Rattlesnake). Some rattlesnakes are very small (e.g., pygmy rattlesnakes, *Sistrurus* spp.) while the larger species (e.g., diamondback rattlesnakes, *C. adamanteus* and *C. atrox*) may exceed 2 m in length.

Old World pit vipers contain about 50 species including the Japanese Mamushi (*Gloydius blomhoffi*) and Habu (*Protobothrops flavoviridis*) (fig. 1.30), Malayan Pit Viper (*Calloselasma rhodostoma*), three species of Sri Lankan hump-nosed pit vipers (*Hypnale* spp.), and the beautiful Chinese Moccasin (*Deinagkistrodon acutus*) (see chapter 7). There are 31 species of *Trimeresurus* confined to Asia and numerous islands in the western Pacific, and some of these are arboreal (figs. 1.31, 5.6). New World pit vipers other than rattlesnakes include snakes of the genus *Agkistrodon* (Copperheads and Cottonmouths, fig. 1.32) and numerous species of several genera distributed in Middle America and South America. The latter include more than 30 species of terrestrial lanceheads (*Bothrops* spp.), the feared bushmaster (*Lachesis* spp.) (fig. 1.33), seven species of palm vipers (*Bothriechis* spp.) (fig. 1.34), seven species of forest pit vipers (*Bothriopsis* spp.), and nine species of thick-bodied hog-nosed pit vipers (*Porthidium* spp.) (fig. 1.35). Three species of jumping pit vipers (*Atropoides* spp.; fig. 1.36) are extremely stout-bodied, approaching the relative girth of the African *Bitis*.

Functional attributes of viperids will be discussed elsewhere in this book, but there is one more viperid species that merits mention before leaving a general introduction to this group of snakes. Fea's Viper (*Azemiops feae*) is an interesting species native to the mountainous regions of Southeast Asia. It has a decided non-viper-like appearance with colorful bands, smooth scales, relatively large head plates, and a somewhat rounded head (fig. 1.37). This species

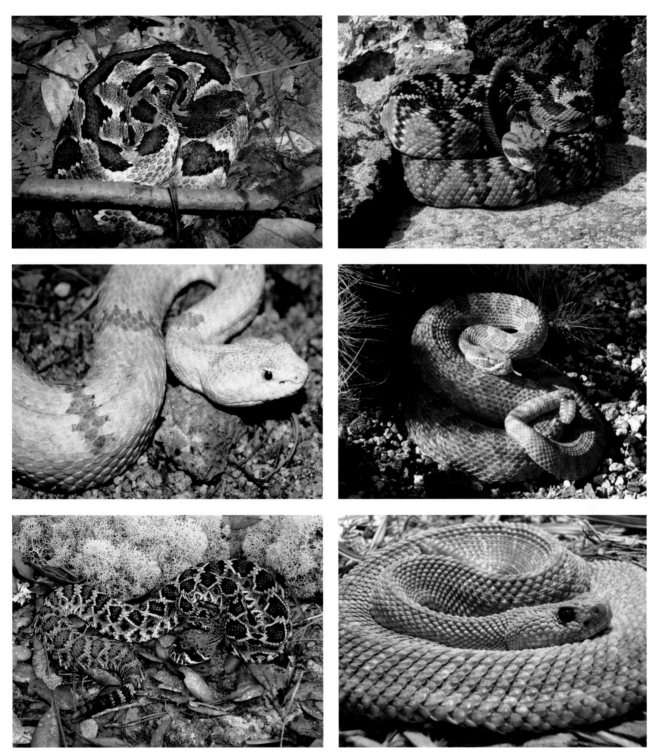

Figure 1.29. Some North American rattlesnakes. **Upper left:** Timber Rattlesnake (*Crotalus horridus*) at Roan Mountain, Virginia. **Upper right:** Black-tailed Rattlesnake (*Crotalus molossus*). **Middle left:** An unusually light specimen of Rock Rattlesnake (*Crotalus lepidus*). **Middle right:** A Hopi Rattlesnake, subspecies of the Prairie Rattlesnake (*Crotalus viridis nuntius*). **Lower left:** A juvenile Eastern Diamondback Rattlesnake (*Crotalus adamanteus*). **Lower right:** Aruba Island Rattlesnake (*Crotalus durissus unicolor*). The Timber Rattlesnake and Eastern Diamondback Rattlesnake were photographed by Dan Dourson. All other photographs were taken by the author.

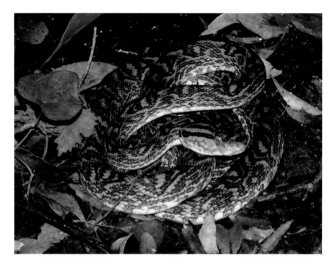

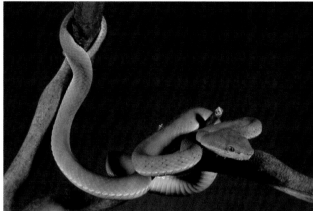

Figure 1.31. A female Chinese Green Tree Viper (*Trimeresurus stejnegeri*) in Taiwan. This species is highly arboreal and has a more slender body form than is typical of ground-dwelling viperid species. The green color also is cryptic, for the snake occurs typically in green tropical vegetation. Photograph by Ming-Chung Tu.

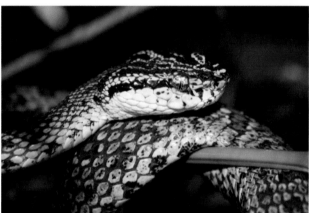

Figure 1.30. The often feared Habu (*Protobothrops flavoviridis*) is a pit viper found in Japan and the Ryukyu Islands (**upper photo**). It is the largest member of its genus and grows to a length of nearly 230 cm (7.5 ft). The body is relatively slender, and the head is quite long. This species has a toxic venom and inflicts numerous snake bites on humans living on certain islands. Many Habus are collected and used to make strong liquor called awamori, which is alleged to have medicinal properties. Photograph by Akira Mori. The **lower photo** features a Jerdon's Pit Viper (*Protobothrops jerdoni*), also called Red-spotted Pit Viper. This is a captive-bred snake from individuals originating in Vietnam. Photograph by the author.

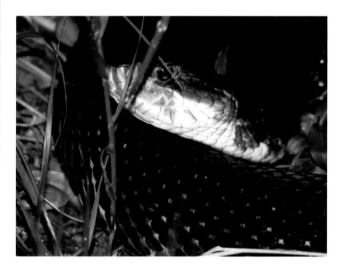

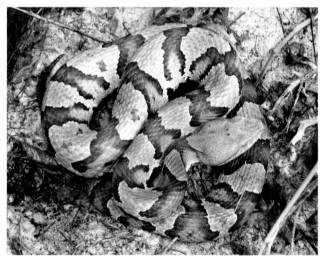

appears to be closely related to pit vipers, but it was once considered to be the most "primitive" (basal) living viper. Recent molecular data place this snake in a separate sub-family, Azemiopinae, which is sister to the Crotalinae.

Elapids: Cobras, Coral Snakes, Mambas, and Sea Snakes

The family Elapidae includes familiar terrestrial species of snakes such as cobras, mambas, coral snakes, kraits, and extensive radiations of Australian-Papuan snakes and marine species we call sea snakes. The elapids are characterized by fixed, hollow fangs located in the front of the mouth, and these are relatively short in the majority of species (chapter 2).

Figure 1.32. Upper photo: An adult Florida Cottonmouth (*Agkistrodon piscivorus conanti*) rests within vegetation while photographed by the author on an island near the Gulf coast of Florida. The **lower photo** features an adult Northern Copperhead (*Agkistrodon contortrix mokasen*) photographed by Dan Dourson in Kentucky.

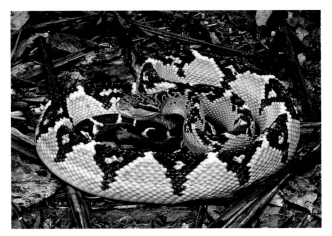

Figure 1.33. The South American Bushmaster (*Lachesis muta*) is the longest pit viper in the Western Hemisphere. The longest recorded specimen measured a little over 3.5 m (about 12 feet) in length. This specimen was photographed by Laurie J. Vitt in Mato Grosso, Brazil.

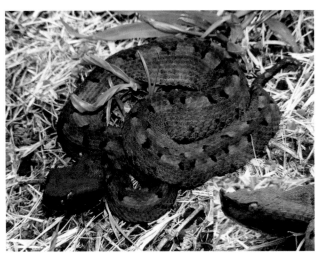

Figure 1.35. An adult Hognosed Pit Viper (*Porthidium nasutum*) in Costa Rica. This species is found in mesic lowland broadleaf forest or rainforest. This snake was photographed by the author at the Instituto Clodomiro Picado, University of Costa Rica, in San José.

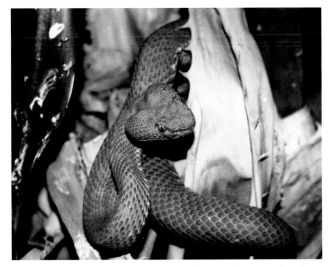

Figure 1.34. A Blotched Palm-pitviper (*Bothriechis supraciliaris*), arboreal and endemic to Costa Rica. This species was once thought to be a subspecies of the Eyelash Pitviper, which it resembles superficially. The color pattern varies, and specimens from most parts of Costa Rica are variably blotched in dorsal coloration. This is a captive individual that belonged to Carl Franklin and was photographed by the author.

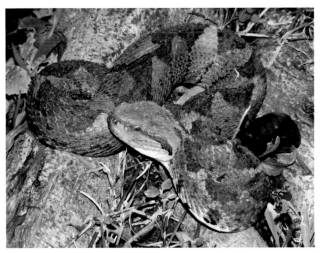

Figure 1.36. Central American Jumping Pit Viper (*Atropoides mexicanus*). This species is found from Mexico south to Panama, and it occurs on the Pacific slopes of Costa Rica, where this specimen was found. It is ground-dwelling, well camouflaged, and has a stout body. The common name of this genus—jumping pit viper—is attributable to energetic defensive strikes that sometimes lift the snake off the ground as if it was "jumping." This specimen was photographed by the author in Costa Rica.

All elapids are venomous, but some are far more dangerous than others. Extremely toxic venoms are characteristic of mambas, some cobras, and sea snakes as well as certain larger terrestrial species inhabiting Australia. There are more than 270 species of elapids worldwide, and they occur throughout a diversity of habitats including warm, tropical oceans and some of the world's driest deserts. Most terrestrial species are oviparous, but viviparity is characteristic of some African and many Australian forms. Other species (e.g., Australian Red-bellied Black Snake, *Pseudechis porphyriacus*) give birth to young that are enveloped in transparent fetal membranes, from which they escape over the course of a few days (see chapter 9).

Elapids are represented in the Americas by coral snakes, which are brightly colored with patterns of bands and rings that are commonly mimicked by harmless species with overlapping ranges (figs. 1.51, 1.52, 5.19). There are about 65 species of coral snakes, primarily neotropical in distribution. Most coral snakes eat other reptiles, including snakes, and such dietary specialization also is characteristic of various other elapids inhabiting the Old World.

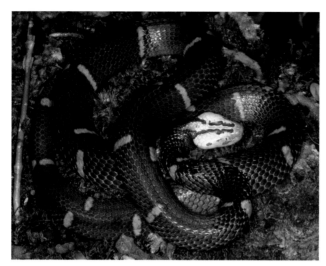

Figure 1.37. An adult Fea's Viper (*Azemiops feae*) from Cao Bang province, Vietnam. Photograph by Dr. Nikolai L. Orlov, Russian Academy of Sciences.

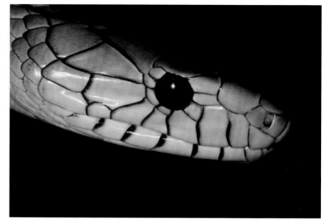

Figure 1.38. The head of a Jameson's Mamba (*Dendroaspis jamesoni*), a highly arboreal species of elapid that is common throughout central Africa. Photograph by John C. Murphy.

Cobras and their relatives such as kraits and mambas occur over extensive regions of Africa and Asia. Mambas (*Dendroaspis* spp.) are native to sub-Saharan Africa where they pose a particular hazard to humans because of their arboreal habits, swift movements, and aggressive defenses. Because a mamba might be well concealed while resting in a shrub or low tree one or more meters above the ground, accidental encounters might involve an aggressive bite received at the head or chest level (fig. 1.38). Cobras are common throughout much of Africa and Asia, posing potential dangers to humans, but the perception of danger is exaggerated by the spectacular behaviors of rising erect while spreading the neck region into a hood and emitting loud and abrupt hisses (fig. 1.39). The hoods of cobras often bear markings that resemble eyes and have startling effects. Several species of cobras have evolved the habit of spitting venom toward an intruder, often aiming for the eyes (see fig. 2.29). A number of Australian elapids also exhibit hooding behaviors, but the neck is seldom flattened as extensively or consistently as in cobras. One of the more spectacular species of cobra is the King Cobra (*Ophiophagus hannah*) of southern and southeastern Asia (fig. 1.39). Some specimens reach a length of 5 m, and all feed on other snakes, which is the basis of the generic name. The King Cobra is the longest venomous snake living today.

Other Asian elapids include 13 species of terrestrial kraits (*Bungarus* spp.), which are brightly colored, nocturnal species that prey on other snakes and often bite persons while they sleep on the ground or in huts (fig. 1.40). Like coral snakes, kraits often live sympatrically with harmless or mildly venomous colubrid snakes that mimic them. Two species of *Boulengerina* (called water cobras) frequent rocky shorelines of lakes where they feed primarily on fish. Various other elapids are arboreal, and others of varying habits resemble New World coral snakes. Among the latter are seven species of African garter snakes (*Elapsoidea* spp.), so-called Asian coral snakes (*Calliophis* spp.; fig. 1.41), and two peculiar species of the genus *Maticora* having exceptionally elongate venom glands measuring up to one-third of the body length! These are also called coral snakes. Many coral snakes, including all the Old World species, may raise their tail when disturbed and display brilliant colors on the underside of the body.

More than a fourth of the world's elapid snakes are represented by the diverse radiation of species inhabiting Australia, New Guinea, and nearby islands. It is interesting to become acquainted with these snakes, as many species have evolved similarities with counterparts in other snake families by the process called *convergent* evolution. Thus, there are large and swift terrestrial species of elapids that are very similar in behaviors and movements to colubrid whipsnakes and racers; others resemble secretive or burrowing species such as ringneck snakes, ground snakes, and Asian coral snakes; and still others are similar to arboreal species of colubrids, and so forth. A very impressive convergence of body form and behavior involves three species of Australian death adders (*Acanthophis* spp.), which resemble some terrestrial vipers (fig. 1.42). The similarities include cryptic coloration, stout body with triangular head, ambush method of capturing prey, and luring of prey by wiggling an elevated tail. Death adders also have evolved relatively long fangs that fit into fleshy sockets in the floor of the mouth. The sockets are receptacles for the fangs, which like other elapids are fixed in place but, like vipers, have some mobility and are relatively long for snaring and envenomating mammals and birds. Other large, swift, and dangerous elapids playing counterpart role to mambas, cobras, and large, diurnally active colubrid snakes include two species of taipan (*Oxyuranus* spp.), brown snakes (*Pseudonaja nuchalis* and *P. textilis*), tiger snakes (*Notechis* spp.), and the Red-bellied Black Snake (*Pseudechis porphyriacus*).

Two radiations of elapids have evolved marine habits (independently) and are collectively called "sea snakes." These were formerly sometimes classified into two separate families, but here are treated as two clades within the Elapidae. This latter classification scheme seems most widely accepted at the present time. Sea snakes known generally as sea kraits (Laticaudini) include eight species of amphibious elapids that are oviparous and spend varying amounts of time in humid, near-shore environments such as rocky shores and limestone crevices of islands in the western Pacific Ocean (fig. 1.43). These snakes spend much time at sea, however, where they feed on fishes, largely or exclusively eels.

The other sea snakes—roughly 60 species (Hydrophiini)—are entirely marine and give birth to live young at sea. The Yellow-bellied Sea Snake (*Pelamis platurus*) is uniquely pelagic in habits and is the only species of marine elapid to have reached the Americas, being quite common along the Pacific coast from Baja California to Ecuador (fig. 1.44). Elsewhere it is the world's most widely distributed snake, ranging from the southeast coast of Africa across the Indo-Pacific to the Americas. Recently, Kate Sanders and colleagues have suggested that the Yellow-bellied Sea Snake and several other mostly monotypic genera be recognized as a single genus, *Hydrophis*, based on their studies providing an improved phylogenetic framework and evolutionary timescale for hydrophiine sea snakes. I believe this suggestion is adequately supported and justified, but I will retain the name *Pelamis platurus* in this book simply because of its long-standing historic familiarity.

Numerous other hydrophiine species occur generally on coral reefs, where they prey on fishes or fish eggs. Some sea snakes have a generalist diet, consuming a variety of fishes, while others are more specialized with prey often restricted to eels or gobies. Three species specialize on fish eggs and forage by probing the head into crevices and burrows. These egg specialists have reduced fangs and relatively blunt faces.

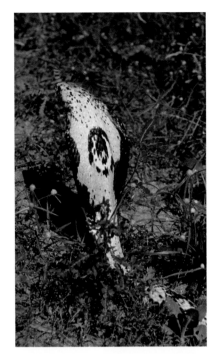
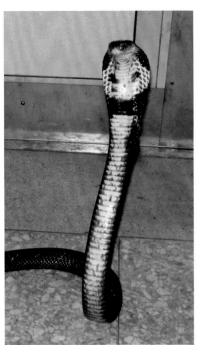
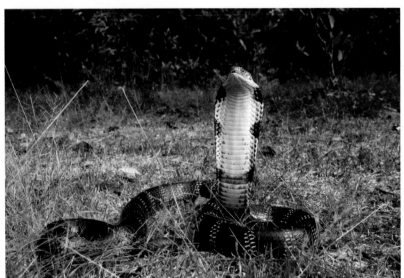

Figure 1.39. Cobras with defensive hoods on display. The **upper left** photo features a dorsal view of an Indochinese Spitting Cobra (*Naja siamensis*) photographed by the author in Thailand. The **upper right** photo shows a ventral view of a raised Chinese Cobra (*Naja atra*), photographed by Coleman Sheehy III in Taiwan. The **lower photo** displays the hood of a King Cobra (*Ophiophagus hannah*) photographed in India by Gowri Shankar.

Most hydrophiine sea snakes are moderate in size, measuring usually between 0.5 and 1 m, while the largest species (Stokes' Sea Snake, *Astrotia stokesii*) reaches lengths near 2 m. Stokes' Sea Snake has a massive and muscular body and broad snout, and its fangs are long enough to pierce a wetsuit (fig. 1.45). These snakes have been reported to sometimes drift in the thousands together on slicks in the Strait of Malacca.

Sea snakes as a group (both clades, or subfamilies) are generally distributed throughout tropical marine and usually

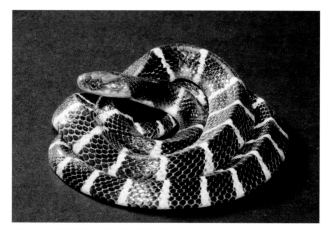

Figure 1.40. Many-banded Krait (*Bungarus multicinctus*) photographed by Ming-Chung Tu in Taiwan.

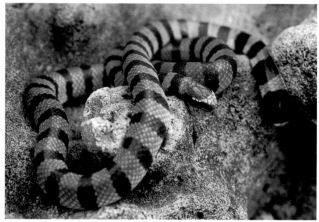

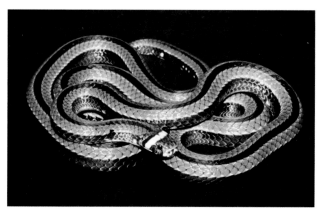

Figure 1.41. Oriental Coral Snake (*Calliophis sauteri*), photographed in Taiwan by Ming-Chung Tu.

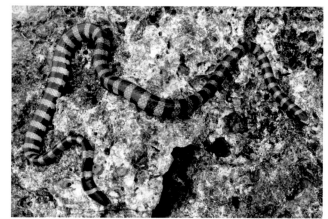

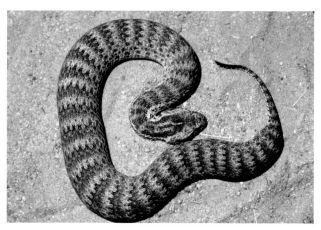

Figure 1.42. Common Death Adder (*Acanthophis antarcticus*) photographed by the author in Victoria, Australia. Note the superficial resemblance to vipers, in terms of the stout body and triangular-shaped head. This species also has elongated fangs compared with other elapid snakes, and some of its behaviors resemble those of vipers (e.g., ambush foraging on prey). The resemblance of this species to vipers is a marvelous example of convergent evolution.

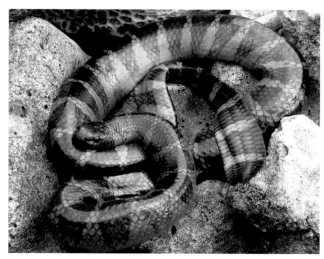

Figure 1.43. Upper photo: Yellow-lipped Sea Krait (*Laticauda colubrina*). **Center photo:** Blue-banded Sea Krait (*Laticauda laticaudata*). **Lower photo:** Chinese Sea Krait (*Laticauda semifasciata*). All snakes were photographed in Taiwan. Note the paddle-shaped tails, which assist swimming. All three species are predominantly marine, but tendencies to spend time on land increase from bottom to top. The upper and lower photographs are by Ming-Chung Tu, and the center photograph is by Coleman M. Sheehy III.

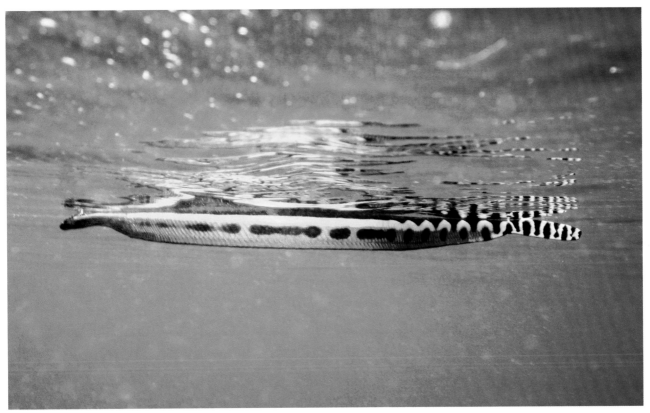

Figure 1.44. An exceptionally colorful Yellow-bellied Sea Snake (*Pelamis platurus*) photographed from beneath the ocean surface off the Pacific coast of Costa Rica. This snake depicts a typical "float-and-wait" posture that is used when these snakes lie at the ocean surface, where they feed on relatively small pelagic fishes. Photograph by Joseph Pfaller.

nearshore waters with greatest species diversity in the Australasian region. Australia has an especially rich fauna of marine snakes, which include over half of the world's species. The genus *Hydrophis* contains by far the most species, which is around 50 percent of the world's total. All sea snakes—both hydrophiine and laticaudine species—characteristically have flattened, paddle-shaped tails (figs. 1.43–1.45; see also chapter 3) and nostrils with valve-like structures that can close the external openings (see figs. 6.10 and 7.14). During swimming, the body also is flattened in a dorsoventral plane as an aid to more efficient locomotion (see chapter 3). Some species dive as deep as 100 m (*Hydrophis*), but most live in relatively shallow waters ranging generally from 20 to 50 m in depth. The skin of sea snakes that have been carefully investigated is modified to exchange a substantial fraction of respiratory gases and also to vent nitrogen as an aid in preventing the Caisson disease (known as "the bends"). More information on the diving adaptations of these remarkable snakes is given in chapter 6.

Colubrids: Common, Diverse, and Familiar Snakes

Many of the familiar and common "harmless" or rear-fanged snakes belong to the family Colubridae, which contains approximately 320 genera and more than 1,800 species distributed throughout the New and Old World land masses. At least seven subfamilies are recognized. It is difficult to describe these snakes in general terms, and the subfamilies are not easily assigned to single common names. It is worth pointing out that the family Colubridae is not the same thing as the larger, more inclusive taxon Colubroidea.

Snakes belonging to the subfamily Natricinae (more than 200 species) are a familiar element of the snake fauna of North America and include the water snakes (*Nerodia* spp.; *Natrix* in the Old World), garter and ribbon snakes (*Thamnophis* spp.), and related species (e.g., Queen Snake and crayfish snakes, *Regina* spp.; Swamp Snake, *Seminatrix pygaea*) (fig. 1.46, 147; see also figs. 4.2 and 4.8). Counterparts to the North American species are represented by other genera distributed largely in Europe, Asia, and Africa. Natricine snakes are semiaquatic or amphibious, but none are completely aquatic like the elapid sea snakes. The diets are varied, but most feed on fish and amphibians. Reproduction varies within this group, as North American species tend to give birth to live young, whereas the majority of Old World species lay eggs.

More than 650 species considered to be "typical" colubrids have worldwide distribution and are classified in the subfamily Colubrinae (fig. 1.48). Some of the more familiar species

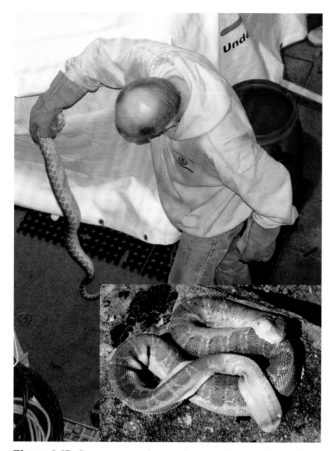

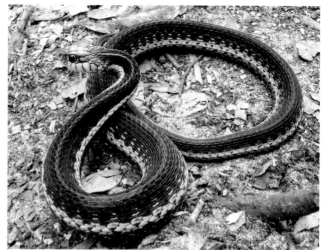

Figure 1.46. A Bluestriped Garter Snake, *Thamnophis sirtalis similis*, photographed in Levy County, Florida by Dan Dourson.

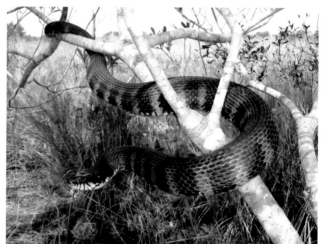

Figure 1.45. Some species of sea snakes grow large and bulky. At the left, Arne Rasmussen holds a large adult *Hydrophis ornatus*, captured in the seas near Sulawesi (photograph by Erik Frausing). The inset shows a specimen of the largest sea snake species, *Astrotia stokesii*, captured on the Australian Great Barrier Reef by Robb Dockerill and photographed by the author.

include king snakes and milk snakes (*Lampropeltis* spp.), rat snakes (*Elaphe* and *Pantherophis* spp.), racers and whipsnakes (*Coluber*, *Drymobius*, and *Masticophis* spp.), various smaller species of secretive ground-dwelling snakes (e.g., *Tantilla* spp.), large indigo snakes (*Drymarchon* spp.), rear-fanged mangrove, tree, or cat snakes (*Boiga* spp.; the Brown Tree Snake *Boiga irregularis* being known for having invaded Guam and decimated parts of the native bird fauna), specialized feeders such as the African egg-eating snakes (*Dasypeltis* spp.; see chapter 2), swift-moving arboreal species (*Thelotornis*, *Dendrelaphis*, *Opheodrys*, spp. and others) including the remarkable Asian flying snakes (*Chrysopelea* spp.; see chapter 3). The latter have evolved morphological and behavioral specializations for gliding. Many of the colubrine snakes are a conspicuous and common element of North American vertebrate fauna and well known to may persons residing on that continent. Interestingly, there is a parallel dominance of numerous species of venomous elapids that are equally familiar to residents of Australia, where terrestrial colubrids are largely

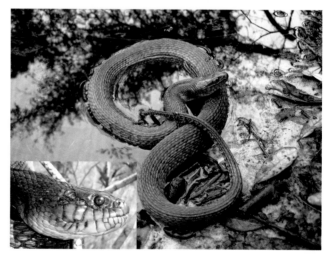

Figure 1.47. Two species of water snakes common to Florida. The **upper photo** features the Florida Banded Water Snake (*Nerodia fasciata pictiventris*), and the **lower photo** shows the Florida Green Water Snake (*Nerodia floridana*). An enlargement of the head is shown in the inset. Both snakes were photographed in Levy County, Florida, by Dan Dourson.

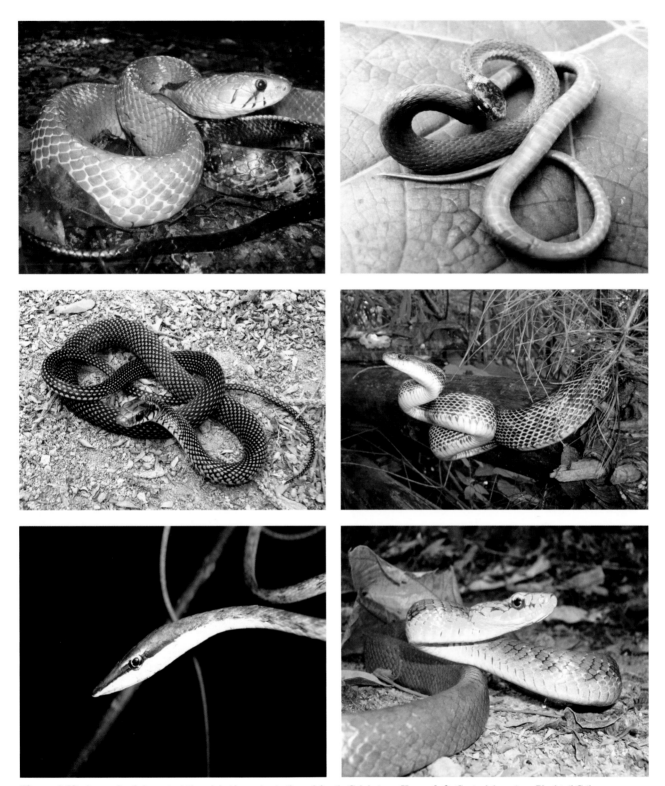

Figure 1.48. A sample of characteristic colubrid species in the subfamily Colubrinae. **Upper left**, Central American Blacktail Cribo (*Drymarchon melanurus*), photographed in Belize by Dan Dourson. **Upper right**, Florida Redbelly Snake (*Storeria occipitomaculata obscura*), photographed in Gainesville, Florida by the author. **Middle left**, Central American Speckled Racer (*Drymobius margaritiferus*), belonging to a clade of snakes also known as Neotropical racers. This individual was photographed in Belize by Dan Dourson. **Middle right**, Black Rat Snake (*Pantherophis obsoletus*), photographed in Florida by Dan Dourson. **Lower left**, Brown Vine Snake (*Oxybelis aeneus*), photographed in Belize by Dan Dourson. **Lower right**, Puffing Snake (*Pseustes poecilonotus*) named for its defensive display of laterally compressed neck. This specimen was photographed in Belize by Dan Dourson.

absent. The two respective faunas—elapids in Australia and colubrines in North America—exhibit numerous convergences in habitats that are structurally and climatically similar. Diets of the various colubrine species are remarkably diverse, and the large majority of species are oviparous with some laying large numbers of eggs (40 or more).

The subfamily Xenodontinae is a monophyletic taxon that contains about 300 species of medium to large (1.3 m) terrestrial snakes found in a diversity of habitats in North, Middle, and South America. This group includes all of the endemic colubrids of the West Indies and the Galapagos Islands. Some of the false coral snake species belong to this group, as well as the familiar North American hognose snakes (*Heterodon* spp.; fig. 1.49), which specialize on eating toads. Ringneck snakes (*Diadophis* spp.) and Mud Snakes (*Farancia abacura*) are also xenodontines (fig. 1.50). The three species just mentioned belong to a subfamily Carphophiinae, which also includes the genera *Carphophis* and *Contia*. A number of the tropical species are swift and racer-like in appearance with arboreal or semiarboreal habits.

Other species are fossorial or aquatic. Xenodontines prey on a range of animals, mostly vertebrates. Some are rear-fanged but with relatively mild venom. Most xenodontines lay eggs, but viviparity occurs in some species.

A clade of snakes formerly defined as Central American xenodontines are now considered to be a subfamily called Dipsadinae and a sister group to the Xenodontinae. The Dipsadinae include about 350 species of mostly small to medium-sized snakes having diverse habits and diets, mostly in Central and South America. Blunt-headed vine snakes (*Imantodes* spp.) are extremely slender and arboreal and feed on lizards (fig. 1.51). Many dipsadine snakes, however, specialize on invertebrates such as earthworms or gastropods, and include the interesting snail-eating snakes (e.g., *Dipsas*, *Sibon* spp.; fig. 1.52). Nearly all of the dipsadine species are oviparous.

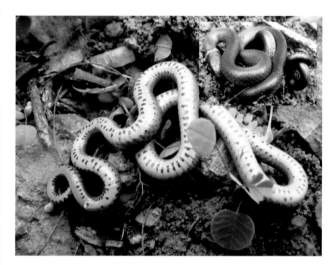

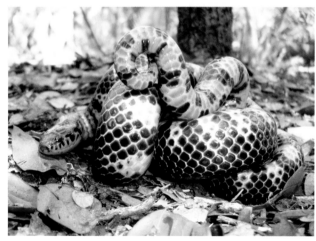

Figure 1.50. Two North American xenodontine snake species, both featured in a defensive posture with the tail elevated to display the colorful underside. The **upper photo** with inset features a Prairie Ringneck Snake (*Diadophis punctatus*) photographed in Kansas by the author. The **lower photo** shows a Mud Snake (*Farancia abacura*) photographed in Florida by Dan Dourson. Both species are secretive and display the red to orange underside of the tail when disturbed.

Figure 1.49. Western Hognose Snake (*Heterodon nasicus*). These photographs feature the upturned and heavily cornified snout used as an aid in burrowing. Other features of this snake superficially resemble a viper. Photographs by the author.

Gastropod Feeders in the Old World

There are about 20 species of Old World snail- and slug-eating snakes, ecologically equivalent to the neotropical genera *Dipsas* and *Sibon*, that belong to a separate family Pareatidae. The New and Old World gastropod feeders were once thought to be closely related, but the similarities are now known to be attributable to convergence. The Asian snakes belong to the genera *Aplopeltura*, *Asthenodipsas*, and *Pareas* distributed through Southeast Asia and the Sunda Shelf. Many of the species are arboreal and, like arboreal counterparts in some of the other subfamilies, extremely slender with broad, blunt heads and large eyes (fig. 1.53). These snakes are primarily nocturnal, and all are oviparous.

The Homalopsidae: Snakes of Mud and Water

Another group of colubroid snakes with partial to strong aquatic tendencies comprises the family Homalopsidae, which is a well-defined lineage containing about 40 species distributed largely in Southeast Asia and Australasia (fig. 1.54). Many of these species live in shallow water habitats, and they have valved nostrils and dorsally directed eyes situated on the top of the head (fig. 7.6). One species, the Keel-bellied Watersnake (*Bitia hydroides*), superficially resembles the true sea snakes in attributes of body form, including reduced ventral scales, relatively enlarged posterior body, and a feebly compressed tail.

All homalopsids have enlarged fangs at the rear of the mouth, which serve to envenomate prey usually consisting of amphibians or fish. Some species (e.g., *Fordonia* and *Gerarda* spp.) consume invertebrates, including hard-shelled animals such as crabs or other crustaceans, which the snakes

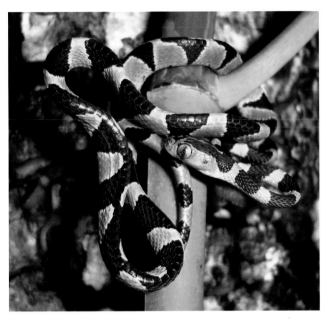

Figure 1.51. A Blunt-headed Tree Snake (*Imantodes cenchoa*) shown in its natural habitat of rainforest in Belize. Photograph by Dan Dourson.

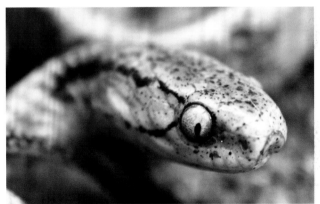

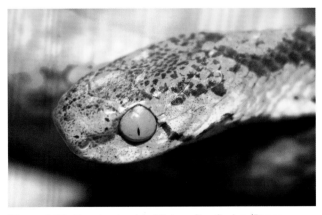

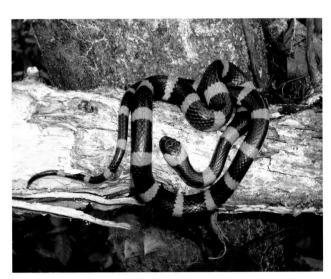

Figure 1.52. A Terrestrial Snail Sucker (*Tropidodipsas sartorii*) photographed in its native habitat in Belize by Dan Dourson.

Figure 1.53. Two closely related Taiwan Slug Snakes (*Pareas formosensis*) illustrating very different eye colors. Both snakes were photographed in Taiwan and have been considered to be a single species, although current unpublished studies may divide the species into three. This species of the family Pareatidae is ecologically and behaviorally convergent with various dipsadine colubrid snakes in the New World. These snakes were photographed in Taipei by the author.

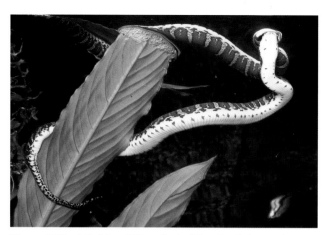

Figure 1.54. A Puff-faced Water Snake (*Homalopsis buccata*) as seen from below when air-breathing in shallow water. Photographed at Kota Samarahan, Sarawak, Malaysia by Indraneil Das.

amazingly rip apart into smaller pieces to swallow. Some members of this family occupy freshwater habitats such as lakes, swamps, or streams (e.g., numerous species of *Enhydris*), whereas others are estuarine and occur in shallow coastal marine waters (e.g., Dog-faced Water Snake, *Cerberus rhynchops*). One very unusual species, popular among some herpetoculturists, is the aquatic Tentacled Snake (*Erpeton tentaculatum*) from southeastern Asia (fig. 7.14). This snake has two fleshy "tentacles" on its snout, which are sensory and are likely an aid to navigation in murky water as well as provider of information from mechanical stimuli such as the disturbance to water when a swimming fish is nearby (fig. 2.10). It appears that all homalopsids give birth to live young, and some may reach incredibly high population densities. In some habitats, *Cerberus rhynchops* can reach densities up to three individuals per square meter!

Toward a Phylogeny of Snakes

Confusion over the evolutionary history and taxonomic classification of snakes has stimulated both debate and controversy among scientists for decades. The works of Bogert, Cope, Dowling, Duméril, Dunn, Hoffstetter, Jan, Underwood, and others provided the classical foundations for snake phylogeny, while more recent historical reviews of the progress made have been offered by Burbrink, Cadle, Crother, Greene, Rieppel, Pyron, Vidal, Wiens, Wilcox, Zaher, and others. Knowledge of morphology continues to be helpful to evaluate phylogeny, and molecular studies have provided large quantities of data that have advanced the understanding of ophidian evolution rapidly. Numerous scientists are now contributing molecular studies and adding new insights concerning phylogenetic relationships at all levels, including specific and limited assemblages as well as higher level taxa. Ultimately, consensus of a comprehensive phylogeny of

snakes will be achieved through improved understanding of both morphological and molecular data. At the time of this writing, however, molecular studies are appearing so rapidly that taxonomic revisions are not always adequately evaluated by the broader community of systematists before other studies appear and keep moving. This is sometimes confusing to the novice for whom it is not always clear what is what.

In spite of the controversy over details, a generalized phylogeny for snakes seems pretty well known and can be qualified without too much debate. So here I shall present what is simply a broad pattern of phylogenetic relationships of snakes that is based in consensus insofar as possible. The following discussion is with reference to a consensus phylogeny that is illustrated in figure 1.55.

What are called lepidosaurs include the ancient but still living New Zealand tuataras and the squamates, which are sister taxa (fig. 1.10). Sister taxa (or groups) are derived from an ancestral species not shared by any other taxon, and they appear on a cladogram as lineages that arise as branches from a single divergence node. Lepidosaurs are a sister group to the branch of reptiles that gave rise to the birds and crocodilians, as illustrated in figure 1.10. The squamates are further subdivided into lizards, amphisbaenians, and snakes. The snakes collectively comprise the suborder Serpentes, which is sometimes called Ophidia. Snakes are considered to be monophyletic but have diverged considerably from ancestral conditions. They have diversified to form a rich assemblage of species within the squamates.

Here you will see a simplified phylogeny of snakes based in consensus from a number of studies including both morphological and molecular data (fig. 1.55). The early or basal divergence of snakes occurred between the Scolecophidia and all other snakes comprising the Alethinophidia. The henophidian snakes are polyphyletic and diversified relatively early into many taxa including the evolution of boas and pythons. The placement of acrochordids (Acrochordidae, or Acrochordoidea) was long considered to be problematic, but recent taxonomic arrangements consider the only three species of acrochordids to be a lineage that is sister to the Colubroidea. Within the latter group, the viperid snakes are sister to the collective taxa of elapids, lamprophiids, homalopsids, and colubrids. The reader may consult recent descriptive taxonomic and phylogenetic literature for more details regarding the classification of higher snakes, much of which is still unresolved or in dispute. One recent molecular phylogenetic analysis places acrochordids, pareatids, and xenodermatid snakes as basally divergent from other caenophidians, and suggests that viperid snakes comprise a successive sister clade to all remaining caenophidians. The fairest thing I can say is that one may regard all current phylogenetic trees as "fluid" hypotheses about evolutionary events that are becoming increasingly, but not entirely, understood.

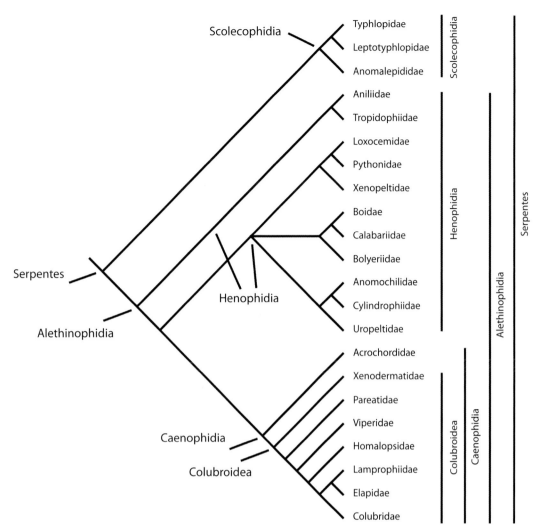

Figure 1.55. A phylogeny of snakes illustrating the author's interpretation of current consensus among herpetological systematists, all of whom do not agree on the details of the relationships. Any such phylogeny should be considered "fluid" (or a hypothesis) and is expected to change as new work is done based on molecular and other methods. The phylogeny illustrates relationships among the principal families of snakes that are listed as terminal branches at the right of the figure. Higher taxa, or groupings of families, are bracketed with bars at the right, each corresponding to principal branchings that are identified within the phylogenetic tree. Drawing by Coleman M. Sheehy III and the author.

Returning to our earlier question—What is a snake?—a summary definition might be given as follows. A snake is a squamate reptile of the suborder Ophidia (or Serpentes), characterized by having a cylindrical, limbless, and scaled body with fused eyelids and no external ear. The jaws are modified for capturing and swallowing relatively large prey, and numerous species in various taxa are venomous. Other attributes will become better understood and more appreciated as the reader explores the remaining chapters in this book.

Additional Reading

Adalsteinsson, S. A., W. R. Branch, S. Trape, L. J. Vitt, and S. B. Hedges. 2009. Molecular phylogeny, classification, and biogeography of snakes of the family Leptotyphlopidae (Reptilia, Squamata). *Zootaxa* 2244:1–50.

Alfaro, M. E., D. R. Karns, H. K. Voris, C. D. Brock, and B. L. Stuart. 2008. Phylogeny, evolutionary history, and biogeography of Oriental-Australian rear-fanged water snakes (Colubroidea: Homalopsidae) inferred from mitochondrial and nuclear DNA sequences. *Molecular Phylogenetics and Evolution* 46:576–593.

Cadle, J. E. 1987. Geographic distribution: Problems in phylogeny and zoogeography. In R. A. Seigel, J. T. Collins, and S. S. Novak (eds.), *Snakes: Ecology and Evolutionary Biology*. New York: Macmillan, pp. 77–105.

Cadle, J. E. 1994. The colubrid radiation in Africa (Serpentes: Colubridae): phylogenetic relationships and evolutionary patterns based on immunological data. *Zoological Journal of the Linnean. Society* 110:103–140.

Caprette, C. L., M. S. Y. Lee, R. Shine, A. Mokany, and J. F. Downhower. 2004. The origin of snakes (Serpentes) as seen through eye anatomy. *Biological Journal of the Linnean Society* 81:469–482.

Cohn, M. J., and C. Tickle. 1999. Developmental basis of limbless-ness and axial patterning in snakes. *Nature* 399:474–479.

Greene, H. W. 1997. *Snakes: The Evolution of Mystery in Nature.* Berkeley: University of California Press. 351 pp.

Gutberlet Jr., R. L., and M. B. Harvey. 2004. The Evolution of New World Venomous Snakes. In J. A. Campbell and W. W. Lamar (eds.), *Venomous Reptiles of the Western Hemisphere*, vol. 2. Ithaca, NY: Comstock (Cornell University Press), pp. 634–682.

Head, J. J., J. I. Bloch, A. K. Hastings, J. R. Bourque, E. A. Cadena, F. A. Herrera, P. D. Polly and C. A. Jaramillo. 2009. Giant boid snake from the Palaeocene neotropics reveals hotter past equatorial temperatures. *Nature* 457:715–718.

Heatwole, H. 1999. *Sea Snakes.* Malabar, FL: Krieger Publishing.

Hedges, S. B. 2008. At the lower size limit in snakes: Two new species of threadsnakes (Squamata: Leptotyphlopidae: *Leptotyphlops*) from the Lesser Antilles. *Zootaxa* 1841:1–30.

Heise, P. J., L. R. Maxson, H. G. Dowling, and S. B. Hedges. 1995. Higher-level snake phylogeny inferred from mitochondrial DNA sequences of 12S rRNA and 16S rRNA genes. *Molecular Biology and Evolution* 12:259–265.

Highton, R., S. B. Hedges, C. A. Hass, and H. G. Dowling. 2002. Snake relationships revealed by slowly-evolving proteins: Further analysis and a reply. *Herpetologica* 58:270–275.

Hoso, M., T. Asami, and M. Hori. 2007. Right-handed snakes: Convergent evolution of asymmetry for functional specialization. *Biology Letters* 3:169–172.

Keogh, J. S. 1998. Molecular phylogeny of elapid snakes and a consideration of their biogeographic history. *Biological Journal of the Linnaean Society* 63:177–203.

Knight, A., and D. P. Mindell. 1994. On the phylogenetic relationships of Colubrinae, Elapidae and Viperidae and the evolution of front fanged venom systems in snakes. *Copeia* 1994:1–9.

Kraus, F., and W. M. Brown. 1998. Phylogenetic relationships of colubroid snakes based on mitochondrial DNA sequences. *Zoological Journal of the Linnean Society* 122:455–487.

Lee, M. S. Y. 2005. Molecular evidence and marine snake origins. *Biology Letters* 1:227–230.

Lee, M. S. Y., A. F. Hugall, R. Lawson, and J. D. Scanlon. 2007. Phylogeny of snakes (Serpentes): Combining morphological and molecular data in likelihood, Bayesian and parsimony analysis. *Systematics and Biodiversity* 5:371–389.

McDowell, S. B. 1987. Systematics. In R. A. Siegel, J. T. Collins, and S. S. Novak (eds.), *Snakes: Ecology and Evolutionary Biology.* New York: Macmillan, pp. 3–50.

Pough, F. H., R. M. Andrews, J. E. Cadle, M. L. Crump, A. H. Savitzky, and K. D. Wells. 2004. *Herpetology.* 3rd edition. Upper Saddle River, NJ: Pearson Prentice-Hall. 544 pp.

Pyron, R. A., and F. T. Burbrink. 2011. Extinction, ecological opportunity, and the origins of global snake diversity. *Evolution* 66:163–178.

Pyron, R. A., F. T. Burbrink, and J. J. Wiens. 2013. A phylogeny and revised classification of Squamata, including 4161 species of lizards and snakes. BMC *Evolutionary Biology* 13:93.

Pyron, R. A., F. T. Burbrink, G. R. Colli, A. N. Montes de Oca, L. J. Vitt, C. A. Kuczynski, and J. J. Wiens. 2011. The phylogeny of advanced snakes (Colubroidea), with discovery of a new subfamily and comparison of support methods for likelihood trees. *Molecular Phylogenetics and Evolution* 58:329–342.

Sanders, K. L., M. S. Y. Lee, Mumpuni, T. Bertozzi, and A. R. Rasmussen. 2012. Multilocus phylogeny and recent rapid radiation of the viviparous sea snakes (Elapidae: Hydrophiinae). *Molecular Phylogenetics and Evolution* 66:575–591.

Scanlon, J. D., and M. S. Y. Lee. 2011. The major clades of snakes: Morphological evolution, molecular phylogeny, and divergence dates. In R. D. Aldridge and D. M. Sever (eds.), *Reproductive Biology and Phylogeny of Snakes.* Vol. 9 of *Reproductive Biology and Phylogeny,* B. G. M. Jamieson, series editor. Enfield, NH: Science Publishers, pp. 55–95.

Shine, R. 2009. *Australian Snakes: A Natural History.* Frenchs Forest, New South Wales, Australia: Reed New Holland.

Slowinski, J. B., and J. S. Keogh. 2000. Phylogenetic relationships of elapid snakes based on Cytochrome b mtDNA sequences. *Molecular Phylogenetics and Evolution* 15:157–164.

Townsend, T. M., A. Larson, E. Louis, and J. R. Macey. 2004. Molecular phylogenetics of squamata: The position of snakes, amphisbaenians, and dibamids, and the root of the squamate tree. *Systematic Biology* 53:735–757.

Vidal, N. 2002. Colubroid systematics: Evidence for an early appearance of the venom apparatus followed by extensive evolutionary tinkering. *Journal of Toxicology: Toxin Reviews* 21:21–41.

Vidal, N., and S. B. Hedges. 2002. Higher-level relationships of snakes inferred from four nuclear and mitochondrial genes. *Comptes Rendus Biologies* 325:977–985.

Vidal, N., and S. B. Hedges. 2002. Higher-level relationships of caenophidian snakes inferred from four nuclear and mitochondrial genes. *Comptes Rendus Biologies* 325:987–995.

Vidal, N., and S. B. Hedges. 2004. Molecular evidence for a terrestrial origin of snakes. *Proceedings of the Royal Society of London B (Suppl.)* 271:S226–S229.

Vidal, N., S. G. Kind, A. Wong, and S. B. Hedges. 2000. Phylogenetic relationships of Xenodontine snakes inferred from 12S and 16S ribosomal RNA sequences. *Molecular Phylogenetics and Evolution* 14:389–402.

Wiens, J., and J. L. Slingluff. 2001. How lizards turn into snakes: A phylogenetic analysis of body-form evolution in anguid lizards. *Evolution* 55:2303–2318.

Wiens, J. ., C. A. Kuczynski, S. A. Smith, D. G. Mulcahy, J. W. Sites Jr., T. M. Townsend, and T. W. Reeder. 2008. Branch lengths, support, and congruence: Testing the phylogenomic approach with 20 nuclear loci in snakes. *Systematic Biology* 57:420–431.

Zaher, H., F. G. Grazziotin, J. E. Cadle, R. W. Murphy, J. C. de Moura-Leite, and S. L. Bonatto. 2009. Molecular phylogeny of advanced snakes (Serpentes, Caenophidia) with an emphasis on South American Xenodontines: A revised classification and description of new taxa. *Papéis Avulsos de Zoologia* (Museu de Zoologia da Universidade de São Paulo) 49:115–153.

Zug, G. R., L. J. Vitt, and J. P. Caldwell. 2001. *Herpetology.* 2nd edition. San Diego: Academic Press. 630 pp.

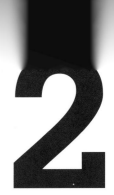

FEEDING, DIGESTION, AND
WATER BALANCE

There are many and ridiculous stories about the swallowing feats of the big snakes. The tales relating to giant pythons engulfing animals as large as an ox are utterly fallacious, nor do the big snakes ever wantonly attack large mammals. The limit of their swallowing capacity would be a moderate-sized antelope—an animal about the size of an American white-tailed deer—and nothing but an unusually large specimen could engulf such prey. A twenty-foot python has been observed by the writer to swallow a forty-pound pig and the process was by no means an easy one.

—*Raymond L. Ditmars*, Reptiles of the World *(1943), p. 140*

Feeding is one aspect of snake behavior that generally fascinates people. There are perhaps two root causes that elicit both interest and awe in the feeding habits of snakes. First, the animals are limbless and must overpower their prey by such unusual means as constriction or envenomation. Second, snakes are intermittent feeders, and most of the common and usually larger species that are familiar to people consume prey that is larger in girth than the mouth of the snake. Many persons are fascinated that snakes swallow relatively large prey and manage to do so by what appears to be amazing elastic properties of the jaws (figs. 2.1, 2.7). The skin also stretches an amazing amount as the prey item is swallowed beyond the jaws.

A snake is basically a long tube and possesses an elongated digestive system (fig. 2.2). Thus, a snake could more or less continually process numerous small items, such as insects or small eggs, or it could feed intermittently on larger items that are accommodated by stretch of the gut, body wall, and skin. Most snakes utilize the second option and swallow the prey entire because they have not evolved teeth that are specialized for tearing, shredding, breaking, or mashing the food into smaller pieces. It is interesting to consider the evolutionary reasons why snakes have evolved the feeding habits they employ, and to ask: What is unique about snakes that constrain or limit the prey they exploit and the manner in which they feed? On the other hand, one can ask: What attributes of snakes have provided evolutionary opportunities for employing the exceptionally effective means by which they capture and utilize prey? Aspects of these questions have fascinated people for centuries (fig. 2.3).

Constraints Related to a Limbless and Elongate Body Form

The following discussion is essentially speculative, but it provides a conceptual basis from which to launch considerations of feeding and digestion in snakes. Fundamentally, because snakes are lacking arms and legs, they cannot catch, handle, and manipulate prey in the same manners that are employed by many other animals. Moreover, without an effective "anchor"—or means of stable stance—it is somewhat problematic or difficult for an animal to browse or graze on vegetation. So what are the most likely foods that are available to snakes?

Insofar as snakes are elongate creatures without limbs, we may consider them to be a long tube with a head at the front end and a tail at the rear. There are three ways in which such an animal might capture food: (1) seize it with the mouth, (2) wrap the body around it, or (3) wrap the tail around it. Two further considerations are important. First, the head is at the end of the animal that first encounters the environment. Second, regardless of the manner of capture, the prey object must be seized by the mouth before swallowing. For these reasons, it seems reasonable to expect the head end of the snake to evolve a mouth with associated

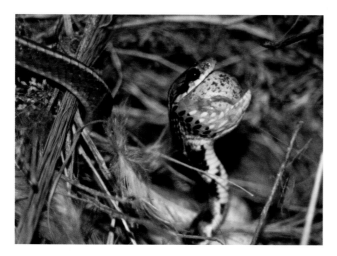

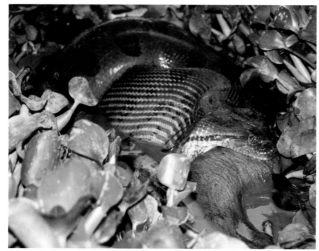

Figure 2.1. Photos illustrating the distensibility of jaws and skin when snakes ingest relatively large objects. In the **upper photo** an Indian Egg-eating Snake (*Elachistodon westermanni*) swallows a bird egg, with amazing stretch of both mucosal tissue and scales on the lower jaw. The **lower photo** illustrates a Green Anaconda (*Eunectes murinus*) swallowing a deer. The upper photo is courtesy of Parag Dandge; the lower photo is courtesy of Jesús A. Rivas.

jaws and teeth that are adapted for seizing prey, in contrast to cutting or masticating prey. Also, we must remember that snakes evolved from lizard-like ancestors and thus inherited lizard-like attributes both of dentition and gape.

Snakes as a group exhibit a propensity to grasp prey items using the mouth, and this involves having an appropriate gape and a good set of recurved teeth. Without having appendages for grasping, holding, and manipulating prey, the teeth must hold the prey firmly, or there must be an alternative means to immobilize the prey. Immobilization is achieved either by injecting the prey item with toxic venom, enwrapping the prey item in body coils, or holding the item firmly within the mouth. Whatever the reasons, the

evolutionary radiation of snakes involved a diversification of feeding specializations for capturing animal prey ranging in size from smaller organisms such as insects, fish, frogs, or lizards to larger avian and mammalian prey having a range of body sizes. Because of the central role of the head in capturing prey, snakes evolved either venoms or constricting mechanisms that subdue prey rapidly in order to avoid potential harm that might be inflicted by the prey. This is especially important for the capture of larger species that are capable of inflicting considerable damage to a snake.

Snakes are well adapted for swallowing relatively large prey entire, without reduction to smaller pieces. There is, however, at least one documented exception to this statement. Gerard's Water Snake (*Gerarda prevostiana*), a homalopsid species, eats crabs by tearing them apart and ingesting the individual pieces. Reducing the prey to pieces is accomplished by holding a crab by the mouth and pulling it through a loop of the body that is formed around it, thereby straining the joints of the crab and causing them to separate. This behavior was reported by Bruce Jayne, Harold Voris, and Peter Ng, but it is rare as far as we know.

The majority of snakes are characterized by comparatively high mobility of the jaws and a large gape size. More basal groups of snakes feed primarily on elongate prey such as earthworms, lizards, or invertebrates, whereas innovations of the feeding apparatus enabled larger snakes to consume heavier and bulkier prey, particularly mammals. Furthermore, snakes or other animals that specialize on eating particular prey typically possess behavioral and morphological traits that facilitate successful foraging. These are generally less important in snakes that have a relatively broad diet, and especially ones that might include carrion as well as living prey.

The Kinetic Skull and Prey Transport

Many persons have witnessed dramatic scenes of snakes swallowing animals that are larger around than their head, and it is well known that these prey are swallowed whole and then moved to the stomach by muscular actions called *peristalsis*. The swallowing of prey is called *prey transport* by functional morphologists, and it is accomplished in snakes only because of unusual mobility of various elements of the skull and jaws. The term, of course, implies movement of prey and also includes "transport" through the esophagus to the stomach.

The skulls of snakes are derived from those of lizards and have been further modified for *kinesis* (joint mobility) and a functional need to better enclose the brain cavity. Anyone who has watched a snake swallow a prey item such as a mouse appreciates the mobility of jaws and skull that are necessary for the animal to manipulate the prey without having arms or hands, and to swallow something that is large in terms of its relative girth. In living reptiles except for turtles, the skull has two postorbital or temporal openings (termed *fenestrae*), known as a *diapsid* condition. Thus, bony elements of the skull form two temporal arches, one below the lower opening and one between the lower and upper opening. Most lizards have lost the lower temporal arch, whereas snakes have lost both of the temporal arches (fig. 2.4). This feature lightens the skull and increases the potential for mobility (fig. 2.5).

Some of the skull bones form movable joints with one another. Typically, the quadrate bone articulates loosely to join the lower jaw with the skull above

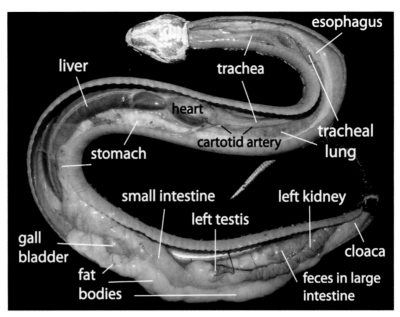

Figure 2.2. Internal anatomy of a young Florida Cottonmouth (*Agkistrodon piscivorus conanti*). Photograph by the author.

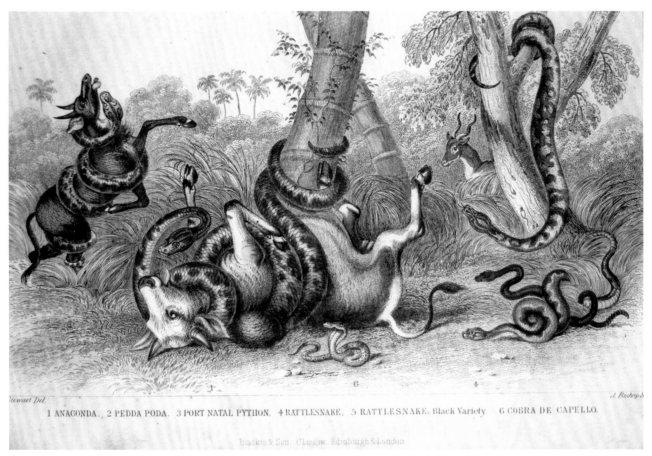

1 ANACONDA. 2 PEDDA PODA. 3 PORT NATAL PYTHON. 4 RATTLESNAKE. 5 RATTLESNAKE, Black Variety. 6 COBRA DE CAPELLO.

Figure 2.3. Historic drawing depicting large constrictors subduing large mammals, which are imaginary exaggerations of the snakes' abilities to swallow large prey. This antique print was originally from *History of the Earth and Animated Nature*, by Oliver Goldsmith (1774), and used in a later edition *A History of the Earth and Animated Nature*, by Oliver Goldsmith, published by A. Fullarton (1850) and Blackie and Son (1862).

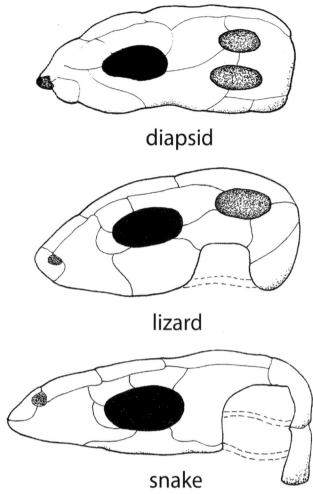

diapsid

lizard

snake

Figure 2.4. Fenestrae (openings) in the bony skull of representative diapsid reptiles. The **upper drawing** illustrates a primitive diapsid condition in which there are two complete temporal fenestrae, with each fenestra bounded by a bony temporal arch. This is characteristic of some primitive reptiles (e.g., dinosaurs) and the living tuatara. The **middle drawing** illustrates the skull of a lizard, representing secondary loss of the lower temporal fenestra. The **lower drawing** illustrates the skull of a snake with secondary loss of both the upper and lower temporal fenestrae. The evolutionary changes illustrated here eventually allowed extreme reduction of bone mass and the associated flexibility of the snake skull that is used during feeding. Drawings by Dan Dourson.

it. The condition of a movable quadrate is called *streptostyly*, and this condition allows the quadrate to move forward and rearward and, to a lesser extent, mediolaterally with respect to the braincase. Streptostyly is associated with the loss of the temporal arches, and this allows the quadrate to swing on a complex articulation between its upper end and the side of the skull. Compared with lizards, the quadrate bone has extraordinary movement in snakes (fig. 2.5).

There is also some degree of motion between the quadrate and the supratemporal bone, and between the supratemporal bone and the braincase. These generate a three-joint system that facilitates lowering the lower jaw and increasing the size of the gape. Other movable bones include the ectopterygoid, maxilla, and prefrontal (figs. 2.5, 2.6). In other reptiles these skull bones are fixed to the braincase or have restricted movement, whereas in snakes these form a linkage of bones having extensive motion relative to the braincase. The parts are joined by ligaments and muscles, characteristically with greater mobility than is seen in lizards. The mechanical linkages include many units, and a variety of movements is possible. Collectively, these permit the capture and ingestion of relatively large prey, which must be swallowed entire. The elements are loosely joined together and operate independently on each side of the head.

For all the movement and potential harm that could be inflicted by the prey, the brain must be protected. The brain of snakes is enclosed in a rigid structure that is formed by downward extensions of the frontal and parietal elements which are sometimes fused and articulate extensively with bone that lies below the brain (fig. 2.6). These structures form a rather solid braincase protecting the brain, and also provide much of the surface area for the attachment of muscles that power much of the movements that are involved in feeding.

The conversion of much of the skull into a rigid box necessitated the losses of certain hinges in the roof of the skull that were present in lizards. The only movable part of the skull roof of snakes is in the facial region where the nasal bones are hinged to the frontal elements (fig. 2.6). In the majority of living snakes the snout can move about this joint, and the condition of having a kinetic joint anterior to the eyes has been termed *prokinesis*. The palatomaxillary elements are movably attached to each other and to the snout and prefrontal, which are capable of movement relative to the braincase. Additionally, however, in natricine snakes (*Nerodia* and *Thamnophis*), there are four movable elements in the snout, and these impart a special condition of mobility that has been termed *rhinokinesis*. In these snakes, movements of the snout bones themselves allow the teeth of the right and left sides to separate further, thereby increasing the extent of movement involved in each cycle of swallowing (see below). Mobility of the nasal elements accounts for the unusual rotations of the snout tip that are sometimes seen during swallowing movements made by garter snakes.

The most uniquely important feature of kinesis in snakes is its association with unilateral mobility of the jaws. Independent movements of the two sides of the lower jaw, coupled with the fact that skin and other tissues connecting them are distensible, permit swallowing of prey that are much larger than the normal size of the snake's head (fig. 2.1

and below). Most snakes transport prey through the mouth using ratcheting movements of the upper jaws, each jaw on right or left side of the head alternately moving over the prey. Characteristically, a snake works prey (and that is *whole* prey) into its mouth by alternately advancing and retracting each of the jaws. During a unilateral cycle of movement, the braincase of the snake is advanced over the prey, rather than the prey being "pulled" into the mouth. The teeth-bearing elements of the upper jaws are "walked" over the prey by alternating shifts of their position, and the prey is never free of grip during the swallowing process. In most snakes the lower jaws have little direct role in transporting prey, but they serve to control the position of the prey in the mouth and to press it against teeth of the overlying palatine and pterygoid bones (fig. 2.6). A detailed example of a snake swallowing prey is shown in fig. 2.7.

Basal or earlier-evolved snakes generally have more limited unilateral extension of the jaws, and the transport of food appears to be the role of the maxillary bone as well as the palatopterygoid bar. However, feeding movements in the basal (scolecophidian) thread snakes belonging to the Leptotyphlopidae exhibit a unique feeding mechanism in which the anterior tooth-bearing elements of the lower mandibles (lower jaws) rotate synchronously in and out of the mouth, thereby dragging the prey into the mouth and esophagus. The prey is transported exclusively by movements of the lower jaw, and such a transport mechanism is unusual among vertebrates. The authors of the study in which this mechanism was reported—Nathan Kley and Elizabeth Brainerd—named these feeding movements *mandibular raking*. Two joints in each lower jaw have unusual mobility and allow their distal half (splenial) to rotate backward into the mouth, something like swinging doors. In most other snakes these joints conform passively to the shape of the prey being swallowed and thus maximize the "fit" of the gape to the prey item. In contrast, mandibular raking in *Leptotyphlops* involves active flexion of these joints. Moreover, there is a rather wide dorsal gap between the anterior splenial bone and the posterior

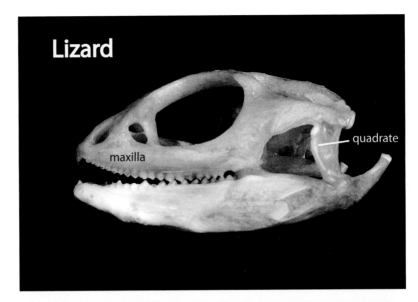

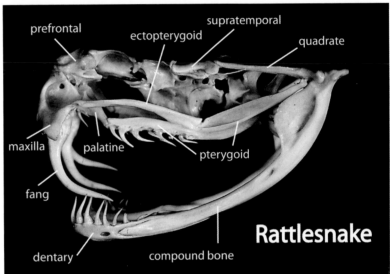

Figure 2.5. Skull of a Bearded Dragon lizard (*Pogona vitticeps*, **upper photo**) compared with a skull of an Eastern Diamondback Rattlesnake (*Crotalus adamanteus*, **lower photo**). The quadrate is movable in both animals, but much more so in the rattlesnake. Note that many elements of the rattlesnake skull are longer, and the skull is lighter, compared with the lizard. Each maxilla of the rattlesnake bears a long fang, and there is an additional replacement fang also in view. The rostral end of the pterygoid functions as a lever during erection of the fangs. Photos courtesy of Elliott Jacobson; skulls courtesy of Jeanette Wyneken (lizard) and Michael Sapper (rattlesnake).

angular bones, which renders the joint between these elements extremely mobile.

Thread snakes feed primarily on the larvae and pupae of social insects and often face dangers during foraging because large, aggressive ants defend their nests tenaciously and can easily kill small snakes. Mandibular raking allows these snakes to feed quickly and to minimize the time they are exposed to potential attack. Studies show that cycles of mandibular protraction and retraction occur at frequencies that can exceed 3 Hz (cycles per second). This represents

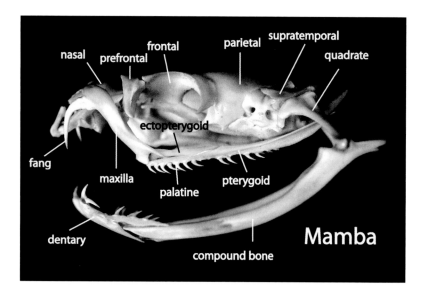

Figure 2.6. Skull and mandibles of a Black Mamba (*Dendroaspis polylepis*). The fangs are supported by the maxillae, which are relatively long compared with vipers and pit vipers. As shown here, the maxillary and palatine bones are capable of erecting the fangs. Note the solid braincase formed by downward extension of the frontal and parietal bones. The photograph is by Elliott Jacobson, and the skull was provided by Michael Sapper.

exceptionally rapid feeding movements in a snake, and thereby reduces the "handling time" involved in swallowing the prey.

Another example of feeding in which the mandibles have a primary role in transporting prey involves evolutionary modifications in advanced, rather than basal, snakes. Several species of tropical colubrid snakes are specialized for feeding on snails. These snail eaters cannot crush the shell, so they must extract the soft body of the snail from its shell. The snake carefully targets the soft body of a snail, grasps it, and then uses its mandibles to extract the fleshy body from its hard shell (fig. 2.8). The mandibles are inserted into the interior of the snail's shell and pull the animal into the mouth using movements that are at least superficially similar to those involved in mandibular raking.

Research has shown that snail-eating snakes have evolved specializations that maximize the effectiveness with which snails are extracted from their shells. The snail body is asymmetric, and the shell of a snail opens either to the right- or the left-hand side. There is a simple genetic basis for whether a shell is "right" or "left-sided." Examination of snake's mandibles reveals that they differ in the number of teeth on the right or left side. This asymmetry is present in all 12 snail-eating specialists in the Pareatidae whereas the jaws of two non-snail-eating species in the same subfamily are symmetric. The asymmetry of the snail eaters matches the "sidedness" of the snails that predominate in their habitat, and it is easier for "right-mandibled" snakes to extract "right-sided" snails from their shells, and they experience more difficulty if a snail is "left-sided."

Feeding on gastropods has evolved independently numerous times among colubrid snakes. These species have vernacular names that include slugsnakes, slug-eating snakes, snail-eaters, and snail-eating snakes—terms that apply especially to the neotropical dipsadine genera *Dipsas*,

Sibon, and *Sibynomorphus* (also called tree snakes), to the Asian pareatine genus *Pareas* and *Aplopeltura*, and to the African genus *Duberria*. Additionally, there are many species of natricine snakes that occur *sympatrically* with slugs and include them in their diet.

Kinesis of the skull and jaws presumably enables more effective apprehension of food by use of jaws in the absence of using the tongue. The tongue has assumed predominantly sensory functions in snakes and is not used to subdue or handle prey. Mobility of the jaws has another important consequence. Transport of food in more specialized (less "primitive") colubroid snakes has shifted to varying extents from the maxillary bones to the more medial pterygoid bones (fig. 2.5). This uncoupling of structure and function allowed for further evolutionary "innovation" involving uses of the maxillary bone in prey capture and the parallel evolution of specializations for the injection of venom. These consequences for prey capture are discussed in the next section.

Modes of Capturing and Subduing Prey

There are several ways in which snakes capture and subdue prey. In nearly all cases, the head is all important and first meets the prey. One exception occurs in the file snakes, particularly the Little File Snake *Acrochordus granulatus*, which capture fish using looping movements of the body trunk or tail. I have watched this behavior many times in captive snakes. Usually these snakes are rather sluggish in many of their movements, and they are inclined to crawl around on a muddy substratum at the bottom of a water column rather than swim rapidly in the open water column. This is fitting, as this species lives largely in shallow coastal waters such as mangroves. When a fish swims near

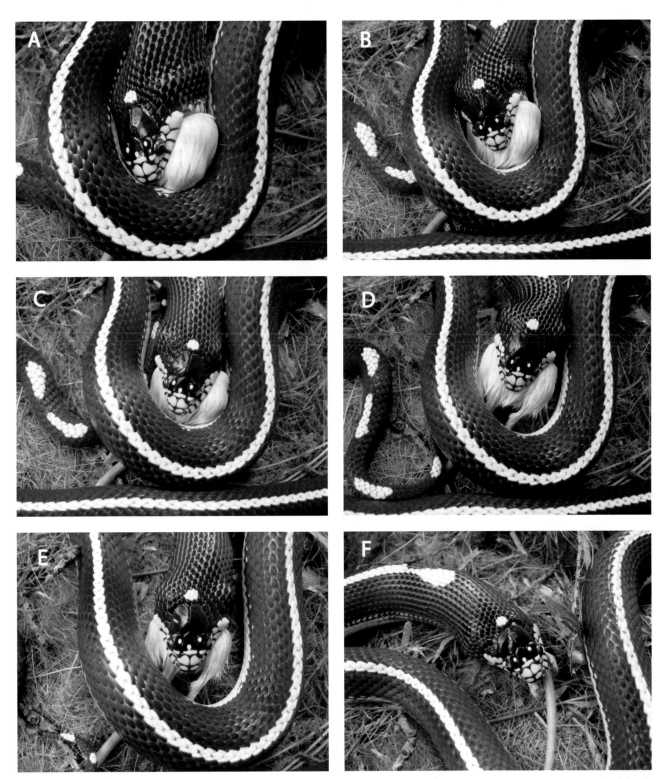

Figure 2.7. Sequence of jaw movements by a California King Snake (*Lampropeltis californiae*) swallowing a mouse that has been immobilized by constriction. The jaw movements progress in sequence from left to right, each stroke advancing the upper jaw and skull of the snake over the mouse (**A** through **E**). Note also the mouse is positioned within a loose coil of the snake, thereby "anchoring" the prey so that it does not shift away from the snake during advances of the jaws. Except for the tail and the rear limbs, the entire mouse is within the neck of the snake in **F**. At all stages, stretching of the skin between the scale rows can be seen. Photographs by author.

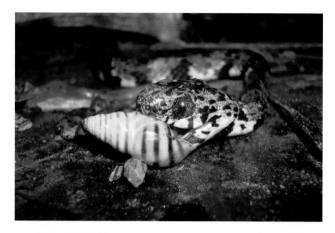

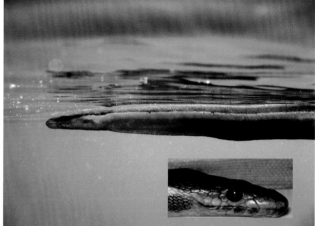

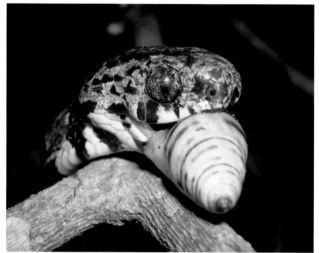

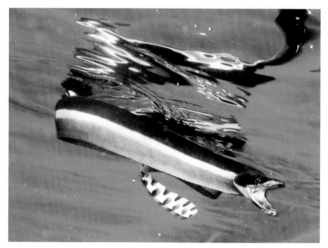

Figure 2.8. A Cloudy Snail Sucker (*Sibon nebulatus*) in Belize extracting a snail from its shell. The mandibles are inserted deeply into the shell, and the recurved teeth are used to extract the snail while the upper jaws grasp the shell. Photographs by Dan Dourson.

Figure 2.9. A Yellow-bellied Sea Snake (*Pelamis platurus*) lies near the ocean surface in a "float-and-wait" posture, waiting to capture a small fish when it swims nearby (**upper photo**). The inset illustrates the relatively long jaw that characterizes this species. In the **lower photo**, a snake is shown with the mouth open to illustrate the gape associated with the elongated jaws, effective for snaring small fishes from the water. These snakes were photographed on the Pacific coast of Guanacaste, Costa Rica by Joseph Pfaller and Coleman Sheehy III (inset).

the snake and disturbs the water in a characteristic way, the snake rapidly throws part of its body around the fish, entrapping it with its spiny-keeled scales (see chapter 5). These snakes often cruise in shallow waters of low tides, hunting for fish that have become concentrated and more easily captured because of the confinement of shallow water. In one instance I observed a snake that was swallowing a fish while holding a second one it had captured within a loop of its trunk at midbody. While swallowing and holding the second fish, it rapidly captured a third fish by means of rapid coiling movements of its tail. Wow! Three fish at a time!

Other snakes possibly employ a similar strategy in using loops or coils of the body to restrain a prey item—or at least slow its escape—while the head of the snake zeros in for a bite. *Nerodia clarkii*, the Gulf Salt Marsh Snake, for example, forage for fish in shallow waters similarly to *Acrochordus*, but in all circumstances where I have observed these snakes capture their prey, the fish are grabbed by swift lateral

movements of an open mouth. Small fishes are captured somewhat similarly by the pelagic Yellow-bellied Sea Snake, *Pelamis platurus*. These snakes lie floating on the ocean surface using what has been called a "float and wait" strategy for snaring small fishes. When a fish swims nearby, the snake captures it in its jaws by rapid sideward swiping movements of the open mouth (fig. 2.9).

Recent studies by Kenneth C. Catania have demonstrated that Tentacled Snakes (*Erpeton tentaculatum*), which are aquatic homalopsids, can take advantage of their prey's escape response by startling fish with their body before striking them. During float-and-wait foraging, a snake assumes a position with the head end forming a J-shaped position and the head forming the base of the J. The snake waits for a fish

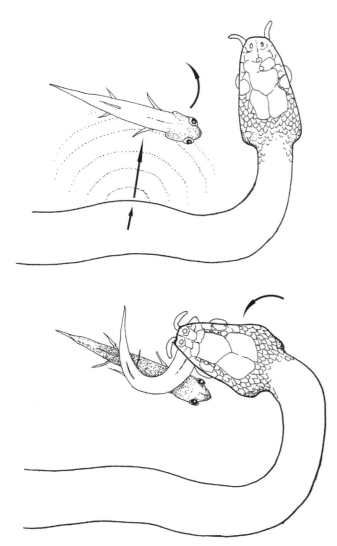

Figure 2.10. Schematic representation of a Tentacled Snake (*Erpeton tentaculatum*) capturing a fish in water. When a fish approaches the snake (**upper drawing**), the snake jerks part of its neck (arrow) such that a segment of the body disturbs the water and sends a compressional wave (arrow) toward the fish. This movement disturbs the fish, which in turn moves its head to begin swimming away from the snake (curved arrow). The snake anticipates the movement of the fish and rapidly captures the fish in its jaws (**lower drawing**). The strike of the snake (arrow) is guided by vision and by water movements (especially at night). The scaled tentacles are sensitive mechanoreceptors that respond to water movements. The stippled fish in the lower figure shows the original position of the fish before it engages in the escape movement. Drawing by Dan Doursen (after fig. 2 in K. C. Catania, Born knowing: Tentacled snakes innately predict future prey behavior, *PLoS ONE* 5:1–10, 2010).

to approach, and when a fish is nearby—usually within the concave region between the head and the snake's body—the snake startles it with jerky movements of the body that initiate an escape response by the fish (fig. 2.10). The snake then strikes to capture the fish and adjusts the strike to the future location of the fish as it moves rapidly in an escape trajectory that is judged quite accurately by the sensory system of the

snake. The tentacles of these snakes are sensitive mechanoreceptors that respond to nearby movements in water (see chapter 7). Vision also is important, but the tentacles provide additional sensory information that becomes increasingly important when vision is diminished by nightfall or turbid water.

Generally, the more commonly employed methods that are used to capture and subdue prey include the following: (1) biting and swallowing; (2) constriction; and (3) envenomation. Of course, the first method is always part of prey capture at some stage of the process. Many snakes simply grasp a prey item and swallow it. The examples of this behavior are far too numerous to mention, but primarily these include snakes that feed on smaller ectothermic prey such as insects or other invertebrates, eggs, carrion, and small vertebrates such as frogs or lizards. Larger, swiftly moving snakes such as racers and whipsnakes, indigo snakes, and even some garter snakes, may capture endothermic prey such as mice or smaller bird species by grasping with the mouth and swallowing the prey directly. I have watched captive Central American indigo snakes (Blacktail Cribo, *Drymarchon melanurus*) chase full-grown mice around in cages, simply grabbing each one with the mouth and rapidly swallowing the animal while it kicked and attempted to bite the snake. Once past the mouth, muscular movements of the neck quickly moved the still-live and wiggling mouse toward the stomach, and one could still see movements of the mouse as it passed posteriorly within the esophagus. One after the other, the snake would swiftly swallow each of several mice in rapid succession. Indigo snakes have a broad, generalist diet and probably capture many small animals in this manner as they move through their habitat in the wild. What I am left to wonder is how many cuts or scratches are inflicted on the snake's internal soft parts as these live animals pass through the snake's mouth and esophagus! Of course these ingested animals will suffocate rather quickly once they are inside the gut.

And this brings us to a very important consideration. As snakes evolved feeding behaviors that included increasingly larger and dangerous prey (in the sense of inflicting serious damage to a snake in self-defense), there arose a dire need for parallel evolution of means to subdue such prey while minimizing the possibility of harm. Also, remember the snake is without limbs and must overcome larger animals without the use of arms or legs—no easy feat if the prey is relatively large! There appear to be no measurements of biting force in snakes, but observations suggest that indigo snakes and some other species that neither constrict nor envenomate their prey have strong jaws and can bite with considerable force. Ophiophagous snakes often kill their prey by using powerful jaws to hold and subdue them

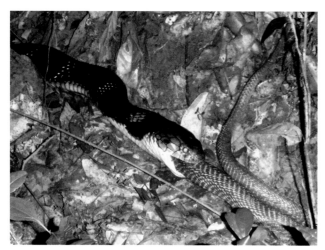

Figure 2.11. A King Cobra (*Ophiophagus hannah*) shown eating a rat snake it has captured and subdued with strong biting prior to ingestion. This snake was photographed in India by Dhiraj Bhaisare.

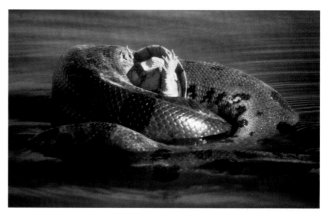

Figure 2.12. A Green Anaconda (*Eunectes murinus*) constricting a turtle. Photographed in Hato el Cedro, Venezuela, by Jesús A. Rivas.

(fig. 2.11). Clearly, there are limitations to this method of immobilizing prey considering the range of sizes and the dangers posed by various prey in comparison with the sole mouth of the predator. The problem of subduing potentially harmful and larger prey was solved in a historical sense by the evolution of constriction or venom as a central part of the prey acquisition process in different lineages of snakes (fig. 2.3). Generally, these two means of prey capture are exclusive. That is, snakes that constrict their prey do not envenomate them, and vice versa.

Constriction is an important means of subduing large or potentially harmful prey, prior to swallowing the item (fig. 2.12). Harry Greene and Gordon Burghardt—two herpetologists who are interested in natural history and behavior—have emphasized this is a key behavioral innovation that evolved during the early history of snakes. Constriction is characteristic of relatively more basal snakes, and has been lost in many of the advanced snakes. If one thinks about it, constriction is a rather obvious means by which a limbless animal might subdue and kill prey, especially if the head is relatively small. Earlier views supposed that the prey animal was crushed by the act of constriction, but it is now widely accepted that the coils that tighten about an animal either kill it or render it unconscious by means of suffocation or blockage of adequate blood flow to the brain. It is possible, of course, that some prey might be crushed faster than they are suffocated when falling victim to large constrictors, but this might also depend on one's subjective definition of the word "crushed."

Constriction is considered to be generally more effective in overcoming endothermic birds and mammals than it is for ectothermic prey. Perhaps this is because of the higher metabolic rate of the former, which succumb quickly if

subjected to inadequate oxygen or blood flow to the brain, whereas ectothermic prey require less oxygen for lower metabolic rates and also are more tolerant of oxygen deficiency at the brain. Snakes that are specialized for constriction have generally thick bodies and move relatively slowly. Perhaps in part because of these characters, envenomation evolved as a very effective alternative means of subduing large prey (see below).

Foraging Behaviors

There are various means by which snakes seek out and capture prey. So-called *active foragers* move through the environment searching for prey, which they attempt to capture at the moment of encounter. There are many examples of this behavior, and it is characteristic of probably most snake species—at least to some degree. Many natricine snakes patrol the edges of streams or ponds seeking frogs, or sometimes enter the water to hunt for fish. Sea snakes are fish specialists, and many species move slowly over coral reefs probing holes and crevices for eels or other fish. Some probe bottom substrates in search of fish eggs. Various species that are called racers or whipsnakes move through terrestrial terrain alert to the movements of lizards or other small vertebrates, striking or chasing them with rapid movements. Similar behaviors characterize various species of elapids. Coral snakes and many other species search for, and follow, the scent trails of small animals using head movements and tongue flicking to locate chemical cues that are left behind by the recent movement of potential prey. Florida Cottonmouth snakes, *Agkistrodon piscivorus conanti*, are attracted to dead and rotting fish that are located by airborne chemical cues possibly from considerable distances (fig. 2.13).

Many snakes seek out particular microenvironments where prey is likely to be concentrated. Examples include cobras, rat snakes, and other species with abilities to climb trees, where they seek out bird nests. Florida Cottonmouth

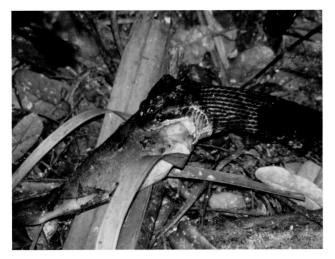

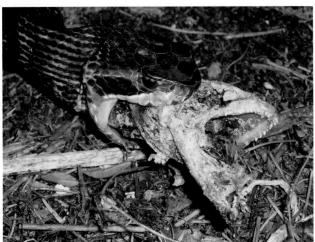

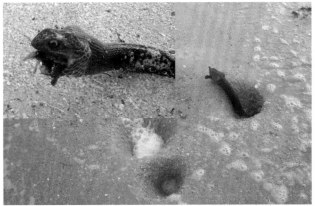

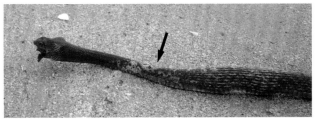

Figure 2.14. Unusual photographs of an Eastern Coachwhip (*Masticophis flagellum flagellum*) foraging on hatchling Loggerhead Sea Turtles (*Caretta caretta*) at St. Lucie Inlet State Park, Florida. The **upper photos** show the snake with a hatchling in its mouth (inset) while emerging from the beach sand in which the turtle eggs were laid. The **lower photo** shows the snake's body, which clearly reveals the snake has swallowed several individual hatchlings. The arrow indicates a point of peristalsis where body muscles were being used to push the prey further along the gut. Photographs are courtesy of Irene Arpayoglou.

Figure 2.13. Florida Cottonmouth snakes (*Agkistrodon piscivorus conanti*) swallowing dead fish on which they forage beneath bird rookeries at the Gulf island of Seahorse Key. In the **lower photo** a snake attempts to swallow a long-dead and dried toadfish. Photographs by the author.

snakes living on some Gulf islands forage beneath bird rookeries where fishes are dropped or regurgitated by colonial nesting sea birds (fig. 2.13). These same snakes, as well as various natricine, homalopsid, and acrochordid species, are attracted to dried-down pools, or shallow waters that are created by low tides, where fishes are likely to be concentrated during drought. Rattlesnakes, Bullsnakes, rat snakes, and many other species seek rodent nests where young as well as older occupants might be found. And many snakes in various taxa enter burrows, where they seek out prey items that might be hiding or living within. The elongate body form of snakes enables them to be very effective predators on burrow- or soil-dwelling animals (fig. 2.14).

Akira Mori and his colleagues have documented an unusually interesting foraging behavior in the colubrid snake *Dinodon semicarinatum*, which exploits the eggs and hatchlings of sea turtles. These snakes actively crawl around the

beach and prey on hatchling sea turtles moving to the sea; they also ambush hatchlings by lying on the sand just above the nest point where the tiny turtles emerge; and they poke their head into the sand and capture hatchlings just before emergence, or eggs before hatching. Similar behaviors have been observed recently involving an Eastern Coachwhip (*Masticophis flagellum*) at a beach in Florida (fig. 2.14).

In contrast with active foragers, *ambush foragers* are snakes that literally lie in ambush for prey, usually at locations where unsuspecting animals are likely to appear. Various pit vipers, for example, coil in positions at the side of rodent trailways or at the base of trees or logs where small mammals might pass. Studies in which the activity and movements of snakes have been assessed usually employ radiotelemetry methods whereby an animal with an implanted radio transmitter can be located using radio signals that are picked up with a receiver (see fig. 4.5). Ambush foraging pit vipers have been noted to spend much of their time at a single location without moving. For example, Harry Greene studied a bushmaster in Costa Rica that spent only 1 percent of alert time moving about during a period of 35 days in which the snake rested for various times at three locations. This snake ate a meal on the 24th night of observation.

Generally, the size of prey increases as the body size of a snake increases during growth to adult size. It might seem self-evident that snakes switch prey items as they grow from very small babies to much larger adults, and these changes are sometimes associated with alterations of foraging behaviors. Some of the better studied examples of *ontogenetic* prey switching (changing prey with growth) are various species of vipers and pit vipers, which may switch from consuming largely ectothermic prey (e.g., lizards) as juveniles to endothermic prey (e.g., small mammals) as adults. The Common Death Adder, *Acanthophis antarcticus* (an elapid species) also switches from ectothermic lizards to small mammals when juvenile snakes grow to adulthood. This is particularly interesting because this species of elapid shares many characters in common with vipers as a result of convergent evolution (fig. 1.42).

Shifts in prey type are also particularly evident in populations of snakes living on islands. For example, Australian tiger snakes, *Notechis* spp., living on the mainland feed principally on frogs, whereas conspecifics on islands consume mostly mammals and birds. Insular water snakes (*Nerodia sipedon*) and Cottonmouths (*Agkistrodon piscivorus*) feed largely on fish, whereas conspecifics consume more amphibians and other prey on the mainland. Most examples of such dietary differences reflect differences in the prey that are available on an island versus mainland.

Gape and Striking

Many persons are somewhat familiar with the striking behavior of snakes, due in part to the tendency of filmmakers usually to feature snakes that are engaged in defensive behaviors. Indeed, while snakes might exhibit alternative defensive behaviors, one is often greeted with biting or striking if he or she approaches a wild snake and attempts to touch or handle it against its will. These circumstances can vary a lot, however. Many harmless snakes can, in fact, be handled without biting if they are approached slowly and without aggressive movements. Placid behaviors also characterize some venomous snakes, although no one should ever make this assumption and handle a venomous snake with bare hands! This being said, there are a number of species of sea snakes that rarely or never bite in defense of being handled. I have watched children at Suva Harbor in Fiji fearlessly playing with Yellow-lipped Sea Kraits, *Laticauda colubrina*, which appear never to inflict any harm to their exuberant captors (see also fig. 2.15).

We must distinguish two categories of striking by snakes. A *defensive strike* is often more a display and may not be directed at an intruder as accurately or rapidly as is a *predatory strike* that is intended to capture prey. Defensive

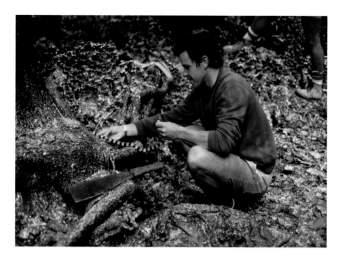

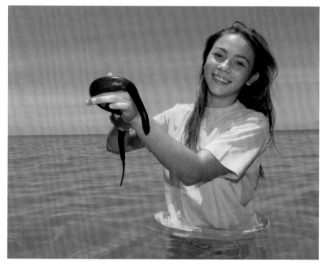

Figure 2.15. Many sea snakes are not inclined to bite when handled or in contact with humans. In the **upper photo** Micheal Guinea gently extracts a Yellow-lipped Sea Krait (*Laticauda colubrina*) from limestone rocks on a small Pacific island. The snake is handled gently and does not attempt to bite. Photographed in Fiji by the author. The **lower photo** features Julia Bonnet holding a Turtle-headed Sea Snake (*Emydocephalus annulatus*) which gently accommodates to the contact. Photographed in Nouméa by Xavier Bonnet.

strikes can involve hissing, gaping of the mouth, and startling but undirected movements intended to frighten off a person or other animal without making actual contact or inflicting a bite. On the other hand, predatory strikes are more carefully executed and more accurately directed at an animal that is intended to be captured for a meal (fig. 2.16). While these differences are well evident to persons who have observed snakes carefully, the details and mechanisms involved in the two categories of strikes have proven difficult to demonstrate and to quantify.

Predatory strikes that might be very carefully executed by a snake also may not be perfect. Strikes can be flawed in various ways, and in some studies David Cundall found that up to 47 percent of strikes by rattlesnakes result in neither

Figure 2.16. A predatory strike executed by an Amazon Tree Boa (*Corallus hortulanus*) in a laboratory setting. The kinematic sequence of the strike is illustrated with progression of photos from top to bottom. In the **upper photo** the body of the snake is drawn into several S-shaped loops in preparation for striking the mouse, while vision and thermal cues play key roles in aligning the snake's strike trajectory from the position of its head to the mouse on the platform at the left. The **middle photo** illustrates the "propulsive" force produced by the muscle actions of the snake, which creates an equal "reaction" force acting in the opposite direction to accelerate the snake's head and forebody in the forward direction. The reaction force is essentially equal to the force of friction, which acts opposite to the propulsive force and is dependent on both the mass (weight) of the snake and the nature of the surface with which it interacts. In the **middle** and **lower photos**, note the gape of the snake's mouth as its lower jaws engage the mouse and the head moves forward to bite forcefully and immobilize the prey. The images are taken from a video sequence produced by Phil Nicodemo.

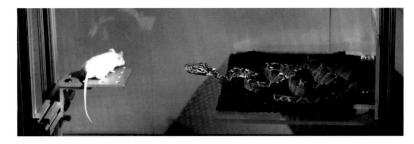

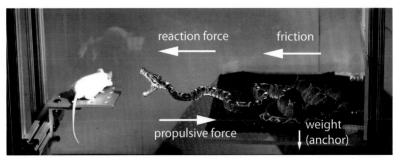

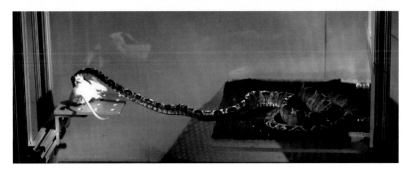

fang penetrating the prey. The probability of missed fang contact or penetration increases with the distance of the strike. This might explain why snakes are observed to strike only when prey animals come into very close range.

Predatory behaviors that involve striking by snakes include (1) visual, mechanical, or chemical location of prey, (2) preparation for the strike—usually by means of intense sensory focus on the prey item and drawing the neck into S-shaped curves, (3) rapidly extending the body during the strike, (4) grasping the prey item with the mouth upon contact, followed by either (5a) continuing to bite or grasp the prey while subduing it with constriction, envenomation, or biting force, or (5b) releasing envenomated prey and trailing it for later ingestion following its death or paralysis. Kenneth Kardong and others have shown that the trailing behaviors of rattlesnakes (*Crotalus* spp.) following a strike can be induced by the strike itself, after which the struck prey is discriminated from others using a distinctive chemosensory profile during trailing. Subtle as it might seem, the odor of the struck prey is changed by the fang penetration and the injection of venom. Envenomation is the most important factor contributing to the chemosensory "image" of the prey following the strike.

The trailing behaviors of rattlesnakes and other viperid species following envenomation of prey are even more complex and fascinating than one might suppose. Recent studies by Eli Greenbaum, David Chiszar, and others have demonstrated that rattlesnakes and Copperheads can recognize prey that is envenomated by conspecific animals and prefer it to non-envenomated prey. However, prey that is envenomated by a distantly related species is not preferred over non-envenomated prey or prey that is envenomated by another individual of the same species. The behavior of sensing and trailing envenomated prey enables a snake to distinguish an animal, say a mouse, from trails that are made by other mice living in the vicinity. This leads the snake to the animal that will succumb to the venom instead of wasting time and energy following other trails. An envenomated rodent can move considerable distances before succumbing to venom, so anything that facilitates the task of finding the prey is likely to be adaptive. Thus, phylogeny, genetic differences between snake species, and the evolution of venom composition might all interact in complex but meaningful ways.

Observations of anatomy and analysis of filmed movements by Thomas Frazetta, Kenneth Kardong, David Cundall, and others have revealed some general similarities of striking in pythons and in several species of vipers. Predatory strikes are extremely rapid. The reaction times involved for the head and trunk muscles to activate or deactivate during striking movements are less than 15 msec, and possibly half that time. As a snake strikes, both mandibles are lowered and the palatomaxillary arches are moved upward while the head is rapidly accelerated toward the prey. The pterygoids move forward with the ectopterygoids, raising the maxilla and pushing the prefrontals forward. This flexes the snout and braincase upward and tends to slant the teeth forward in a stabbing motion. Movements of the head are considered to be important for erection of the fangs, while the mandibles are the first elements to contact the prey. These movements are reversed as the jaws close, bringing the teeth-bearing bones closer and engaging the teeth in the prey. The lower jaw is thrust forward during the strike and is retracted as the mouth closes.

The total duration of typical predatory strikes that have been studied in viperid snakes varies from 150 to 500 ms, and the time between the beginning of a strike to making contact with the prey is typically about 50 to 100 ms. These times can vary as a function of the size of the snake and its prey. One should always remember that however slowly some of these snakes move during routine movements and other nonfeeding behaviors, their strike can be lightning fast!

In some crotaline snakes (e.g., *Crotalus horridus*), rotation of the prefrontal bone around its attachment to the frontal bone elevates the snout and helps to elevate the fang base relative to the braincase during the extension phase of the strike (fig. 2.5). Elevation of the prefrontal decreases the distance between the tip of the fang and the roof of the mouth, which better enables each fang to be carried over the dorsal surface of the prey before it impales the animal. The fangs are brought down on the prey's surface and often penetrate during the contact or bite phase of the strike when the jaws are below their maximum displaced positions. If the prey is released following envenomation, the maximum gape involving displacements of both mandibles and the fangs is usually achieved after envenomation when the prey is released.

In the case of venomous snakes, there is a tendency for larger species possessing elongated fangs to envenomate and quickly release the bite of the prey if it is large and potentially dangerous. This is especially true for mammalian prey that can struggle vigorously, bite, tug, and scratch. If the prey item is relatively small or innocuous, however, the snake often maintains a grasp on the animal and holds it firmly in the mouth (before swallowing) until the prey ceases to struggle. Indeed, the biting tactics of snakes are dependent on the nature of their prey.

Cottonmouths are an excellent example of striking variability, insofar as these snakes have a generalist diet and take a wide range of prey. If the prey is a dead or small fish, a frog, or even a baby mouse, the items are swallowed immediately upon being bitten, whereas larger rodents are struck and envenomated, then released to be followed and eaten later. This latter behavior appears to be a common strategy among viperid snakes that prey on larger rodents or small mammals that might inflict considerable harm if they are not immobilized. Another example of "bite and release" is the tactic employed by sea kraits (e.g., *Laticauda colubrina*) to envenomate dangerous fishes like moray eels while minimizing the probability of being harmed. These snakes search for moray eels by entering holes among corals, and if one is found the snake quickly bites and envenomates the eel, then quickly withdraws and waits for the venom to act. The snake reenters the hole somewhat later to swallow the eel after it has succumbed to the venom.

On the other hand, nonvenomous constrictors such as boas and pythons necessarily retain a bite on their prey, which must be quickly enveloped and subdued with constricting coils. Arboreal snakes that eat birds tend to bite and hold because it would be difficult to follow the prey if it was released. Finally, rear-fanged snakes (see below) tend to hold onto prey items that must be worked to the posterior aspect of the open jaws in order to inject venom. These snakes often bite with much force and may "chew" or close hard on the prey for some while in order to effectively envenomate the prey (fig. 2.17).

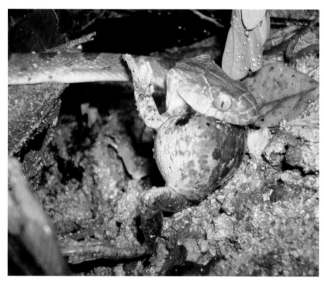

Figure 2.17. A Cat-eyed Snake (*Leptodeira septentionalis*) eating a tree frog (*Smilisca baudinii*) in Belize. The frog inflates its lungs to enlarge the body in an effort to prevent being swallowed. The snake, in turn, patiently "chews" on the frog to impale the posterior maxillary teeth, which function as fangs to envenomate the frog. The venom eventually causes paralysis and deflation of the lung, so the frog can be pulled further into the mouth and eventually swallowed. Photograph by Dan Dourson.

The striking and biting behaviors of snakes can be very different when we consider species that are adapted to foraging in different media. Whereas various prey items on terrestrial surfaces are generally struck head-on, fishes in water are often struck by lateral movements of the open mouth. Studies of Cottonmouths have demonstrated that terrestrial strikes exhibit higher angular velocities during closure of the mouth and higher angles of gape during the retraction phase of a strike when the head pulls back from the prey, compared with strikes when the snakes are in water. Shawn Vincent and colleagues have demonstrated that the success of strikes is considerably greater in terrestrial situations than in water.

The size of the prey that can be swallowed depends, of course, on the gape of the mouth, and this varies among different taxa of snakes. Fundamentally, snakes exhibit very large gape compared with other vertebrates owing to several features of the jaws and skull (figs. 2.9, 2.18). The two mandibles are fused by a rigid joint in most amniotes, but in snakes the distal tips of the jaw are connected by ligaments and can move independently of one another. Moreover, each mandible can bow outward and adjust to the shape of the prey owing to a joint at or near its center (where the dentary meets the compound bone of the lower jaw) and to the kinetic attachment of the quadrate, which connects the lower jaw with the skull (figs. 2.5, 2.18). The muscles that move the various skull and jaw elements are complexly elongate, representing conditions that favor a large gape and mobility of the teeth-bearing bones. The extreme gape of snakes is perhaps best seen and appreciated when a snake swallows a rigid-shelled egg of a bird (figs. 2.1, 2.19).

Vipers, in particular, exhibit morphological specializations that enhance the ability to capture and swallow relatively large prey. These include a stout body, relatively large head with elongate jaws, long fangs, and comparatively small-size scales on the head that favor kinesis. The anterior and posterior excursions of the palate and maxillary bones in vipers exceed those that have been recorded for any other major clade of snakes. Such movements are related to features of the floor of the braincase and its attached constrictor muscles. The upper-jaw movements of some rattlesnakes can exceed those in nonviperid snakes by a factor of two. One measure of how these features translate into swallowing performance and efficiency is that vipers use fewer cycles of jaw movements than do colubrids to transport prey through the mouth, if the prey are equivalent in terms of relative mass.

The mechanics of striking varies with the size and shape of a snake. Two considerations are most important. First, either high inertia or some amount of anchoring is required for snakes to avoid inaccurate or totally flawed strikes. Consequently, on horizontal surfaces resistance to unwanted movement attributable to propulsive forces (fig. 2.16) can be provided by anchoring against irregularities in the substrate or by the inertia attributable to large mass, or both. Striking performance might be assisted in large-bodied snakes such as vipers through relatively large posterior mass, which also increases the frictional resistance to movement. More

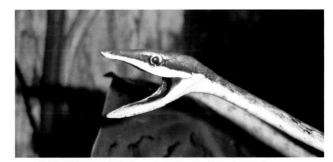

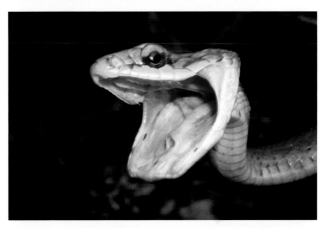

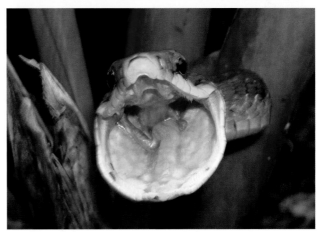

Figure 2.18. Defensive displays illustrating the large gape of snakes. The **upper photo** illustrates a Brown (or Mexican) Vine Snake (*Oxybelis aeneus*) with open mouth that is specialized for snaring lizards or small birds. The **middle** and **lower photos** depict a Neotropical Bird Snake (also called Puffing Snake) (*Pseustes poecilonotus*) which displays a menacing mouth, showing the extreme width while the tips of the mandibles are separated. The open glottis (entry to trachea) can be seen in the middle photo. Dan Dourson photographed these snakes in Belize.

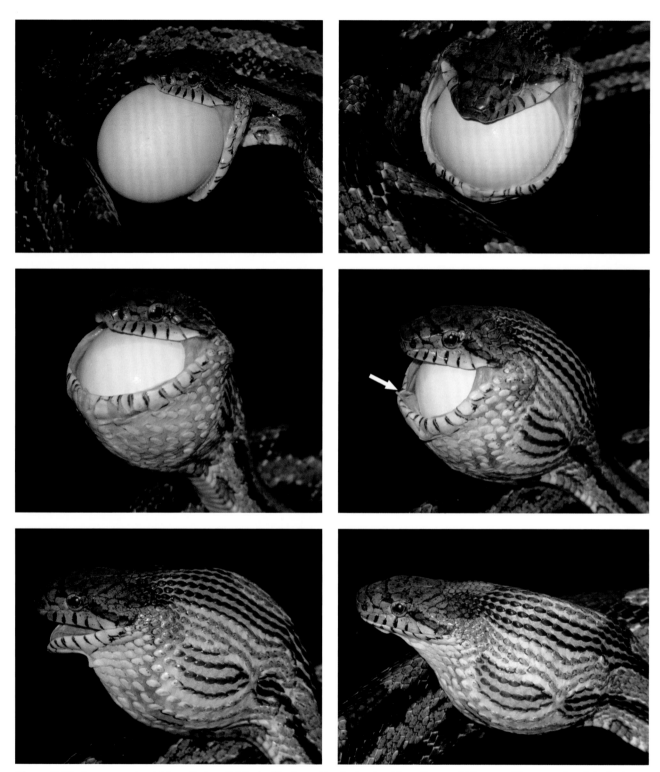

Figure 2.19. A sequence in which an Eastern Rat Snake (*Pantherophis alleghaniensis*) swallows a chicken egg. The rows of teeth in the lower jaws can be seen at the margins of the mandible in the **upper two photos**. In the photograph at **right-center**, note the glottis is open and protruded from the mouth (arrow) to enable breathing while the egg is in the mouth. Photographs by the author.

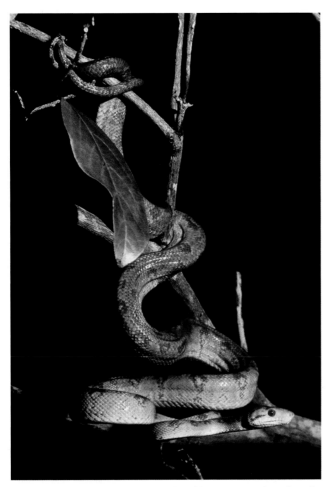

Figure 2.20. A Grenada Bank Tree Boa (*Corallus grenadensis*) on the island of Grenada, shown in a striking position while its body is anchored on a tree branch. Note how the prehensile tail anchors the snake to a part of the tree branch. Photograph by Richard Sajdak.

gracile species—for example, many arboreal snakes—can also anchor by coiling a prehensile tail or part of the trunk around a branch or other object (figs. 1.31, 2.20).

David Cundall has suggested that the body form of snakes has been adapted to optimize striking in relation to momentum of the head and anterior body. The mass of the head is accelerated and increases momentum as it propels toward the prey. If the momentum is too high, there will be a tendency for the head to continue beyond the point of contact with the prey. This might explain why many snakes, especially vipers, have a reduced mass at the anterior trunk in addition to attributes of the head that increase shock-absorbing ability. These adjustments are especially important for larger-size snakes. Generally, larger species exhibit relatively greater mass and velocity of their heads.

One question that has intrigued biologists and snake specialists alike is whether a character such as predatory gape is "plastic" and can be induced to change with an experimental change in the size of prey. There are mixed

answers to this question. In some cases, experimental manipulation of prey size during the growth of young snakes does not result in any differences in growth of the head skeleton, for example in the Boa Constrictor (*Boa constrictor*). On the other hand, the jaw length of Australian tiger snakes (*Notechis* spp.) living on islands is different from conspecifics that live on the mainland, and the difference appears to be controlled both by genes and by the environment. Neonates of the insular tiger snakes have larger heads than do counterparts living on the mainland, despite similar body sizes. This geographic difference is apparent at birth and presumably reflects genetic adaptation to different diets, the insular snakes feeding on relatively large chicks of nesting birds and the mainland snakes feeding mainly on frogs. Moreover, the relative size of the jaws of insular snakes that feed on large prey (large mice) increases during growth to become larger than those of siblings that are fed on smaller prey (small mice). These tiger snakes appear to be highly adaptable predators that can track prey resources by means of a complex response that involves genetically "hard-wired" traits as well as developmental plasticity of these traits.

The growth of head shape in Cottonmouths (*Agkistrodon piscivorus*) is especially interesting. The size of prey generally increases with body size of Cottonmouths, as occurs in other snakes generally, but shifts of prey type during ontogeny have not been detected. Cottonmouths undergo a developmental change in head shape, in which juveniles tend to have relatively broader and higher, but shorter, head shapes compared to adults. Relatively small head size appears to characterize the adults, in which the gape scales with negative allometry relative to body size according to a recent study by Shawn Vincent and coworkers. That is, the head becomes relatively smaller as the body grows larger. The authors of this study suggest that the gape and head shape characteristics of Cottonmouths likely reflect the generalist nature of their diet. My own studies of Florida Cottonmouths on islands emphasizes that dietary breadth exhibited by these snakes increases the probability of encountering usable energy resources in situations where these can be ephemeral, transitory, and variable in quality and quantity. Specialization of diet or strongly selective foraging behaviors could be disadvantageous in such environments, whereas the acceptance of a range of prey increases the foraging opportunities.

Teeth and Fangs

Teeth are very important for the capture and swallowing of prey by snakes. The dentition of the earliest reptiles is poorly known, but appears to have consisted usually of simple, conical teeth that correlated with a carnivorous or

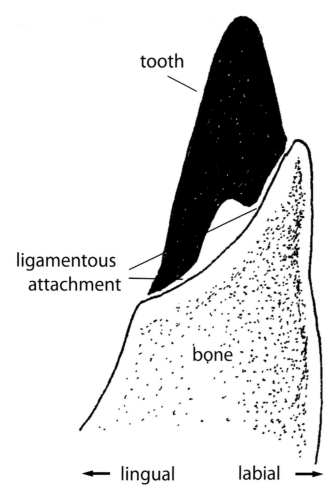

Figure 2.21. A schematic image showing a pleurodont condition of tooth attachment. The tooth does not have a "root" but is anchored by fibrous attachment largely to the inner (lingual or medial) wall of the bone and within a groove of the bony element on which it is supported. Drawing by Dan Dourson.

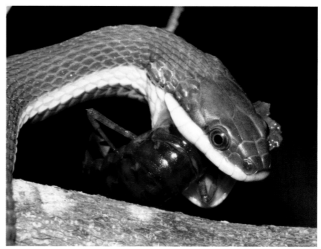

Figure 2.22. A Crayfish Snake (*Regina rigida*) swallowing a crayfish in Florida. This species lives in swampy, low, wetland areas where it specializes on eating crayfish. It has chisel-shaped teeth that help to ingest this hard-shelled prey. However, these snakes have a preference for crayfish that have recently molted and are therefore relatively soft-bodied compared with animals in which the cuticle has mineralized. Photograph by Joseph Pfaller.

piscivorous (fish) diet. These evolved in snakes to become adapted for seizing prey. In most snakes the teeth are long, thin, sharp, and recurved—ideal for piercing and grasping (figs. 2.5, 2.6). They are firmly anchored to the jaw and are often set in deep grooves, but usually against a higher "outer" (labial) than "inner" (lingual) wall (fig. 2.21). This is known as a *pleurodont* condition of tooth attachment, which is characteristic of lizards and snakes. The maxillary teeth are attached to the jawbone by mineralized tissue, and the attachment morphology is known as *ankylosis*.

There are exceptions to this basic form. Highly specialized tubular teeth evolved in elapid and viperid snakes to deliver venom (figs. 2.5, 2.6). Teeth are reduced in both size and number in the egg-eating snakes, *Dasypeltis* and *Elachistodon*, so the eggshell is more easily enveloped by a mouth having an interior that is very "fleshy." And there are several genera of snakes including the primitive genus *Xenopeltis* (a

xenopeltid) and at least five genera of colubrids that have hinged teeth adapted for feeding on hard-bodied and nondeformable prey such as skinks. These lizards are covered with stiff, strongly cycloid scales underlain by osteoderms. Such armor poses dangers of breakage to long, sharp, and firmly anchored teeth. Therefore, the teeth of these snakes are attached to bone by flexible connective tissue fibers, and they fold backward against the jaws. The teeth are also modified to be typically small, numerous, flattened at their ends, and extremely smooth on their leading surfaces. There are also other modifications of the head in these snakes, which, together with the teeth, enable them to grasp and to swallow very hard prey. There are exceptions to these statements, and numerous snakes swallow both soft- and hard-bodied prey depending on the relative size (fig. 2.22).

Replacement

The dentition of snakes is not static, but rather the functional teeth are continually being replaced. Hence, new teeth take the place of older ones that are lost or damaged. The replacement process begins very early in life and continues throughout the life of the animal. The organization of teeth begins early in the embryo where precursors of teeth appear on bands of specialized epithelium. The earliest formed teeth are often reabsorbed at a rudimentary stage of development. Subsequently, teeth form as new buds, often in successive waves along the length of the jaw. The teeth continue to grow until they become full size, at which time they attach to bone and become functional. After some time, the teeth begin to undergo reabsorption and are replaced, a process that is not dependent on wear. The pattern of replacement usually is such that the teeth undergoing replacement are flanked by new, more or less intact, teeth that develop at the bases of the functional teeth and will contribute the next generation. The replacement occurs in "waves" except in some taxa.

Visible evidence of the replacement process for teeth is the common occurrence of one or more smaller "replacement" fangs just behind the functional fang of a viperid snake (fig. 2.5). The paired fangs are replaced alternately, and the new fang becomes anchored and connected to the venom duct before the functional fang is shed. Such shed fangs are frequently found undigested in the feces of these snakes! Hmm . . . Certain enterprising persons might not have realized they could use this as a renewable source of fangs to be used for jewelry, rather than killing snakes for their fangs.

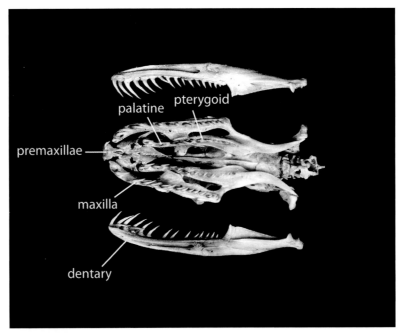

Figure 2.23. Palatal view of the skull and medial profiles of the mandibles of a Reticulated Python (*Broghammerus reticularis*) illustrating the teeth-bearing bones. The outermost elements in the photograph (dentary) represent the lower jaw, which articulates with the upper jaw shown in the center. Note that some replacement teeth can be seen at the end of the lower dentary. Photograph by Elliott Jacobson; skull courtesy of the Florida Museum of Natural History.

Patterns of Dentition

The primitive pattern of teeth in snakes evidently consisted of a single row of sharp, conical teeth numerously distributed on the premaxilla, maxilla, dentary, pterygoid, and palatine bones. This pattern of distribution is observed in living pythons (fig. 2.23). It has generally been conserved, except for the evolution of long, recurved teeth, reductions or expansions of tooth number, and the development of grooved or tubular fangs on the maxilla in various lineages of snakes (figs. 2.5, 2.6).

In the majority of living snakes the premaxilla is reduced and without teeth, except in boas and pythons. Teeth have persisted on the pterygoid and palatine bones (palate), but are reduced in size or number in certain colubrid species. Teeth are present on the dentary in most snakes, but they may be absent, reduced in number, or limited to the anterior part of this element in some taxa.

The structure and dentition of the maxilla is very important in snakes, and maxillary characters have been very useful for interpreting phylogeny. In the more basal snakes, the maxilla bears rather simple and uniformly shaped teeth. In scolecophidians, the dentition is specialized in relation to the burrowing habits of these animals. In *Typhlops*, the maxillary teeth are small, slightly compressed, simple cones, and there are no teeth on the dentary. The maxilla of *Leptotyphlops* is without teeth, and the dentary bears only a few small teeth. Uropeltid snakes have a limited number of teeth on the maxilla and dentary, none on the premaxilla, and rarely on the palate. Boas and pythons, on the other hand, have a moderately large number of teeth on all of the usual teeth-bearing bones (fig. 2.23). The teeth are usually long, recurved, and lacking compression. In various more derived lineages, the maxillary teeth become regionally enlarged, anteriorly or posteriorly, either as part of a continuous series of teeth or with gaps in dentition where teeth are absent. The enlarged teeth are solid, grooved, or tubular in various groups of snakes (figs. 2.5, 2.6).

Colubrid snakes have undergone extensive adaptive radiations, reflected in part by variation of dentitions. All colubrids lack teeth on the premaxilla, but there are usually well-developed teeth on the dentary and in a long row on the palatine and pterygoid. The maxillary teeth are rather uniform and form a fairly long row of simple conical structures. Elapid snakes vary in the arrangement of dentition on the maxilla, some having a series of teeth that become reduced in size posteriorly (front to rear), whereas others exhibit well-developed tubular fangs on a greatly abbreviated maxilla. In mambas (*Dendroaspis*), the maxilla usually bears but a single prominent fang, and there is an enlarged tooth on the anterior end of the dentary (fig. 2.6). The elongated fangs and anterior teeth of mambas are likely to be adaptations for securing prey without dropping it, insofar as these snakes are arboreal. In vipers and pit vipers, the maxilla is highly specialized as a reduced bone that is short and hinged, bearing an elongate fang that rotates with movement of the element (fig. 2.5).

Feeding on slugs and snails (malacophagy) has arisen independently in several lineages of colubroid snakes, most notably the Asian pareatids and the neotropical dipsadines and xenodontines (fig. 2.8). Long, slender teeth tend to be typical on the anterior dentary and posterior maxilla of malacophagous snakes and are hypothesized to be specializations for gripping the slippery, mucus-covered skin of the prey. However, Eric Britt and his colleagues could not demonstrate such features in certain garter snakes (*Thamnophis* spp.) when their teeth were compared with congeneric species having different dietary preferences. Numerous teeth that are narrow and prominently recurved tend to be characteristic of fish specialists, which often have elongated jaws (figs. 2.9, 2.24).

Examples of greatly reduced dentition include the colubrid egg-eating snakes, *Dasypeltis*, and the elapid sea snake *Emydocephalus*. *Dasypeltis* has at most four or five very small curved teeth on the maxilla, three or four teeth on the palatine, and another three at the extreme rear of the dentary. The reduction of teeth is associated with the habit of eating eggs, which have relatively flat and hard surfaces (figs. 2.1, 2.19). Sea snakes belonging to the genus *Emydocephalus* are specialized for feeding on fish eggs and also exhibit extreme reduction of teeth. The dentary and palate both lack teeth, and the maxilla bears no teeth except for the fangs.

Fangs

Fangs evolved to inject venom into the prey of various snakes that possess them. The term *fang* refers to a grooved or tubular tooth that is used to inject venom, although numerous teeth could well serve the same purpose in species in which the fangs are small and venom secretions are dispersed during chewing actions on the prey. Fangs are functionally best developed in representatives of the Elapidae (e.g., cobras) and Viperidae (e.g., rattlesnakes) (figs. 2.5, 2.6). The fangs of viperids are the largest and most effective structures that have evolved in nature for injecting venom (fig. 2.25).

Snakes that possess completely tubular fangs are referred to collectively as *solenoglyphs*. During development, these fangs begin as conical teeth with a pulp cavity. As they develop, one wall of the tooth pushes inward and the side walls grow over it to form a tube. Each fang is erected by rotation of a reduced maxilla on the prefrontal bone (fig. 2.5). The maxilla bears no teeth other than the hollow,

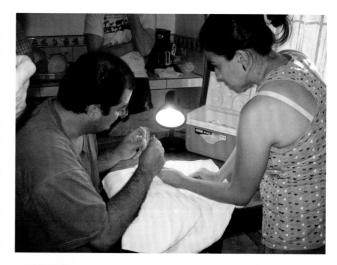

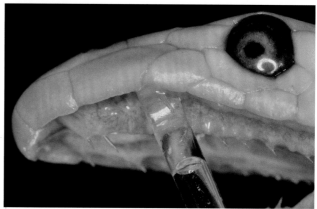

Figure 2.24. Prof. Mahmood Sasa and Jazmín Arias, University of Costa Rica, extract venom from the fang of a Yellow-bellied Sea Snake (*Pelamis platurus*). Note in the **lower photograph** how the teeth are elongated and recurved for snaring fishes, and the fang is equivalent in size to other teeth on the maxilla. Clear venom can be seen in the upper part of a capillary tube that covers the left fang of the snake. Photographs by Coleman Sheehy III (upper) and Philipp Figueroa (lower).

tubular fang. When the fang is not erected, it folds against the roof of the mouth. Snakes with such fangs include the viperid and atractaspidine species. In the viperids, the tips of the fangs are directed toward the prey during striking and effectively "spear" it, rather than biting prey in a downward movement. Unlike the viperids, stiletto snakes (*Atractaspis*) envenomate prey by moving a fang sideward out of one side of a closed mouth and slashing it sideways or backward into the prey. The fang movements are very agile and considered to be adaptations for envenomating prey that are encountered inside earthen burrows. These fangs are relatively long and associated with a relatively short maxilla. Other species of atractaspidine snakes curiously exhibit every known type of fang dentition, some having fangs resembling those of elapids and others having grooved posterior fangs. One species (*Aparallactus modestus*) appears to lack grooved fangs altogether (*aglyphous* condition) and may not produce venom.

The fangs of viperid snakes are exceptionally long, hollow teeth that rotate through extremely large angles due to mobile connections between the upper jaws and the braincase. Recent analysis of video records by David Cundall indicate that vipers representing 86 species in 31 genera reposition fangs after they contact the prey in more than a third of 750 recorded strikes. A snake may reposition a fang when it misses the prey entirely, or when it initially contacts prey regions that do not permit adequate penetration. Repositioning is prevalent even in species that normally release prey following a strike. The rapidity of fang repositioning suggests there is extraordinary development and sensitivity of the neuromuscular system that controls the fang movement, including sensitive detection of fang penetration and very rapid modulation of antagonistic muscle contractions.

Elapid snakes possess single, hollow, or grooved fangs at the anterior end of each maxilla, which is relatively long (fig. 2.6). Each fang is fixed and does not fold back because of the relative immobility of the maxillary unit. This condition is known as *proteroglyph*. In many species the fangs of elapids are relatively short, sometimes hardly distinguishable from the other teeth (fig. 2.24). If one looks inside the mouth of many elapid snakes (not recommended), it is difficult to imagine the snake is dangerous in comparison with the appearance of fangs in viperid species. In Australian death adders (*Acanthophis* spp.), however, the fangs are quite long and represent one of the morphological characters of these snakes that are convergent with those of viperids.

Various colubroid snakes possess posterior maxillary teeth that are enlarged or grooved to function as fangs. In *Boiga*, for example, the maxilla bears a pair of alternately functioning fangs, preceded by a series of relatively small and simple anterior teeth. In this and other opisthoglyphous colubrids, there may be a few small teeth behind the fangs and a gap between the fangs and the more anterior teeth.

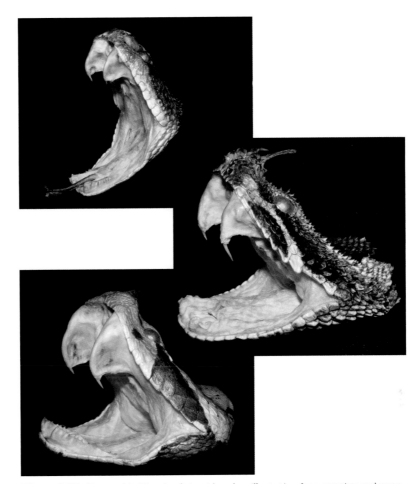

Figure 2.25. Freeze-dried heads of viperid snakes illustrating fang erection and gape in three species: **top**, Southern Pacific Rattlesnake (*Crotalus oreganus helleri*); **center**, Rhinoceros Viper (*Bitis nasicornis*); **bottom**, Gaboon Adder (*Bitis gabonica*). There is a fleshy sheath that covers each fang, normally folded flat against the roof of the mouth when not erected. The Gaboon Adder has the largest relative fang size of any species of snake. Photographs are of freeze-dried heads and taken by the author.

Venom

One cannot adequately consider the mechanisms and strategies of feeding in snakes without discussing the subject of venom. *Venom* is a term that is used to describe some form of potentially toxic secretion produced by one organism to the detriment of another. The secretion is delivered to another animal through some form of specialized structure—in the case of snakes, a fang. Venoms are often confused or categorized with *poisons*, but the latter must be ingested to alter the physiology of the consuming organism. The principal difference between venom and poison is that venomous animals actively deliver their toxic secretions (through a fang or stinger), whereas poisonous animals generally rely on passive means of afflicting another organism.

Venoms also should not be confused with *toxins*. These are chemicals of biological origin that can adversely alter the physiology of an organism. Toxins are pure substances, whereas venoms are mixtures of biologically active and inert substances. Both venoms and poisons generally contain toxins. The oral secretions of snakes that contain toxins and are used to immobilize prey are considered to be venoms. There is debate, however, concerning whether similar oral secretions that are not known to have an ecological role should be considered venoms. Recent publications have championed the view that all oral secretions having biologically active compounds and arising in specialized glands should be considered venoms. There is little question that many snake species that are now considered to be "harmless" may eventually prove to have venom. A tragic instance of such reclassification occurred when Dr. Karl P. Schmidt of the Field Museum of Natural History in Chicago was killed from the bite of a Boomslang (*Dispholidus typus*), which previously had been considered to be harmless.

Snake venoms occur only within the families of snakes comprising the Colubroidea. Thus, it is generally held that venom arose in the ancestor(s) of this clade and subsequently underwent modifications in composition, glandular morphology, and tooth shape as the basal snakes of this group radiated and speciated. However, venoms are found in multiple lizard families, and perhaps only the type of modified venom apparatus, and not venom itself, is of unique origin in the Colubroidea. Bryan Fry, an Australian venom specialist, has suggested that venom had an earlier reptilian origin than was previously supposed.

Generally, snake venoms consist largely of soluble polypeptides in water, but may also include carbohydrates, lipids, metal ions, and other organic compounds such as amines. Polypeptides comprise about 90 percent of the dry weight of most venoms, and many of these have enzymatic activity. Enzymes vary in their specificity and have catalytic properties that induce biochemical transformations without themselves being modified. Various components of venom affect a wide range of physiological functions. The numerous actions of venoms include effects on cells and cell membranes, transmission of nervous signals, muscular contraction, blood pressure, blood components and coagulation, inflammation, and necrosis.

Historically, venoms have been considered to be either *hemotoxic*, affecting the blood, or *neurotoxic*, affecting the nervous system. However, these terms do not adequately describe the variation and complexity of venom, and specific venoms may contain compounds that produce both effects. Although the potency of venoms varies, recent studies (e.g., Susanta Pahari, Stephen Mackessy, and Manjunatha Kini) suggest that there is greater compositional similarity among advanced snakes than has been previously recognized. The many effects of venom are diverse, and they vary among taxonomic group, ecology, diet, population, and even within individuals. Some of the important components of venom follow.

- *Proteolytic enzymes* (*proteases*) are components of venom that degrade structural proteins into component peptides or amino acids, often leading to damage in the walls of blood vessels. They are involved in the tissue destruction that is present in *necrosis*, and many have important actions on blood coagulation. They are found in the venoms of all known venomous species, and the concentrations are particularly high in the venoms of viperid snakes.
- *Hyaluronidases* are commonly called "spreading factors" because they degrade hyaluronic acid, which is a ubiquitous component of the extracellular matrix of tissues and helps to cement cells together. When hyaluronic acid is degraded by hyaluronidase, the remaining venom components are more easily spread throughout tissues, including blood vessels that are rendered to be "leaky." This enzyme is common in most snake venoms.
- *Phospholipases* hydrolyze phospholipids, which are important components of cell membranes. These can weaken cell walls and lead to numerous physiological effects including edema and damage to muscle. These enzymes are found in nearly all snake venoms.
- *Acetylcholinesterase* is an enzyme that hydrolyzes acetylcholine, a chemical that is important for mediating the transmission of nerve signals. This enzyme is a common component of elapid snake venoms and contributes to the neurotoxic actions of those venoms.
- *Toxins* are proteins of variable molecular weight, but generally smaller than that of enzymes. They are highly variable in structure and function, but most affect the nervous system by altering the transmission of nerve signals at the neuromuscular junction. The venoms of elapid snakes are particularly rich in toxins.
- *Nerve growth factors* are proteins that stimulate growth of nerve cells and are found in elapid and viperid venoms. The actions and biological function of these components of snake venom are not well understood.
- *Disintegrins* are peptides found in viperid venoms, and they act to inhibit integrins. These are proteins in membranes that transfer messages across cell membranes to the intracellular cytoplasm.
- A large variety of other factors display a range of actions, including inhibition or activation of enzymes, vasodilation of blood vessels, destruction of cells and receptor sites, lowering of blood pressure, and cessation of breathing.

The efficacy of venoms and the diversity of their pharmacological properties have fascinated humans since the

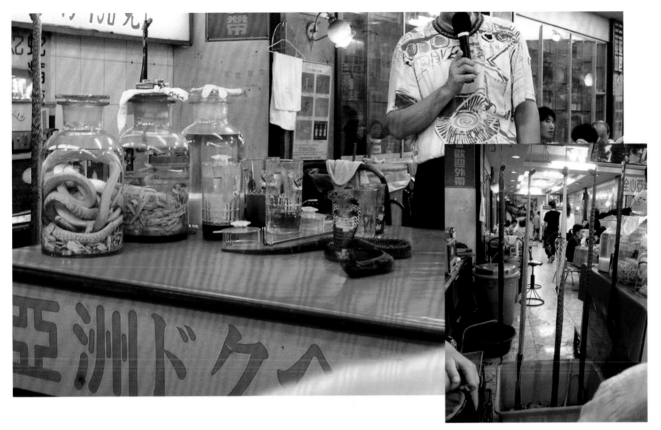

Figure 2.26. A snake shop in Taiwan where the proprietor and a cobra entertain people who visit and purchase snake products that are sold for various supposed health benefits. A live Chinese Cobra (*Naja atra*) is displayed on the table next to jars containing snake parts and fluids. To the left one can see two snakes that are suspended while blood is being drained from a cut tail. The photo to the **lower right** features other snakes—rat snakes and a cobra—that are having their skin removed. The skin of each snake, as well as other internal organs, is used for commercial products. Photographs by the author.

time of Aristotle, and the ancients developed many snake products—including venom, blood, and viscera—that were used in various medical remedies of the time. Some of these practices are still thriving in parts of Asia, and treatments using snake venom are still an important part of mystical healing and folklore (fig. 2.26). Today components of snake venoms are used in basic research, pharmacology, diagnostics, and therapeutics. Venom properties have enabled scientists to achieve numerous advances in medical diagnosis and treatment related to hypertension, vascular disease, muscular dystrophy, cancer, hemorrhage, congenital neuropathies, and many other disease states. They have also contributed useful applications for such things as surgical sutures and enhancement of drug delivery. The famous biologists James Watson and Francis Crick used nucleotidase enzymes from cobra venom to help elucidate the structure of the DNA molecule.

Venom Delivery Systems

The production and effective use of venom depends on the *venom delivery system*, which consists of the venom itself, an associated gland that produces and stores the venom,

and specialized teeth that are used for delivery of the venom (fig. 2.27). The evolutionary origin of venom presumably involved a co-opted salivary gland, modifications of teeth, and natural selection for improved abilities to capture and subdue prey. Most evidence suggests that venoms are most important for aiding the capture of prey, although other uses of venom include defense and the possible enhancement of digestion. Indeed, it is conceivable that a digestive function could have led to increasing toxicity of salivary secretions that secondarily became effective in capturing prey.

Venom injected into prey reduces the time that a snake is in contact with something that is alive, either because the animal is struck, released, and followed later to its point of death, or because the envenomated animal ceases struggling while being held in the snake's mouth. The reduction of contact time with living prey is important because struggling and biting prey can be injurious or even lethal to a hungry snake. A reduction of prey handling time reduces the energy involved in subduing the prey and significantly decreases the potential for injury to the snake. This is almost certainly the reason that so many snake venoms are

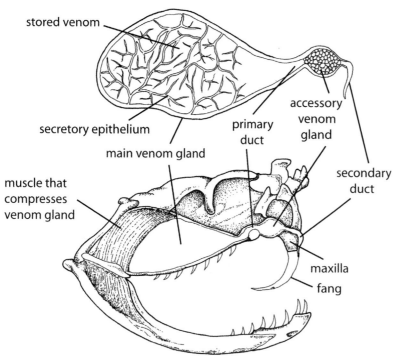

stored venom

secretory epithelium

main venom gland

primary duct

accessory venom gland

secondary duct

muscle that compresses venom gland

maxilla

fang

Figure 2.27. Schematic illustration of the venom delivery apparatus in a viperid snake. The **upper drawing** is an enlargement featuring details of the venom gland and ducts, shown in association with the skull and fang in the **lower drawing**. Drawings by Dan Dourson, after fig. 13.36 in K. V. Kardong, *Vertebrates: Comparative Anatomy, Function, Evolution*, 4th ed. (McGraw-Hill, 2006).

very potent: they have evolved to paralyze or kill prey quickly, and the potential harm to humans who might be bitten by a snake acting defensively is a secondary factor in relation to the evolution of venom properties. The more dangerous the prey item of a snake, the more likely the tendency for the snake to strike and envenomate the animal, release it, and consume it later after it has died. Some species have a demonstrated capacity to track envenomated prey by sensing and following trails that bear chemical cues related to the unique chemical signatures of the venom.

Since the origin of a rudimentary venom gland, the morphology of the gland has been altered in different lineages. Generally, differences in the morphology of venom glands can be categorized in four general types: (1) the atractaspidine type; (2) the colubrid type, historically referred to as Duvernoy's gland; (3) the elapid type; and (4) the viperid type. The more consistent gland structures are found in the Elapidae and Viperidae, whereas there is more variation in the atractaspidine and colubrid species.

The atractaspidine type of venom gland generally is large, tubular, and elongated posteriorly behind the eye (extending beyond the head in some species). These glands consist of largely unbranched tubules radiating from a central lumen. The terminal duct of the gland typically empties venom into anterior, tubular fangs, and venom appears to be forcibly

ejected through the compressive action of an adductor muscle that extends from the parietal bone around the posterior end of the gland to the corner of the mouth.

The venom (or Duvernoy's) gland of colubrids, when present, is relatively small in most species and located posteriorly and ventrally to the eye. This gland is somewhat oval, laterally compressed, and considered to be the ancestral state of the Colubroidea. In *Boiga irregularis* (one of the few colubrid species in which the venom gland has been examined), the gland is multilobed with secondary branching within each lobe. The Duvernoy's gland contains either purely serous cells or a mixture of serous and mucosal cells in different species. There is a small central cistern analogous to the lumen of other venom glands, but is generally greatly reduced in comparison. A single primary duct empties the central cistern into the oral epithelium near the corner of the mouth. Usually there are no compressor muscles associated with the gland.

Elapid snakes possess an oval-shaped serous gland that is associated with a mucous-secreting accessory gland. The main gland is located ventrally and posterior to the eye and is composed of tubules with simple or complex branching patterns. These tubules empty into a narrow lumen that is surrounded by the accessory gland. Venom is discharged to the anterior fangs after passing through the accessory gland, powered by muscular compression of the dorsal and ventral aspects of the gland. It appears that in elapid species of snakes the venom is stored mostly within cells, rather than in the lumen of the gland.

The viperid venom gland is the most intensely studied and appears to have a rather consistent morphology (fig. 2.27). The gland is large, triangular in profile, and divided into several lobules by folds in the surrounding tissue. There is a large lumen that is fed by multiple, complexly branched tubules. The lumen connects by means of a primary duct to a mucosal accessory gland, which in turn leads to a secondary duct that empties into large, tubular fangs at the anterior end of the mouth. The viperid venom gland stores large quantities of venom, which are ejected by a complex pattern of muscle sometimes referred to as the *compressor glandulae*.

Venoms that are produced by the various glands are delivered to prey by means of specialized teeth that aid in rupturing of the skin and/or conducting the venom by means of dental grooves or canals. These include (1) *aglyphous* (small, ungrooved) teeth throughout the oral cavity (many

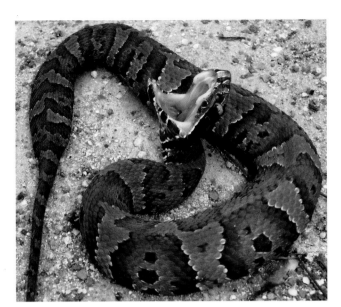

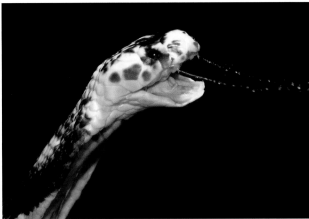

Figure 2.29. Jets of venom being "spat" by an Indochinese Spitting Cobra (*Naja siamensis*). The venom can be rapidly expelled from the fangs and aimed at the eyes of a threatening animal at distances up to about 3 meters. Photograph by Guido Westhoff.

Figure 2.28. A young Florida Cottonmouth (*Agkistrodon piscivorus conanti*) gaping its mouth in a defensive display. The common name is attributed to the white appearance of the fleshy mouth that is shown during these defensive gaping behaviors. Photographed in Florida by Dan Dourson.

colubrids); (2) *opisthoglyphous* (grooved) teeth located in the dorsal, posterior aspect of the mouth (many colubrids and some atractaspidines); (3) *proteroglyphous* fangs fixed to the anterior maxilla (all elapids and some atractaspidines); and (4) large, rotating *solenoglyphous* fangs located on the anterior maxilla (viperids and some atractaspidines).

The various venom delivery systems represent a progression from simpler teeth and less specialized venom delivery to more specialized fangs and venom glands that are capable of delivering large volumes of highly toxic venom in species of snakes that feed on larger and more dangerous prey. The latter are capable of inflicting considerable damage to envenomated prey, and to potential predators!

An interesting problem is how the venom gland can synthesize and store a suite of toxins that can be mobilized almost instantaneously to subdue prey, yet can be stored without the components of venom harming the snake or destroying each other. Several mechanisms are protective during storage, including acidic pH of the venom and the presence of components that inhibit enzymatic activity during storage of the toxins. However, the toxins are activated spontaneously upon their being injected into prey. Venom glands are structurally complex, and the accessory gland might be a site where venom components are activated.

Spitting Venom

Venom is used defensively during bites inflicted when a venomous snake defends itself and bites an attacker or threatening animal. Even better for the snake, however, if

it can keep its adversary at bay without contacting it. This is the reason that snakes have evolved concealing coloration or behaviors, and stereotyped threatening displays such as inflating the neck, hissing, or gaping the mouth (fig. 2.28). Unfortunately, humans sometimes misinterpret these displays as aggressive actions or attacks because they can be frightening. Chances are, however, the snake prefers simply to be left alone rather than to strike or bite.

Spitting venom is a highly specialized behavior that has evolved multiple times in species of African and Asiatic cobras. The term "spitting" refers to the expulsion of venom as a pressurized horizontal stream, usually aimed at the eyes of a harasser or predator (fig. 2.29). Some cobras can spit venom as far as 3 meters and can "aim" the spit quite accurately. During spitting, muscle contractions rotate the maxilla and elevate the palatomaxillary arch, which moves the fang sheath dorsally and removes a physical barrier of soft tissues to the expulsion of venom. Simultaneously, contraction of muscles associated with the venom gland increases pressure on the venom within the gland and forces the venom through the venom duct and fang. The elevated venom pressure propels the venom as an airborne stream beyond the orifice of the fang, but only after physical displacement of the fang sheath allows venom to flow through the fang. The fang opening of a spitting cobra has a more circular aperture than does that of nonspitting cobras, which assists the venom stream to exit forward rather than downward (fig. 2.29).

The Allocation of Venom

The amount of venom that a snake injects into a target (or spits at a target) can vary with the size of a snake, whether the situation is defensive or predatory, the size and nature of the target, and a variety of other factors. There is disagreement regarding whether snakes have the ability to control, or "meter," the expenditure of venom, or whether the expenditure of venom is related more to the nature of a "strike" and the features of the surface of the target. There appears to be rather good evidence supporting the abilities of snakes to meter the quantity of venom they expel. William Hayes and colleagues have demonstrated that spitting cobras, for example, expend larger quantities of venom during biting than during spitting, related to a capacity for regulating the contraction of the venom gland according to the context. It seems likely that such regulation is widespread in snakes and that selection favors behavioral or physiological mechanisms that expel the appropriate amount of venom depending on the target and the context.

Factors Affecting the Variation and Evolution of Venom

The variability of snake venoms is widely known and has been reported since antiquity, based on the observations of snakebite victims and confirmed more recently using molecular and immunological techniques. Research has demonstrated there is much variation in venom composition and toxicity at multiple taxonomic levels and within a single species. There are important variations in venom within a population—even within a small group of related individuals. In some snake species certain components have been found in individuals of one sex but not the other. There is usually stability of various components throughout the age of an individual, but some studies have shown there are changes in venom properties during aging. For example, the venom of juvenile *Bothrops jararaca* was shown to have a higher toxicity for frogs than that of adults, and this difference correlates with the diet of young snakes including frogs and lizards, which are not eaten by the adults. It has also been noted that certain proteins appear, disappear, or become modified during the life span of an individual snake.

In many cases the reasons for variation in the chemical components of venom are not well understood, and there is tremendous variation that needs to be explained. However, in well-studied examples the properties of venom have been shown to correlate with variation in the local diet, genetic relatedness, and geographic location (including *genetic drift* related to random mutations following the isolation of snake populations on islands). In one case it was shown by Jenny Daltry and coworkers that variation in the composition of venom in different populations of the Malayan Pit Viper (*Calloselasma rhodostoma*) correlated strongly with the nutritional status of the population. These results suggest that the availability of certain prey species could exert selection pressures on the composition

of the venom. The manner in which venoms evolve differences has been debated, and clearly venom composition can be influenced by different modes of evolution including natural selection, patterns of gene flow, and genetic drift. In some cases it has been proposed that some variation of venom composition might simply have no adaptive value.

The toxin components of snake venom evolve with relative rapidity, and this is usually viewed as an adaptation related to feeding. However, molecular research indicates that proteins of opossums that counteract the effects of snake venom have evolved rapidly in species of this mammal that eat venomous snakes. This suggests that venom has a defensive role as well as one related to prey capture. Recent data published by researchers associated with the American Museum of Natural History now support the hypothesis that there is a biochemical "arms race" between venomous animals and their prey.

The variability in the biochemical composition of venom can, of course, alter the immunological sites that are recognized by antibodies that are used in the treatment of snakebite. Thus, the effectiveness of a given antivenin might vary depending on the geographic location where a particular snakebite occurred. Further, the random mixing of venoms that are obtained from different populations of snakes has been found to be an insufficient solution to the problem. Envenomation of humans by snakes continues to be a global problem, especially in developing tropical countries of Africa, Asia, and Latin America. However, the actual frequencies of snakebite and their severity throughout the world remain largely unknown.

Digestion

Gut Structure and Function

Digestion refers to the mechanical and chemical breakdown of food prior to the absorption of the resulting nutrients for further modification and distribution to the body. The organ that functions in the digestion of food is called the *digestive tract, alimentary canal, gastrointestinal tract,* or simply *gut* (fig. 2.2). The digestive tract of snakes is fundamentally similar in its anatomical features to that of other vertebrates. The food is passed (transported) from the mouth through the *esophagus,* which connects the throat, or pharynx, with the stomach. The prey item is transported through the esophagus by muscular contractions involving the trunk muscles of the neck, which "push" the prey into the stomach (fig. 2.30). Salivary secretions from the mouth and mucous secretions in the esophagus lubricate the prey and help it to "slide" through the esophagus in front of the wave of muscle contraction. From the stomach food passes through the small intestine to the large intestine, and

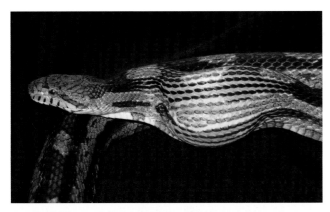

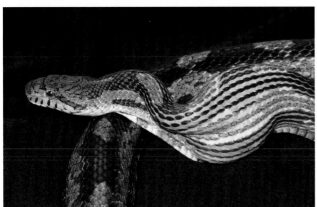

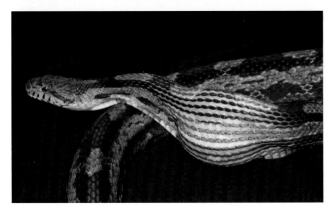

Figure 2.30. A sequence wherein an Eastern Rat Snake (*Pantherophis alleghaniensis*) moves an egg through its neck toward the stomach. Contraction of the body muscles create a wave where first the left side of the neck pushes against the egg (**upper photo**), followed by the right side of the neck pushing against the egg (**middle photo**). Photographs by the author.

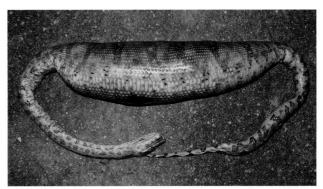

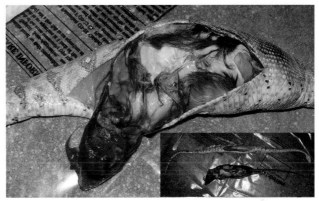

Figure 2.31. A partially digested rat as it was found in the stomach of a juvenile Mexican Boa Constrictor (*Boa constrictor*). The digestion of the animal is in its very early stages. The **upper photo** and the **inset** in the **lower photo** illustrate the size of the rat in relation to that of the snake, internalized and externalized respectively. This snake was found freshly dead from unknown causes in Puerto Angel, Mexico. Photographs by Coleman Sheehy III.

finally to the *cloaca*, where the feces are formed and evacuated from the animal via the cloacal opening.

Generally, snakes swallow their prey entire and do not chew or otherwise tear and break the items into smaller pieces. Therefore, when the prey reaches the stomach where chemical digestion begins, the digestive enzymes must act on the prey from the outside to in. As humans, we appreciate our parents' advice to "chew our food" so that it is broken into smaller pieces, thereby increasing the surface area for the action of digestive enzymes and thereby enhancing the efficiency of the process. Because prey items are swallowed whole by snakes, digestion generally takes longer than it does in humans or many other mammals depending on the exact nature of the food (fig. 2.31). The injection of venom into animals that fall prey to venomous snakes introduces a cocktail of enzymes to the internal body, where they are distributed by "spreading factors" of venom and blood circulation. Thus, some herpetologists speculate that enhancement of digestion might have been one of the early factors in natural selection that helped to promote the evolution of venom and venom delivery systems. Recent studies by Marshall Mc-Cue have shown, however, that injection of venom into mice that are fed to rattlesnakes does not speed up or facilitate their digestion. Thus, some persons may well doubt that venom facilitates the breakdown and digestion of food.

Stomach

The swallowed prey item passes from the esophagus into the stomach, which is the first (or most anterior) expanded part of the digestive tract. Its walls are highly distensible, and its expanded size helps to accommodate large food items during the initial period of digestion (figs. 2.31, 2.32). In cases where multiple, very large, or especially long prey such as fish are eaten by a snake, the swallowed items are accommodated only partly within a greatly stretched

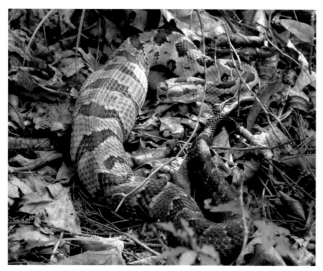

Figure 2.32. A Timber Rattlesnake (*Crotalus horridus*) rests while engorged with a recently ingested small mammal (likely a squirrel, chipmunk, or rat). The prey item has greatly distended the stomach and surrounding body wall. This snake was photographed in Arkansas by Steven Beaupre.

stomach and partly within the esophagus rather than entering the intestine (fig. 2.33). Of the two compartments, however, only the stomach has capacity for digestion. When the stomach is not distended with food, its wall relaxes into folds called *rugae*—something after the manner of an accordion. These folds, as well as generally thickened tissue relative to the esophagus, help to delineate the stomach portion of the digestive tract (fig. 2.34).

The epithelium lining the inner wall of the stomach is glandular and characterized by the presence of gastric glands (*gastric* refers to stomach). Various of these gastric glands secrete mucus, hydrochloric acid, or proteolytic enzymes. The enzymes digest the food with aid from the acid medium. The food eventually becomes a liquefied and partially digested soup-like slur (called *chyme* or *digesta*) before entering the intestine. The lowermost part of the stomach that meets the intestine is called the *pylorus*, and the entry of chyme into the intestine is regulated by a pyloric valve.

The gastric pH that is maintained during digestion ranges from 1.5 to 4 in several species of snakes that have been studied. Unlike mammals, which maintain an acidic stomach environment between meals, after food leaves the stomach of snakes the pH increases to around 7 to 7.5. The duration of gastric acid and enzyme production is a function of body temperature and both the size and composition of a meal. The duration of gastric pH and enzyme

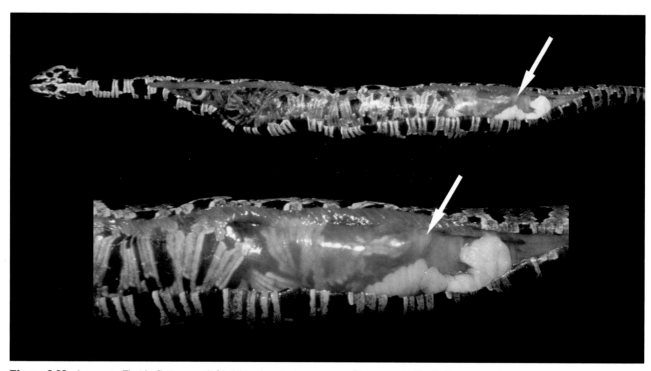

Figure 2.33. A neonate Florida Cottonmouth (*Agkistrodon piscivorus conanti*) has cannibalized a littermate of approximately the same size. The ingested littermate has been curled back on itself, and the stomach of the predatory snake has been stretched exceptionally thin to accommodate the meal. The **lower** photograph shows a closer view in which the ingested snake can be seen abutting against the duodenum of the intestine (arrows). Photographs by the author.

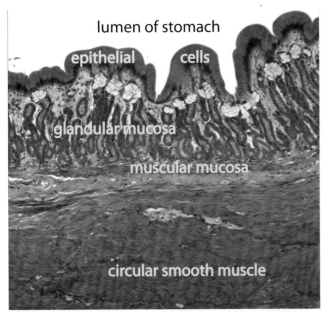

lumen of stomach

epithelial cells

glandular mucosa

muscular mucosa

circular smooth muscle

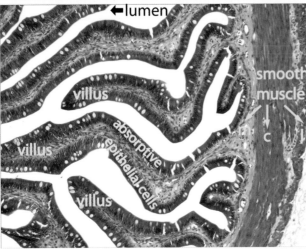

←lumen

smooth muscle

villus

villus

absorptive epithelial cells

villus

Figure 2.34. Photomicrographs illustrating histological sections through portions of the stomach (**upper photo**) and small intestine (**lower photo**) of a Dumeril's Ground Boa (*Acrantophis dumerili*). The absorptive epithelial cells of the mucosa are arranged on mucosal folds (stomach) or villi (intestine), and the latter especially increase the absorptive surface area. Arrows point to the layers of smooth muscle in the intestine. The smooth muscle of the mucosa is thin and consists of a single cell layer in the intestine (m). The outer smooth muscle is circular in arrangement (c), with outer longitudinal muscle (l) being thinner and shown only for the intestine. The histological stain is Masson's trichome. Photomicrographs by Elliott Jacobson.

secretion increases with the size and structural composition of food. Digestion is prolonged at lower temperatures and is critically slowed or ceases altogether if the temperature falls below about 10°C. The precise temperature threshold varies in different species (see chapter 4).

Intestine

The intestine is a very important segment of the gut where the final digestive breakdown of food occurs, and the resulting products are absorbed into the blood circulation. The surface of the intestinal mucosa bears numerous fingerlike strictures called *villi* (*villus* singular), and the mucosal cells covering the surfaces of individual villi are in turn covered with numerous smaller projections, termed *microvilli*—perhaps several thousand per individual cell (fig. 2.34). Collectively these greatly enlarge the absorptive surface area that is exposed to the chyme within the lumen. The membrane of the microvilli has embedded enzymes that act strictly in the local environment of the microvilli. The anterior part of the intestine also receives digestive enzymes via a small duct that conveys these enzymes from the pancreas. The liver secretes bile, which is stored in the gall bladder and conveyed by a duct to the intestine, where it serves to emulsify lipids, or fats (fig. 2.2). Collectively these various secretions neutralize the acids from the stomach, break fats apart, and further digest the chyme within the lumen of the intestine. Because snakes are carnivores, many of the digestive enzymes—both in the stomach and in the intestine—are proteases that digest protein.

The chyme is broken, mixed, and moved in a net posterior direction by the peristaltic actions of smooth muscle in the intestinal wall. The arrangement of these muscles involves an inner circular layer and an outer longitudinal layer (fig. 2.34). Contraction of the circular layer and simultaneous relaxation of the longitudinal layer both constricts and elongates the intestinal tube. Alternately, relaxation of the circular layer coordinated with active shortening of the longitudinal layer results in shortening and distension of the intestinal tube.

The intestine consists of two principal regions, the anterior *small intestine* and the posteriormost segment called the *large intestine*. The large intestine is much shorter than the small intestine and usually has an enlarged diameter. Following the acidic phase of digestion in the stomach, the final stages of digestion and mixing occur in the small intestine. Absorption of the digestive products, including water, occurs largely within the large intestine. The undigested parts of the chyme that are not absorbed are formed into feces, which become increasingly more solid in composition due to the intestinal absorption of water. The feces also contain large amounts of bacteria that are passed along from the upper parts of the gut where bacterial populations flourish and participate in digestion.

The feces empty into the cloaca, which is the most posterior segment of the gut (fig. 2.35). It is a common chamber that receives digestive products from the intestine and urinary products from the kidney, and is also a passageway for products from the reproductive tract. As such, the cloaca typically contains the feces together with a slurry of *uric acid* and *urates* from the kidney. Urates are salts of uric acid. Together these form a crystalline waste product of nitrogen metabolism, which is excreted by the kidney. Uric acid is poorly soluble in water and can be eliminated in a precipitated form, which is

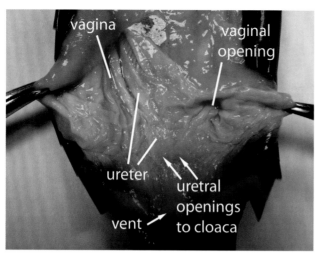

Figure 2.35. Cloaca of a Florida Cottonmouth (*Agkistrodon piscivorus conanti*). This is the posteriormost aspect of the digestive tract and receives the digestive wastes from the intestine, fetuses from the paired oviducts, and urine from paired ureters. Each oviduct connects to one of the paired ovaries, and where the terminal segment enters the cloaca it is termed *vagina* or *vaginal pouch*. The vagina at the left has been cut to reveal the ureter that runs alongside of it. One also sees the mucosal folds where sperm can be stored. Each of the paired ureters communicates with one of the kidneys. This snake died from unknown causes and was frozen until the tissues were observed following thawing. Photograph by the author.

the familiar white to yellow solid material that is seen together with the fecal elimination of snakes. If a snake is in good water balance both the feces and the urates might appear quite soft or fluid, especially if these are eliminated after the snake has had a good drink of water. On the other hand, if a snake is partially dehydrated and has not drunk recently, the feces and the urates appear more solid and can actually be very hard and compressed. This is due to extra water absorption, which probably occurs in the cloaca as well as the small intestine. Occasionally, excess water absorption from a large volume of feces can result in a compaction that forms a blockage and is not easily passed by the snake. Thus, access to water is important with respect to adequate digestive function in snakes.

The various enzymes, venom toxins, acid secretions, and bacteria chemically reduce the food to elemental components of carbohydrates, proteins, and lipids, which are absorbed into the blood circulation across the wall of the intestine. The digestive tract can be regarded as an input-output system, with food entering the mouth and feces exiting the cloacal opening (vent), while water and nutrients are taken up and distributed to the body from the digestive regions that lie between these "in" and "out" terminal points of the gut. The mechanical motions attributable to smooth muscle are coordinated largely by nerves that activate the smooth muscles in the wall of the gut. The simultaneous coordination of digestive secretions is controlled by the physical presence of food in the gut, and by gastrointestinal hormones secreted from endocrine cells in the walls of the stomach and intestine. Compared with some other vertebrates (especially mammals), very little is known about the control of digestive secretions in snakes, although it is assumed to be quite similar.

Periodic Feeding

Snakes are characterized as *discontinuous*, *intermittent*, or *periodic* feeders. Because rates of metabolism, and therefore energy requirements, are relatively low, snakes do not require a lot of food—at least in comparison with endothermic birds and mammals (see chapter 4). Further, because many snakes have the capability for feeding on comparatively large prey, which they swallow entire, snakes do not need to feed often. However, one other consideration is very important. The period of annual time that is available for feeding and growth is variously limited in temperate climates, because snakes are dormant or inactive during the colder months and cannot digest food at low temperatures. Therefore, there are circumstances in which many species of snakes do not eat as frequently as their digestive systems might otherwise permit. The requirement for energy varies with many factors including temperature, activity, growth, and reproduction.

Generally, snakes ingest about 6 to 30 meals per year, totaling 55 to 300 percent of their body mass, to meet their overall energy needs according to estimates by Harry Greene. Very little is known about the frequency of feeding by wild snakes in their natural environment, and whether prey is sufficiently abundant for a given snake population or whether it is limited. Studies in which rattlesnakes (*Crotalus atrox* and *C. horridus*) were artificially fed supplemental food demonstrated that such food supplementation led to increased rates of growth and reproduction. Of course the foraging success of individual snakes in a wild population will vary, and some may do very well while others may become emaciated and die from malnutrition. Here we can appreciate the advantage of the low metabolic rate, however. If mammals cannot find food, generally they will perish within a few days or weeks, whereas some species of snakes in captivity can survive for more than a year without a meal. Some rattlesnakes can survive without food for periods up to two years. Further, if we consider only the energy required for routine maintenance, a 50 g garter snake in Michigan requires only the equivalent of one 44 g frog to sustain itself for an entire year according to estimates by Warren Porter and C. Richard Tracy. In another study, Marshall McCue and I estimated that an insular adult Cottonmouth in Florida requires only 1 kg of fish for annual maintenance and activity. This would be equivalent to only a few small to medium-size fish. In a study of foraging modes comparing a "lie and wait" Sidewinder Rattlesnake

(*Crotalus cerastes*) with a widely "active foraging" Coachwhip (*Masticophis flagellum*), Stephen Secor and Kenneth Nagy found that the more active Coachwhip consumed prey energy at a rate about 2.1 times greater than did the less active sidewinder.

The digestive tract is a highly dynamic organ that responds dramatically to changes in the quantity and quality of food. Different sections of the gut become immediately active upon the arrival of food or chyme. Additionally, the demands for digestion related to feeding lead to changes in morphological and physiological features of the gut, including increases in metabolic activity and changes in the mass and shape of the epithelial lining that double or triple the absorptive surface area. Simultaneously, there is an increase in the capacity to secrete digestive enzymes and for molecular "transporters" to take up nutrients across the intestinal wall. Such a response to feeding is termed *up-regulation* and may occur within 24 to 48 hours of ingesting a meal. The responses are fully reversible, and *down-regulation* occurs in the absence of food or during voluntary fasting. Extended periods of fasting are characterized by reductions in metabolic rate and in the atrophy of the digestive tract.

The responses to feeding have been especially well studied in the Burmese Python, *Python molurus*, by Stephen Secor. Within one to three days after ingesting a meal, the intestinal capacity for nutrient uptake increases from 11 to 24 times that of fasting levels, while the intestinal mucosa more than doubles in mass (fig. 2.36). There are also considerable increases in the masses of other organs, such as the liver, that are active in processing nutrients. The up-regulated condition of the intestine returns to fasting levels by the time of defecation at 8–14 days. Similar up-regulation occurs in the digestive responses of snakes that feed infrequently (four- to six-week intervals).

In contrast, snakes that feed more frequently (one- to two-week intervals) exhibit very little changes in the intestinal mass or capacities for nutrient uptake. Consideration of digestive costs suggests that saving energy has probably driven the evolution of low mass and low activities of the digestive organs during fasting, and of large up-regulated responses to ingestion of a meal in species that feed infrequently. Generally, the dichotomy of responses I have described is seen between ambush foraging snakes (mostly pythons, boas, and vipers) and actively foraging snakes that feed relatively more frequently in the wild (e.g., many colubrid and elapid snakes).

Rates, Costs, and Efficiency of Digestion

Rates of Digestion

Rates of digestion in snakes vary considerably depending on both the external and internal conditions of the animal. Generally, digestion increases with temperature, but

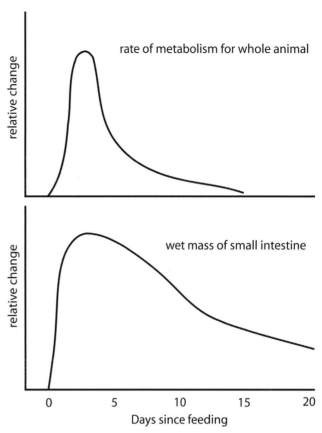

Figure 2.36. Relative increases in metabolic rate and wet mass of the small intestine, measured as mean changes in Burmese Pythons (*Python molurus*) following the ingestion of rodent meals. The original units were measured as rates of oxygen consumption and grams, respectively. These graphs are approximations of the original data and are intended only to show relative changes through time (see references for Stephen Secor and Jared Diamond). Drawing by the author.

only up to some limit. Thus snakes at low body temperatures digest more slowly than do those at higher temperatures, other factors being equal. Further, it seems intuitive as well as based in observation that for a given temperature, it takes a snake longer to digest a large meal (remember, swallowed whole) than it does to digest a smaller meal. But within certain limits the size of prey seems not to affect digestion rates in some species of snakes (e.g., *Thamnophis elegans*, *Vipera aspis*). However, the nature or composition of the prey can definitely influence the digestion rate. Softer prey such as a frog or fish is digested quite rapidly, within 36 to 72 hours depending on size, whereas harder items such as crustaceans or hard-shelled insects take longer. Mammals and birds are digested more slowly than are fish or frogs owing to the presence of hair, feathers, claws, or beaks (figs. 2.31, 2.37). Hard, keratinous proteins are more difficult to digest than are softer tissues, and these are typically passed and eliminated intact in feces.

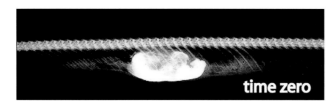

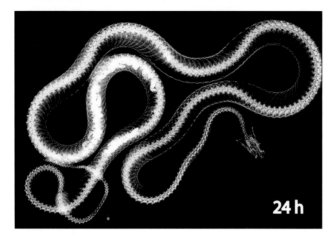

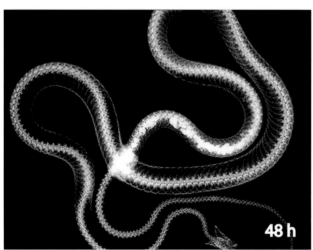

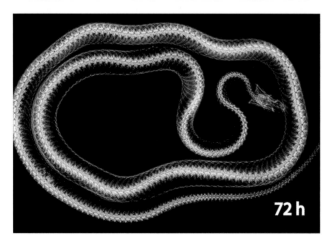

Figure 2.37. Radiographs of a Black Rat Snake (*Pantherophis obsoletus*) digesting a chick that was injected with barium. The **uppermost** image shows the position of the chick in the stomach shortly after being swallowed. The descending images that follow illustrate the condition of the chick during sequential times following ingestion. Photographs by Elliott R. Jacobson.

Digestive Efficiency

Scientists usually quantify the "efficiency" of digestion in terms of the net energy that is absorbed into the body by the digestive tract. That is, digestive efficiency can be expressed as the ratio of the absorbed energy to the total energy that is present in the intact prey before digestion, expressed as a decimal fraction or as a percentage. The energy that is neither digested nor absorbed is what appears as feces, together with some added bacteria. Generally, digestive efficiencies of most squamate reptiles that have been studied approach or exceed 90 percent. The few measurements in snakes are generally between 85 to 95 percent and vary with species, individuals, meal size, and temperature. If the indigestible hair component is excluded from calculations, the digestive efficiencies can be extremely high—between 99.3 and 99.8 percent! Perhaps the high digestive efficiencies are important in species with long intervals between feeding and reflect the longer passage times for feces in these species (see below).

The high efficiencies of digestion have some important implications for how snakes increase their acquisition of energy when there is need. Because the amount of energy extracted from meals is relatively high, there is not much room for improving the energy gain per meal. Further, some studies indicate that digestive efficiency varies little with temperature. Therefore, the manner by which snakes are able to increase their input of chemical energy is to increase the rate of feeding and passage of feces, rather than to increase the amount of calories that are absorbed from individual meals. That is, increasing energy gain from food is a game of increasing *rate* rather than *efficiency* of extraction.

The efficiency achieved depends on the composition of the prey. Fur, feathers, and mineralized structures such as teeth and some bones are indigestible, as are most plant materials. Plants with thin and relatively soft cellular walls can be digested by some species, however (fig. 2.38).

Fecal Passage Time

The formation, storage, and evacuation of feces are important features of the digestive processing of food. If we consider the relatively large size of meals that are eaten by snakes, the time that feces are held within the lower digestive tract adds a potentially considerable component to the overall mass of a snake. The time elapsed from ingestion to defecation, known as the gut *passage time*, typically varies from a few hours or a few days in birds and mammals to several weeks or longer in other species of vertebrates. However, snakes are clearly champions when it comes to the range and maximum passage time for fecal matter.

Stout and heavy species of terrestrial snakes, especially ground-dwelling viperid and boid species, retain and accumulate fecal material for periods of months while on a regular

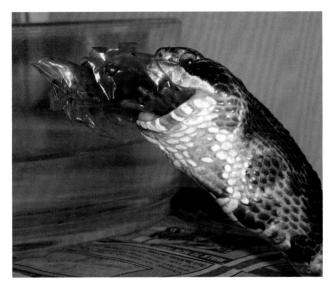

Figure 2.38. A captive Florida Cottonmouth (*Agkistrodon piscivorus conanti*) eating marine algae (*Ulva lactuca*) that was tainted with fish odor. This alga species has soft cell walls and is digestible by the snake. Such consumption of plant material probably rarely happens, but is possible when Cottonmouths forage along island beaches and consume dead fishes that might be washed ashore along with other objects including much marine plant material. Photograph by the author.

feeding schedule. My investigations of the Gaboon Adder, *Bitis gabonica*, indicate that these snakes accumulate feces to what appears to be a maximum of storage capacity regardless of the rate of feeding. Thus, at slower feeding rates the passage time can be as long as a year or more, whereas at faster feeding rates the passage time is reduced to about 1.5 months. In either case, feces are accumulated to the extent they represent about 5 to 20 percent of the total mass of the snake. The maximum defecation interval that has been observed in the Gaboon Adder is 420 days! Other maxima include 174 days in *Python molurus* and 386 days in *Python curtus*.

In contrast to the heavy-bodied species just mentioned, slender arboreal species of snakes are characterized by relatively rapid passage times—the known minimum being 23 hours in a Haitian tree snake, *Uromacer oxyrhynchus*, to my knowledge. There is also a trend among snakes for more active species to have shorter passage times than do sedentary species. It appears to make sense for more active species to void excess fecal mass and thereby lighten the load in locomotion. This appears to be especially important in arboreal species that climb within, or over, foliage that might provide weak and unstable support.

There is one possible penalty that snakes might pay when they retain fecal mass, especially without adequate intake of water. Compacted fecal matter can form an intestinal obstruction if the mass of material is large, and/or if the material is very dense and hard due to removal of water (that is taken up by the gut). Gastrointestinal obstructions

are known in various captive snakes, and have been reported, albeit rarely, in wild-caught animals.

In summary, the storage of fecal mass in snakes varies positively with the structural body mass of species, which in general reflects their habitat and foraging mode. For whatever reasons arboreal species have evolved slender body shape with low mass, the frequent defecation exhibited by these species helps to keep the mass low. On the other hand, for whatever reasons the stout, ground-dwelling, ambush predatory vipers and pythons have evolved heavy bodies, the accumulation of feces adds to the structural body mass especially at the posterior end of the animal. The posterior trunk of these snakes usually remains on the ground as an important anchor during striking, and perhaps this is nature's reason for the evolution of extremely long passage times. Thus, extremely prolonged retention of feces possibly functions as metabolically inert ballast in the heavier species, while simultaneously enhancing the maximum uptake of water and nutrients. Voiding a large mass of feces that might be stored in this way is potentially risky and is greatly facilitated by access to drinking water.

The Energy Cost of Digestion

When snakes consume a prey item and digest it, there is an energetic cost that is reflected in an increase in the rate of metabolism (fig. 2.36). The increment of metabolism above normal resting levels is called *specific dynamic action* (abbreviated *SDA*), *postprandial metabolic response*, *postprandial thermogenesis*, or *postprandial calorigenic response*. SDA represents the sum total of energy that is expended on the ingestion and processing of a meal. These energy costs reflect the mechanical and biochemical processes involved in digestion and the assimilation of digestive products.

The digestion of an intact meal is an expensive undertaking, especially for snakes that consume large prey items. For example, SDA responses of Burmese Pythons characteristically involve 5- to 44-fold increases in the rate of metabolism measured in these snakes. Stephen Secor estimated that in Burmese Pythons activities of the stomach contributed about 55 percent of SDA, protein synthesis contributed another 26 percent, gastrointestinal up-regulation contributed about 5 percent, and other activities about 14 percent.

Characteristically, the postfeeding rate of metabolism increases rapidly within 24 hours after feeding, and then declines more slowly. The response peaks early, usually within 24–48 hours, and declines to normal after about 4–12 days depending on the species and prey item (fig. 2.36). Generally, species of snakes that feed infrequently have lower rates of metabolism when fasting but greater increases of metabolism in SDA, longer durations of elevated metabolism, and higher total extra energy expenditure in SDA than do species that feed relatively frequently. Stephen Secor and Jared Diamond found that in various species, SDA represents from 13 to 33 percent of the total energy that is ingested with a meal and tends to be higher in infrequent feeders compared with frequent feeders. Evidently, however, down-regulation of the gut (fig. 2.36) and other organs following feeding contributes to the low rates of fasting metabolism and saves long-term energy during the periods between meals in the infrequent feeders. Arguably, it appears there has evolved an association between natural feeding intervals and the regulation of gut performance in snakes.

Water Balance in Snakes

Water is an essential resource for snakes, just as is food or energy. Like other vertebrates, it is important for snakes to maintain an appropriate content of body water so that the composition of cells and body fluids are kept within a range that is compatible with living processes. Generally, the tissues of snakes consist of about 65 to 80 percent water, and dehydration below this range can be deleterious or lethal. Therefore, snakes require water for living just as they do food.

There are three sources of water available to snakes (or any other animal). First, there is a certain amount of preformed water that is available in the food that is eaten. This is called *dietary water*. Second, small amounts of water are formed during the metabolism of food, after it is broken down during digestion and assimilated into tissues. This is called *metabolic water*. The third source of water is free water in the environment, which ultimately comes from rainfall. All three sources of water are part of a snake's "water budget," but most species depend to some degree on drinking fresh water in the environment in order to maintain water balance.

To remain in water balance, an animal must replenish water that is lost from the body. Hence, averaged over time, the input of water must equal the summed outputs or losses of water, just as the same is true of energy inputs and outputs with respect to the food that is required for fueling an animal's metabolism. The inputs of water for a snake include dietary water, metabolic water, water that is obtained by drinking from the environment, and water that might leak across the skin or other membranes from the environment. The latter is potentially quite important for aquatic animals, which also accidentally ingest water that "leaks" through the mouth during the process of swallowing food. This latter water has been referred to as "incidental drinking." On the output side, the losses of water include water that is lost in feces and urine, and water that

leaks across the skin surfaces either in evaporation, or in the case of aquatic animals, water that leaks across the skin or exposed membranes in response to osmosis. The latter can be potentially important for marine animals. These inward and outward fluxes of water are summarized in figure 2.39 and are discussed in more detail in the sections that follow.

The Kidney

The kidneys of snakes are paired structures located in the dorsal body cavity with the right kidney more anterior in location than the left kidney (figs. 2.2, 6.5). The kidneys filter the blood and remove waste products. They are simpler than those of mammals, and they cannot produce urine that is more concentrated than the body fluids. Snakes do not have a urinary bladder, and the urine is carried by ducts from the kidneys and empties directly into the cloaca.

With respect to water balance, urine is liquid derived from blood plasma and therefore contains water. Thus, excretion of wastes in urine requires losses of water. However, water can be a waste product in need of excretion if it is present in excess amount. In this case, the urine will be less concentrated and greater in volume to remove body water. On the other hand, if water is in short supply the urine will be more concentrated and produced in smaller quantities to conserve water. Once urine enters the cloaca it can be further modified by the uptake of water—either in the cloaca or hindgut—and held for some while or excreted with less water. Also, snakes produce *uric acid* as the principal form of nitrogenous wastes that result from the metabolism of protein. The white or yellow mass associated with urine or feces consists of urates, and these may be present as a slurry of soft material or as a solid mass, sometimes nearly stonelike. The differences in fluidity depend on how much water has been reclaimed from the urine and urates before their elimination. Thus, a dehydrated snake will eliminate solid and very dry urates (and also feces) as a result of water retention prior to elimination. Uric acid is an advantageous form of nitrogenous excretion because it easily precipitates and can be eliminated with minimum loss of water (compared with the other forms of nitrogenous waste, urea and ammonium).

As a husbandry issue, adequate water is important for the normal elimination of feces and urates. If a snake becomes dehydrated, these products tend to form a more hardened mass that can sometimes create a blockage that can be harmful or even lethal to a snake. It can be surmised that there are very effective mechanisms for conserving water by withdrawing and retaining water that is normally eliminated with urine and feces, and this occurs in the hindgut and cloaca. These processes are not well studied in snakes, however.

Salt Glands

Salt glands are excretory structures that are accessory to the kidney and have the capability to secrete concentrated salt solutions. These have evolved in various taxa of tetrapods that live in dry habitats and are lacking a kidney with a capacity to excrete very concentrated urine, which include birds and various reptiles. Among snakes these occur in various lineages of marine species living in habitats where ingestion of excess salt creates an osmotic problem and compounds the tendency to lose water to a salty environment. The salt concentration in the body fluids of snakes, including marine species, is only about one-third or less of that present in seawater. Thus, marine snakes will tend to lose water and gain salt from the environment, which can greatly disturb water balance. Salt glands help to alleviate this dual problem, but they are variously effective in different species depending on the size of the glands and their rate of secretion.

The salt glands of snakes are relatively small structures that are located in the lower jaw beneath or anterior to the tongue casing (acrochordids, laticaudines, and hydrophiines), or in the case of homalopsids there is a premaxillary location. In other taxa of tetrapods, salt glands are associated with other locations in the head, including nasal, orbital, and oral cavities.

The presence of salt glands in marine snakes may help to confer the ability of these animals to live in seawater. Indeed, François Brischoux and his colleagues have demonstrated that species residing in ocean water of higher salinity generally possess salt glands that have been shown to secrete salts at higher rates than do those of other species inhabiting lower salinity water. However, some species of marine snakes (*Acrochordus granulatus*, *Laticauda* spp. and *Pelamis*) require fresh water to avoid dehydration, so in these species salt glands might help to regulate salt balance and slow the rate of dehydration, but they are not sufficient alone to maintain water balance. These subjects need to be investigated more thoroughly in a broader range of species.

Water Flux across the Skin

The skin is a complex organ that has many functions, including regulation of the amount of water that moves across the skin, either as a bidirectional osmotic flux (e.g., aquatic species) or as evaporation from skin surfaces to surrounding air (fig. 2.39). These movements of water—either in or out of the skin—are regulated in large part by a

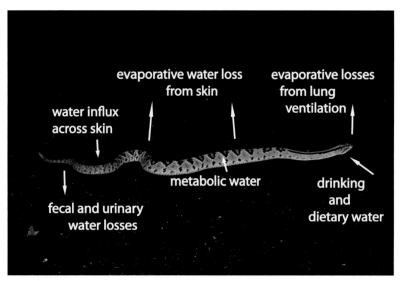

Figure 2.39. Hypothetical water fluxes in and out of a Central American Rattlesnake (*Crotalus simus*). The net exchange (over time) determines whether the snake will be in positive or negative water balance. This rattlesnake was crossing a road in Guanacaste Province, Costa Rica. Photograph by Shauna Lillywhite.

permeability barrier consisting of layered lipids sandwiched in between alternating layers of keratin inside the stratum corneum of the epidermis (see chapter 5). Within the skin, lipid bodies (termed *lamellar granules*) are secreted from differentiating α-cells and subsequently become organized into lamellar "sheets" that fill the extracellular spaces.

Both the quantity and organization of these lipids generally correlate with the aridity of the habitat in which a species lives. The drier the environment, the greater the quantity of lipids that occur in the permeability barrier. This appears to be the mechanistic basis for the generalization that species of snakes living in drier terrestrial habitats tend to have lower rates of cutaneous evaporative water loss, compared with those living in more mesic habitats. Among sea kraits (*Laticauda* spp.), studies by the author and his colleagues have demonstrated that rates of water loss across the skin are much lower when snakes are in seawater than when they are in air. Sea kraits are partly terrestrial, however, and species that spend more time on land tend to have lower rates of evaporative water loss than do those that are more thoroughly aquatic. Finally, those species of sea kraits that are relatively more aquatic tend to have lower rates of water loss across the skin when in seawater than do the species with more terrestrial tendencies. In other words, the properties of the skin tend to be "adjusted" for conserving water relative to the habitat in which a species spends more of its time.

In the embryos of egg-laying species of snakes, the embryonic epidermis tends to slough within the egg, and a permeability barrier of partial competence is formed within the epidermis prior to the snake's hatching. The resistance of the skin to evaporative water loss improves with subsequent skin-shedding events, which indicates there is some capacity for the skin to improve its barrier effectiveness. There is some indication that the effectiveness of the permeability barrier can be improved or "adjusted" during ecdysis in response to the aridity of the environment. Further research is needed on this subject before it can be generalized, however.

Drinking Behaviors of Snakes

Many persons who have maintained snakes in captivity have noted that occasionally certain individuals will stop feeding, and that some species are reluctant to eat at all. However, a thirsty snake will always, in my experience, drink water. The voluntary "will" to drink implies a snake is thirsty, and the sensation of thirst implies there is a physiological signal related to dehydration and negative water balance. In wild populations, snakes have various opportunities to drink. These include standing bodies of water such as ponds or lakes, freshwater streams, rainfall, and water that might collect on the body of a coiled snake, or on leaves, small depressions, and so on, during rainstorms and persist for some while thereafter. If water is not available, for example during a seasonal drought, snakes might go for long periods without a drink. In these circumstances, dehydrating snakes might become reclusive and remain down burrows or in other places where evaporative losses are mitigated and body water is conserved. Generally, snakes that are living in arid environments have a suite of adaptations to conserve water and/or tolerate a considerable degree of dehydration. Some species might be able to depend largely, or perhaps exclusively, on dietary and metabolic water. However, such ability has not yet been demonstrated for snakes.

Terrestrial species of snakes will generally drink water on a somewhat regular basis whenever water balance becomes slightly negative. In some cases the consumption of water increases following feeding. Digestion requires water, followed by production of urine to eliminate nitrogenous wastes that result from the metabolic processing of the absorbed food products. If snakes have access to water, feces are eliminated in a moist or wet condition, which also reflects these water losses. In contrast, recent studies by the author and his associates have demonstrated that sea snakes are reluctant to drink fresh water unless they have been dehydrated to a considerable extent (10 to 20% or more loss of body mass in several species). This probably reflects an evolutionary suppression of the drinking stimulus related to the influence of other traits that conserve body water and increase the tolerance to dehydration as these snakes adapted to marine existence.

David Cundall and his colleagues have investigated the biomechanics of drinking in snakes. Many advanced species of snakes drink by sucking water into the mouth followed by compression of the mouth cavity that forces the water into the esophagus. However, some of these species are capable of drinking without sealing the margins of the mouth, which implies that water can be ingested without being dependent on buccal pumping. Opening and closing movements of the jaws are variable, as is the volume of water that is ingested with each cycle of jaw movements. Snakes drink using a variety of movement patterns, and the jaws might be variably "sealed" (or not) in different circumstances. In addition to the use of periodic buccal pumping, mucosal folds in the mouth of snakes act like a sponge to trap water or attract water by capillarity. Cundall and his colleagues have proposed a second model for drinking—termed the "sponge model"—in which water is moved by the rhythmic squeezing and relaxation of parts of the mouth having channels or surfaces with sponge-like properties. Some of the adhering water can move in an anterior direction, but water that moves in a posterior direction goes toward the esophagus. The rear part of the mouth cavity contains expanded regions that are sponge-like and overlain by muscles. Complex movements of these and other muscles drive the water.

The mucosal folds in the mouth that entrap and move water are features that likely evolved in relation to the stretching of mouth parts around relatively large prey. The function of these features in drinking is therefore likely to represent a secondary use of anatomical traits having another, perhaps principal, function related to feeding.

Additional Reading

Aubret, F., R. Shine, and X. Bonnet. 2004. Adaptive developmental plasticity in snakes. *Nature* 431:261–262.

Bedford, G. S., and K. A. Christian. 2000. Digestive efficiency in some Australian pythons. *Copeia* 2000:829–834.

Bels, V., and K. V. Kardong. 1995. Water drinking in snakes: Evidence for an esophageal sphincter. *Journal of Experimental Zoology* 272:235–239.

Bonnet X., and F. Brischoux. 2008. Thirsty sea snakes forsake refuge during rainfall. *Australian Ecology* 33:911–921.

Brischoux, F., R. Tingley, R. Shine, and H. B. Lillywhite. 2012. Salinity influences the distribution of marine snakes: Implications for evolutionary transitions to marine life. *Ecography* 35:994–1003.

Britt, E. J., A. J. Clark, and A. F. Bennett. 2009. Dental morphologies in gartersnakes (*Thamnophis*) and their connection to dietary preferences. *Copeia* 43:252–259.

Catania, K. C. 2009. Tentacled snakes turn C-starts to their advantage and predict future prey behavior. *Proceedings of the National Academy of Sciences* (USA) 106:11183–11187.

Catania, K. C. 2010. Born knowing: Tentacled snakes innately predict future prey behavior. *PLoS ONE* 5:1–10.

Chippaux, J.-P. 2006. *Snake Venoms and Envenomations*. Malabar, FL: Krieger Publishing.

Chiszar, D., A. Walters, and H. M. Smith. 2008. Rattlesnake preference for envenomated prey: Species specificity. *Journal of Herpetology* 42:764–767.

Corbit, A. G., C. Person, and W. K. Hayes. 2013. Constipation associated with brumation? Intestinal obstruction caused by a fecalith in a wild Red Diamond Rattlesnake (*Crotalus ruber*). *Journal of Animal Physiology and Animal Nutrition*. doi:10.1111/jpn.12040.

Cox, C. L., and S. M. Secor. 2007. Effects of meal size, clutch, and metabolism on the energy efficiencies of juvenile Burmese pythons, *Python molurus*. *Comparative Biochemistry and Physiology* A 148:861–868.

Cox, C. L., and S. M. Secor. 2008. Matched regulation of gastrointestinal performance in the Burmese python, *Python molurus*. *Journal of Experimental Biology* 211:1131–1140.

Cundall, D. 2000. Drinking in snakes: Kinematic cycling and water transport. *Journal of Experimental Biology* 203:2171–2185.

Cundall, D. 2002. Envenomation strategies, head form, and feeding ecology in vipers. In G. W. Schuett, M. Höggren, M. E. Douglas, and H. W. Greene (eds.), *Biology of the Vipers*. Eagle Mountain, UT: Eagle Mountain Publishing, pp. 149–161.

Cundall, D., E. L. Brainerd, J. Constantino, A. Deufel, D. Grapski, and N. J. Kley. 2012. Drinking in snakes: Resolving a biomechanical puzzle. *Journal of Experimental Zoology* 317:152–172.

Cundall, D., and A. Deufel. 2006. Influence of the venom delivery system on intraoral prey transport in snakes. *Zoologischer Anzeiger* 245:193–210.

Cundall, D., and H. W. Greene. 2000. Feeding in snakes. In K. Schwenk (ed.), *Feeding: Form, Function, and Evolution in Tetrapod Vertebrates*. San Diego: Academic Press, pp. 293–333.

Daltry, J. C., W. Wüster, and R. S. Thorpe. 1996. Diet and snake venom evolution. *Nature* 379:537–540.

De Queiroz, A., and J. A. Rodríguez-Robles. 2006. Historical contingency and animal diets: The origins of egg eating snakes. *American Naturalist* 167:682–692.

Deufel, A., and D. Cundall. 2003. Feeding in *Atractaspis* (Serpentes: Atractaspididae): A study in conflicting functional constraints. *Zoology* 106:43–61.

DeVault, T. L., and A. R. Krochmal. 2002. Scavenging by snakes: An examination of the literature. *Herpetologica* 58:429–436.

Dmi'el, R. 1998. Skin resistance to evaporative water loss in viperid snakes: Habitat aridity versus taxonomic status. *Comparative Biochemistry and Physiology* 121A:1–5.

Fry, B. G., W. Wüster, S. F. R. Ramjan, T. Jackson, P. Martelli, and R. M. Kini. 2003. Analysis of Colubroidea snake venoms by liquid chromatography with mass spectrometry: Evolutionary and toxinological implications. *Rapid Communications in Mass Spectrometry* 17:2047–2062.

Fry, B. G., N. Vidal, J. A. Normal, F. J. Vonk, H. Scheib, S. F. R. Ramjan, S. Kuruppu, K. Fung, S. B. Hedges, M. K. Richardson, W. C. Hodgson, V. Ignjatovic, R. Summerhayes, and E. Kochva. 2006. Early evolution of the venom system in lizards and snakes. *Nature* 439:584–588.

Furry, K., T. Swain, and D. Chiszar. 1991. Stike-induced chemosensory searching and trail following by prairie rattlesnakes (*Crotalus viridis*) preying upon deer mice (*Peromyscus maniculatus*): Chemical discrimination among individual mice. *Herpetologica* 47:69–78.

Gartner, G. E. A., and H. W. Greene. 2008. Adaptation in the African egg-eating snake: A comparative approach to a classic study in evolutionary functional morphology. *Journal of Zoology* 275:368–374.

Greenbaum, E., N. Galeva, and M. Jorgensen. 2003. Venom variation and chemoreception of the viperid *Agkistrodon contortrix*: Evidence for adaptation. *Journal of Chemical Ecology* 29:1741–1755.

Greene, H. W. 1983. Field studies of hunting behavior by bushmasters. *American Zoologist* 23:897.

Greene, H. W., and G. M. Burghardt. 1978. Behavior and phylogeny: Constriction in ancient and modern snakes. *Science* 200:74–77.

Hayes, W. K. 2008. The snake venom-metering controversy: Levels of analysis, assumptions, and evidence. In W. K. Hayes, K. R. Beaman, M. D. Cardwell, and S. P. Bush (eds.), *The Biology of Rattlesnakes*. Loma Linda, CA: Loma Linda University Press, pp. 191–220.

Hayes, W. K., S. S. Herbert, J. R. Harrison, and K. L. Wiley. 2008. Spitting versus biting: Differential venom gland contraction regulates venom expenditure in the Black-Necked Spitting Cobra, *Naja nigricollis nigricollis*. *Journal of Herpetology* 42:453–460.

Herbert, S. S., and W. K. Hayes. 2008. Venom expenditure by rattlesnakes and killing effectiveness in rodent prey: Do rattlesnakes expend optimal amounts of venom? In W. K. Hayes, K. R. Beaman, M. D. Cardwell, and S. P. Bush (eds.), *The Biology of Rattlesnakes*. Loma Linda, CA: Loma Linda University Press, pp. 221–228.

Jackson, K. 2003. The evolution of venom-delivery systems in snakes. *Zoological Journal of the Linnean Society* 137:337–354.

Jackson, K., N. J. Kley, and E. L. Brainerd. 2004. How snakes eat snakes: The biomechanical challenges of ophiophagy for the California King Snake, *Lampropeltis getula californiae* (Serpentes: Colubridae). *Zoology* 107:191–200.

Janoo, A., and J.-P. Gasc. 1992. High speed motion analysis of the predatory strike and fluorographic study of oesophageal deglutition in *Vipera ammodytes*: More than meets the eye. *Amphibia-Reptilia* 13:315–325.

Jansa, S. A., and R. S. Voss. 2011. Adaptive evolution of the venom-targeted vWF protein in opossums that eat pitvipers. *PLoS ONE* 6:e20997.doi:10.1371/journal.pone.0020997.

Jayne, B. C., H. K. Voris, and P. K. L. Ng. 2002. Snake circumvents constraints on prey size. *Nature* 418:143.

Kardong, K. V. 1974. Kinesis of the jaw apparatus during the strike in the cottonmouth snake, *Agkistrodon piscivorus*. *Forma et Functio* 7:327–354.

Kardong, K. V., and V. Bels. 1998. Rattlesnake strike behavior: Kinematics. *Journal of Experimental Biology* 210:837–850.

Kardong, K. V., and H. Berkhoudt. 1998. Intraoral transport of prey in the reticulated python: Tests of a general tetrapod feeding model. *Zoology* 101:7–23.

Kardong, K. V., P. Dullemeijer, and J. A. M. Fransen. 1986. Feeding mechanism in the rattlesnake, *Crotalus durissus*. *Amphibia-Reptilia* 7:271–302.

Kardong, K. V., and J. E. Haverly. 1993. Drinking by the common boa, *Boa constrictor*. *Copeia* 1993:808–818.

Kardong, K. V., and T. L. Smith. 2002. Proximate factors involved in rattlesnake predatory behavior: A review. In G. W. Schuett, M. Höggren, M. E. Douglas, and H. W. Greene (eds.), *Biology of the Vipers*. Eagle Mountain, UT: Eagle Mountain Publishing, pp. 253–266.

Kley, N. J., and E. L. Brainerd. 1999. Feeding by mandibular raking in a snake. *Nature* 402:369–370.

Kley, N. J., and E. L. Brainerd. 2002. Post-cranial prey transport mechanisms in the black pinesnake, *Pituophis melanoleucus lodingi*: An x-ray videographic study. *Zoology* 105:153–164.

Lahav, S., and R. Dmi'el. 1996. Skin resistance to water loss in colubrid snakes: Ecological and taxonomic correlations. *Ecoscience* 3:135–139.

Lavin-Murcio, P., B. G. Robinson, and K. V. Kardong. 1993. Cues involved in relocation of struck prey by rattlesnakes, *Crotalus viridis oreganus*. *Herpetologica* 49:463–469.

Lillywhite, H. B. 2006. Water relations of tetrapod integument. *Journal of Experimental Biology* 209:202–226.

Lillywhite, H. B., L. S. Babonis, C. M. Sheehy III, and M.-C. Tu. 2008. Sea snakes (*Laticauda* spp.) require fresh drinking water: Implication for the distribution and persistence of populations. *Physiological and Biochemical Zoology* 81:785–796.

Lillywhite, H. B., F. Brischoux, C. M. Sheehy III, and J. B. Pfaller. 2012. Dehydration and drinking responses in a pelagic sea snake. *Integrative and Comparative Biology* 52:227–234.

Lillywhite, H. B., P. de Delva, and B. P. Noonan. 2002. Patterns of gut passage time and the chronic retention of fecal mass in viperid snakes. In G. W. Schuett, M. Höggren, M. E. Douglas, and H. W. Greene (eds.), *Biology of the Vipers*. Eagle Mountain, UT: Eagle Mountain Publishing, pp. 497–506.

Lillywhite, H. B., J. G. Menon, G. K. Menon, C. M. Sheehy III, and M.-C. Tu. 2009. Water exchange and permeability properties of the skin in three species of amphibious sea snakes (*Laticauda* spp.). *Journal of Experimental Biology* 212:1921–1929.

Mackessy, S. P., and L. M. Baxter. 2006. Bioweapons synthesis and storage: The venom gland of front-fanged snakes. *Zoologischer Anzeiger* 245:147–159.

McCue, M. D. 2005. Enzyme activities and biological functions of snake venoms. *Applied Herpetology* 2:109–123.

McCue, M. D. 2007. Prey envenomation does not improve digestive performance in Western Diamondback Rattlesnakes (*Crotalus atrox*). *Journal of Experimental Zoology* 307A:568–577.

McCue, M. D. 2007. Western Diamondback Rattlesnakes demonstrate physiological and biochemical strategies for tolerating prolonged starvation. *Physiological and Biochemical Zoology* 80:25–34.

McCue, M. D., and H. B. Lillywhite. 2002. Oxygen consumption and the energetics of island-dwelling Florida Cottonmouth snakes. *Physiological and Biochemical Zoology* 75:165–178.

McCue, M. D., H. B. Lillywhite, and S. J. Beaupre. 2012. Physiological responses to starvation in snakes: Low energy specialists. In M. D. McCue (ed.), *Comparative Physiology of Fasting, Starvation, and Food Limitation*. Berlin: Springer-Verlag, pp. 103–131.

Mori, A., H. Ota, and N. Kamezaki. 1999. Foraging on sea turtle nesting beaches: Flexible foraging tactics by *Dinodon semicarinatum* (Serpentes: Colubridae). In H. Ota (ed.), *Tropical Island Herpetofauna: Origin, Current Diversity, and Conservation*. New York: Elsevier Science, pp. 99–128.

Pahari, S., S. P. Mackessy, and R. M. Kini. 2007. The venom gland transcriptome of the Desert Massasauga Rattlesnake (*Sistrurus catenatus edwardsii*): Towards an understanding of venom composition among advanced snakes (superfamily Colubroidea). *BMC Molecular Biology* 8:115.

Pope, C. H. 1958. Fatal bite of captive African rear-fanged snake (*Dispholidus*). *Copeia* 1958:280–282.

Porter, W. P., and C. R. Tracy. 1974. Modeling the effects of temperature changes on the ecology of the garter snake and leopard frog. In J. W. Gibbons and R. R. Sharitz (eds.), *Thermal Ecology Symposium*. AEC Symp. Ser. Conf-739505, Oak Ridge, pp. 594–609.

Pough, F. H., and J. D. Groves. 1983. Specializations of the body form and food habits of snakes. *American Zoologist* 23:443–454.

Reinert, H. K., D. Cundall, and L. M. Bushar. 1987. Foraging behavior of the timber rattlesnake, *Crotalus horridus*. *Copeia* 1984:976–981.

Rodriguez-Robles, J. A., C. J. Bell, and H. W. Greene. 1999. Gape size and evolution of diet in snakes: Feeding ecology of erycine boas. *Journal of Zoology* (London) 248:49–58.

Roberts, J. B., and H. B. Lillywhite. 1980. Lipid barrier to water exchange in reptile epidermis. *Science* 207:1077–1079.

Roberts, J. B., and H. B. Lillywhite. 1983. Lipids and the permeability of epidermis from snakes. *Journal of Experimental Zoology* 228:1–9.

Schuett, G. W., D. L. Hardy Sr., R. L. Earley, and H. W. Greene. 2005. Does prey size induce head skeleton phenotypic plasticity during early ontogeny in the snake Boa constrictor? *Journal of Zoology* (London) 267:363–369.

Secor, S. M. 1995. Ecological aspects of foraging mode for the snakes *Crotalus cerastes* and *Masticophis flagellum*. *Herpetological Monographs* 9:169–186.

Secor, S. M. 2003. Gastric function and its contribution to the postprandial metabolic response of the Burmese python *Python molurus*. *Journal of Experimental Biology* 206:1621–1630.

Secor, S. M. 2009. Specific dynamic action: A review of the postprandial metabolic response. *Journal of Comparative Physiology* B 179:1–56.

Secor, S. M., and J. M. Diamond. 1995. Adaptive responses to feeding in Burmese Pythons: Pay before pumping. *Journal of Experimental Biology* 198:1313–1325.

Secor, S. M., and J. M. Diamond. 1998. A vertebrate model of extreme physiological regulation. *Nature* 395:659–662.

Secor, S. M., and J. M. Diamond. 2000. Evolution of regulatory responses to feeding in snakes. *Physiological and Biochemical Zoology* 73:123–141.

Secor, S. M., and K. A. Nagy. 1994. Energetic correlates of foraging mode for the snakes *Crotalus cerastes* and *Masticophis flagellum*. *Ecology* 75:1600–1614.

Shine, R. 1980. Ecology of the Australian death adder *Acanthophis antarcticus* (Elapidae): Evidence for convergence with the Viperidae. *Herpetologica* 36:281–289.

Smith, T. L., G. D. E. Povel, and K. V. Kardong. 2002. Predatory strike of the tentacle snake (*Erpeton tentaculatum*). *Journal of Zoology*, London 256:233–242.

Taub, A. M. 1967. Comparative histological studies of Duvernoy's gland of colubrid snakes. *Bulletin of the American Museum of Natural History* 138:1–50.

Taylor, E. N., M. A. Malawy, D. M. Browning, S. V. Lemar, and D. F. DeNardo. 2005. Effects of food supplementation on the physiological ecology of female Western diamond-backed rattlesnakes (*Crotalus atrox*). *Oecologia* 144:206–213.

Tu, M.-C., H. B. Lillywhite, J. G. Menon, and G. K. Menon. 2002. Postnatal ecdysis establishes the permeability barrier in snake skin: New insights into lipid barrier structures. *Journal of Experimental Biology* 205:3019–3030.

Vidal, N. 2002. Colubroid systematics: Evidence for an early appearance of the venom apparatus followed by extensive evolutionary tinkering. *Journal of Toxicology, Toxin Reviews* 21:21–41.

Vincent, S. E., A. Herrel, and D. J. Irschick. 2004. Ontogeny of intersexual head shape and prey selection in the pitviper *Agkistrodon piscivorus*. *Biological Journal of the Linnean Society* 81:151–159.

Vincent, S. E., A. Herrel, and D. J. Irschick. 2005. Comparisons of aquatic versus terrestrial predatory strikes in the pitviper, *Agkistrodon piscivorus*. *Journal of Experimental Zoology* 303A: 476–488.

Young, B. A., A. Aguiar, and H. B. Lillywhite. 2008. Foraging cues used by insular Florida Cottonmouths, *Agkistrodon piscivorus conanti*. *South American Journal of Herpetology* 3:135–144.

Young, B. A., K. Dunlap, K. Koenig, and M. Singer. 2004. The buccal buckle: The functional morphology of venom spitting in cobras. *Journal of Experimental Biology* 207:3483–3494.

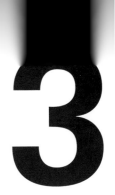

LOCOMOTION: HOW SNAKES MOVE

There has been much conjecture about the methods of locomotion of serpents. The speed, strength and agility of many species appears astonishing. . . . Here is true specialization, presenting a group of creatures which have lost their limbs yet acquired remarkable dexterity with apparently little effort, through no visible means.

—*Raymond L. Ditmars,* Snakes of the World *(1943), p. 16*

Limbless Movement

One of the truly remarkable attributes of snakes is how well these limbless animals move through a variety of landscapes—over, through, or around features of their highly varied habitats. Snakes swim, dive, move rapidly through bushes or across rocks, crawl across featureless sand terrain, climb vertically up trees where they move swiftly through canopy, and, in some species, catapult from great heights and glide through the air to land without harm on the ground below. Even the more usual or common movements over terrestrial landscapes can be extraordinary in their appearances. I recall vividly on several occasions while looking for snakes that might be crossing country roads, when a large, dark-colored snake such as a Southern Black Racer or Southern Pacific Rattlesnake moved on pavement and progressed without interruption to cross to the other side. In many such cases the snake's movement conjured the image of black oil pouring onto the road and flowing, seemingly frictionless, across the road surface. A similar scene was witnessed on numerous occasions while driving slowly and looking for snakes during the evening on paved roads in the California desert. Sidewinder Rattlesnakes, appearing white when illuminated by the headlights of an automobile, appeared to glide across the road as they were watched from a distance. On other snake hunts, off-road, I recall hearing countless "swishes" in dry, summer grasses as racers or whipsnakes moved off rapidly in advance of my walking, never to be seen as they disappeared into the drying vegetation. I was only aware of their presence because of the sounds that were created by undulating, slender bodies moving through stems and leaves of the summer grasses. Once at a beach near Naples, Florida, I heard a distinct sound resembling a low-pitched whirring noise as a magnificent large Eastern Coachwhip snake undulated across damp sand to escape into nearby vegetation. I was surprised, and simultaneously delighted, by the sound that was produced when the belly scales of the snake met the damp sand of the beach. Of course, occasional captures or sightings of snakes confirmed the meaning of these particular sounds, which are available to anyone who is alert to his or her surroundings while enjoying a summer walk.

The more one thinks about how snakes move, and their ability to move rapidly and gracefully over many surfaces, the more we are in awe at the amazing, swift, and seemingly effortless locomotion of snakes when moving without limbs. How do snakes perform the amazing and impressive feats that anyone can witness in the appropriate circumstances? Obviously, we need to learn more about the structure of the snake's body, especially the skeletal elements and their attached muscles with overlying skin.

Muscle and Skeletal Adaptations

The body of a snake is elongated and limbless, and these conditions have evolved many times in various vertebrate lineages—for example fishes, salamanders, and lizards. Snakes, however, exhibit marvelous variation and seeming perfection of these attributes. To simplify matters, one might consider a snake to be a simple tube with elongated organs inside, separated by numerous supporting bones with muscles to move them and a tough but pliable skin covering the outside (figs. 2.2, 6.9, 6.12). Relative to standing quadrupedal vertebrates, snakes have a low center of mass that is close to the ground. The limbless body presents a large area of frictional contact with the ground (but see below), and the mass of the snake is distributed over an extended area, rather than two or four points of contact that are associated with feet, as in mammals.

One obvious problem with elongating the body is the internal organs must be adjusted, reshaped, and reorganized to fit into the narrow body without sacrificing mobility. Thus, many of the internal organs of snakes are elongate in comparison with those of less attenuated animals (fig. 2.2). This condition is especially true for the lung, liver, the kidneys, and the testes. The heart is also elongated and comparatively slender in arboreal species of snakes, many of which are exceptionally thin.

In most snakes the internal organs are contained within an elongated body cavity that is surrounded by skeletal elements above and on both sides. These skeletal elements consist of vertebrae and attached ribs. The latter in most cases are curved outward and downward, with their free ends positioned at or near the ventrolateral edges of the snake just above the ground (fig. 1.3). The belly plates are underlain within the snake by connective tissue and muscle, so the ribs and vertebral column surround the internal organs except for the ventral aspect of the animal. In many terrestrial snakes the ventral boundary of the internal body cavity is relatively wide, but in some other groups, for example, sea snakes, the body is considerably compressed in the vertical plane for swimming and the tips of the ribs on each side of the body lie relatively closer together (figs. 3.1, 5.7). In any event, the evolutionary elongation of a limbless body has resulted in an extended vertebral column with many well-developed vertebrae. Humans, for example, have 12 vertebrae articulating with ribs that enclose the thoracic cavity, and these elements are absent from much of the body length (if the legs are included). Many species of fish typically have 30 to 60 vertebrae, including the body and the tail. In contrast, snakes usually have more than 100 vertebrae in the body alone, and some species have more than 400 vertebrae extending from the neck to near the tip of the tail. As a result, snakes are extremely flexible. Ribs are distributed along the length of the body, but not the tail (fig. 1.3).

The number of vertebrae possessed by a snake is related to its maximum length, and it therefore appears that the number of vertebrae has evolved in response to selection on body size. Studies by Lars Lindell also show, however, that the number of vertebrae can be related to behavior and ecology, apart from being affected by body size. For example, constricting species have more vertebrae per unit of size than do nonconstricting species, and burrowing species tend to have fewer vertebrae per unit of size than do species that occupy other habitats. The number of vertebrae

can also affect the locomotion of snakes. Snakes with more vertebrae are generally slower than those having fewer.

All movements of snakes are dependent on the interactions between the elongate skeleton and the muscles that attach to them. A common feature that is present in most (but not all) patterns of snake locomotion is that vertebral bending is used in various ways to generate propulsive forces. Commonly, undulating forms of locomotion depend on waves of lateral bending that are propagated from head to tail. The vertebrae of snakes have many accessory elements that resist torsion, and the various parts are aligned such that lateral bending is generally easier than is bending in the dorsal-to-ventral plane. Exceptions are the ability of the neck to bend during displays of the well-known "hood" of cobras (fig. 1.39), and the prehensile tails of various arboreal species such as rat snakes, vine snakes, and many boas (fig. 2.20).

Many aquatic and fast-moving terrestrial species of snakes possess vertebrae with articulating parts called *zygapophyses* that are prominently broad with lateral extension (fig. 3.2). Presumably, this increases the effectiveness of the lever systems involved with muscles that flex the vertebral column laterally. In these snakes the articulating surfaces also tend to be relatively small, and the vertebrae tend to be long and narrow. In arboreal species of snakes, the structure of the zygapophyses provides a bony shelf on which attachments of muscles can act to lock the otherwise flexible vertebral column into a rigid beam to facilitate the snake extending the unsupported body considerable distances when it climbs from one branch of a tree to another.

The axial musculature of snakes is extremely complex with many muscles and tendons that have origins and insertions at various locations with respect to the axial skeleton (fig. 3.3). Collectively, these muscles have segments that form longitudinal columns and span many ribs. If one thinks about it, the central nervous system of a snake must do an amazing job of integrating information about the landscape across which it moves, and simultaneously activate the requisite muscles in an appropriate pattern all along the length of the body. For long-bodied species, especially, this requires superb neural control to ensure that the appropriate muscles are activated with precise timing at variable distances from the brain, which serves as a "command center."

Various muscles act as coherent units. For example, the *spinalis-semispinalis*, *longissimus dorsi*, and *iliocostalis* consist of overlapping segments that form longitudinal columns (fig. 3.3). These are *epaxial* muscles and have been shown to be activated to provide most of the power and control that are required for the undulatory movements of snakes. The various muscle actions cause bending of the body and also stabilize the ribs against pulling when the

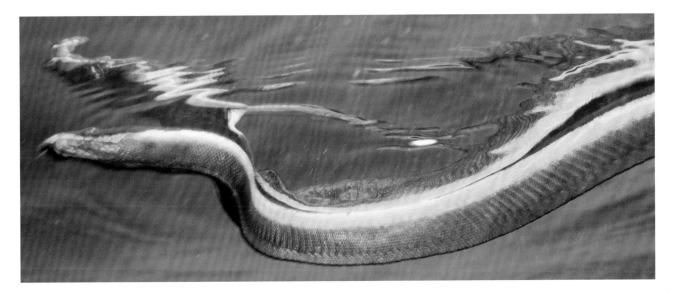

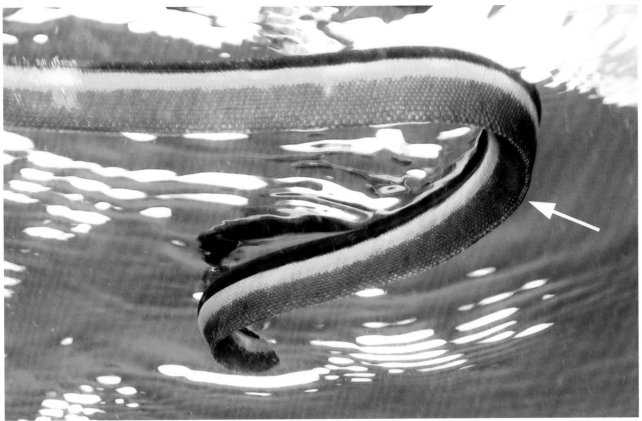

Figure 3.1. Underwater views of the Yellow-bellied Sea Snake (*Pelamis platurus*) illustrating the vertically flattened body when the snake is swimming or floating in the ocean. Individual ribs can be seen in the **upper photo**, and the absence of broad ventral scutes can be seen in the **lower photo** (arrow). The skin below the ribs is flattened into a ventral body keel. These snakes were photographed in Costa Rica by Joseph Pfaller.

body bends laterally. Some of the axial muscles extend over large numbers of vertebrae, and elongated tendons form connections between these muscles (fig. 3.3). In fast-moving species, the distances spanned by some muscle-tendon chains extend over 40 consecutive ribs (or vertebral units), whereas in slower species the same muscle units may span fewer than 9 vertebral units. Relatively short muscle units are thought to facilitate the force of constriction, which tends to be associated with slower-moving snakes. Constrictors are relatively less "stiff" and have greater flexibility than many faster-moving snakes. The evolution of vertebral number and, in some cases shorter muscle segments, seems to account in part for this difference. In contrast, the longer muscle-tendon units characteristic of the faster snakes

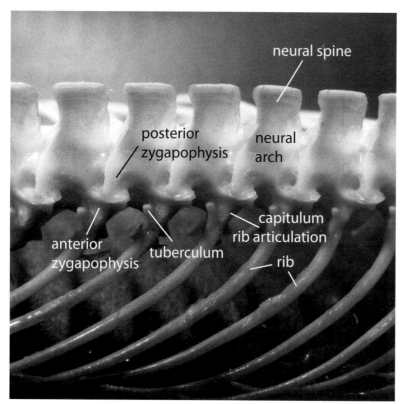

Figure 3.2. A segment of the vertebral column of a Cottonmouth snake (*Agkistrodon piscivorus*) showing several vertebrae with articulating ribs. The head of each rib (*capitulum*) articulates with a single vertebra. The *zygapophyses* provide surfaces for articulation between successive neural arches, allowing some degree of horizontal (and lesser vertical) movement but preventing undue torsion. Skeleton courtesy of the Florida Museum of Natural History and photographed by the author.

might enable a snake to utilize longer undulations, theoretically with more efficient use of power due to having fewer points of force application and dissipation of energy in overcoming lateral resistance (see below). A point of force application (from snake to a physical feature in the environment) is called a *resistance site* (fig. 3.4). Elongated tendons add length to a contractile unit while minimizing the muscle involved, which has greater mass. Generally, studies have demonstrated that much of the variation in segmental length of the locomotor muscles is related to habitat, body form, and the manner of movement (see below).

Locomotion: How Do Snakes Move?

A simple game that one can engage to illustrate the amazing locomotor adaptations of snakes is to lie on the floor with arms held straight back against the side of the body and, while holding this position, try to move forward without using arms, hands, or feet. This sounds simple and probably silly, but after some while during serious attempts at moving without the use of arms or legs, one begins to realize that appropriate forces are necessary and missing due

to the inadequate structure and function of the human skeleton and the muscles attached to it. Similarly, one can also try this in water. Again, after a short time making serious attempts to glide forward like a snake, one appreciates the fact that the human body, while capable of bending at the waist, is not designed for effective undulating movements that are capable of creating forward propulsion in water. But we are limbed creatures, so we swim using our arms and legs. Following these simple and entertaining games, watch a snake carefully as it moves, and think about the amazing movements you see in context of the features that are described in this chapter.

Aquatic Locomotion: Swimming in Water

All living aquatic reptiles—including crocodilians, turtles, and lizards, as well as snakes—are secondary swimmers, insofar as these aquatic species evolved from terrestrial ancestors. Interestingly, all snakes can swim—some better than others—and all species have the ability to undulate in water, usually with the head held up while floating due to inflation of the elongated lung. Sometimes, the conscious and purposeful aquatic tendencies of snakes are surprising. For example, Eastern Diamondback Rattlesnakes, *Crotalus adamanteus*, often enter marine waters voluntarily, and they are regularly sighted as they swim between islands in the coastal waters of Florida. Indeed, some of the more plentiful, remaining populations of this species are on the coastal keys of Florida's Gulf coast or the East coast intracoastal waterway. Some rattlesnakes have been sighted more than 10 miles from shore in the Gulf of Mexico. In Southern California, Red Diamond Rattlesnakes, *Crotalus ruber*, are occasionally washed down rivers during periods of high rainfall. Subsequently, they can be seen swimming in offshore ocean waters or crawling onto beaches. Unlike rattlesnakes in the eastern United States, however, these are not likely to be in the ocean water out of choice.

All aquatic snakes swim by movements called *undulation*, regardless of the type of locomotion their terrestrial relatives might have used on land. This is the most ubiquitous form of swimming and occurs in representatives from all classes of vertebrates except birds. Snakes undulate with lateral movements, in contrast with specialized marine

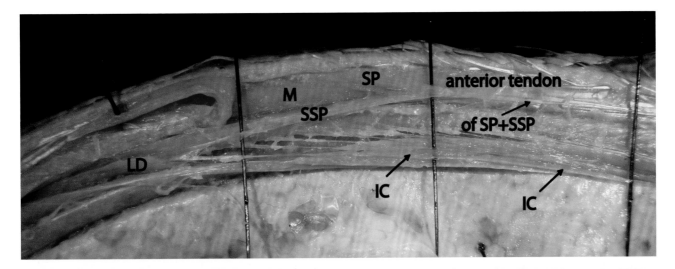

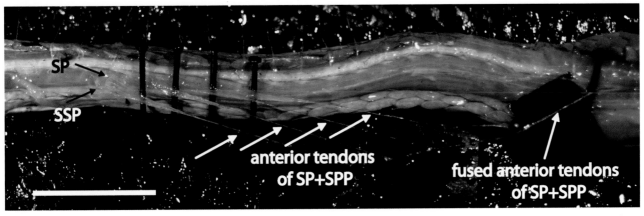

Figure 3.3. Axial muscles of snakes, used in locomotion. The **upper** photograph illustrates a dissection of the axial muscles in a preserved rat snake (*Pantherophis obsoletus*). The **lower** photograph illustrates fine dissection of a preserved *Ahaetulla prasina*, illustrating fused and elongate tendons (arrows) associated with the anterior *spinalis semispinalis* muscles. Note the individual muscle units associated with each tendon to the left of each respective element in the figure. This illustrates an unusual morphology located in the trunk near the head, and is not typical. The scale bar at the lower left of this photograph equals 1 cm. Abbreviations: IC, *iliocostalis*; LD, *longissimus dorsi*; M, *multifidus*; SP, *spinalis*; SSP, *semispinalis*. Dissections and photographs by Phil Nicodemo.

mammals, which undulate in a vertical plane. Undulatory locomotion can be illustrated by the swimming movements of a sea snake. In smooth propulsive movements, the body is bent into a wave that travels backward along the body (fig. 3.5). Each body segment moves from side to side as successive waves move from head to tail. As each undulating wave travels backward, water is accelerated to the side and toward the rear by the rear-facing segment of the body, which produces a propulsive force by pushing against the water. Almost immediately the water is acted on by the next propulsive segment of the wave.

The amplitude of lateral movements and the tendency for undulating body segments to act more directly backward (opposite to forward movement) with propulsive force against the water tend to increase toward the tail. That is, the angle of the body relative to the overall direction of swimming tends to increase and thereby accelerate the water rearward. Eventually, after being influenced by all the propulsive

segments of the entire body, water is "discharged" into a wake beyond the tip of the tail or body (fig. 3.5). These aspects of the locomotion may not be obvious to a casual observer who watches a snake swim rapidly across a pond or a stream.

The swimming behavior of Yellow-bellied Sea Snakes (*Pelamis platurus*) has been studied by a team of investigators led by Jeffrey Graham at the Scripps Institution of Oceanography. The swimming movements are very much like that of an eel (termed *anguilliform* swimming). During near-surface swimming there are four half-waves present along the body having amplitudes that increase toward the tail. Routine swimming velocities ranged up to 20 cm/s when snakes were near or at the surface, while swimming velocities were lower at 1–8 cm/s when snakes swam below the surface. During subsurface swimming the snake typically assumes a posture in which the tail is elevated—also characteristic of other sea snakes—and the posterior part of

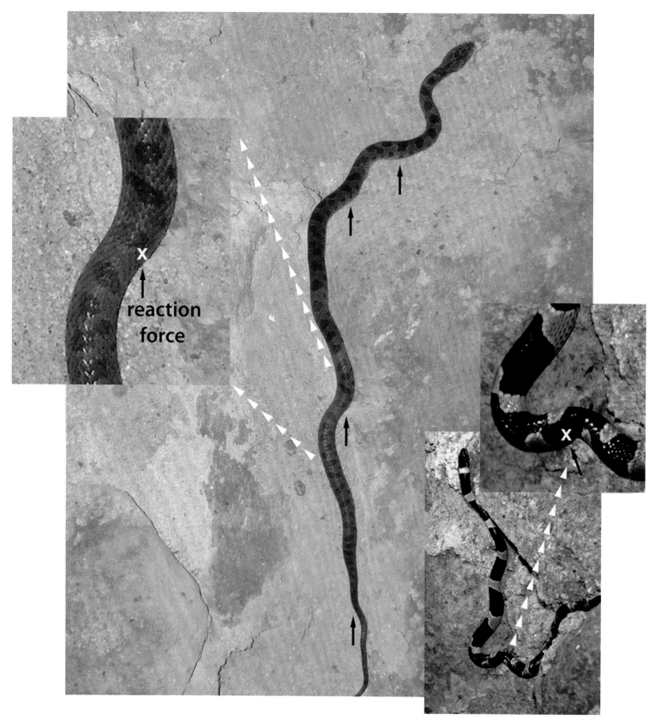

Figure 3.4. A Cat-eyed Snake (*Leptodeira annulata*) crawling vertically up a rock face in Guanacaste, Costa Rica. Points of force application, called *resistance sites*, are indicated by the solid black arrows. These are places where a physical irregularity in the rock surface provides a "catch" where the snake's body pushes and creates propulsive force as an undulation passes the point. The summed reaction forces at these points provide the force vector that moves the snake forward, or upward, on the rock face. The resistance site near the center of the photograph is shown with enlargement to its **left**. The white "x" indicates the point where the body is pushing maximally against the resistance site. Notice how the snake's body is "tightened" at this point to exert force against the rock. At the **lower right** a second snake (*Leptodeira nigrofasciata*) is shown crawling up a rock face. Here a prominent resistance site (x and arrow) is illustrated where there is a distinct projection on the rock face. This feature is shown with magnification in the projected enlargement (follow broken white arrowheads). Snakes were photographed in Guanacaste, Costa Rica: *L. annulata* by Coleman Sheehy III; *L. nigrofasciata* by Shauna Lillywhite.

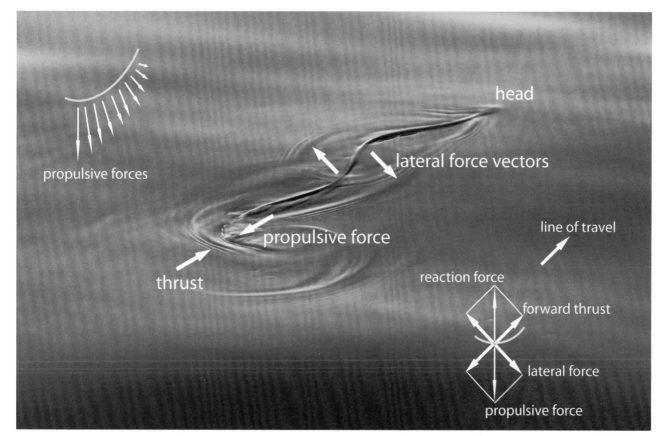

Figure 3.5. A swimming Yellow-bellied Sea Snake (*Pelamis platurus*) near the Guanacaste coast of Costa Rica illustrates the forces that contribute to its movement through water. The muscles of the snake create waves of undulation that move backward along the body, progressing from the neck to the paddle-shaped tail. Each undulating wave presses against the water to produce a *propulsive force*. The water in turn creates a *reaction force*, which acts in the opposite direction and produces forward *thrust*. The directions of the propulsive forces generated by a hypothetical body segment (yellow) are indicated by arrows at the left, including component vectors that act laterally or sideways at right angles to the direction of movement. The magnitude of each force is indicated by the length of the respective arrow. The collective forces act more or less equally on each side of the body as waves progress from the head to tail. Therefore, the lateral force vectors cancel and add nothing to the thrust that moves the snake forward. The vector components are further illustrated in the lower diagram to the right of the snake, where the edge of a body segment is represented by the yellow curved line. Similarly, at the left-hand side of the snake one sees that both the direction and magnitude of the propulsive forces change in relation to the curvature of the body, again represented by the yellow curved line. Only a single force vector is illustrated in more detail to the right of the snake. The wavelets that are evident in the water adjacent to the snake are produced by the undulating waves of the snake's body pushing against the water. Note that these are greater and broader near the tail end of the snake, where the larger components of thrust are produced by the tail, which can be seen in this photo to be "pushing" more in the backward direction than sideward against the water. Photograph and labeling by the author.

the body assumes a nearly vertical orientation. Swimming in this posture involves torsional and rolling motions rather than simple undulations, and these may contribute to thrust. Swimming speeds measured in other species of both laticaudine and hydrophiine sea snakes by Richard Shine and his coworkers range between mean values of 23 and 141 cm/s, with males swimming faster than females. Amphibious sea snakes swim faster in water than they crawl when they are on land.

Thrust is the forward-acting force on the animal and equals the sum of all contributions of the propulsive segments (imagine the length of the snake being divided up into as many segments as you like, each interacting against the surrounding water at variable angles). The various propulsive

segments do not contribute equally to thrust. The more posterior body segments move with greater amplitude; hence, the posterior parts of the body move faster through greater distances and "push" against the water with vectors of propulsive force that act more directly toward the tail. Therefore, the greater forces are more nearly aligned with the direction of movement. This principle is illustrated in fig. 3.5.

The propulsive force depends on the mass of the water affected by each propulsive segment, which depends, in turn, on body shape. The depth, or width, of the body increases the propulsive force. Because the more posterior parts of the body contribute more to thrust, forces are maximized when the greatest depth of the body is posterior. This is precisely the way the body is designed in many of the fully aquatic sea snakes (fig. 3.6). However, there are nearly always exceptions to general rules in nature, and the Yellow-bellied Sea Snake (*Pelamis platurus*) undulates its body to move backward as well as forward. This species is pelagic and spends time floating on the surface of the sea, waiting to capture fishes that attempt to hide beneath objects including the snake. Swimming backward seems to be a maneuvering strategy, which might explain the more uniform body shape that characterizes this species (fig. 1.44).

The swimming performance of an aquatic animal depends not only on thrust propelling it forward, but also on overcoming forces that resist the forward motion. Such forces are, collectively or individually, referred to as *resistance*. The origins of resistance are complex but can be divided into several components. First is an *inertial* component due to mass of the animal and the enveloping water around it. The inertial force predominates when an animal has large size and relatively low velocity. Second is a *drag force* attributable to viscosity of the water, which is equivalent to friction. Third is a *vertical force* attributable to gravity. If an animal is negatively

buoyant, or has a tendency to sink in water, this decreases the total resistance when an animal is swimming toward the bottom, and, conversely, it increases the resistance when the swimming is toward the surface. Fourth, if an animal is turning, *centrifugal acceleration* adds to the resistance. This force acts at right angles to the forces resisting forward movement. The relative magnitudes of the resistance forces vary with the type of swimming. When inertial forces dominate drag forces, then an object will usually continue to move for a considerable distance after it stops producing thrust, as occurs when boats shut off their engines.

Of the forces mentioned, the drag force is the most complex. It arises primarily from viscous effects in the *boundary layer*, which refers to a thin film of water that immediately surrounds the moving snake. In physical terms, the boundary layer is the region of water adjacent to the animal's surface where the velocity of water relative to the snake decreases from near zero (at the body surface) to that of surrounding, undisturbed water (called the "free stream" velocity) with increasing distance away from the snake (fig. 3.7). In other words, there is a gradient of velocity extending outward in water away from the snake's surface. Energy is dissipated in shearing forces that resist a distortion of the adjacent "layers" of water. Stated another way, there is frictional dissipation of energy as adjacent layers of water try to "slide" past each other. Here friction is related to the "stickiness" of fluid in the adjacent interacting layers of water. (In this description the reader must imagine a layer of water to consist of a three-dimension sheet, which includes all the water of a particular velocity and extends as a continuous envelope around the snake. The next adjacent sheet, or layer, moves at a slightly different velocity, as long as one is within the boundary layer, and so on.)

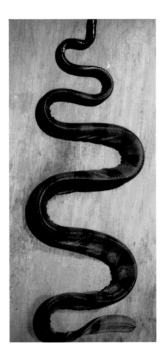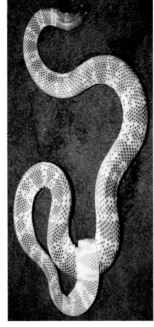

Figure 3.6. A Black-headed Sea Snake (*Hydrophis melanocephalus*) photographed on a board to illustrate the overall body morphology (**left**). Note that the body increases in depth toward its posterior end where the tail terminates in a broad "paddle." The smaller head and neck are related to feeding habits that involve probing the head into small holes or crevices in the sea floor or coral. This specimen was photographed at Heron Island on the Great Barrier Reef of Australia. The snake on the **right** is another species of *Hydrophis* (*H. elegans*) collected near Weipa on the Gulf of Carpentaria. The two snakes illustrate variability in the body form of these related species. Not all sea snakes exhibit the extreme morphology of *H. melanocephalus*, which is used here simply to illustrate some of the features that are discussed in the text. Photographs by the author.

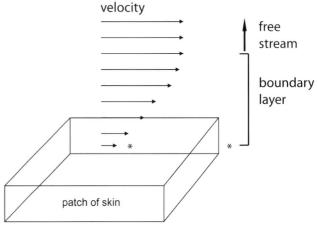

Figure 3.7. Illustration of a boundary layer of fluid next to a hypothetical patch of skin. The length of the horizontal arrows represents the velocity of the fluid, which increases with distance away from the skin surface (*). The boundary layer ends where the velocity becomes constant with further distance, which is called the "free stream." Drawing by the author.

The magnitude of the drag force depends on the frictional properties of skin, the area that is in contact with water, and how the boundary layer interacts with the rest of the flow around the animal. During high rates of acceleration, the boundary layer gradually increases in thickness. Initially, although acceleration is high, the speed or actual velocity of movement is low. Therefore, the frictional drag is small during fast starts, and the resistance to movement is dominated largely by inertial forces. This can be very important, as we will see in the following discussion.

With respect to periodic or intermittent (stop-and-go) swimming, it is advantageous for the propulsive segments to maximize thrust. Because the frictional drag is relatively small during accelerations, a propulsive segment with large area has a relatively small penalty in terms of drag. The principal source of resistance for intermittent swimming is the mass of the system, or more correctly the nonmuscular "dead weight." Adaptations of morphology that reduce the dead weight and increase the proportion of body represented by force-producing muscle increase the capacity for acceleration. On the other hand, drag increases with the square of swimming speed and is the principle source of resistance for prolonged or sustained swimming at moderate speeds.

Both thrust and the theoretical "efficiency" of locomotion can vary with the speed of swimming. Insofar as drag increases with swimming speed, thrust must also be increased to enable forward movement. This increase in thrust is achieved by an increase in either the frequency or the amplitude of undulations, or both. In a recent study of swimming in sea kraits (Laticauda spp.), a team of investigators led by François Brischoux attached accelerometers to snakes and determined that swimming speed was related to a combination of increase in frequency and amplitude of the sway undulations produced by the swimming muscles. These observations confirmed previous studies that were based more strictly on analysis of motion. These and previous data also confirm that the amplitude of the body undulation increases progressively from head to tail, which implies that the speed of propagation of the propulsive wave also increases from head to tail.

The various factors affecting thrust and the resistance to motion during acceleration and turning can be summarized in terms of a hypothetical optimal morphology, which can be defined to maximize performance. These features are, first, a relatively large body with area of body increasing toward the tail. A second important feature is an appropriately flexible body so that the amplitude of swimming undulations can be maximized. This is also a property of swimming snakes. A third feature is a large ratio of muscle mass relative to body mass. *Power* is proportional to the volume (more strictly, cross-sectional area) of muscle, whereas drag is proportional to the area of the object that interacts with water. Therefore, power increases relative to drag if the body

mass consists largely of muscle. These combined features appear to be present in the body design of a number of sea snakes, illustrated by *Hydrophis* spp. (fig. 3.6). Considering all species of snakes, however, some experts will realize there are exceptions to these generalizations.

Sea snakes tend to flatten the entire body medially or vertically (midsaggital or vertical plane) when swimming, which enlarges the area of contact with water to produce thrust (fig. 3.1). Such vertical flattening also is characteristic of the extremely supple-bodied file snakes (*Acrochordus* spp.) as well as some highly aquatic colubrid snakes while swimming. Some aquatic species also flatten the skin below the tips of the ribs to produce a ventral body keel (e.g., *Pelamis platurus*, figs. 3.1, 5.7). Moreover, the tail of sea snakes is laterally flattened into a paddle-like structure that comprises most of the tissue posterior to the vent (fig. 3.8). Presumably, this feature increases the capacity for posterior thrust when swimming, and more powerful swimmers have larger "paddles" with greater area in the vertical plane, in addition to greater muscle mass (fig. 3.8). Recent studies by Kate Sanders and her colleagues have demonstrated that the fully aquatic hydrophiine sea snakes have evolved specialized extensions of the caudal vertebrae that help to support the laterally compressed tail in these marine species. Considering this principle in broader terms, one may note that evolutionary shifts from terrestrial to aquatic habitats has produced laterally compressed "paddles" on the feet, fins, or tails of a variety of vertebrates.

Curious to investigate this phenomenon further, Fabien Aubret and Richard Shine conducted studies in which artificial paddles were affixed to the tails of juvenile tiger snakes (*Notechis scutatus*, a terrestrial species), and they demonstrated that relatively small paddles on the tail (35 percent of tail length) increased swimming speeds by 25 percent, but decreased crawling speed on land by 17 percent. Surprisingly, a larger paddle (84 percent of tail length) was less than half as effective for increasing swimming speed as was the smaller paddle. Of course, these were artificial structures that no doubt increased the stiffness of the tail. Evidently, the larger paddles of sea snakes are only effective following adaptive modification of the musculoskeletal systems that generate propulsion (fig. 3.8). While swimming is almost certainly the key adaptation of the paddle-shaped tail of sea snakes, other additional functions are also possible. On several occasions I have observed sea kraits (*Laticauda semifasciata*) near the ocean surface slap the water violently with the tail just before diving to escape. Perhaps this is a behavior that communicates a threat to other snakes, or that acts to startle or confuse potential predators. This statement is admittedly pure speculation, and the "slapping" might simply be the inadvertent result of a snake attempting to dive rapidly.

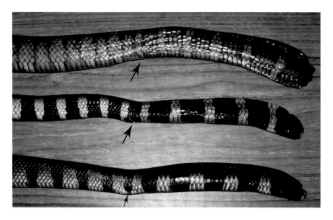

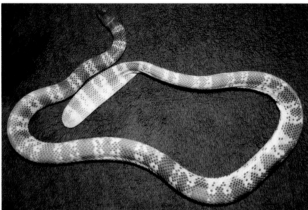

Figure 3.8. Paddle-shaped tails of three species of sea kraits having different aquatic tendencies are shown in the **upper photo**. From top to bottom these are *Laticauda semifasciata*, highly aquatic; *Laticauda laticaudata*, somewhat amphibious; *Laticauda colubrina*, amphibious, but spending considerable time on land. Note that the more highly aquatic species (*L. semifasciata*) has a somewhat broader tail in the dorsoventral plane, and it appears more muscular, presumably to power swimming (see chapter 1 for further description of habits). The arrows point to the vent (cloacal opening) of each snake. Photograph was taken at Orchid Island, Taiwan, by Coleman M. Sheehy III. The **lower photo** illustrates a relatively broader tail in a fully aquatic sea snake, *Acalyptophis peronii*, photographed by the author in Australia. The sea kraits are partly terrestrial, whereas this latter species is a "true" sea snake and is entirely marine. The sea kraits and true sea snakes represent two independent lineages, so the similar paddle-shaped tails in the two groups represent a nice example of *convergent evolution* (see reading by Sanders et al., 2012).

Bruce Jayne has compared swimming performance between an amphibious, nonconstricting semiaquatic snake (*Nerodia fasciata*) and a constricting terrestrial snake (*Elaphe, = Pantherophis, guttatus*). This comparison is of interest because of differences in habits, number of ribs (*Elaphe* has 50 percent more total vertebrae than *Nerodia*), and other anatomical features. Both species swam with similar waveform and maximum speed, which ranged from 103 to 155 cm/s in the larger snakes. The maximum forward velocity increased positively with increasing length of a snake in both species. Also in both species the amplitude and wavelength of lateral

undulations increased from anterior to posterior along the length of the body. Many of these parameters were quite similar to those of swimming eels.

In another study, Fabien Aubret and coworkers investigated locomotion in young tiger snakes (*Notechis scutatus*) that they raised for five months in either an aquatic or terrestrial environment. The snakes raised in water were able to swim 26 percent faster, but crawled 36 percent slower, than did their siblings that were raised without water for swimming. Thus, swimming performance can be *phenotypically plastic* in these snakes, which are closely related to sea snakes. Some have suggested that such plasticity might have accelerated large-scale evolutionary transitions like those from terrestrial to aquatic or marine environments.

Terrestrial Locomotion: Moving over Varied Landscapes

The movements of swimming snakes are also quite relevant to terrestrial locomotion, but the lack of buoyancy and nature of the substrate add variation to the principles that are involved. Gravity pulls downward on the mass of the animal, and the resulting inertial forces and frictional interaction with the substrate must be overcome in order to achieve forward movement. It is amazing how effortless this appears when snakes of various species are observed while moving in their native habitats. There are several fundamental patterns of movement that are observed in snakes, referred to as "modes" of locomotion, and most species are capable of switching their manner of movement depending on the particular features of the environment or, sometimes, the speed required. The movements of snakes are complex and may involve more than one manner of movement in different circumstances, or sometimes simultaneously in different regions of the body. There is recent evidence that progression of speed with movement can involve changes in the mode of movement, similarly to changes of gait in terrestrial vertebrates with limbs, notwithstanding the biomechanical differences.

Lateral Undulation

The more commonly familiar form of serpentine locomotion is termed *lateral undulation* or *horizontal undulatory progression*. Some might also refer to this mode of movement as "slithering," for the body of the snake moves continuously relative to the ground or substrate. This behavior makes for effective escape reactions and also adds fun and challenge to the act of catching snakes!

During lateral undulation the mass of the animal is supported by forces that are transmitted by means of the ventral and lateral body surfaces, which are continually in contact with the ground and associated objects. The propulsive forces, however, are exerted via the sides of the trunk.

Beginning at the head, a series of undulant or wavelike curves passes from front to rear, and the backward facing surfaces contact and push against irregularities in the ground surface (fig. 3.4). Whenever a bend of the body contacts a surface object such as a rock or small hillock of soil, it deforms locally to fit more closely around it and exerts force against it (fig. 3.4). If the surface over which a snake moves lacks these irregularities and has extremely low friction, the snake cannot move forward and simply thrashes back and forth in vain! However, most natural surfaces contain irregularities, and even very small ones that may not be obvious to human observers will work. The entire body of the snake slides past these sites, and the resistance forces are exerted at these points (fig. 3.4). These are variously called *contact zones*, *reaction sites*, *push points*, or *sites of resistance*.

During lateral undulation the head of the snake pushes off an uneven part of the ground, and each succeeding body part follows where the head left off. Each part of the body progressively follows the direction of the head. The snake travels forward, each point along the body moving at constant speed following a more or less sinusoidal path. The snake produces thrust by bending continuously around each point of contact, thereby shifting it to more posterior segments of the body. The waves of bending are propagated posteriorly such that they push laterally and posteriorly against the reaction sites on the surface of the substrate. When a snake pushes against multiple reaction sites simultaneously, the vectors of force that act laterally cancel each other, and the resultant vector propels the snake forward. That is, the summation of these reactive forces produces a net forward thrust (figs. 3.4, 3.9, 3.10). Each bend pushes against an object, and then slides out of contact with it.

The lateral undulations are created by alternating waves of muscle contraction that progress from the neck toward the tail. Such movement requires precise neuromuscular coordination. The propulsive forces due to the snake pushing against the resistance sites are generated by the axial muscles (fig. 3.3). Such forces pass perpendicular to the contact surfaces. Because all of the body is in constant motion, frictional forces at the resistance sites and the substratum induce forces that oppose the forward motion. Therefore, progression by means of lateral undulation is facilitated by low-friction surfaces so long as there are points for resistance contact. The ventral scale surfaces are designed with a morphology and orientation to reduce friction that opposes the direction of forward movement (see figs. 5.9, 5.13). This aspect of a snake's scale design is evident if one runs a hand both forward and backward along the belly of a snake and compares the frictional resistance with similar movements over the back of the snake. The hand slides more easily in the front-to-rear direction along the belly.

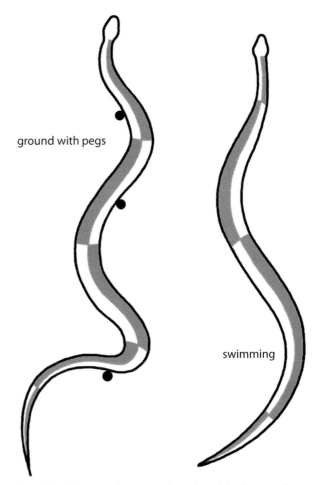

ground with pegs

swimming

Figure 3.9. Schematic illustration of muscle activity (gray color) during lateral undulation in snakes. The snake at the **left** is crawling on a smooth surface with pegs provided for resistance sites (dark circles). The snake to the **right** is swimming in water. The undulations are traveling from head to tail, and the onset and offset of activity is indicated by the posterior and anterior boundaries of the shaded areas, respectively. The drawings are based on information from electromyography of major epaxial muscles. For both types of lateral undulation, muscle activity is propagated posteriorly, and at a given longitudinal location muscle activity occurs only on one side of the body in an alternating fashion between the left and right sides. For terrestrial locomotion, the muscle activity along the entire length of the snake begins at maximal convexity and ends at maximal concavity with respect to the side of the active muscle. By contrast, during swimming the timing of muscle activity relative to bending shifts along the length of the snake because the speed of propagation of muscle activity exceeds the speed of propagation of lateral bending (as also occurs in the swimming of fishes). Drawings by Jason Bourque, Florida Museum of Natural History, after fig. 18 in B. C. Jayne, Muscular mechanisms of snake locomotion: An electromyographic study of lateral undulation of the Florida Banded Water Snake (*Nerodia fasciata*) and the Yellow Rat Snake (*Elaphe obsoleta*), *Journal of Morphology* 197:159–181, 1988.

As the animal moves, it senses irregularities while it is in motion, and the curves of the body are forced into contact with variously spaced resistance sites wherever they are encountered. In many cases, the head of the snake is elevated

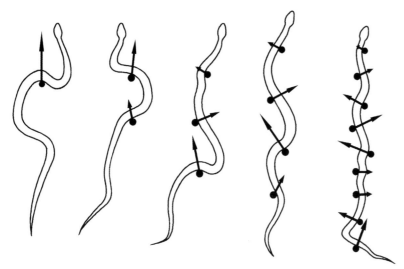

Figure 3.10. Forces generated by snakes using variable numbers of pegs for lateral undulation movement across a flat surface. Each arrow represents the reaction force exerted by the peg against the body of the snake, which is equal and opposite to the force exerted by the body of the snake against the peg. The length of each arrow indicates the relative magnitude of the reaction force. The sum of the reaction forces has a net forward component that contributes to the forward progression of the snake. With increasing number of pegs, the energy lost to lateral forces increases. Longer snakes have a greater array of contact sites to utilize and should be able to contact three or more points more often than can shorter relatives. Hypothetically, there is likely to be an optimal number of contact points for any particular size snake that maximizes the forward movement for any output of energy. Drawing by Jason Bourque, Florida Museum of Natural History, and after fig. 9.5 in J. L. Edwards, chapter 9 in M. Hildebrand, D. M. Bramble, K. F. Liem and D. B. Wake (eds.), *Functional Vertebrate Morphology* (Cambridge: Belknap Press of Harvard University Press, 1985).

and carried off the substrate as the body moves. Raising the head involves a cantilevering action, and the axial musculature shifts the weight of the elevated part toward the region of the body that remains in contact with the ground.

Studies of snake locomotion generally involve a combination of motion analysis (called *kinematics*) and measurements of the electrical activity of muscles (called *electromyography*, abbreviated EMG). The latter is accomplished by means of placing electrodes in specific muscles and recording the timing and intensity of their activity. Most of these studies have involved snakes that are moving by means of lateral undulation. In such movements, the epaxial muscles are activated sequentially along the body such that waves of muscle activity propagate along the trunk in a posterior direction. The timing of such muscle activity is consistent with the shortening of muscle units and the formation of bends in the snake.

Some studies of snake locomotion have employed snakes that are observed while moving over a flat, smooth surface with vertical pegs that are provided as the sole resistance sites (fig. 3.9). When snakes are moving among pegs, muscle activity on the side of the animal opposite the point of contact pushes the snake's body against the peg. The activity of the muscles causes the vertebral column to bend around the

peg and reverse its curvature anterior to it (fig. 3.9). Most of the force that is directed against a peg is produced by the muscles in the bend of the body contacting the peg, rather than by the muscles in distant bends. The extent of bending around a peg and the reversal of curvature anterior to the peg determine the direction of force exertion and the consequent movement that results.

The mechanical features of the snake's body result in relatively low curvature (that is, a long radius) of the vertebral column around each peg, while the body wall exhibits greater (short radius) but asymmetric curvature around the peg. The sharp bends around resistance sites involve complex movements produced largely by the epaxial muscles. The higher curvature of the body wall around the anterior surface of each resistance site appears to involve a suite of factors including the vertebral curvature, possibly axial torsion, and movements of the ribs and body wall.

The forces exerted by a laterally undulating snake must be sufficient to bend the body laterally, push its sides against vertical surfaces at reaction sites, and overcome resistance due to lateral and ventral *sliding friction* (roughly equal to the mass of the snake multiplied by the *coefficient of friction*). The term *sliding friction* refers to a resistance to motion that is generated at a point (or area) of contact between two surfaces that are in motion. The body curvature and the activity of muscle units increase in response to increased resistance to forward motion that might be acting on a snake. Experimentally, the addition of mass to a snake increases the resistance it must overcome to move itself forward, and therefore increases the force that is required for propulsion. The increased force that is exerted by the snake can be judged from the increased muscle activities indicated by the EMG. One other feature of muscle activity seems to be important. The axial muscles are activated immediately before, or when, they become stretched to maximum, and they are deactivated when they reach either resting length or maximal shortening.

Early studies suggested that progression by lateral undulation is most stable with at least three contact points, hence posteriorly directed vectors. More recent studies have shown that the mechanism of propulsion by lateral undulation also works with one or more contact points, although parts of the body can tend to slip sideways more when there is just a single contact point. Situations in which snakes cannot find one or more stable contact points cause the snake to shift to a different mode of movement, such as *sidewinding* or *concertina* locomotion (see below). Increasing the number of contact points increases both friction and the laterally directed forces relative to the forward directed forces. However, investigations involving snakes that are crawling on a smooth surface having intermittent vertical pegs indicate there are two advantages associated with multiple points for propulsive contact. First, contact with multiple pegs enables the cancellation of lateral force vectors over an extended length of the body, and this stabilizes the body against lateral slippage. Second, contact with multiple pegs reduces the curvature around each individual peg (fig. 3.10). These two effects seem to facilitate higher speeds of travel with less lateral slippage, but to a limit. When the contact points are very numerous, the lateral vectors become relatively larger and the friction increases—which means losses of energy and a reduction in speed. Fast-moving snakes such as racers and whipsnakes characteristically move with fewer long and shallow bends in the body, rather than numerous shorter and deeper bends.

Recently, David Hu working with collaborators in mathematics has investigated undulating locomotion ("slithering") of snakes on strictly flat surfaces. The team used video, mathematical models, and measurements of the frictional properties of snake skin to evaluate the mechanics of slithering locomotion. When a snake is undulating over a smooth, flat surface, it dynamically distributes its weight so that its belly presses against the substrate and periodically "loads" its weight at specific points of contact where the ventral scutes press against the surface. These points of weight loading are where the body has zero curvature. The snake's body may remain in contact with the substrate all along its length, but the weight distribution is nonuniform. During more rapid locomotion, segments of the body are alternately lifted off and then onto the substrate. Whereas the body undulates from side to side, the center of the snake's mass moves constantly in the forward direction as sliding friction is used to generate propulsive forces and exceeds the inertial forces by an order of magnitude. The inertial forces attributable to the sideward undulations are balanced by the sum of sliding frictional forces in addition to the forces generated by the internal muscles of the body. One important property of ventral scales that Hu and his team discovered is that friction, or resistance to movement, is highest when a snake is sliding sideways, rather than forward. The increased sideways friction seems to be necessary for forward movement across bare terrain that lacks rocks or other objects as push points. Other biomechanical studies have demonstrated that nanoscale geometric surface features of scales impart low friction for forward movement, but are an effective stopper for backward motion (see also chapter 5).

I believe it is fair to conclude that the movements of undulating snakes in many habitats arise from a combination of features that are observed when a snake in the laboratory moves among pegs or when it slithers over a featureless terrain. Some functional morphologists also speculate that snakes might dynamically change their frictional interactions with the surfaces over which they crawl by actively adjusting the attitude or orientation of the belly scutes.

Lateral undulation is commonly employed by numerous terrestrial species of snakes and is often used in combination with other modes of locomotion. Undulating movements are seen in the graceful and dramatic crawling of swiftly moving species such as racers, whipsnakes, or brown snakes, and are also used by snakes such as mambas and vine snakes to climb over objects or to move in three-dimensional habitats of bushes and trees. The slender appearance of many terrestrial and arboreal species is well suited to undulatory progression, but this mode of movement likely becomes less efficient and more difficult in stouter and heavier species. While snakes that are undulating appear to move very quickly and may well escape someone who is in pursuit, the maximum velocities measured in swiftly crawling snakes such as racers and mambas are around 12–13 km/h (3.33 to 3.61 m/s) and somewhat less in other species such as garter snakes. Research investigations by Bruce Jayne and Albert Bennett have shown that rapid but usually brief locomotion (called "sprint") increases in speed (m/s) with increasing body length of snakes, except for the larger snakes tested. These same investigators also demonstrated that the inherent sprint speed of individual garter snakes is correlated with their survival in nature, except during the first year of life.

Lateral undulation in snakes appears to be highly specialized and provides a unique propulsive system that uses marvelous control of body muscles. Limbless lizards, in comparison, cannot as effectively maintain contact with a push point or resistance site as the body travels forward sliding along a push point. Lizards often push against the resistance site for a short distance and then slip laterally out of contact with it, whereas snakes can keep the body in contact with, and pushing against, the resistance site until they push off of it with the tail. The local adjustment of curvature around an object or point of contact represents exquisite sensory control of muscles and appears to be a unique characteristic of snakes.

Concertina Locomotion

This mode of snake locomotion utilizes stationary body parts as anchors to push or pull the remaining body forward (fig. 3.11). *Static friction* associated with the stationary part is used as the reaction force to enable forward progression. This arrangement works so long as muscular-induced forces do not exceed the static friction force. Therefore, neuromuscular control during concertina locomotion is very important. The

Burrow   **Ground surface**

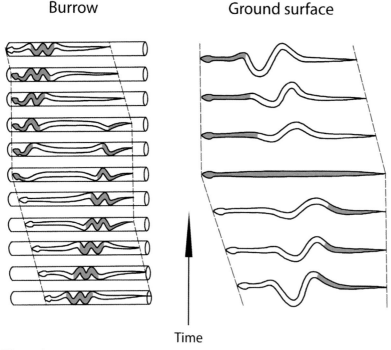

Time

Figure 3.11. Schematic representation of hypothetical snakes engaged in concertina locomotion, one inside a tube or burrow (**left**) and one moving over a flat surface (**right**). In each case the snake progresses from right-to-left (anterior direction) by anchoring part of the body against the interior of the burrow of against the ground surface, extending the body anterior to the anchored segment of snake, then anchoring the anterior part of the body and pulling the posterior body toward the newly anchored segment. The shaded part of each snake represents the anchored segment of body. Sequences are stopped in time progressively from bottom to top of each drawing (arrow). Progression of the snake in the burrow involves bending of the internal axial skeleton. Drawings by Jason Bourque, Florida Museum of Natural History, after fig. 9.7 in J. L. Edwards, chapter 9 in M. Hildebrand, D. M. Bramble, K. F. Liem and D. B. Wake (eds.), *Functional Vertebrate Morphology* (Cambridge: Belknap Press of Harvard University Press, 1985).

While moving forward, a snake using concertina movement alternates anchoring with folding, then anchoring with extension, and so on. One part of the body anchors against the substrate or tunnel wall while a body segment immediately behind folds like an accordion to "pull" that part of the snake forward. Once forward, a part of the snake posterior to the original anchor being considered then again anchors the body and the segment immediately in front extends the folded body forward. These actions are repeated along the length of the snake and alternately in time. The snake alternately pulls its body into bends and then straightens out the body forward from the bends. Some have compared this locomotion to snakes taking steps. Mean velocities associated with concertina locomotion are around 0.1 km/h (2.78 cm/s) or less depending on the attributes of the environment (tunnel width relative to snake, etc.).

Concertina movement can be used in three dimensions and is often used by arboreal snakes on tree limbs or branches, as well as by fossorial or terrestrial species moving in burrows. Having one part of the body anchored can be a very advantageous thing when crawling over objects that are thin, capable of movement, and potentially unstable. Also, the static friction

force of friction is related to the product of the friction coefficient (characteristic of the properties of the substrate) multiplied by the mass. Therefore, the mass of the snake must be sufficient to induce an adequate reaction force. On the other hand, as the body mass increases, so does the sliding friction associated with the moving part of the snake, and so does the effort that is required to lift the body. When a snake is moving through an earthen tunnel, or burrow, the snake actively pushes against the sides of the tunnel to provide a static anchor. Considerable muscular force might be generated in anchoring the body against the walls of the burrow, so the energetics of concertina locomotion inside a burrow is likely to be different from that of a snake that is moving on a flat surface. Concertina locomotion on a flat surface outside a burrow is often mentioned or illustrated in review articles and books, but in fact it is rarely observed. Recently, Matthew Edwards and the author uncovered a secretive blind snake (*Leptotyphlops ater*) beneath a stone in Guanacaste, Costa Rica. This small snake made repeated attempts to crawl away using concertina movements.

force can be increased by muscular effort as in constricting around branches (fig. 2.20). When crawling in burrows, snakes can use multiple sites for anchoring the body, and static friction can be employed by lateral as well as ventral surfaces of the snake. The confining space limits the amplitude of flexions, and therefore a greater number of flexions are typically used. This could be energetically more expensive and diminishes the endurance of the snake when crawling distances through subterranean tunnels.

Both concertina and lateral undulation locomotion are probably difficult for snakes that are both short and stout. In these cases, either *rectilinear* or *sidewinding* locomotion usually compensates for the disadvantages.

Rectilinear Movement

This term refers to straight-line motion, which in snakes involves comparatively slow forward progression powered by muscles and movements of the belly scales. Such movement relies on flexibility of the integument and the use of muscles that are bilaterally symmetric (fig. 3.12). The belly scales are alternately lifted somewhat from the substrate and pulled forward, then positioned downward and pushed backward. When the ventral scales are in static contact with the substrate, the body is actually pulled forward over them. The cycle repeats when the body has moved far enough forward to stretch the scales. Thus, groups of ventral scales are alternately placed in static contact with the ground followed by local active stretching that extends the ventral body wall somewhat like that of an inchworm. These movements occur simultaneously at several points along the body. The dorsal surface of the snake progresses at a constant velocity, and the continual movement of mass conserves momentum. But the movement is slow and typically characteristic of heavy-bodied snakes such as vipers, boas, and pythons, although probably all snakes are capable of such progression. Instead of the body undulating gracefully back and forth across the ground, the snake moves in a nearly straight line and appears to be powered by some unseen force. The progression of the animal can be very precise, quiet, and rather amazing to watch.

The principal muscles employed in rectilinear locomotion involve the *costocutaneous* muscles that run between the ribs and the skin (fig. 3.12). One set of inferior muscles at a particular point along the body pulls on the ventral scales and anchors them to the ground, thereby providing a pivot point against which other muscles can act. Similar muscles immediately posterior to this point pull the vertebral column forward and simultaneously add their affected ventral scales to the pivot site. Another set of superior muscles anterior to the pivot site acts simultaneously to lift the local scales off the substrate and pulls them forward of the

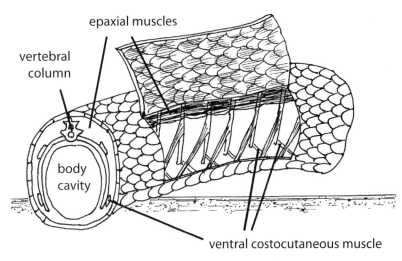

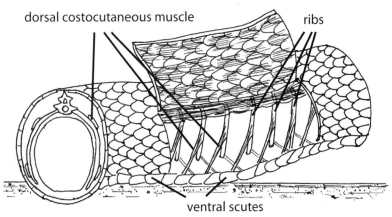

Figure 3.12. Schematic illustration of features in rectilinear locomotion by a hypothetical snake. The costocutaneous muscles connect the ribs with skin and impart forces involved in moving the snake forward from left to right in the figure. The ventral costocutaneous muscles anchor the ventral scutes in contact with the ground, and successive scutes are recruited in this manner to the region of ground contact (**upper** to **lower** figure). These scutes provide a zone of resistance points against which the muscles can act to move the snake forward. The ventral costocutaneous muscles associated with the contact zone act to pull the ribs and vertebral column forward, while the dorsal costocutaneous muscles act to lift the ventral scutes in advance of the contact zone and to pull them forward. The actions of both sets of muscles impart a continuous momentum to the vertebral column, and the dorsal body of the snake moves steadily forward. Several different ventral parts of the snake alternately fix to the substrate, then lift out of contact and quickly accelerate forward to "catch up" with the dorsal part of the body. The ventral scutes are alternately lifted and pulled forward, then pulled downward and backward. The flexibility of the skin is important to these actions. Drawing by Dan Dourson, modified from fig. 3.34 in C. Gans, *Biomechanics. An Approach to Vertebrate Biology* (Philadelphia: J.B. Lippincott, 1974).

pivot site. The result is that each of several pivot sites moves posteriorly along the body of the snake. The sequential contractions of the muscles impart a continuous momentum to the vertebral column, imparting the steady forward movement of the dorsal body of the snake. Simultaneously, the ventral part of the snake alternately fixes to the substrate, then lifts out of contact and quickly accelerates forward to catch up with the dorsal side of the body. The belly

scales are alternately lifted and pulled forward, then pulled downward and backward. Flexibility of the skin is of paramount importance here. As in the other modes of locomotion, if one observes a snake crawling in this fashion—and especially a heavy snake—it can be seen that the ventral scutes and segments of the snake respond to irregularities in the substrate such that the detailed pattern of the scute movements is dynamic and variable.

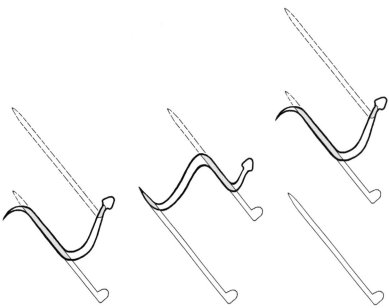

Figure 3.13. Schematic illustration of the progressive movements of a Sidewinder Rattlesnake (*Crotalus cerastes*), moving by sidewinding in a direction toward the top of the illustration. The shaded portions of the body are in contact with the substrate (sand), and the open portions of the body are lifted above the substrate. At any moment, the snake typically has two parts of its body in contact with the substrate and two parts lifted above the substrate. See text for further explanation. Drawing by Jason Bourque, Florida Museum of Natural History, after fig. 9.8 in J. L. Edwards, chapter 9 in M. Hildebrand, D. M. Bramble, K. F. Liem, and D.B. Wake (eds.), *Functional Vertebrate Morphology* (Cambridge: Belknap Press of Harvard University Press, 1985).

Sidewinding

This form of locomotion is well known and has been somewhat romanticized in context of western movies and various tales of life challenges in the desert. One immediately thinks of the Sidewinder Rattlesnake (*Crotalus cerastes*), but other desert vipers of Africa and Asia (as well as some other species) also employ sidewinding as a means of moving over flat, smooth, or slippery surfaces. Homalopsid snakes, for example, might employ sidewinding to move over mudflats, and various diurnal snakes can behave similarly when lifting the body off of excessively warm ground. Various surfaces can be of either lesser or greater frictional resistance, and sidewinding locomotion can still be employed.

Sidewinding progression involves a snake lifting the head and moving the anterior body forward, placing it in static contact with the substrate. While both head and tail are anchored in static contact with the ground, the middle section of the body is lifted forward and essentially "rolls out" against the substrate from that point. The neck is then curved, lifted, and moved forward again to repeat the action (fig. 3.13). During these movements the trunk of the snake may become bent in more than a single plane. The mechanism of movement involves static friction and irregularities in the substrate, which are either present as a passive feature of the physical environment or are created by the snake

as its body pushes sand into a small ridge, for example (fig. 3.14). Movement of the snake creates vertical and posteriorly directed pressure against the ground, which produces the reaction force and moves the snake forward without slippage or sliding.

Sidewinding movements utilize axial muscle units in ways that are fundamentally similar to those studied in lateral undulation, except that some muscles are activated bilaterally in the regions of trunk that are lifted off the substrate. A key aspect of sidewinding locomotion is the ability of the snake to transfer the support of its mass to the body segments that progressively contact the substrate. Such actions depend on exquisite control of the axial musculature. Compared with other snakes, species that specialize in sidewinding (e.g., *Crotalus cerastes*) possess fewer vertebrae and shorter segments of axial musculature, and are relatively small and moderately stout with short tails.

Because sidewinding involves lifted segments of the body, the laterally directed forces produced at each contact site are unbalanced and the snake moves laterally as well as forward. Sidewinding snakes leave characteristic tracks that appear as a series of short separated impressions set at roughly 30° angles from the direction of movement. The ends of the individual impressions consist of a "J" on one side, formed by the head and neck, and a "T" on the other side, formed by the tail. The direction of movement is indicated by the hook of the J, and fresh impressions allow one to easily follow the movements of a snake (fig. 3.14).

Studies by Bruce Jayne and Stephen Secor have confirmed a long-held conjecture that sidewinding is mechanically proficient and conserving of energy. Probably all midsized snakes are capable of sidewinding, but only desert vipers and certain homalopsid species appear to be specialized to routinely employ this mode of locomotion. Maximum speeds of sidewinding snakes are around 3.7 km/h (about one m/s).

Slide-pushing

This is a mode of terrestrial locomotion that involves vigorous undulations and sliding of the body. It is functionally intermediate between lateral undulation and sidewinding, and is also similar to undulating motions of snakes when swimming in water. The term is attributable to Carl Gans, who described this as a separate mode of locomotion although it may well employ elements of the other two modes just mentioned. An

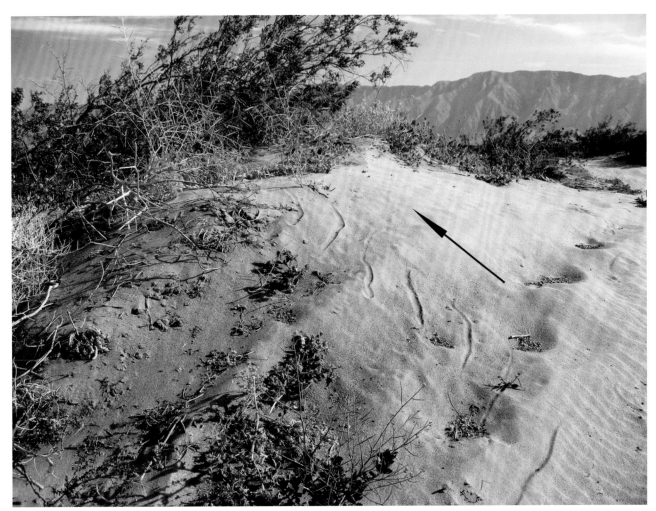

Figure 3.14. Tracks in sand made by a Sidewinder Rattlesnake (*Crotalus cerastes*) that moved up a mound of sand in the direction of the arrow. The snake was found coiled beneath a shrub at the top of the mound. These tracks are particularly deep as the snake had to exert considerable force against the sand in order to sidewind uphill. This trackway was photographed by the author in the Anza-Borrego Desert of Southern California.

alternative and very descriptive name for this movement is *slipping undulation*. Picture a snake that is attempting to crawl either by lateral undulating movements or by sidewinding movements, except that the substrate has very low friction and the body of the snake slides backward as it attempts to push against reaction sites. What happens is the posterior contact zones slide backward relative to the ground at several times the forward velocity. The snake does move forward, but at a slow rate. The head and neck travel forward at a relatively steady pace, while the head swings back and forth less so than the trunk.

The propulsive forces used in slide-pushing involve local force application by rapidly traveling waves of the snake's body. As the surfaces contact the ground, sliding friction is induced, but with an asymmetry. Anteriorly, the scales of the ventral body contact the ground. Posteriorly, there is torsion of the body and the ground contact also involves the sides of the trunk. The dorsolateral scales have a higher coefficient of friction and experience somewhat less slippage at right angles to the longitudinal axis of the body. The resistance to slippage is proportional to the product of the friction coefficient and the mass, which are both usually greater at the posterior end of the snake. Slowly this moves the snake forward over a low-friction surface, often at an angle to the direction it is facing. The principal difference between this mode of movement and that of lateral undulation is that the posterior reaction zones are fixed in an "undulating snake," but they move backward in the case of slide-pushing.

Slide-pushing is comparatively inefficient, for it involves many more undulating movements per unit of forward progression than occurs in a lateral undulating snake. Rather than considering this to be a specialized, evolved mode of movement, it should perhaps be regarded simply as an exaggerated attempt at movement when conditions of the substrate become poorly suitable for limbless locomotion. This mode of movement is used by various snakes when moving on slippery surfaces, or during initial attempts to rapidly escape a potential threat. An example might be the terrifying sight for some people who might encounter a snake in their house, and when disturbed the poor animal attempts to escape by wriggling and slipping across a slick floor such as linoleum. Such a snake appears frantic and probably much larger than it actually is when the story is told to a neighbor. Or the misunderstood animal is interpreted as attacking the resident, should the observer accidentally get between the snake and the shelter it is seeking.

Other Specialized Behaviors in Terrestrial Locomotion

Burrowing

Many snakes live in burrows or utilize subterranean tunnels for refuge from weather and predators. A variety of cavernous underground spaces are used for "denning" or overwintering when snakes seek refuge individually, or they form social aggregations consisting of tens or hundreds of individuals. In many cases, snakes share burrows with other animals, or they construct their own. Snakes that truly burrow usually exhibit a number of morphologic specializations including modified heads and rostral scales, shovel-like snouts, and tails with roughened or spiked scales (fig. 3.15; see also figs. 1.11–1.16, 1.20, 1.24, 1.49). Burrowing is accomplished by "wiggling" or "plowing" through loose soil and sometimes scooping dirt laterally with the enlarged rostral scale. The rough tail is used to anchor the body during these movements, or to plug the burrow and prevent the entry of unwanted guests. Head modifications usually involve reinforced buttressed skulls to absorb the forces that are generated during digging.

Certain snakes such as uropeltid and probably typhlopid species employ a special type of concertina locomotion in burrows and crevices only slightly larger in diameter than the body of the animal. These snakes bend the vertebral column separately from the outer parts of the body, which can be expanded to contact the wall of the burrow or crevice. Such contact provides sites of stable support, allowing the axial core of the body to move forward (or backward) relative to the contact sites which, in turn, are repositioned to produce forward movement (fig. 3.11).

Snakes that occur in habitats with desert sands either utilize burrows made by other animals (e.g., Sidewinder Rattlesnakes use rodent burrows) or move beneath the sand in a manner that resembles swimming. *Sand swimming* enables snakes to move through sand without forming a tunnel due to the loose nature of the collective sand grains. This manner of movement is not well studied but

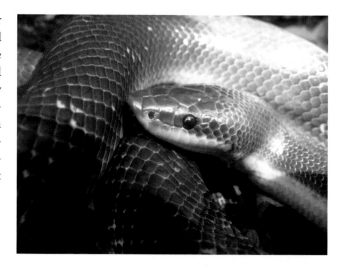

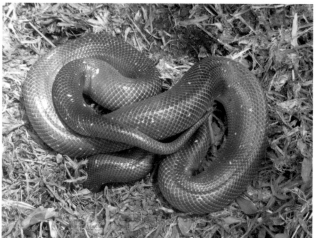

Figure 3.15. The head of the Mexican Burrowing Python, *Loxocemus bicolor*, exhibits a strong, countersunk jaw (**upper photo**) that is used for burrowing in tunnels and animal burrows. The **lower photo** shows the snake with its head and neck in soil as it begins to burrow. This species enters tunnels and nesting sites of iguanas where it feeds on their eggs. Both snakes are different specimens that were photographed by the author in Guanacaste, Costa Rica.

involves propulsion by means of reaction forces attributed to all surfaces of the animal that might contact sand grains during undulating movements, as in swimming. Snakes that engage in this behavior with regularity possess valvular nostrils to prevent the entry of particles when breathing, and concave bellies that prevent the filling of spaces around the snake so the body can expand and contract during lung inhalation and exhalation of air. Breathing by means of vertical movements is common in sand-swimming reptiles and also in rock-dwelling forms. Kenneth Norris and Lee Kavanau investigated burrowing behaviors of the Western Shovel-nosed Snake (*Chionactis occipitalis*) and observed that during active burrowing the head was bent slightly downward, and the overhanging rostral scale created a cavity that was free of sand. This snake breathes while in

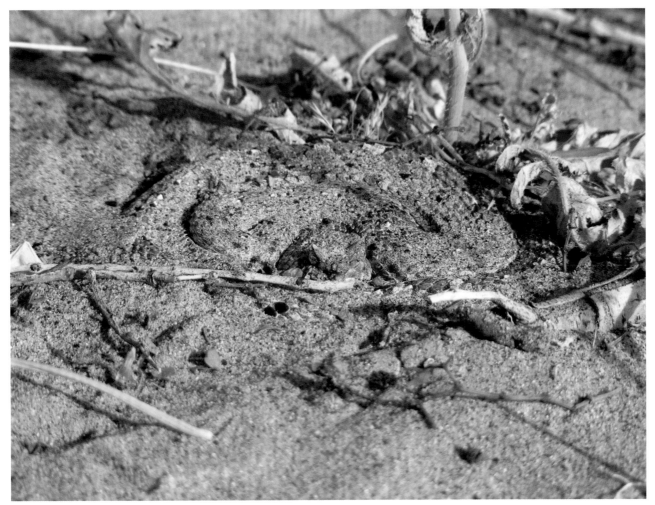

Figure 3.16. A Sidewinder Rattlesnake (*Crotalus cerastes*) partially cratered in desert sand beneath a creosote bush at Borrego Valley, California. Note the close camouflage match between the snake and the surrounding sand. The "horns" over the eyes keep them free of sand when the snake is buried more deeply. This is a common "ambush" behavior of this species of snake, which feeds on rodents and lizards. Photograph by the author.

sand by vertical movements of the gular region that is located in this sand-free cavity near the head.

A modified mode of burrowing occurs in a behavior that has been termed "cratering." Desert vipers will coil on the surface of sand and, by continually moving the body while remaining in a coiled posture, gradually displace the sand beneath while the snake "sinks" gradually downward into the substrate. With enough effort such snakes can bury themselves completely, but they usually leave the eyes exposed and may use the position as an advantage for ambushing prey that might wander near unknowingly (fig. 3.16). Cottonmouths and probably other snakes sometimes crater themselves deeply into leaves or other debris in response to cool or falling temperatures.

Jumping

Amazing as it sounds, although snakes are without limbs some species or individuals can actually "jump" during certain defensive actions. The behavior is not common, as most snakes prefer to anchor the body when striking at prey or a potential predator. An actual "jump" involves a vigorous strike in which the momentum of the accelerated head and anterior trunk carry the attached body momentarily off the ground. Sometimes particularly agitated snakes will slide or jump forward during strikes that occur while the animal is on unstable or down-sloping substrate. Some species such as African Horned Adders (*Bitis caudalis*) and jumping pit vipers (*Atropoides* spp.; fig. 1.36) characteristically spring forward into the air during vigorous strikes that comprise a defensive strategy. In other cases, smaller snakes may catapult into the air during frantic strikes or escape behaviors, and some arboreal species may purposely leave their substrate during launches into aerial descents (see below).

A very interesting aspect of snake behavior is that some species and individuals may exhibit exaggerated aggression if someone is in the way of a snake that is escaping from disturbance in a particular direction. Bruce Means has termed this "blocked-flight" aggression, during which a snake may raise its head, flatten its body, mouth-gape, strike, and sometimes "jump" toward a person if he or she is blocking the flight path of the animal.

Life in the Canopy: Climbing and Gliding

Life and movement in arboreal habitats is challenging for a variety of reasons. Probably the majority of snake species that are said to be *arboreal* also move on the ground during foraging, nesting, dispersing, and other behaviors; therefore the presence in a canopy is transient or cyclic, but not permanent. However, some species of snakes are highly arboreal and are typically found (most of the time) above ground in shrubbery or trees. On the other hand, there are numerous snakes that are terrestrial and ground-dwelling, but readily climb into vegetation for a variety of reasons including basking, foraging, escape from predators, and so on. In the New World, a variety of whipsnakes, racers, and rat snakes readily take to trees and can move swiftly through above-ground vegetation. Similarly, Old Word rat snakes, mambas, and some cobras perform similar feats. There are a number of snake species in which the young are highly arboreal, but switch to a more ground-dwelling existence as they grow older and longer. The switch could be related to predator avoidance, prey-switching, or the fact that vertical postures are less stressful on the cardiovascular system if the body—hence blood column of the major arteries and veins—is short rather than long (see chapter 6).

In terms of locomotion, movement through vegetation or upon branches requires precise neuromuscular coordination and the ability to sense whether smaller, unstable branches can support the mass of the climbing snake. A variety of movements is used, primarily lateral undulation in combination with concertina and, more rarely, rectilinear progression. Currently, detailed investigations of climbing behavior and mechanics in snakes are being carried out in the laboratory of Bruce Jayne at the University of Cincinnati. Some of the new findings indicate that Corn Snakes (*Pantherophis guttatus*) and Boa Constrictors (*Boa constrictor*) characteristically perform a variant of concertina locomotion with periodic stopping and gripping when moving horizontally or uphill on cylindrical perches. If pegs are present on cylindrical perches, the added resistance sites elicit lateral undulation and increased speed of movement. Maximal speeds are greatest on perches of intermediate diameter that approximate the width of the snake. The forward velocity decreases when either the incline or diameter of a perch increases, and the snakes are not able to move, either uphill or downhill, when large-diameter perches are experimentally inclined to 45° or 90°. These studies indicate that balance, grip, and the "fit" to a perch all can limit the ease of climbing on perches.

Many terrestrial snakes, and arboreal species in particular, have a remarkable ability to *cantilever*, or to extend the anterior body horizontally without support. Some gracile and arboreal species (e.g., vine snakes and the like, figs. 1.48, 1.51) are able to extend the body to more than 50 percent of its length when bridging gaps in vegetation or substrate (fig. 3.17). Amazingly, one of the recent observations from Bruce Jayne's laboratory is that some individual Brown Tree Snakes (*Boiga irregularis*) are able to support nearly 90 percent of their snout-vent length in air above a supporting perch before making contact with a second destination perch directly above the supporting perch! Studies in Jayne's laboratory have shown recently that snakes are able to cross larger gaps when there is a vertical component of the gap distance relative to strictly horizontal distance. When the gap has a vertical component (i.e., higher or lower than the level of the snake's starting perch), gravity acts over a relatively shorter horizontal distance, and this enhances a snake's ability to produce sufficient muscular force to prevent buckling.

Juvenile snakes are able to cantilever better than can adults of the same species, presumably due to a lower mass relative to the length of body. While features of muscle and

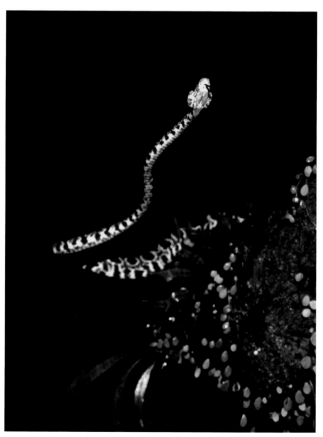

Figure 3.17. A Grenada Bank Tree Boa (*Corallus grenadensis*) illustrating a dramatic extension of the body in air, while the posterior tail and body are anchored to a tree. Photographed in Grenada by Richard Sajdak.

skeletal features of a snake's vertebral column are generally conserved in evolutionary terms, several modifications of vertebrae and associated epaxial muscles and their tendons appear to be related to cantilever performance. Arboreal snakes are generally slender with low relative mass and a compressed body form compared with strictly ground-dwelling relatives (figs. 1.31, 1.48). A large number of arboreal species are relatively short compared with nonarboreal relatives, and the body exhibits lateral compression (fig. 1.51). Additionally, some arboreal boas and vipers possess ribs that are directed downward rather than outward, thereby rendering the body to be narrow, yet deep, in cross-section. These features assist a snake to extend its body horizontally without undue downward displacement of muscle to form a dorsally convex vertebral arc.

Aspects of arboreal locomotion have also been studied recently by Ron Rozar at the University of Miami. He investigated movement behaviors and performance in eight pairs of taxonomically related species having terrestrial and arboreal relatives. He demonstrated that the arboreal species were generally superior in their abilities to bridge gaps and to traverse narrow-diameter perches. The arboreal species were also found to have greater climbing endurance than their terrestrial relatives; that is, they could sustain climbing movement for longer periods of time. Overall, the arboreal snakes were superior to their terrestrial relatives in climbing abilities, but the terrestrial species won out when it came to crawling performance over horizontal ground. Rozar suggests that there might be "trade-offs" in the proficiency of locomotion in the two habitats related to the specialized morphology that is characteristic of many arboreal species of snakes.

Straight Up and Down

Probably in most circumstances snakes climbing or moving through vegetation are nearly horizontal and use "switch-backs" (like roads coursing up a mountainside) to change elevation. However, there are instances where snakes climb using a fully vertical posture. One example is the climbing by New World rat snakes straight up the trunks of pine trees. These snakes might climb vertically to heights in the tens of meters, and one reason for such ascent is to forage for eggs or chicks in bird nests. The fully vertical position of the snake challenges the blood circulation, and this is discussed further in chapter 6. Additionally, the snake must find irregularities on the tree surfaces where it can engage resistance sites for production of thrust.

People have sometimes asked me how such climbing snakes come *down* from the tree. The answer to this question

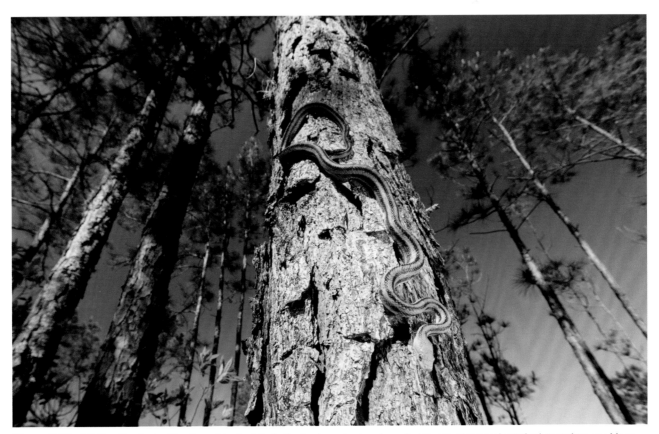

Figure 3.18. A Yellow Rat Snake (*Pantherophis obsoletus*) clinging to a pine tree in central Florida. It is not clear whether snakes are able to proficiently move downward on such a tree trunk, or whether they simply fall (purposely) to the ground. Photograph by Mac Stone.

is not clear. It is possible for snakes to climb down trees using the same features of the tree surfaces that are used in upward movement, or sometimes snakes simply fall to the ground (fig. 3.18). No one knows the intentions of snakes in these circumstances, but purposeful "dropping" could have been a behavioral precursor to the launches of gliding snakes that are discussed next.

Gliding

Perhaps the most remarkable behavior of moving snakes is that of *gliding*. While numerous cylindrical animals swim through water, "flying" snakes of the genus *Chrysopelea* are the only limbless animals that glide through air. Most animal gliders, such as flying squirrels or tree frogs, use static structures such as paired, outstretched "wings" to generate lift during gliding, but snakes have no appendages to create the wings or to assist with control during aerial movements. Yet gliding that has been studied in the Paradise Tree Snake (*Chrysopelea paradisi*) is on par with that of other gliders and demonstrates remarkable control over the direction of descent. This snake is a colubrid species that lives in tropical forests of Southeast Asia. Evidently, it engages flight primarily for escape, or to chase prey, or simply to glide from tree to tree (fig. 3.19). Remarkably, Paradise Tree Snakes can take off by jumping, maintain a stable glide path, maneuver while in gliding flight, and land safely without injury.

The *kinematics* of this "flying snake" was investigated in detail by John ("Jake") Socha while he was a graduate student at the University of Chicago. He determined the entire three-dimensional gliding trajectory of wild-caught *Chrysopelea* that were videotaped when jumping from a horizontal branch at the top of a 10-meter-high tower in an open field at the Singapore Zoological Gardens. The snake prepares for "take-off" by hanging from a branch with the anterior body looped into the shape of a J. It then jumps by accelerating up and away from the branch; simultaneously it straightens and flattens the body dorsoventrally. The body width nearly doubles, and the ventral surface becomes slightly concave in shape. Dorsoventral flattening is one of the key features of the gliding behavior of snakes (fig. 3.19).

As the snake pitches downward and increases in speed, the head and tail are drawn laterally toward the midpoint into the shape of an S, and the snake begins to undulate laterally and to generate lift. In mid-glide, the anterior body orients parallel with the ground while the posterior body cycles up and down in the vertical plane. The aerial lateral undulation appears to be a modified form of typical terrestrial locomotion, although the frequency of undulations is about one-third lower, while the amplitude is higher. The feat is probably more complex than terrestrial locomotion because the snake maintains a ventrally concave shape while undulating. The combination of movement and postural regulation

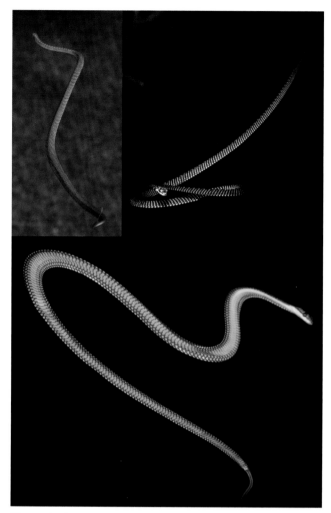

Figure 3.19. Photographs of a Paradise Tree Snake (*Chrysopelea paradisi*) in various stages of gliding. The **upper left** photo shows a dorsal view of a snake just after it has "launched" itself from an arboreal perch. The other images illustrate the extremely flattened shape of the snake during gliding, both dorsal and ventral views. Photographs are by Jake Socha.

presumably requires neuromuscular control that is quite specialized. John Socha has suggested that mobility and control of rib movements that are necessary for holding body shape during undulation might have originated in relation to fine grip control that is involved in climbing vegetation. The high amplitude undulations might serve to maximize the body length that is available for generating lift and might also function to control instabilities related to pitch and roll.

A gliding Paradise Tree Snake is amazingly adept at maneuvering while in air. Unlike many fliers, the snake can turn sharply without banking. A turn is made by moving the anterior body while the head is moving toward the direction of the turn. One snake that was being filmed turned sharply to avoid a tree during mid-glide. Typically, the flights of these snakes indicated the airspeed along the trajectory of glide averaged 8.1 m/s, or 29.2 km/h. The minimum glide angles of snakes averaged 28° and ranged from 13° to 46°. In more practical terms, the gliding ability of these snakes is roughly equivalent to that of other gliding vertebrates.

The Energetic Costs of Snake Locomotion

A limbless condition has evolved independently in several groups of vertebrates, including salamanders, amphisbaenians, and lizards, in addition to the snakes. Earlier speculations based solely on biomechanical considerations presumed that the energetic cost of such locomotion was lower than that for vertebrates with limbs. Some of the arguments favoring low energy expenditure during limbless locomotion include no cost for vertically displacing the center of gravity (as occurs in a walking or running human), no cost for accelerating or decelerating limbs (there are none!), and a relatively low cost for supporting the body. Subsequent investigations have shown, however, that the actual energetic costs of locomotion in snakes can vary considerably depending on the species and the mode of locomotion that it employs.

Contrary to earlier expectation, the net energetic cost of a racer (*Coluber constrictor*) moving by lateral undulation is equivalent to that of running in many limbed animals such as lizards, arthropods, and mammals. Energy costs are often compared using a measure called the *net cost of transport*, which specifies the amount of energy that is used to transport a given mass of an animal (say a gram) a given distance (for example, per kilometer). Such energy costs associated with locomotion vary significantly with the mode of movement. Thus, it was found that the energetic cost of concertina locomotion is about seven times greater than is that for lateral undulation. The greater cost associated with the concertina mode of locomotion possibly relates to the greater frequency of movements, the smaller distance traveled per cycle of movement, and the summed contributions of both sliding plus static frictional resistances. If the same snake is moving by either mode, it travels less distance per cycle during concertina locomotion compared with lateral undulation, and the cost per cycle of movement is higher during concertina movement. The anchoring aspect of concertina locomotion requires that part of the trunk must be at rest, so acceleration of body segments alternates with deceleration during the movement cycles. Theoretically, such loss of momentum with each cycle of progression costs energy.

In contrast, a Sidewinder Rattlesnake (*Crotalus cerastes*) that is moving by sidewinding exhibits a net cost of transport that is somewhat less than half that of a racer (*Coluber constrictor*) that is moving by lateral undulation. It appears that the lifting of the body during sidewinding movements is energetically more economical than is the combined work that is involved in overcoming the ventral and lateral sliding frictional forces that are inherent in lateral undulation. It is unclear whether the reduced cost of sidewinding also is related to the specialized anatomical features that are found in proficient sidewinders such as *Crotalus cerastes*. Of course, the energy cost of locomotion depends on the nature of the substrate and the incline of the path of movement (see fig. 3.14).

In spite of the differences in energy costs, the endurance of locomotion is not very different between a laterally undulating racer and a sidewinding rattlesnake. The term *endurance* refers to how long a given level of locomotion effort can be sustained. If the two snakes mentioned above are moving at a speed of 0.6 km/h, the mean endurance is about 73 minutes.

Snakes as Robots

Snakes have provided an interesting subject for robotics in context of military, medical, and sundry other applications where movement over complex terrain or narrow spaces is important. Robotic snakes have been made small enough to maneuver around organs that are inside the human chest cavity, while larger ones are able to carry a camera and transmit views from a treetop after crawling or swimming to a tree and climbing it (fig. 3.20). Robotic snakes have been called *snakebots*. Some of the advantages of snakebots over other types of robots include (1) ability to maneuver over rough terrain; (2) ability to climb steps; (3) ability to move over soft or thick materials; (4) ability to span gaps; (5) ability to fit or squeeze into tight or narrow spaces; (6) a segmental structure in which similar segments can be replaced easily; (7) ability to change body shape; and (8) advantages in hostile environments in which exposed and projecting surfaces such as limbs are easily damaged. Some disadvantages of snakebots relate to control problems, limitations of transporting loads, temperature control, and operating speeds that are slower than those of robot vehicles having wheels. The numerous advantages, however, render snakebots to be potentially quite useful.

It is important to realize that no snakebot can accurately or completely mimic the actual locomotion of live snakes, but these robots can be made in various shapes and sizes and perform a large variety of tasks that would be difficult otherwise. One example of a very clever use of snakebots is an application in animal control. A snakebot can pursue dangerous or invasive animals (a rabid raccoon, for example) and assist with their capture. Many such animals will attack a snakebot when it comes close, and the potential contact will result in the snakebot emitting an electrical shock that paralyzes the aggressive animal. Snakebots are currently being developed for search and rescue applications at a Biorobotics Laboratory at Carnegie Mellon University, and are being investigated as a new type of interplanetary probe by engineers at the NASA Ames Research Center. Thumbs

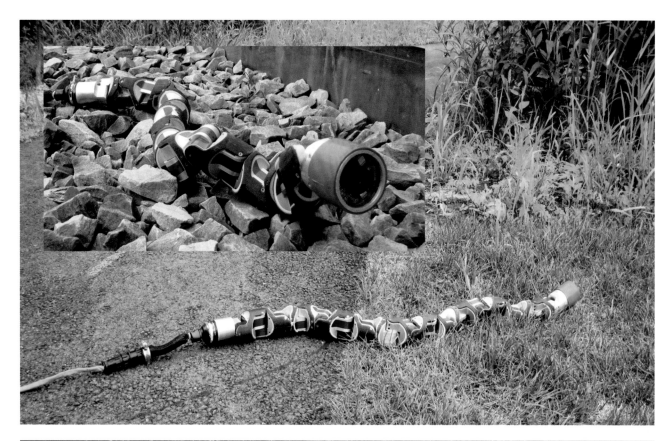

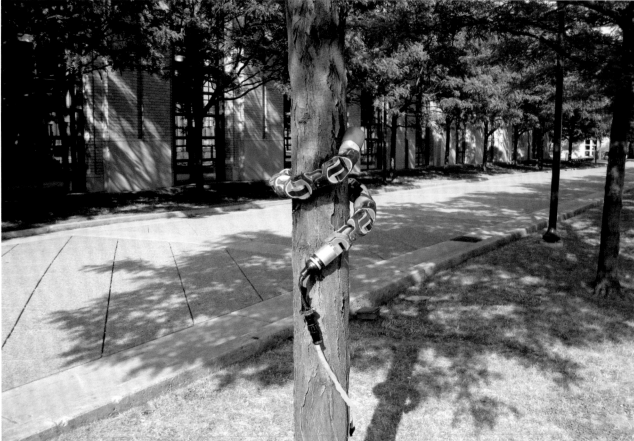

Figure 3.20. Robotic snakes, or "snakebots," illustrated crawling over various surfaces, and climbing a tree. Each snakebot has a camera mounted in front. Photos are courtesy of Howie Choset, a professor at Carnegie Mellon University's Robotics Institute who was named as one of the top 100 innovators in the world under the age of 35.

up for real snakes being the inspiration for such innovative research!

Additional Reading

Aubret, F., and R. Shine. 2008. The origin of evolutionary innovations: Locomotor consequences of tail shape in aquatic snakes. *Functional Ecology* 22:317–322.

Aubret, F., X. Bonnet, and R. Shine. 2007. The role of adaptive plasticity in a major evolutionary transition: Early aquatic experience affects locomotor performance of terrestrial snakes. *Functional Ecology* 21:1154–1161.

Brisçhoux, F., A. Kato, Y. Ropert-Coudert, and R. Shine. 2010. Swimming speed variation in swimming sea snakes (Laticaudinae): A search for underlying mechanisms. *Journal of Experimental Marine Biology and Ecology* 394:116–122.

Byrnes, G., and B. C. Jayne. 2010. Substrate diameter and compliance affect the gripping strategies and locomotor mode of climbing boa constrictors. *Journal of Experimental Biology* 213:4249–4256.

Cundall, D. 1987. Functional morphology. In R. A. Seigel, J. T. Collins, and S. S. Novak (eds.), *Snakes: Ecology and Evolutionary Biology*. New York: McGraw-Hill, pp. 106–140.

Dial, B. E., R. E. Gatten Jr., and S. Kamel. 1987. Energetics of concertina locomotion in *Bipes biporus* (Reptilia: Amphisbaenia). *Copeia* 1987:470–477.

Gans, C. 1974. *Biomechanics: An Approach to Vertebrate Biology*. New York: Lippincott.

Gans, C. 1984. Slide-pushing: A transitional locomotor method of elongate squamates. *Symposium of the Zoological Society of London* 52:12–26.

Gasc, J.-P., D. Cattaert, C. Chasserat, and F. Clarac. 1989. Propulsive action of a snake pushing against a single site: It's combined analysis. *Journal of Morphology* 201:315–329.

Graham, J. B., W. R. Lowell, I. Rubinoff, and J. Motta. 1987. Surface and subsurface swimming of the sea snake *Pelamis platurus*. *Journal of Experimental Biology* 127:27–44.

Gray, J. 1946. The mechanism of locomotion in snakes. *Journal of Experimental Biology* 23:101–120.

Hazel, J., M. Stone, M. S. Grace, and V. V. Tsukruk. 1999. Nanoscale design of snake skin for reptation locomotions via friction anisotropy. *Journal of Biomechanics* 32:477–484.

Hirose, S. 1993. *Biologically Inspired Robots: Snake-Like Locomotors and Manipulators*. Oxford: Oxford University Press.

Hu, D. L., J. Nirody, T. Scott, and M. J. Shelley. 2009. The mechanics of slithering locomotion. *Proceedings of the National Academy of Sciences* (USA) 106:10081–10085.

Jayne, B. C. 1982. Comparative morphology of the semispinalis-spinalis muscle of snakes and correlations with locomotion and constriction. *Journal of Morphology* 172:83–96.

Jayne, B. C. 1985. Swimming in constricting (*Elaphe g. guttata*) and nonconstricting (*Nerodia fasciata pictiventris*) colubrid snakes. *Copeia* 1985:195–208.

Jayne, B. C. 1986. Kinematics of terrestrial snake locomotion. *Copeia* 1986:915–927.

Jayne, B. C. 1988. Muscular mechanisms of snake locomotion: An electromyographic study of lateral undulation of the Florida Banded Water Snake (*Nerodia fasciata*) and the Yellow Rat Snake (*Elaphe obsoleta*). *Journal of Morphology* 197:159–181.

Jayne, B. C. 1988. Muscular mechanisms of snake locomotion: An electromyographic study of the sidewinding and concertina modes of *Crotalus cerastes*, *Nerodia fasciata* and *Elaphe obsoleta*. *Journal of Experimental Biology* 140:1–33.

Jayne, B. C., and A. F. Bennett. 1990. Selection on locomotor performance capacity in a natural population of garter snakes. *Evolution* 44:1204–1229.

Jayne, B. C., and A. F. Bennett. 1990. Scaling of speed and endurance of garter snakes: A comparison of cross-sectional and longitudinal allometries. *Journal of Zoology* (London) 220:257–277.

Jayne, B. C., and J. D. Davis. 1991. Kinematics and performance capacity for the concertina locomotion of a snake (*Coluber constrictor*). *Journal of Experimental Biology* 156:539–556.

Johnson, R. G. 1955. The adaptive and phylogenetic significance of vertebral form in snakes. *Evolution* 9:367–388.

Kelley, K. C., S. J. Arnold, and J. Gladstone. 1997. The effects of substrate and vertebral number on locomotion in the garter snake *Thamnophis elegans*. *Functional Ecology* 11:189–198.

Lillywhite, H. B., J. R. LaFrentz, Y. C. Lin, and M.-C. Tu. 2000. The cantilever abilities of snakes. *Journal of Herpetology* 34:523–528.

Lindell, L. E. 1994. The evolution of vertebral number and body size in snakes. *Functional Ecology* 8:708–719.

Means, D. B. 2010. Blocked-flight aggressive behavior in snakes. *IRCF Reptiles and Amphibians* 17:76–78.

Moon, B. R., and C. Gans. 1998. Kinematics, muscular activity and propulsion in gopher snakes. *Journal of Experimental Biology* 201:2669–2684.

Norris, K. S., and J. L. Kavanau. 1966. The burrowing of the Western Shovel-nosed Snake, *Chionactis occipitalis* Hallowell, and the undersand environment. *Copeia* 1966:650–664.

Ruben, J. A. 1977. Morphological correlates of predatory modes in the coachwhip (*Masticophis flagellum*) and rosy boa (*Lichanura roseofusca*). *Herpetologica* 33:1–6.

Sanders, K. L., A. R. Rasmussen, and J. Elmberg. 2012. Independent innovation of paddle-shaped tails in viviparous sea snakes (Elapidae: Hydrophiinae). *Integrative and Comparative Biology* 52:311–320.

Secor, S. M., B. C. Jayne, and A. F. Bennett. 1992. Locomotor performance and energetic cost of sidewinding by the snake *Crotalus cerastes*. *Journal of Experimental Biology* 163:1–14.

Shine, R., H. G. Cogger, R. N. Reed, S. Shetty, and X. Bonnet. 2003. Aquatic and terrestrial locomotor speeds of amphibious sea-snakes (Serpentes, Laticaudidae). *Journal of Zoology* (London) 259:261–268.

Shine, R., and S. Shetty. 2001. Moving in two worlds: Aquatic and terrestrial locomotion in sea snakes (*Laticauda colubrina*, Laticaudidae). *Journal of Evolutionary Biology* 14:338–346.

Socha, J. J. 2002. Gliding flight in the paradise tree snake. *Nature* 418:603–604.

Socha, J. J. 2011. Gliding flight in *Chrysopelea*: Turning a snake into a wing. *Integrative and Comparative Biology* 51:969–982.

Walton, M., B. C. Jayne, and A. F. Bennett. 1990. The energetic cost of limbless locomotion. *Science* 249:524–527.

TEMPERATURE AND ECTOTHERMY

Of the hundreds of variables that can shape the phenotype of an organism, temperature has undoubtedly captured more than its share of attention.

—*Michael J. Angilletta Jr.,* Thermal Adaptation: A Theoretical and Empirical Synthesis *(2009), p. 1*

Heat Exchange with Long Bodies and No Limbs

Like most other reptiles, snakes are exemplary of *ectotherms*—animals that rely on the external environment for sources of heat to elevate the body temperature. This condition is fundamentally different from the physiology of birds and mammals, which generate internal heat production by means of relatively high rates of metabolism (energy expenditure attributed to all the living processes within cells). The condition in birds and mammals is termed *endothermy*, in contrast to that of snakes, which is termed *ectothermy*. The higher rates of metabolism of endotherms confer relatively more freedom from the variation of external conditions related to geography and climate, but it comes with a cost. Endotherms must take in more energy as food in order to run their heat-generating machines, whereas ectotherms require less energy per time, in many cases approaching a full order of magnitude less than what is required by an endotherm. Thus, endotherms—especially smaller animals such as hummingbirds and rodents—must eat on a daily or even hourly basis, whereas some snakes have survived more than a year without food. Considering ecological communities, Harvey Pough of Cornell University estimated that reptiles can produce as much biomass annually as do the resident birds and mammals, even though they consume a much smaller fraction of the net primary production in their environment. The comparatively low rates of metabolism of snakes conserves energy relative to that expended by birds and mammals, but it does not produce sufficient heat to elevate the body temperature significantly. Thus, if a snake is to warm itself, it must seek sunlight or warmer parts of the microenvironment in order to elevate its body temperature (but see below).

The attenuate and limbless body form of snakes has important consequences with respect to the manner in which these animals are influenced by their physical environment and the behaviors by which they interact with it (fig. 4.1). First, an elongated body has a relatively large surface-to-mass ratio and does not accumulate and store heat as easily as is the case for a more spherical shape and centrally positioned mass. Of course, this limitation can be offset temporarily when the length of a snake is drawn into a tight coil, as shown in fig. 4.1. But when moving, the mass of the snake exchanges heat with the environment along its length, and there is less "thermal inertia" in a snake than there is in, say, an armadillo of similar mass. Furthermore, the long body is subject to more regional variation of body temperature and heat exchange than would be the case for a more compact body form.

Second, because snakes have no limbs, their body is in continuous contact with the ground or other surfaces upon which it crawls. Therefore, the exchange of heat is influenced strongly by conduction to and from the substrate, in contrast with, let's say, a lizard that can erect its limbs and stilt its trunk off the ground (fig. 4.2). Both animals are subject to radiative and convective heat exchange due to wind or air movement, but the snake is relatively more influenced by conductive exchange of heat with the ground upon which it crawls. When a desert lizard runs across hot sandy surfaces (sometimes bipedally!), only the hands or feet have minimal and intermittent contact with the ground, whereas a crawling snake on the same hot substrate conducts heat into its body over a much larger area of contact.

I was very surprised on two separate occasions to find snakes that were moving at midday in full summer sun across an open field. The setting was a field of dried grass in

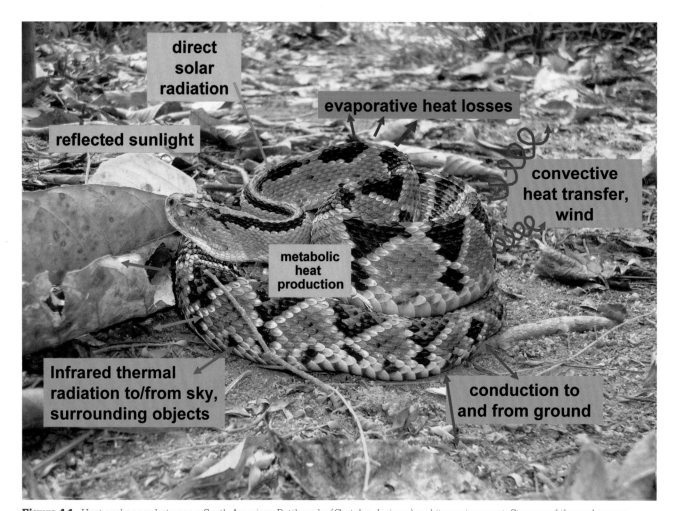

Figure 4.1. Heat exchanges between a South American Rattlesnake (*Crotalus durissus*) and its environment. Streams of thermal energy radiating to the snake include direct solar radiation, indirect long-wave radiation from sky and surrounding objects, and possibly conduction from the ground. The snake, in turn, radiates long-wave radiation to the environment, may conduct heat to the substrate, and loses heat by convection and evaporation of water. Pathways (or modes) of heat transfer represented by **red** arrows indicate heat transfer from the environment to the rattlesnake (plus metabolic heat production); pathways of heat transfer represented by **blue** arrows indicate heat transfer from the rattlesnake to the environment; and pathways of heat transfer represented by **brown** arrows indicate bidirectional heat exchange to or from the environment depending on which object is warmer. If it is a very warm day with air temperatures greater than the snake's surface temperature, the snake might gain heat by convection. The direction of net heat exchange depends on the difference in absolute temperature between the snake, the ground, and other objects in the snake's environment. All objects having a temperature above absolute zero radiate long-wave infrared radiation, and the net exchange of such radiation between the snake and any object in its environment depends on the difference in temperature. The snake's body temperature depends on the balance between input and output of the various streams of energy flow. This snake was photographed in Belize by Dan Dourson.

the Laguna Mountains of San Diego County, California. These snakes were likely moving from one area of chaparral or shaded oak woodland to another, but each was traversing an open field that was in between. I captured each of these snakes on the two occasions—one a Southern Pacific Rattlesnake and the other a San Diego Gopher Snake—and took the body temperature of each, which felt warm to my hands. The body temperature of the rattlesnake was 39.5°C, and that of the gopher snake was very near the same value. Both temperatures were quite close to the upper lethal limit of temperature tolerance. If either snake had not found a hole or shelter, or had not been captured by me, it might

have met its death in the open field. These were two events that stimulated my thinking about the ease of overheating in snakes that find themselves on heated ground surfaces during very warm days (fig. 4.3).

Lawrence Klauber during the 1930s recognized that temperature limited the activity of snakes, and soon thereafter both Walter Mosauer and Raymond Cowles became influential in promoting further thoughts about body temperature and its control in squamate reptiles. Studies by these two herpetologists, and by Charles Bogert, established that both lizards and snakes have rather specific preferences for body temperature. These early investigations stimulated what

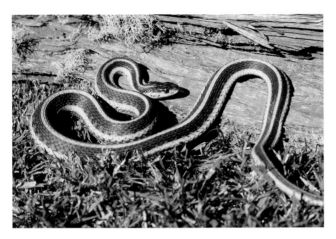

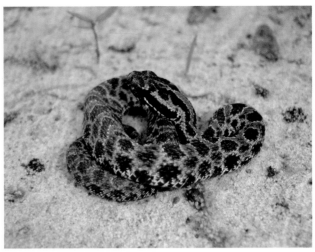

Figure 4.3. A Dusky Pygmy Rattlesnake, *Sistrurus miliarius barbouri*, will potentially overheat if it remains too long in open, sunlit sand during hot days in northern Florida. Photo by Dan Dourson.

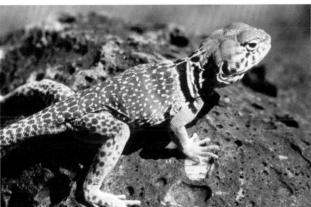

Figure 4.2. A Red-sided Garter Snake (*Thamnophis sirtalis parietalis*) basks with its body flattened, remaining largely in contact with the substrate on which it lies (**upper photo**). The body temperature therefore is influenced to a large extent by the temperature of the ground or objects on which it lies. In contrast, a Collared Lizard (*Crotaphytus collaris*) (**lower photo**) can minimize the influence of the substrate by raising its body off the ground or above the object on which it rests. Many lizards do this when the substrate becomes too warm, whereas the snake must crawl to a cooler substrate if it is threatened by an excess rise in its body temperature. The snake was photographed in Kansas, and the lizard was photographed in Nevada by the author.

later became a long-lasting interest in *behavioral thermoregulation* and the importance of temperature in the ecology and life history of reptiles. Lizards have been the principal subjects of these studies, but snakes have provided important additional insights and are uniquely suitable animals for investigating many interesting facets of this subject. The word "thermoregulation" is a shortened form of "temperature regulation" and is commonly used in literature on this subject.

During the several decades following the early studies of Ray Cowles and Charles Bogert, scientists have reported data for body temperatures measured in more than 100 species of snakes representing more than 10 different families. Many of the early measurements were obtained opportunistically using a rapid-registering glass thermometer

(then called a *Schultheis* thermometer, named after its manufacturer) or an electronic thermometer using either a thermistor or thermocouple as a sensor (fig. 4.4). Herpetological humorists have referred to this as "grab and stab" because investigators enthusiastic to obtain body temperatures of animals in the wild would catch an animal (especially lizards) and quickly obtain a cloacal temperature using one of the devices shown in fig. 4.4. It was relatively easy to obtain field data in this way. People eventually realized, however, that interpretations of such data had limitations if there was inadequate information provided about the thermal environment of a snake. Additional limitations related to (1) reporting single instead of repeated measurements from an individual, (2) having a limited number of measurements from conspecific individuals, and (3) introducing a bias due to the time of day that individuals collected measurements according to their own schedule. Thus, the evaluation of thermoregulation and the variation and causes of temperature selection in snakes has been inadequate until the more recent adoption of more sophisticated approaches. These have included continuous or repeated measurements of body temperatures from free-ranging snakes using *radio telemetry* (fig. 4.5), and the correlation of behaviors and physiology with body temperatures of snakes during experimental studies in the laboratory.

Behavioral Thermoregulation

With a few exceptions (see below), ectothermic vertebrates depend on behavioral interactions with their environment in order to regulate body temperature because there is insufficient heat production from metabolism to maintain a warm body temperature continuously in variable environments.

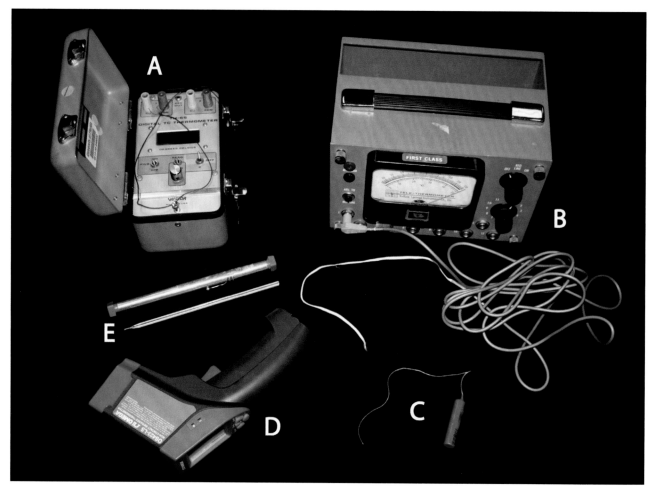

Figure 4.4. Various devices that have been used to measure body temperatures of snakes and other small vertebrates, and the temperatures of their environment. Progressing clockwise from the upper left: (**A**) A Wescor two-channel Digital TC Thermometer, which measures temperature by means of a thermocouple at the termination of two small wires attached to the posts on the instrument. Each channel can utilize a separate thermocouple wire, and the output can be recorded on a computer. (**B**) A Yellow Springs Intruments Co., Inc. 12-channel Tele-thermometer, which measures temperature by means of a thermistor embedded at the end of various cables or leads that are attached to the instrument. The one shown here is a flat disc that is designed to measure temperatures of flat surfaces, or can be used to indicate the temperature of a fully absorbing "black body" if painted black and used to intercept solar radiation. Each of 12 channels can accommodate a separate thermistor probe, and the various outputs can be recorded on a computer. (**C**) A Holohil Systems Ltd. implantable radio transmitter with an attached aerial. This unit can be implanted into the body cavity of a snake, and temperature-dependent signals can be picked up from a distance using an antenna and a calibrated recording device. (**D**) An Omega noncontact Infrared Thermometer, which detects the infrared energy emitted by any material (e.g., an animal surface) and converts the energy factor into a temperature reading. The temperature of the emitting surface must be above absolute zero (0° Kelvin). This instrument enables temperature measurements from a distance without contacting the object that is being measured. (**E**) A Schultheis rapid-registering thermometer is shown lying next to a metal protective carrying case. This small thermometer has a reduced bulb and can rapidly measure temperatures from 0 to 50 °Celsius. The early models of these thermometers were manufactured by Schultheis and Sons of Brooklyn, New York, but are available now from Miller and Weber of Queens, New York. These thermometers are easily carried in the field and have been used to quantify field temperatures for more than 50 years. Photograph by the author.

Endotherms such as birds and mammals can do so primarily due to their high rate of metabolism, combined with insulation (fur, feathers, or blubber in the case of aquatic forms) that sequesters the metabolic heat within the body and retards the losses of heat to cooler surroundings. Snakes, lacking insulation and having an attenuate body form, dissipate heat rather rapidly and thus seek out direct solar radiation and warm microenvironments in order to elevate body temperature (fig. 4.2). The modest rate of metabolic heat production does contribute to the animal's heat load at any given time, and there are physiological attributes such as variations of blood flow that can help to control the rates of heating or cooling. However, behavior is overridingly important because it is used to adjust the net rate of heat flux to and from the physical environment, which determines the rate and direction of body temperature change (fig. 4.1).

There are two aspects of behavior that are of primary importance to thermoregulation in snakes. The first is sometimes

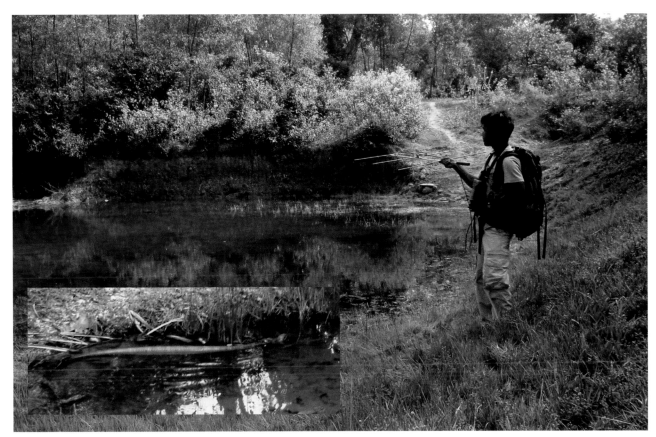

Figure 4.5. Dhiraj Bhaisare radio-tracks a King Cobra (*Ophiophagus hannah*) in the rainforest of the Western Ghats, India. Radio signals allow the tracking antenna and receiver (not shown) to locate the snake, which is some distance away and shown here in the **inset**. A radio transmitter has been surgically implanted into the body cavity of the snake. Such transmitters can be configured to transmit temperature as well as other physiological information (e.g., heart rate), in addition to the location of a free-ranging animal. Photographs by Thimappa, a local tracker.

termed *shuttling* and refers to movements back and forth between warmer or cooler parts of the environment, depending on the need of the animal. Numerous species of snakes living in temperate climates flatten the body to absorb solar radiation following their morning emergence in the spring prior to engaging in movement and activity (fig. 4.2). During hotter periods of the day these same snakes will seek shaded environments to avoid overheating (fig. 4.6). Retreating to subterranean shelters or beneath leaf litter sometimes can retard heat loss and can be important in limiting nocturnal cooling. On the other hand, boa constrictors in tropical climates were shown by investigations of Samuel McGinnis and Robert Moore to maintain body temperature as much as 7°C below shaded ground temperatures by seeking out subterranean environments that were cooler.

The elongate body form of snakes presents a relatively large surface area to the environment, especially if the snake is flattened and fully outstretched. However, when the body is tightly coiled (as in fig. 4.1) the surface-to-mass ratio is greatly reduced and in some species can approach the minimum possible ratio exemplified by a sphere. Such coiling minimizes heat exchange with the environment and

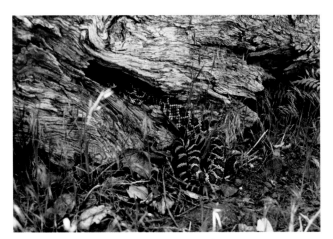

Figure 4.6. A Southern Pacific Rattlesnake (*Crotalus oreganus helleri*) seeks a shaded shelter during midday when environmental temperatures have warmed considerably and the radiant energy from direct sun is relatively intense. This animal was photographed by the author in the Laguna Mountains of Southern California, where the species is largely diurnal but restricts much of its activity to nighttime in the middle of the summer.

increases the likelihood of controlling body temperature by means of cardiovascular adjustments or metabolic heat production. In large constrictors such as boas and pythons, rates of heat loss to the environment are reduced by as much as one-half, although this factor varies with the environment. Social aggregations of snakes can also further modify the environment-body surface interactions. Large overwinter aggregations of snakes tend to occur at northern latitudes, where James Gillingham and Charles Carpenter discovered that the tendency of snakes to form tight aggregations within a den is temperature-dependent. The snakes increasingly aggregate as the temperature falls (fig. 4.7). On the other hand, many snakes with ranges in latitudes having more moderate climates tend to overwinter singly rather than in large aggregations.

Opportunities for active thermoregulation can be somewhat limited in fossorial habitats, aquatic environments, and even some terrestrial environments in the tropics. Thus, some snakes might behave "passively" and merely conform to their thermal environment. Aquatic snakes living in freshwater or marine environments live essentially at ambient water temperature, which might be thermally uniform or variable depending on the particular habitat. However, Richard Shine and Robert Lambeck studied aquatic file snakes (*Acrochordus arafurae*) in northern Australia and found that the variability of body temperature is significantly less than that of the surrounding water in which they live. Much of the year, the body temperature varies by no more than a few degrees Celsius owing to the stability of water temperature and the selection of microhabitats on the part of the file snakes. Snakes living in ponds or streams can alter their body temperature by moving between warmed shallow edge waters and the deeper waters that are nearer midstream (fig. 4.8).

The second aspect of behavior important to thermoregulation involves postural adjustments such as flattening, tilting, coiling, or extending the body. Such behaviors alter the exposure and contour of body surfaces, thereby adjusting the regional exchanges of heat between the snake and its environment. Postural adjustments are a way in which a snake "finetunes" the direction, rate, and location of heat flows to and from the body. On cold mornings, Australian Red-bellied Blacksnakes (*Pseudechis porphyriacus*) flatten the body broadly, somewhat akin to a cobra but including the entire body, and then tilt up on edge so the broad surface is exposed at right angles to the early morning sun. Harold Heatwole and Clifford Ray Johnson studied blacksnakes that were implanted with thermocouples and demonstrated that postural adjustments over a narrow range of body temperature abruptly alter the thermal gradients within the body.

Snakes are long creatures, so there is clearly a likelihood of thermal variation along the length of the body in various circumstances. When snakes are observed to thermoregulate behaviorally in the laboratory using a finite heat source such as heat lamp, there is a pronounced tendency for at least

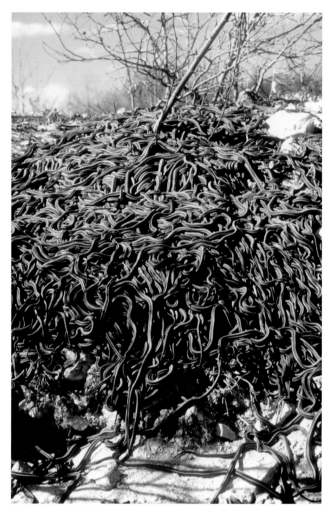

Figure 4.7. Hundreds of Red-sided Garter Snakes (*Thamnophis sirtalis parietalis*) amass together outside the entrance to a den where these snakes overwinter in southern Manitoba, Canada. Large aggregations of snakes are typical at many denning sites in temperate regions having cold winters. Photograph by Tracy Langkilde.

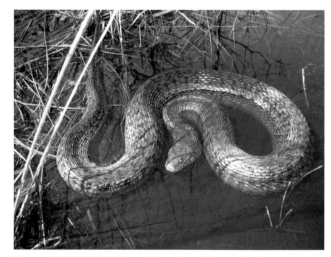

Figure 4.8. A Florida Green Water Snake (*Nerodia floridana*) rests at the edge of a pond where the water has been warmed by the sun. This snake was photographed in Levy County, Florida, by Dan Dourson.

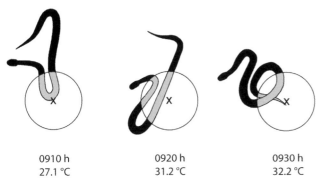

| 0910 h | 0920 h | 0930 h |
| 27.1 °C | 31.2 °C | 32.2 °C |

Figure 4.9. Schematic illustration of a recorded sequence of body positions, noted at 10-minute intervals, for an adult Red-bellied Black Snake (*Pseudechis porphyriacus*) basking beneath an infrared heat lamp. The "x" represents the center of irradiance from the lamp, and the circle indicates roughly the isotherm where irradiance falls off to 50 percent of maximum. The numbers indicate the time and core body temperature of the snake (measured by radiotelemetry). Drawing by Jason Bourque, Florida Museum of Natural History, based on fig. 2 in H. B. Lillywhite, Behavioral thermoregulation in Australian elapid snakes, *Copeia* 1980:452–458, 1980.

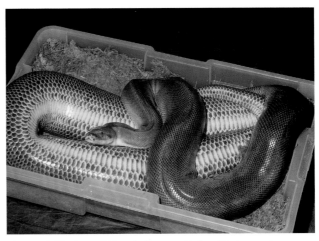

Figure 4.10. A gravid female Burmese Python (*Python molurus bivittatus*) lying in an "upside-down" position with much of the ventral body upright. This snake also features an unusual color morph of this species. Photograph by David Barker.

some individuals to adjust their position such that different parts of the body alternate location beneath the heat lamp. These behaviors suggest the snake is altering the regional heat input through time so as to maintain a more uniform body temperature throughout its length. I discovered this phenomenon while studying the thermoregulatory behaviors of Australian elapid snakes (fig. 4.9). During early observations, I found myself saying simply "Yes, the snake is still under the heat lamp." But upon closer inspection I came to realize that individual snakes were making subtle adjustments in their position. The result was very crudely analogous to grilling meat or kabobs on a barbecue: various parts of the meat or vegetables (body of the snake) must be turned regularly with respect to the heat source if one wishes to cook (warm) the object evenly.

A number of species of pythons have been reported to bask "upside down" by inverting the normal body position such that the ventral side is facing up. Such body inversion is usually limited to the posterior half of the snake, while the head and anterior body remain with a more normal upright posture (fig. 4.10). Such inverted basking postures are more prevalent when a female snake is gravid, possibly functioning to distribute heat to the reproductive tract and incubating embryos. On the other hand, David Barker suggested to me that the position might be related more to the comfort of the female when the body is heavy with young, much as position becomes important to the comfort of a pregnant woman. Basking positions and postures of various snakes also are thought to maximize body temperature of the gut when a recently taken meal is being digested.

Thermal Preferences

The tendency for snakes to maintain their body temperature within a narrow range or at a particular level has been described by various words. The more commonly used terms are *preferred body temperature*, *thermal preferendum*, *mean selected temperature*, or sometimes *preferred range*. For sake of convenience in this chapter I will use the term preferred body temperature (PBT) to indicate the mean of body temperatures that are measured either in active snakes in the wild, or as the mean of body temperatures that are recorded when snakes are allowed to exploit a gradient or mosaic of temperatures in the laboratory. When given a choice of environments with adequate thermal opportunities, many species of snakes select a PBT generally within the range of 29 to 34°C, and usually very close to 30°C. Measurements for numerous species have been summarized in various publications that are listed at the end of this chapter. Diurnal species inhabiting relatively open habitat may regulate body temperature at levels in excess of 30°C, whereas lower temperatures are characteristic of snakes that are nocturnal, fossorial, or occupants of shaded habitats. Some species that have been investigated carefully are capable of regulating body temperature with a very high degree of precision, sometimes varying no more than 1–2°C when a heat source is available.

Charles Peterson of Idaho State University studied garter snakes (*Thamnophis elegans*) using radio telemetry and demonstrated a typical triphasic pattern of thermoregulation. This consisted of (1) a rapid heating phase in the morning when relatively cool snakes emerged and basked in direct sunlight, (2) an extended "plateau" phase while snakes thermoregulated during the day, and (3) a long cooling phase during the late afternoon and night when snakes were secluded in nocturnal retreats (fig. 4.11). Raymond Huey and a

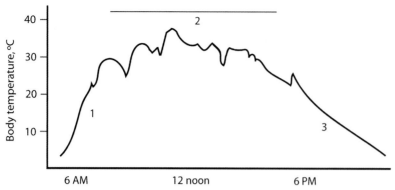

Figure 4.11. Hypothetical but characteristic plot of the daily changes in body temperature of a snake that (**1**) emerges in the morning and heats rapidly during exposure to full sunlight, (**2**) behaviorally regulates body temperature during an extended "plateau" phase when the thermal environment is appropriate, and (**3**) cools slowly when the sun sets and the snake seeks shelter from the cooling environment. Drawing by the author.

team of collaborators studied these snakes at Eagle Lake in northeastern California and found that they retreated beneath rocks of intermediate thickness, which offered the snakes an appropriate variety of thermoregulatory opportunities relative to thinner or thicker rocks. Snakes beneath the selected rocks were protected from overheating, but they could achieve their preferred body temperature for long periods—longer times than if they remained on the ground surface or if they moved up and down within a burrow. One female snake, for example, maintained a body temperature between 27.6 ° and 31.6 °C for 14 hours (the mean or "average" = 30.3°C), and for an entire 24 hours the body temperature never decreased below 23.6°C.

A number of herpetologists have found that temperatures of a snake's head are maintained within more narrow limits than are body temperatures measured elsewhere in the snake, suggesting that relatively more precise regulation of head temperature above that of body temperature might help to optimize functioning of the central nervous system. Some diurnal lizards and snakes have been observed to warm the head before they fully emerge from nighttime retreats.

In a very interesting study of Northern Rubber Boas (*Charina bottae*), Michael Dorcas and Charles Peterson found that diurnally active snakes maintained a warmer head at temperatures below their thermal preference, but they maintained warmer bodies when temperatures were above their thermal preference. In other words, rubber boas regulate their head temperature more precisely than their body temperature during the daytime. Furthermore, rubber boas were shown to exhibit significantly higher head temperatures than body temperatures during the night. The active maintenance of head-body temperature differences (about 2 °C) can be attributed either to behavioral mechanisms such as preferential head warming, or to physiological mechanisms involving blood shunts or countercurrent heat exchangers (see chapter 6).

Whether physiological mechanisms explain the maintenance of regional body temperature differences in snakes is not known (see below).

The preferred body temperatures of snakes may undergo seasonal changes and can be modified by changes in physiological factors or the physical environment. The term *acclimation* refers to a reversible change in a character (including measures of performance such as the speed of locomotion) that results from a prolonged change in the environment, especially temperature. Thus, if an animal that is, let's say, adapted to low temperature experiences warm temperatures for a prolonged period of some days or weeks, a physiological *performance* curve (see below) might gradually shift upscale so that the function is improved to better match the temperature. Such physiological changes usually involve alterations in the quality and quantity of enzymes that are related to alterations of genetic expression induced by the change of temperature. By definition, these changes are reversible, and of course they have limitations. In scientific literature, the term acclimation generally refers to such changes when they are induced in the laboratory, whereas the term *acclimatization* is used to describe such changes that go forward naturally in a wild animal's environment.

Studies of acclimation that occurs when snakes are subjected to different temperatures in the laboratory demonstrate an inverse relationship between the PBT and the acclimation temperature. Such acclimation responses have various interpretations, but they indicate a resetting of thermoregulatory "set points" during prolonged exposure to the temperature changes. A variety of factors in addition to environmental temperature potentially influence PBT set points, including illumination, reproductive condition, feeding, skin shedding, endogenous seasonal or circadian rhythms, age, and sex. Much work remains to be conducted in order to understand the variation of body temperature, both within and between species, and the genetic determinants of the PBT in relation to interactions with forces of natural selection in a species' environment.

Physiological Thermoregulation

Internal Thermogenesis and Endothermy
Although the majority of snakes are likely to be strict ectotherms nearly all of the time, we know of documented circumstances in which internal heat production is capable of elevating body temperature above that of the immediate

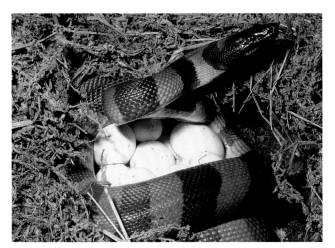

Figure 4.12. A Ringed Python (*Bothrochilus boa*) brooding her clutch of eggs. The egg temperatures are regulated by spasmodic muscle twitches of the female snake, which is similar to muscle "shivering" in humans. Photograph by David Barker.

environment. The most dramatic and well-known example is in connection with the brooding behavior of female pythons. Female pythons gather their eggs into a heap around which the snake coils tightly and encloses the clutch in the center of the coils (fig. 4.12). The female generates heat for transfer to the eggs by means of twitching her body muscles. The means of heat generation is very similar to what occurs when mammals—including humans—shiver to produce body heat in response to cold exposure. Skeletal muscles are activated by nerves, but not in a coordinated way to produce movement. Rather, the muscles twitch sporadically and generate tension without shortening to produce movement. The spasmodic twitching of muscles in the python thus generates heat, which warms the body of the female and transfers heat to the eggs that are located between the body coils.

The controlled production of body heat with significant transfer to elevate the temperature of a brooded clutch of eggs has been shown convincingly in three species of pythons, but many others might be incapable of significant heat production. Isometric muscle contractions have also been noted in rat snakes (*Pantherophis obsoletus*) and Bullsnakes (*Pituophis melanoleucus*) when exposed to low temperatures (10°C and 8°C, respectively). The contribution of such muscle activity to body temperature in these circumstances is not known, however.

The phenomenon of heat generation during brooding by pythons is known as *facultative endothermy* (and in mammals *shivering thermogenesis*). The phenomenon has been studied most completely in Burmese Pythons (*Python molurus*) and was first investigated by Lodewyk H. S. Van Mierop and Susan Barnard. Brooding female Burmese Pythons generate muscular heat when ambient temperatures fall below about 31°C, and the elevated body temperature remains within the general range of 31 to 33°C over an ambient range of at least 10°C. The heat that is generated by the snake maintains the temperature of her brooding eggs close to 30°C when air temperatures range between 23 and 30°C. Thus, brooding female pythons can elevate the temperatures of developing eggs by some 7°C above the temperature of the nest outside the brooding female. These snakes are not only capable of endothermy, but they use it to regulate body temperature and, indirectly, the temperature of the incubating eggs. This brooding behavior is advantageous in pythons whose geographic range extends to mountains where air temperatures can fall to levels that might slow the development and hatching of the species' eggs. Some other pythons (e.g., Water Pythons, *Liasis fuscus*) show facultative maternal brooding behavior, with the genesis of body heat being used to warm the clutch. Richard Shine and others have therefore suggested that a female python's "decision" where to locate her eggs and whether to remain and brood them can have important consequences for the subsequent development and success of the offspring. These are wonderfully "hot" topics in snake biology!

Surprisingly, there are other very interesting examples of endothermy in snakes. One is a condition that I discovered recently in newly hatched California King Snakes. The hatchlings are born with a large amount of yolk that is still present in their digestive tract. For periods up to two weeks, the skin temperature of hatchlings averages 0.6°C above the ambient temperature. This small but significant elevation of body temperature is thought to result from the active absorption and metabolism of the yolk and is therefore analogous to what is called *postprandial thermogenesis* (specific dynamic action; see chapter 2). A group of scientists led by Glenn Tattersall have carefully investigated South American Rattlesnakes (*Crotalus durissus*) and demonstrated that postfeeding elevation of body temperatures can result from internal thermogenesis related to metabolic responses to feeding. The body surfaces of fed rattlesnakes have been shown to elevate 0.9–1.2°C by thermal imaging, so the magnitude of associated changes in deep core temperatures could well be even more pronounced (fig. 4.13). This degree of thermogenesis is sufficient to enhance digestion significantly. More important, however, are voluntary seeking of warmer environments or increased basking to elevate body temperature following feeding. For example, David Slip and Richard Shine found that Australian Diamond Pythons (*Morelia spilota*) select temperatures that are several degrees higher after feeding in order to speed up the digestion of food. Not all snakes, however, elevate their body temperature following feeding.

Larger snakes, by virtue of their mass, can retain heat longer than can smaller individuals and thus have greater thermal inertia, especially when the body is drawn into a

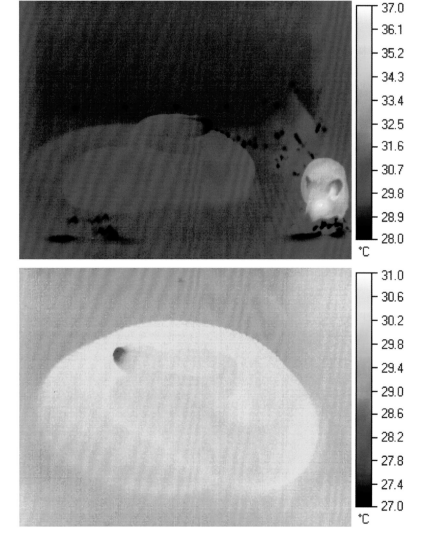

Figure 4.13. Thermal images illustrating postfeeding thermogenesis in a South American Rattlesnake (*Crotalus durissus*). The **upper photo** shows a rattlesnake prior to feeding on a live mouse that can be seen nearby. Note the warm body temperature of the endothermic mouse relative to that of the rattlesnake. The **lower photo** shows the rattlesnake again, 24 hours after it has eaten the mouse. The elevated body temperature of the rattlesnake is due to metabolic heat production related to an up-regulation of metabolism associated with digestion of the mouse. The "cold" spot at the head of the snake is attributable to respiratory evaporative cooling of the nasal passages associated with breathing. The vertical numerical scales to the right of each photo indicate how surface temperature varies according to the colors in the image. Note these scales are different for each image. Photographs by Glenn J. Tattersall.

tight coil. The possibility of endothermic elevation of body temperature is increased further when snakes aggregate in large numbers. Theoretical calculations by Fred White and Robert Lasiewski have suggested that a hypothetical aggregate of 150 denning rattlesnakes could maintain an aggregate body temperature about 15°C above the ambient den site temperature. This level of endothermy is attributable to metabolic heat production relative to an aggregate "effective" surface area that is 40 percent of the summed surface areas of individual snakes if they were in isolation. While

snakes in aggregated situations appear very capable of controlling their rates of heat loss to some extent, there is no evidence that metabolic heat production is actively engaged in thermoregulation as in the brooding female pythons.

Respiratory Heat Transfer Mechanisms

When snakes are exposed to stressfully higher body temperatures, they may increase the rate of lung ventilation and breathe with the mouth open. Evaporation from moist membranes lining the mouth, trachea, and lung cools these surfaces and potentially removes heat from the body. Such *evaporative cooling* can be important to thermoregulation in endothermic birds and mammals, and can stabilize brain temperatures of desert Chuckwalla lizards some 3°C below air temperatures. However, such cooling probably has marginal influence in the body's heat balance of snakes. Thermographic images of temperature differences between the head and body of rattlesnakes have revealed regions of cooling around the mouth and nasal capsule, suggesting that heat loss occurs by means of evaporative cooling in the ventilatory passageways (fig. 4.13). A research team lead by Brendan Borrell demonstrated that the differences in temperature between the head and body increase from about 2°C to about 3°C when rattlesnakes begin rattling. These and other studies suggest that behavioral activities such as locomotion and rattling might change breathing rate and thereby influence cooling of the head relative to the body. How these mechanisms might be activated during heat stress has not been evaluated.

Whether or not snakes actively pant to remove body heat is not well studied (see also chapter 6). The phenomenon is documented in a number of lizards, yet no snake is known to effectively pant. Perhaps panting is less effective in snakes because of the long shape of the body with its heat content being more removed from the region of cooling (at or near the head) than is the case in lizards. The hypothalamus of the brain is an important center for regulating thermoregulatory responses, including behavior, in both mammals and lizards. This is likely to be true in snakes as well.

Why Do Snakes Thermoregulate?

Snakes regulate their body temperature for basically two reasons: (1) to avoid thermal extremes that threaten their existence, and (2) to maximize or optimize bodily functions. At the low end of the temperature scale, snakes and other animals must avoid freezing to death. At the high end, temperature disrupts the structure of proteins and can be especially injurious to enzymes, causing denaturation that impairs the ability of molecules to maintain proper structure and therefore function. One immediate consequence is that coordinated systems such as nerves and muscles lose orchestration and therefore their integrity of response. The result is death as movement, breathing, blood circulation, and other vital activities become disrupted or impaired.

Tolerance Limits to Cold

The temperature at which a cooling snake loses coordination and movement is potentially lethal if the animal cannot escape from that condition. Laboratory determinations of such a temperature is termed the *critical thermal minimum* (CTMin), representing the temperature at which long-term survival is not possible unless the snake escapes from this or lower temperatures. Critical thermal minima have been determined for perhaps about a dozen species and are generally in the range of one to two or several degrees Celsius above freezing. Freezing temperatures are threatening because of the potential damage that occurs to cells from ice crystals that form in the cellular or extracellular fluids and physically disrupt or destroy the cellular membranes and other structures. Freezing of body fluids also increases the osmotic concentration of fluids that result when water is withdrawn from solutes during the formation of ice crystals. This reduces the solvent relative to solutes, and the resulting osmotic concentrations in the remaining fluids disturb cellular function and the distribution of body fluids in the various body compartments. The effect is very similar to dehydration.

Many reptiles and some snakes have the ability to escape the lethal effects of freezing temperatures by "supercooling" the entire body to temperatures that are below the normal freezing point without the formation of ice crystals. Several colubrid, elapid, and viperid species of snakes have been shown by Charles Lowe and his colleagues to supercool to temperatures ranging roughly from –4 to –7°C. Survival following supercooling without the formation of internal ice is widespread among ectothermic vertebrates and is probably quite common among snakes, especially those that manage to survive at high latitudes and high mountains.

Numerous animals living in seasonally cold environments also have the ability to endure the freezing of extracellular body fluids (cells must be protected from freezing). This phenomenon is termed "freeze tolerance" and has been studied and best characterized in several species of frogs and turtles. Garter snakes (*Thamnophis sirtalis*) and boreal vipers (*Vipera berus*) can endure brief exposures to freezing temperatures, but they die when temperatures fall below about –2 to –3°C for more than a few hours. Some peripheral freezing of skin and muscle tissue is probably tolerated, but the penetration of ice to core vital organs such as the heart is not.

The process of freezing has been studied in frogs and in turtles. Formation of ice crystals is initiated at a peripheral site such as the skin, and is propagated inward in a directional manner through the body. Ice forms first in spaces outside the organs, such as the abdominal space; then eventually the organs freeze. During thawing, melting occurs uniformly throughout the body core, and the organs melt before the ice that surrounds them.

In amphibians and some reptiles other than snakes, so-called "antifreeze" proteins inhibit the formation of ice crystals in body fluids, and "ice-nucleating" proteins may initiate and control the formation of ice in the extracellular fluids. A common adaptation is for low molecular weight metabolites such as glucose to accumulate seasonally during cold weather and to provide resistance to freezing of intracellular fluids and the whole body. Studies of turtles have shown that genes responsive to cold produce proteins that help to protect cells from the injurious effects of reduced blood flow and oxygen that results from the freezing of blood plasma during exposure to extreme cold. However, these physiological and biochemical aspects of freeze tolerance have not yet been demonstrated in snakes.

Tolerance Limits to Heat

Temperatures that are high-end counterparts to critical thermal minima are termed *critical thermal maxima* (CTMax). These also have been measured in about a dozen species of snakes and typically range from 37 to 44°C with a mean around 40°C. Death ensues if the body temperature increases just a few degrees higher than this point. Like many other vertebrates, the operational body temperature of snakes is much closer to the upper lethal limit than it is to the lower lethal limit. At least, this is true if the animal is given a choice and has the means to achieve its preferred body temperature. Again, snakes must be very careful to avoid overheating because they crawl with the ventral body surfaces in contact with the substrate. This imposes great difficulty for regulating body temperature if the environmental temperatures are hot. Therefore, the principal defense of snakes against overheating is the behavioral avoidance of microenvironments that might transfer excessive heat to a snake. Such avoidance explains why one does not see snakes crawling around during the hotter daylight hours in open, hot environments such as a low-latitude desert. The snakes are secluded down holes or beneath rocks and other objects where the extreme temperatures of more open environments are avoided.

Thermal Sensitivity, Performance Curves, and Trade-offs

Anyone familiar with chemistry and physics knows that fundamental physical and chemical processes are accelerated by temperature, and that biochemical reaction rates increase with increasing temperature up to some maximum. Therefore, life processes that depend on underlying biochemistry—respiration, digestion, growth, and so on—are sensitive to changing temperatures. This means also that coordinated systems—composed of many parts but acting as a whole—alter in performance with changes in temperature. Most persons familiar with snakes or other ectothermic reptiles have observed comparatively slow movements during locomotion or tongue flicking when the animal is cold, whereas at higher temperatures all the action speeds up considerably.

So-called "performance curves" usually refer to the thermal sensitivity of key tasks or functions, which are quantified in some manner and plotted as a function of temperature. Examples are illustrated in figure 4.14. The concept has become widely used in comparative biology, particularly in context of linking phenotypic traits, performance, and fitness. There is, of course, tremendous variation of performance curves, and they can be expected to vary with species as well as individual acclimation history related to previous thermal exposure. Each performance curve predicts the thermal optimum, or temperature of maximum value, and the *performance breadth* of a given function, which is some measure of the thermal range over which performance has some subjective value to the organism.

Regardless of the underlying mechanism or causation of the thermal sensitivity, adaptation for performance at low temperatures (e.g., locomotion in cold-climate European vipers) usually involves a trade-off with performance at high temperatures, and vice versa (e.g., locomotion in warm-environment tropical file snakes). Put in other words, a genotype or phenotype that performs well at low temperatures usually performs poorly at high temperatures and vice versa. Hence, there are constraints on performance depending on the environment and the adaptive specialization of the animal. However, some "escape" from these constraints is possible owing to acclimation (fig. 4.14).

Another word that is commonly used to express the variation of a phenotype attributable to environmental influence is *phenotypic plasticity*. And the range of phenotypes that are expressed by a given genotype operating under a range of environmental conditions common to an animal's habitat is called *reaction norm*. Fundamentally, all such

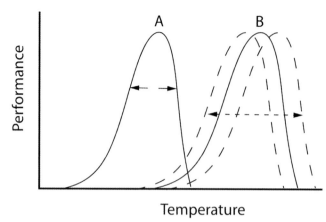

Figure 4.14. Hypothetical *performance curves* depicting how a chosen variable (digestion, for example) changes with temperature. The breadth of each performance curve is indicated by the horizontal arrows, which describe the limits of temperature within which a large percentage of the functional range is expressed (say, 95 percent). **Curve A** depicts a hypothetical performance curve in a species of snake that is adapted to living at low temperatures (e.g., at high altitude or latitude) and is subjected to colder environmental temperatures than is the species represented by **curve B**, which features a performance curve for a species adapted to living at higher temperatures (a warm-environment species). The variation or shifts of the function depicted at curve B (dashed line) represents hypothetical changes that are related to *acclimation* or *acclimatization*. That is, if the animal is subjected to changing temperatures in the environment, the performance shifts upscale (in response to warmer temperatures) or downscale (in response to cooler temperatures) if the environmental change is prolonged. The horizontal dashed line represents the total increase in performance breadth that is attributable to thermal acclimation. These changes in the physiology or performance of the animal in response to environmental variation are called *phenotypic plasticity*. Drawing by the author.

terms relate to the inherent ability (genetic capacity) of a species to alter its structure, function, and behavior for improved survival in response to changing aspects of the dynamic environments in which a species lives.

The sensitivity of life processes to temperature, as well as other resources such as availability of water, limits the activities of snakes both in time and in space. Hence, many snakes that live in temperate climates are active at different times of the day depending on the season and how daily changes in the thermal environment influence the ability of a snake to achieve appropriate body temperatures. A dramatic example of such seasonal change is the switch in behavior of snakes that are diurnal during early spring and become nocturnal during the hotter periods of summer (fig. 4.15).

The variation of body temperature has potentially many consequences for snakes, just as for other ectotherms that also have variable body temperatures. Rates of resting metabolism generally increase exponentially with temperature so that energy requirements are increased at higher temperatures but with the advantage of enhanced muscle performance, foraging

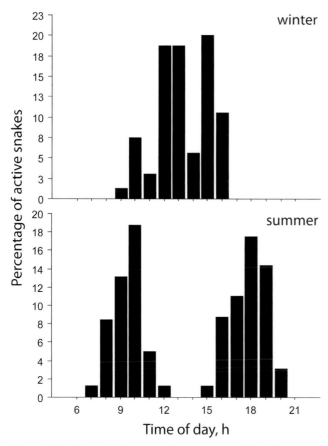

Figure 4.15. Bar graph illustrating the percentage of Black Tiger Snakes, *Notechis ater niger*, that are active in two different seasons, based on studies at the Franklin Islands, South Australia. Note that snakes are more active during midday in winter when the season is cooler, but during the hotter summer the activity shifts to early morning or late afternoon and evening hours. Data are redrawn by the author, from T. D. Schwaner, A field study of thermoregulation in Black Tiger Snakes (*Notechis ater niger*: Elapidae) on the Franklin Islands, South Australia, *Herpetologica* 45:393–401, 1989.

An interesting example of how temperatures that are selected by snakes influence important functions is the behavioral choice of temperature that increases the chemical energy that might be gained following the ingestion of a meal. Using empirical models related to digestion in Chinese Green Tree Vipers (*Trimeresurus s. stejnegeri*), Tien-Shun Tsai and his collaborators demonstrated that selection of elevated body temperatures (about 28°C) for a brief period following eating (see chapter 2) consistently maximized the amount of energy that was gained from the meal.

Herpetologists have recognized that there are costs as well as benefits to thermoregulation in ectotherms such as snakes. The idea has been championed by Raymond Huey and holds that a snake that maintains a high body temperature—by sun exposure for example—might also be more exposed to predators than if it was more reclusive in its behavior. Equally or more important, higher temperatures increase the rate of metabolism so that snakes use more energy when the body temperature is high. This situation is all right provided the foraging success compensates, but if prey items are in short supply it might be a better strategy to conserve energy by spending less time at the higher temperatures. This subject of "trade-offs" becomes even more complicated when one considers the interactions of temperature with evaporative water losses, skin shedding, reproduction, immune responses, and numerous other living processes. There is evidence that some snakes adjust their thermoregulatory strategy according to the status of energy and water balance, reproduction, and other factors. More detailed studies are needed, however, before models of cost-benefit analyses can be generalized. As with many things in nature, we can take satisfaction in knowing that behaviors of snakes are undoubtedly far more complex and interesting than we usually give credit.

Additional Reading

Avery, R. A. 1982. Field studies of body temperatures and thermo-regulation. In C. Gans and F. H. Pough (eds.)., *Biology of the Reptilia*, vol. 12. New York: Academic Press, pp. 93–166.

Bennett, A. F. 1984. Thermal dependence of muscle function. *American Journal of Physiology* 247:217–229.

Borrell, B. J., T. J. LaDuc, and R. Dudley. 2005. Respiratory cooling in rattlesnakes. *Comparative Biochemistry and Physiology* A 140:471–476.

Cowles, R. B. 1939. Possible implications of reptilian thermal tolerance. *Science* 90:465–466.

Cowles, R. B., and C. M. Bogert. 1944. A preliminary study of the thermal requirements of desert reptiles. *Bulletin of the American Museum of Natural History* 83:261–296.

Dorcas, M. E., and C. R. Peterson. 1997. Head-body temperature differences in free-ranging rubber boas. *Journal of Herpetology* 31:87–93.

success, and so on—up to some limits, of course. Some snakes exhibit a "plateau" of the rate of metabolism at temperatures corresponding to the activity range of the species, suggesting there is adaptation to stabilize performance related to energy use at those temperatures that are most favorable for the animal's activity. Temperature also affects growth and development, but there have been surprisingly few studies of these phenomena in snakes. The advantage of higher temperatures for growth is related in part to increased muscle performance, foraging success, and rapid digestion and absorption of ingested food items. In ecological terms, temperature can affect the frequency of feeding, the manner in which snakes forage, the time spent foraging, success of prey capture, processing of ingested energy, reproduction, avoidance of predators, and survivorship. Nocturnal behaviors of snakes during summers, for example, can reduce the exposure of active snakes and therefore the risk of capture by diurnal predators such as hawks.

Gillingham, J. C., and C. C. Carpenter. 1978. Snake hibernation: Construction of and observations on a man-made hibernaculum (Reptilia, Serpentes). *Journal of Herpetology* 12:495–498.

Graham, J. B. 1974. Body temperatures of the sea snake *Pelamis platurus*. *Copeia* 1974:531–533.

Gregory, P. T. 1990. Temperature differences between head and body in garter snakes (*Thamnophis*) at a den in central British Columbia. *Journal of Herpetology* 24:241–245.

Hammerson, G. A. 1977. Head-body temperature differences monitored by telemetry in the snake *Masticophis flagellum piceus*. *Comparative Biochemistry and Physiology* 57:399–402.

Heatwole, H., and C. R. Johnson. 1979. Thermoregulation in the Red-bellied Blacksnake, *Pseudechis porphyriacus* (Elapidae). *Zoological Journal of the Linnean Society* 65:83–101.

Heatwole, H., and J. A. Taylor. 1987. *Ecology of Reptiles*. 2nd edition. Chipping Norton, New South Wales, Australia: Surrey Beatty & Sons,.

Huey, R. B. 1982. Temperature, physiology, and the ecology of reptiles. In C. Gans and F. H. Pough (eds.), *Biology of the Reptilia*, Vol. 12. New York: Academic Press, pp. 76–98.

Huey, R. B., C. R. Peterson, S. J. Arnold, and W. P. Porter. 1989. Hot rocks and not-so-hot rocks: Retreat-site selection by garter snakes and its thermal consequences. *Ecology* 70:931–944.

Huey, R. B., and M. Slatkin. 1976. Costs and benefits of lizard thermoregulation. *Quarterly Review of Biology* 51:363–384.

Klauber, L. M. 1939. Studies of reptile life in the arid Southwest. *Bulletin of the Zoological Society of San Diego* 14:1–100.

Landreth, H. F. 1972. Physiological responses of *Elaphe obsoleta* and *Pituophis melanoleucus* to lowered ambient temperature. *Herpetologica* 28:376–380.

Lillywhite, H. B. 1980. Behavioral thermoregulation in Australian elapid snakes. *Copeia* 1980:452–458.

Lillywhite, H. B. 1987. Temperature, energetics, and physiological ecology. In R. A. Seigel, J. R. Collins, and S. S. Novak (eds.), *Snakes, Ecology and Evolutionary Biology*. New York: Macmillan, pp. 422–477.

Lowe, C. H., P. J. Lardner, and E. A. Halpern. 1971. Supercooling in reptiles and other vertebrates. *Comparative Biochemistry and Physiology* 39A:125–135.

McGinnis, S. M., and R. G. Moore. 1969. Thermoregulation in the Boa Constrictor *Boa constrictor*. *Herpetologica* 25:38–45.

Mosauer, W. 1936. The toleration of solar heat in desert reptiles. *Ecology* 17:56–66.

Naulleau, G. 1983. The effects of temperature on digestion in *Vipera aspis*. *Journal of Herpetology* 17:166–170.

Peterson, C. R. 1987. Daily variation in the body temperatures of free-ranging garter snakes. *Ecology* 68:160–169.

Porter, W. P., and C. R. Tracy. 1974. Modeling the effects of temperature changes on the ecology of the garter snake and leopard frog. In J. W. Gibbons and R. R. Sharitz (eds.), *Thermal Ecology AEC Conference 730505*. Oak Ridge, Tennessee, pp. 595–609.

Pough, F. H. 1983. Amphibians and reptiles as low-energy systems. In W. P. Aspey and S. I. Lustick (eds.), *Behavioral Energetics: The Cost of Survival in Vertebrates*. Columbus: Ohio State University Press, Columbus, pp. 141–188.

Scott, J. R., and D. Pettus. 1979. Effects of seasonal acclimation on the preferred body temperature of *Thamnophis elegans vagrans*. *Journal of Thermal Biology* 4:307–309.

Shine, R., and R. Lambeck. 1985. A radiotelemetric study of movements, thermoregulation, and habitat utilization of Arafura filesnakes (Serpentes: Acrochordidae). *Herpetologica* 41:351–361.

Shine, R., T. R. L. Madsen, M. J. Elphick, and P. S. Harlow. 1997. The influence of nest temperatures and maternal brooding on hatchling phenotypes in water pythons. *Ecology* 78:1713–1721.

Slip, D. J., and R. Shine. 1988. Thermoregulation of free-ranging diamond pythons, *Morelia spilota* (Serpentes, Boidae). *Copeia* 1988:984–995.

Tattersall, G. J., W. K. Milsom, A. S. Abe, S. P. Brito, and D. V. Andrade. 2004. The thermogenesis of digestion in rattlesnakes. *Journal of Experimental Biology* 207:579–585.

Tsai, T. S., H. J. Lee, and M.-C. Tu. 2009. Bioenergetic modeling reveals that Chinese green tree vipers select postprandial temperatures in laboratory thermal gradients that maximize net energy intake. *Comparative Biochemistry and Physiology A* 154:394–400.

Tu, M.-C., H. B. Lillywhite, J. G. Menon, and G. K. Menon. 2002. Postnatal ecdysis establishes the permeability barrier in snake skin: New insights into lipid permeability barrier structures. *Journal of Experimental Biology* 205:3019–3030.

Van Mierop, L. H. S., and S. M. Barnard. 1976. Thermoregulation in a brooding female *Python molurus bivittatus* (Serpentes: Boidae). *Copeia* 1976:398–401.

White, F. N., and R. C. Lasiewski. 1971. Rattlesnake denning: Theoretical considerations on winter temperatures. *Journal of Theoretical Biology* 30:553–557.

5

STRUCTURE AND FUNCTION
OF SKIN

> He who does not find core or substance in any of the realms of being, like flowers which are vainly sought in fig trees that bear none,—such a monk gives up the here and the beyond, just as a serpent sheds its worn-out skin.
>
> —The Worn-out Skin: Reflections on the Uraga Sutta, *translated by Nyanaponika Thera (Kandy: Buddhist Publication Society, 1989)*

Where Body Meets the Outside World

The skin of snakes is a very important organ and one that can be incredibly beautiful, adorned by natural selection with exquisite colors and patterns. The color pattern of the skin, and its sleek appearance, is for many persons the foremost attribute that focuses our attraction to the animal. The word *integument* refers to the covering of an animal, which is the skin and its derivatives such as scales, feathers, fur, or "horns" of various kinds. It is in this broader context that I will use the term "skin" in this book. As such, the skin of a snake is usually the largest organ of its body, at least in terms of mass. It is also of extreme importance, having multiple functions and interactions with the environment. We humans take comfort in the fact that beauty is more than skin deep, but for snakes the beauty we see is virtually all in the skin.

The interest of humans in the skin of snakes, and speculations about the functions of reptilian skin, has had a long history. The disciples of Aesculapius, the Greek god of healing, revered snakes and interpreted their periodic skin-shedding as a symbol of rebirth and renovation (fig. 5.1). Aristotle was interested in the abilities of Old World chameleons to change colors. More recently the idea that reptiles first "conquered" dry land because of their cornified integument has been implied in general textbooks, and some folks still believe that squamate reptiles are essentially waterproof owing to the presence of "scales" on the skin. Herpetoculturists have become fascinated with the many unusual color patterns that are expressed within a species, and they have selected for particular genetic lines that are popular with pet enthusiasts. Unfortunately, many snakes have been killed in various parts of the world and their skins have been tanned to adorn various products of leather or jewelry (fig. 5.2). But let us return to a consideration of skin that is based in structural features and functions that are more relevant to the snake itself.

First and foremost, the integument of any animal provides a barrier between the internal environment and the outside world. It is a mechanical barrier that protects the underlying muscles, blood vessels, and internal organs from abrasion and physical injury. It also functions as a physiological barrier and prevents the excess losses or gains of water, ions, and other components of the body fluids. The skin acts to prevent things from getting in as well as out. Therefore, the skin acts to prevent the entry of unwanted chemicals, especially microbes and toxins.

We see that the skin acts as a barrier, but the barrier is not absolute. Thus, the skin acts to regulate the exchange of some things but does not prevent their passage entirely. For example, respiratory gases—oxygen and carbon dioxide—are exchanged to some extent in aquatic snakes that breathe, in part, across the skin. Simultaneously, skin that is permeable to the respiratory gases must also regulate the exchange of water, ions, and toxins. This is a complicated subject that will be revisited elsewhere in this book. The skin also is a transducing surface, absorbing solar radiation that is converted to heat and very often used to warm the body. (A *transducer* is something that changes the form of energy that impinges on it. See chapter 7 for further discussion.) Another example is when mechanical vibrations are sensed by nerves in the skin, which convert the mechanical energy into bioelectric energy that is used to transmit nerve signals from the skin to the brain. Solar energy impinging on the skin also is used to initiate chemical reactions that lead to the synthesis of Vitamin D.

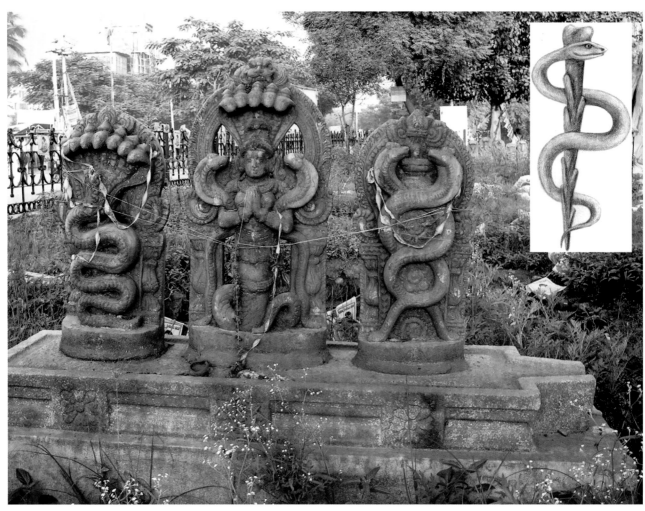

Figure 5.1. Stone carvings depicting various items of snake worship, located on a Hindu temple ground in south India. The stone at the far right resembles a caduceus, or "herald's staff" carried by Hermes in Greek mythology. The same staff was also borne by heralds in general and consists of a staff entwined by two snakes. This symbol was used in astrology and alchemy, and also became recognized as a symbol of commerce. The caduceus is sometimes confused with the traditional medical symbol, which has only a single snake and represents the rod of Asclepius (**inset**). The photograph is courtesy of Romulus Whitaker, and the inset was drawn by Shauna Lillywhite.

As we can judge from this discussion, the skin is an organ having many functions. And there are others. Shedding of skin releases substances that communicate chemical signals between snakes. As an example, female garter snakes of various species shed their skin soon after they emerge from dens or overwintering sites. The new skin bears a substance identified as a methyl ketone, which acts as a chemical attractant for male snakes of the same species. Such a chemical is called a *pheromone*, defined as a chemical substance produced by an individual organism and released into the environment for the purpose of signaling a social response from other individuals of the same species. The pheromone of the garter snake adheres to the ground where they crawl, and males locate the females by trailing them. Thus, the skin mediates communication between individuals by means of releasing pheromones onto trails (see also chapter 9).

Structure of the Dermis and Epidermis

Much of what people know about skin is based in clinical, pharmaceutical, and cosmetic contexts related to human skin, which for most practical purposes is fairly homogeneous (although it is a composite organ). In contrast, the skin of snakes is very heterogeneous and consists of a system of layered membranes. The more complex, outer part of the skin is the *epidermis*, separated from the *dermis* below it by a basement membrane (fig. 5.3). The innermost dermis consists largely of fibrous connective tissue composed mostly of collagen fibers, and is separated from underlying body muscles by looser connective tissue and fat. For reasons not entirely understood, the dermis of some species is applied very tightly to the underlying muscle, whereas in others it is considerably looser. Persons who have skinned snakes are probably aware of these differences. In other reptiles (e.g., crocodilians, turtles, and some

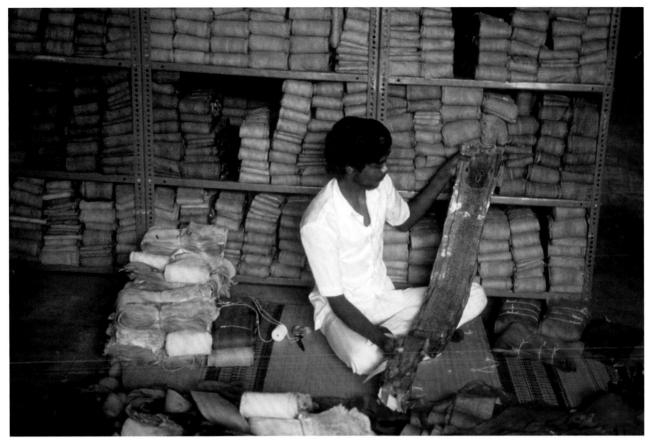

Figure 5.2. Hundreds of tanned snake skins in a warehouse of the Bharat Leather Corporation in Chennai (formerly Madras), India. This was a clearinghouse for snake skins that was established after the ban on snake skin trade was enacted in the 1970s, the idea being to clear existing stocks of snake skins once and for all. Presently there is no legal snake skin industry in India. Photograph by Romulus Whitaker.

lizards) the dermis gives rise to bony plates and other structures that are lacking in snakes. The dermis in snakes adds mechanical strength and thickness, and it is an important underlying support for the epidermis above it.

The epidermis of snakes consists of a layered structure including both dead and living cells. Two principal types of keratin are present, each adding strength and rigidity to the scaled surfaces. Keratins are fibrous proteins that are formed when living cells—keratinocytes—die as they mature and synthesize protein fibers. The resulting matrix of keratin fibers is simply called *keratin*, a word that is also synonymous with *corneous* or *cornified* layers. Whereas mammalian skin has only one type of keratin, α-keratin—which gives rise to nails, claws, and hair—the skin of snakes consists of both α-keratins and β-keratins. The latter resemble the very stiff keratins that are characteristic of bird feathers. These two classes of keratins occur in separate horizontal layers that are arranged vertically in snake skin. All of the keratinized layers of the epidermis—termed the *stratum corneum*—are derived from living cells that proliferate from a basal layer lying above the dermis (figs. 5.3, 5.4).

The more rigid layers of β-keratin overlie the less rigid layers of α-keratin beneath. The outermost keratin is derived from a single layer of β-cells and is termed *oberhautchen*. This is a unique constituent of the epidermis of lepidosaurs and gives rise to the sculptured patterns that adorn the surfaces of scales (see below). Beneath the oberhautchen are several more cell layers of β-keratin. Evidently, the function of the entire β-layer is largely mechanical. The presence of this stiffer type of keratin serves to maintain the shape of a scale (see below) by acting in equilibrium with forces that are generated by the complex arrangement of horizontal struts and vertical columns of collagen fibers within the dermis.

The β-keratin is separated from the α-keratin layers deeper below by a thin layer of strand-like keratin known as the *mesos* layer. The mesos layer is a highly specialized region that is rich in lipids and comprises the barrier to water movement, thus serving as a check against excessive losses of water to the environment. A complex mixture of lipids is secreted from specialized organelles into extracellular spaces where they become organized into flattened layers that envelope, and alternate with, layers of keratin. Several

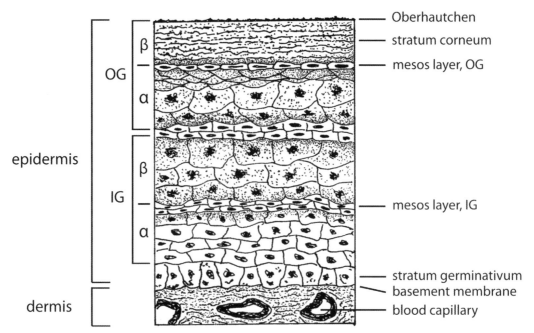

Figure 5.3. Schematic illustration of the generalized skin structure in snakes. Two generations of epidermis are shown, representing the outer generation (OG) of tissue that will be sloughed from the body during skin shedding, and the inner generation (IG), which is new epidermis that is formed before the older OG is shed. The outermost thin layer of beta (β) keratin is termed oberhautchen and bears the microsculpturing that is discussed elsewhere in the text. The mature α- and β-keratin layers collectively comprise the stratum corneum, and are derived from the living layer of stratum germinativum cells below. The stratum germinativum cells lie against a basement membrane, which separates the epidermis from the dermis with its blood capillaries below it. The mesos layer is a layer of specialized cells that separates the β- and α-keratin and contains lipids that comprise the water permeability barrier. Another zone of specialized cells (not labeled) separates the inner and outer generations, which split apart in this region during shedding of the OG. Drawing by Dan Dourson, after fig. 1 in H. B. Lillywhite, Water relations of tetrapod integument, *Journal of Experimental Biology* 209:202–226, 2006.

layers of α-keratin occur immediately below the mesos layer, followed by living immature α-cells yet to undergo keratinization. These α-cells differentiate from the basal layer that marks the inner boundary of the epidermis (fig. 5.4).

Scales

The layered distribution of cell types occurs over the entire body surface, but regional differences of thickness are related to the structure of scales. The skin of snakes and other squamates develops within the embryo as a surface that becomes folded into scales. Each fold, or scale, has an outer and inner surface creating a region known as a *hinge*. The hinge regions are more flexible than either the outer or inner scale surfaces and enable the epidermis to be deformed when the snake moves. They also permit considerable stretching when a swallowed prey item expands the skin. Indeed, when a snake is engorged with a large prey item it has eaten, the area of exposed hinge tissue may exceed that of the scales that occur in between (figs. 2.19, 2.31, 2.32). The epidermal covering of the hinge region is usually thinner than that of the other scale surfaces. Moreover, the β-layer is relatively thin on both the hinge and inner scale surfaces compared with the outer scale surfaces (fig. 5.5).

The size, geometry, and gross structure of scales also vary from species to species, and regionally on the body. Generally, the ventral scales (termed *scutes*) are broad and extend from side to side as one single structure (fig. 5.6; see also fig. 1.6). There are exceptions to this morphology, however, and the ventral scales are much smaller or equivalent to dorsal body scales in file snakes (*Acrochordus* spp.), many sea snakes, and species in some other taxonomic groups (fig. 5.7; see also fig. 3.1). The scales on the remainder of the trunk tend to be rather uniform but variable among species (figs. 5.8, 5.9). The scales on the head also vary considerably depending on the species of snake.

Scales in various taxa have evolved to be small and granular (e.g., as in file snakes, *Acrochordus* spp., and some other marine species), large and flattened (as in boas and pythons, various elapids and colubrids), or thickened with cornified keels, projections, or other structures (various vipers and pit vipers). Scales having a relatively smooth and usually flattened surfaces are termed *smooth* in contrast to scales having a visibly roughened appearance attributable to a small spine or a central longitudinal ridge, which are termed *keeled* (figs. 5.8, 5.9; see also figs. 1.16, 1.26–1.29, 1.33, 1.46–1.48). This terminology refers strictly to the external appearances of scales when these are viewed with the naked eye.

Figure 5.4. Photomicrographs featuring histological features of the skin of Dumeril's Ground Boa (*Acrantophis dumerili*). The **upper image** illustrates cell layers in skin during the resting stage prior to epidermal renewal of a shedding cycle. The alpha (α) and beta (β) keratin layers are separated by the mesos layer, which tends to split as an artifact of preparation due to the presence of lipids that form the permeability barrier against water loss. The stratum germinativum (sg) is a living layer of cells that gives rise to all the keratinized cells above it. The basement membrane of the sg separates the epidermis from the dermis below. The **middle image** features an early stage of epidermal renewal. The α- and β-keratin layers of the outer (o) and inner (i) generation of epidermis are separated by a clear layer that becomes a zone of separation when the old outer epidermis separates from the new inner generation epidermis. The oberhautchen layer (Obi) of cells forming in association with the inner, renewing epidermis is seen just below the clear layer. It will keratinize to become the thin, outermost surface layer of the β-keratin to become the new epidermis. Immature cells that will contribute to the β- and α-keratin of the new generation are seen between the stratum germinativum and the newly keratinizing β-layer of the inner generation (βi). The **lower image** shows a biopsied scale in the late renewal phase approximately two days before shedding of the outer epidermis. Lacunar tissue can be seen just above the region of epidermal separation (clear layer), and the oberhautchen, remaining β-layer, and much of the α-layers of keratin have completed maturation in the inner epidermal generation, so that only a few immature cells can be seen above the stratum germinativum. Photomicrographs by Elliott Jacobson.

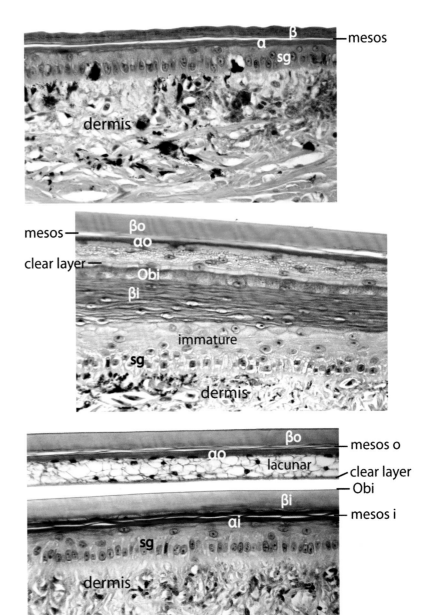

The outermost (oberhautchen) surfaces of snake scales bear microscopic patterns of sculpturing, referred to by various names such as *microornamentation*, *microdermatoglyphics*, *microstructure*, *microarchitecture*, and other terms. The patterns of microsculpture have been revealed by scanning electron microscopy (SEM), which produces enlarged images of minute structures on the surfaces of objects. Scanning electron micrographs have shown that the scale surfaces of various snakes are sculptured in complex patterns of minute ridges, spines, and other protuberances (fig. 5.10). Specific patterns of microsculpturing are characteristic of particular taxa of snakes, and these characters have been proposed for use as diagnostic characters. Less is known about the significance of these features to the lives of snakes that exhibit various sculptured patterns.

Patterns of microsculpturing seem likely to influence the exchange of radiant energy, heat, and evaporation of water, but these possibilities have not yet been rigorously investigated. There is strong circumstantial evidence that the microscopic surface morphology of some burrowing species acts to prevent the adhesion of dirt, and the scale surfaces of many snakes are hydrophobic and repel water (fig. 5.11). The prevention of wetting at the surfaces of snake epidermis may well be important with respect to the potential problem of swelling, which results from hydration of keratinous tissue. Such swelling might physically disrupt the mesos layer and thereby impair the permeability properties of

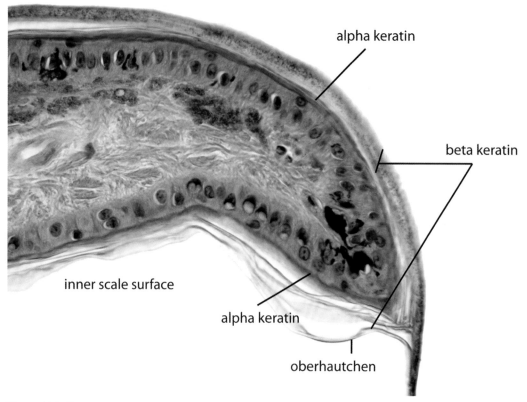

outer scale surface

alpha keratin

beta keratin

inner scale surface

alpha keratin

oberhautchen

Figure 5.5. Photomicrograph of a histological section through the skin of Dumeril's Ground Boa (*Acrantophis dumerili*). The section illustrates both the outer and inner regions of the scale during the resting phase when one generation of the epidermis is present. The beta (*β*) keratin is thicker on the outer scale surface and is represented only by the thin oberhautchen on the inner scale surface. The mesos layer can be seen as strand-like material between the *β*- and *α*-keratin, an artifact of separation especially at the right end of the scale. The cells with bluish nuclei comprise the stratum germinativum. Section was stained with H & E. Photomicrograph by Elliott Jacobson.

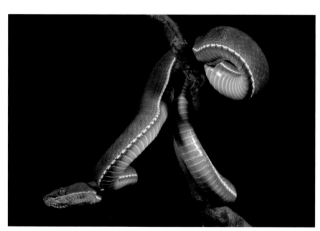

Figure 5.6. A Chinese Green Tree Viper (*Trimeresurus stejnegeri*) rests on a branch, revealing the width of the belly scutes in comparison with the dorsal and lateral body scales. This photo features a Taiwanese specimen and is courtesy of Ming-Chung Tu.

the skin. Numerous snakes are exposed to water for significant periods, especially species that are aquatic or semiaquatic, or that live in areas of high rainfall. Moreover, some natricine species of snakes are known to overwinter in circumstances where they are entirely immersed in water at the blind ends of burrows. The hydrophobic properties of the outer scale surfaces thus might function partly to prevent the inward diffusion of unwanted water that otherwise contacts the skin.

The shape, orientation, and pigmentation of scales might also influence rates of radiative heat exchange and consequently the temperature and evaporation characteristics of the skin. It need not be inferred, however, that the water or thermal relations of snakes are necessarily significant selective forces that have shaped the topography of the integument. On the other hand, nor do the characteristic microsculptured patterns appear to be simply a by-product of the splitting of the corneous layers of old from new epidermis during skin shedding, an idea that has been a subject of some discussion. My own observations have revealed that the outer keratinous surface of the spectacle covering the eye is not sculptured like the other scale surfaces, but

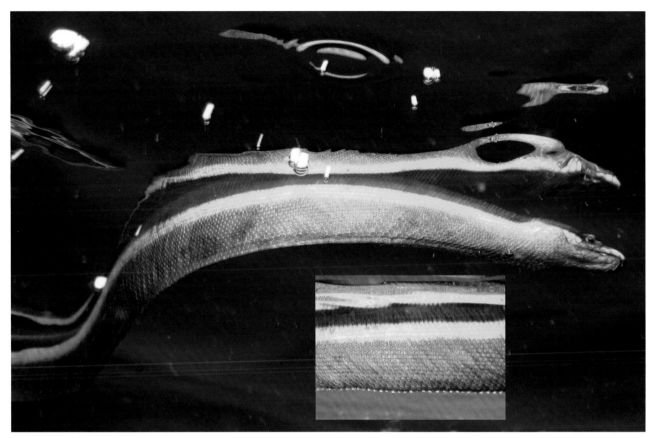

Figure 5.7. Underwater view of a Yellow-bellied Sea Snake (*Pelamis platurus*) illustrating the single row of ventral scales. Broad ventral scutes are simply absent. This is no doubt an adaptation for swimming because the snake flattens its body in the dorsoventral plane, and the lowermost aspect (belly) becomes a flattened keel with rows of scales not greatly different from the rest of the body. The **inset** shows the ventral keel in more detail. This snake was photographed in Costa Rica by Joseph Pfaller.

rather is comparatively smooth to permit the unobstructed entry of light. Therefore, given the regional variation, the microsculpturing patterns on various scale surfaces cannot be a simple nonadaptive product of skin shedding.

There is one feature of the epidermis that appears, however, to be a physical coincidence of the structure. The outer skin of a newly shed snake may be colorful with iridescence that results from the physical interaction of visible-spectrum radiation with the sculptured surfaces. The patterns of microsculpturing act as a diffraction grating and project colors of the spectrum when light is reflected in specific patterns from the opaque edges of the sculpture pattern (fig. 5.12). These appear to be incidental structural colors that are unrelated to any adaptive meaning or significance. The brilliance of these colors is most intense just after shedding and fades as time passes, probably due to the gradual wear or the accumulation of minute debris upon the oberhautchen surfaces.

In at least some species, it has been shown that the sculpturing of scale surfaces differs between the sexes. This subject has been studied in some detail for sea snakes by Carla Avolio, Richard Shine, and Adele Pile at the University of Sydney. They have suggested that sexual differences in the

roughness of scale surfaces is more common in marine than in terrestrial snakes, that the condition is more pronounced in male snakes, and that roughness of scale surfaces might assist the positioning of males during courtship. The rougher surfaces that are characterized by spines or protruding structures are more highly innervated and likely to be sensitive to tactile cues, and they also enhance friction between male and female when the bodies are in contact. The surface structures might also play a hydrodynamic role in modifying water flow over the body. The authors demonstrated that the rougher scale surfaces reduce the boundary layer over the body and create more turbulent flow, which they suggest might enhance the cutaneous exchange of respiratory gases during activities such as courtship.

The nanoscale structures of microsculpturing on scale surfaces also have important implications for locomotion. The surfaces of ventral scales exhibit highly organized arrays of microfibrilar projections or "micro-hairs" that point in the posterior or caudal direction and are separated by sharp grooves (fig. 5.13). Each microfibril is from one to a few hundred nanometers in diameter, based on measurements in boid snakes. These create an asymmetry with

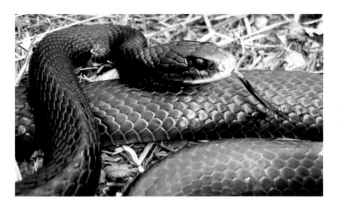

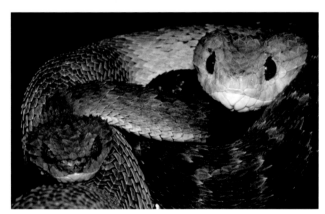

Figure 5.8. Photos featuring the body scales of three species of snakes. The **upper photo** shows a Florida specimen of Eastern or Black Racer (*Coluber constrictor*), which has smooth scales. The **middle photo** reveals the keeled scales of a Florida Green Water Snake (*Nerodia floridana*). In the **lower photo** a male and female Rough-scaled Bush Viper (*Atheris squamiger*) are seen resting together. These snakes have very rough scales with prominent central ridges and spiny tips, especially prominent in the male (at left). The upper and middle photographs are by Dan Dourson, and the lower photograph is by Elliott Jacobson.

respect to the frictional properties of the scales, which exhibit low friction for forward motion relative to backward motion (see also chapter 3).

Finally, there have also been observed systems of micropores penetrating the oberhautchen surfaces. These are speculated to be a possible delivery system for lipids that might provide surface lubrication, enhance resistance to water loss, or expel chemical attractants related to courtship (see chapter 9). The real function of such pits has not been demonstrated, however, and requires further research.

Ecdysis: The Shedding of Skin

Snakes periodically shed their skin, a phenomenon that occurs in all lepidosaurs and is usually referred to as shedding, sloughing, or ecdysis. Skin shedding was well known to the ancients, and there is considerable mythology and folklore related to the subject. Snakes shedding skins have become powerful symbols of rebirth and renewal (fig. 5.14).

It is generally well known that snakes initiate the act by rubbing the snout or head against an object, which loosens the skin and breaks it away from the new skin beneath (fig. 7.4). As the snake crawls forward, it literally crawls out of the old skin, which turns inside out and is left behind in the process. There are certainly subtle variations on this theme, but the procedure is generally similar in all species, and in normal circumstances the old skin is left behind as one entire piece rather than being shed in patches. Some aquatic species of snakes living where rough objects are not generally present to assist skin shedding may tie themselves into loose knots and use their own body to push or pull the old epidermis backward and off the trunk or tail. This behavior has been observed in pelagic sea snakes (*Pelamis platurus*) and in file snakes (*Acrochordus granulatus*) (fig. 5.15).

The shed skin is soft and moist at first, but it soon dries to become relatively brittle. It appears whitish in color and translucent, being quite thin upon careful inspection; for it is only a mature generation of epidermis that is shed, and not the next immature generation of epidermis or the thicker dermis that lies beneath.

Paul Maderson first described in detail the cellular changes that take place in the skin of a snake throughout the shedding cycle. Many subsequent studies have emphasized the wonderful complexity of the cycle especially in the context of the interaction between intrinsic and environmental factors in its control. The entire shedding cycle is surprisingly complex, and the controlling influences are still very much a mystery. Here we shall explore only a brief overview of the relevant morphological changes that occur.

A mature generation of epidermis (*epidermal generation*: figs. 5.3, 5.4) consists of a keratinized layer of β-keratin, with

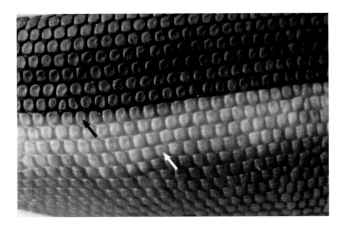

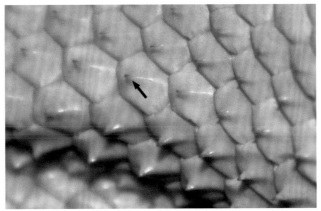

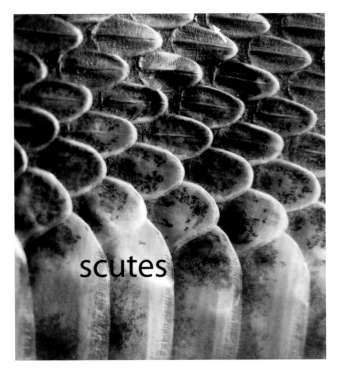

scutes

Figure 5.9. Photographs of skin surfaces of a Yellow-bellied Sea Snake (*Pelamis platurus*) (**upper photo**), Shaw's Sea Snake (*Lapemis curtus*) (**middle photo**), and an Eastern Diamondback Rattlesnake (*Crotalus adamanteus*) (**lower photo**). The scales of *Pelamis* are tuberculate and well separated with flattened surfaces. Note there are small spinules or spots in the middle of the scale surfaces (arrows). These are almost certainly sensory structures, but they have not been studied in detail morphologically or physiologically (see chapter 7). Prominent keels with central spines (arrow) are seen on the lateral scales of *Lapemis*, which is a male and develops such scale roughness during the mating period. The scales of the rattlesnake are keeled, and each dorsal scale has a central ridge, or "keel," running its length. The belly scutes are shown in the lower part of the figure. Note that there are transitional scales between the ventral scutes and dorsal scales that do not have ridges. The direction of orientation with respect to the snake is head-to-tail from left-to-right. The sea snakes were photographed in Costa Rica (*Pelamis*) and Australia (*Lapemis*). The rattlesnake was photographed in Florida. All snakes were living specimens photographed by the author.

sandwiched between alternating layers of lamellar lipids as described above. Keratinized α-keratin occurs beneath the mesos layer, formed from multiple cell layers similarly to the β-layer. Below the α-keratin there is a transitional region wherein mature keratin merges with immature α-cells that are in various stages of keratinization (fig. 5.4). All of the living cells that contributed to these described layers are derived from the *stratum germinativum* at the innermost base of the epidermis, overlying the dermis beneath.

Immediately following ecdysis, the new generation of epidermis is more or less in the state just described, and it may remain that way for some time that is known as the "resting stage." After some while, which can vary from weeks to months, the skin enters a "renewal stage" in which a new *inner generation* of epidermis begins to form beneath the older, mature *outer generation* of epidermis (fig. 5.4). Essentially what happens is that cells proliferate from the basal germinal layer and begin to keratinize as they accumulate between the outer generation and the stratum germinativum. Progressive keratinization of these newly proliferated cells produces a new generation of epidermis that is nearly mature by the time of shedding. Thus, at ecdysis there is a mature outer generation of epidermis that overlies a newly formed, but not quite mature, inner generation of epidermis. The extent of development of the new, inner generation α-layer varies considerably at the time of ecdysis.

One further detail regarding these tissues requires comment. Prior to formation of the new β-layer belonging to the inner generation, several layers of unusual cells form at the base of the outer generation. These cells separate the two generations of epidermis, although technically they are part of the older outer generation because they disappear at the time of shedding. These cells are called "lacunar cells,"

the microsculptured oberhautchen forming the outermost surface contacting the environment. The entire β-layer is derived from multiple cell layers. Beneath the β-layer is the mesos layer, consisting of several thin layers of keratin

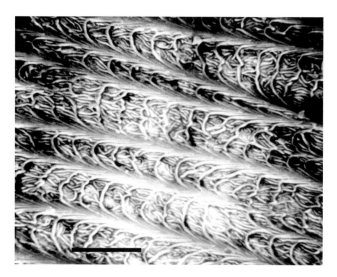

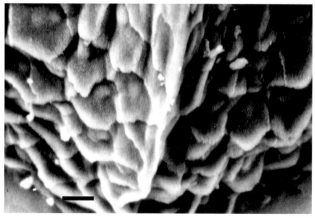

Figure 5.10. Scanning electronmicrographs illustrating microsculpturing on the surfaces of snake scales. The **upper photo** shows part of the dorsal scale from an African Stripe-bellied Sand Snake, *Psammophis subtaeniatus*. The surface oberhautchen in this species illustrates a pattern of ridges separated by shallow crevices sculptured with tertiary spaces and ridges. The rear (or caudal) end of the scale (and snake) is toward the right side of the micrograph. The **lower photo** features the rear part of the dorsal scale from a Russell's Viper, *Daboia russelii*. The oberhautchen scale surfaces in this species consist of elevated knobs or projections, each having a honeycombed surface and being increasingly elevated in the central part of the scale, which forms a "*keel*." The rear of the scale (and snake) is toward the bottom of the micrograph. Each black scale bar is 10 μm, and the lower micrograph is at a higher magnification than the upper one. Micrographs are by the author.

and the single layer of cells overlying the oberhautchen of the new inner generation is called the "clear layer." The tissue of the clear layer interdigitates with the sculptured surfaces of the inner (new) generation of oberhautchen and essentially "unzips" from it during the actual process of shedding when the two generations of epidermis separate. Thus, the shed "skin" that is lost from the snake at ecdysis consists of the outer generation β-layer (including oberhautchen) and α-layers of keratin, including the lacunar cells and clear layer.

The process of shedding is aided evidently by fluids that penetrate these tissues at the time of shedding, but the nature and control of such fluids are not well understood. The "fluid" may contain water and/or lipids and accounts for the generally damp nature of the shed generation of epidermis immediately after it is shed from the snake's body. Enzymes that degrade some of the clear layer and lacunar tissue are also present at the time of shedding.

Periodic shedding occurs in all snakes, and it seems that the general features of epidermal renewal are similar in all species. Characteristically, the renewal and shedding of the epidermis is a synchronized cycle of events that occur simultaneously over the entire body, rather than in patches. The periodicity of shedding, however, varies. Some snakes may shed their skins only once or twice per year, whereas others shed more frequently (sea snakes, for example). Because the keratin in the scales of snakes is a rigid material, shedding is required to permit growth. Thus, shedding can be expected to relate generally to the growth of snakes, and those snakes with the higher inputs of food might be expected to shed more frequently than others, assuming that all other factors are equal.

Other factors, however, can also influence the frequency of shedding, independently of growth per se. Sea snakes shed their skin relatively frequently, sometimes at two- to six-week intervals. One of the reasons is thought to relate to removal of fouling organisms that can tend to grow on the outer surfaces of these snakes. Barnacles, bryozoans, and algae have all been found growing on the skin of sea snakes (fig. 5.16). It is also thought that shedding is important to renew epidermis that might become damaged over time, likely involving minute breaks or fractures in the permeability barrier. Thus, an important function of shedding might also relate to renewal or possibly improvement of the permeability barrier in relation to environmental influences on water balance.

Many snakes shed their skin within a few days following birth or hatching. Working in my laboratory at the University of Florida, Ming-Chung Tu and I discovered that in California King Snakes (*Lampropeltis californiae*) this initial ecdysis results in a doubling of the skin resistance to evaporative water loss, and the resistance increases still further following the second ecdysis. These phenomena might explain some behaviors of newborn snakes, which often remain either with a parent in some viviparous species (e.g., certain pit vipers) or at the site of hatching from eggs until the first ecdysis, after which the young snakes disperse away from the site of birth. Remaining more reclusive right after birth might conserve evaporative losses of body water during the period before the first ecdysis when evidently the permeability barrier to water loss has not yet been established (see chapters 2 and 9).

Skin Color: Causes, Patterns, Significance

Colors are wonderful, and without them snakes would be far less interesting. Imagine if every snake you encountered or saw featured in a film was the same drab color of pink or gray. Boring? But, in fact, snakes have myriad colors and patterns of color in their skin, not all of which is genetically determined by the expression of pigments. First, we shall examine the physical basis of coloration, and then turn to some interesting topics related to its significance.

The Physical Basis of Color

What we call "color" results from the visual perception of specific wavelengths of electromagnetic radiation. Radiation wavelengths between 400 nm and 750 nm comprise what is called the "visible spectrum" of light, with reference to the visual capabilities of the human eye. Other animals, including some snakes, can perceive wavelengths somewhat outside this range. The colors we see are attributable to wavelengths of light that is reflected back from an object (say, skin) to enter our eyes, where it excites visual receptors that are categorically different depending on which wavelengths they are "tuned." This excitation of visual receptors is passed on to the parts of the brain responsible for interpreting visual sensation by means of nerve signals that pass along the appropriate pathway of interconnected neurons (single nerve cells). Wavelengths of light that are either absorbed by the skin or transmitted through it do not contribute to the colors we see. We see only the components of light that are reflected back to our eyes.

Skin color results from complex interactions among the chemical and physical properties of the tissue. What is known as *structural color* is that component of coloration which is attributable to physical features of the skin other than pigments. For example, the microsculpturing patterns on the surfaces of scales create patterns of wavelength interference that produce iridescent colors, especially prominent right after skin shedding, when the skin surfaces are new and clean (fig. 5.12). The physical properties and geometry of keratin organization in the skin can determine what wavelengths of light are selectively absorbed, refracted, or reflected. Fluorescence—the emission of light from a surface after it has absorbed radiation from an outside source—might possibly occur in a

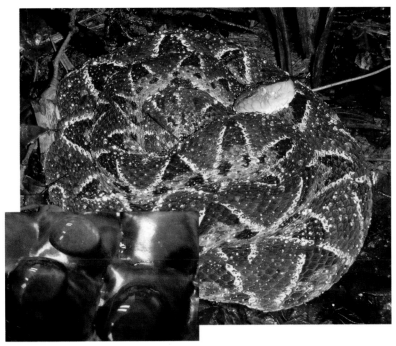

Figure 5.11. Water droplets are shown beaded on the surface of a Fer-de-Lance (*Bothrops asper*) photographed in Belize by Dan Dourson (**upper photo**). A higher magnification of the phenomenon is illustrated on the shed epidermis from a sea krait, *Laticauda semifasciata*, photographed by the author (**lower photo**). The scale surfaces are hydrophobic and repel water; thus the surface tension forces cause the water droplet to assume a near-spherical shape instead of spreading to form a flatter film.

species of blind snake (*Leptotyphlops humilis*), but the suggestion is anecdotal.

Most of the color we see in snake skin, however, is attributable to the presence and pattern of chemical compounds we call *pigments*. Most of the pigments involved are fixed within the skin, but the lighter skin regions of some snakes may turn from pinkish to white depending on the amount of blood that is flowing through the skin. In this case, the pink or reddish coloration is attributable in large part to reflectance of light from hemoglobin within the red blood cells. Hemoglobin is a respiratory pigment and carries oxygen around the body (see chapter 6). Nevertheless, it is called a pigment because of its light-reflecting properties that impart color to it.

Pigments that are fixed within the skin are synthesized within cells called *chromatophores*. There are four principal groups of chromatophores that contribute to the coloration of snakes. The more common, widespread, and better known of these is the *melanophore*, an irregular-shaped cell that contains the pigment *melanin*. Melanin is a dark pigment derived from the oxidation products of tyrosine and dihydroxyphenol compounds. The color can vary from dark red to dark brown or black. Melanins are present in the skin and are also found associated with some of the internal organs of an animal. There are two kinds of melanophores in the skin. Dermal melanophores are broad, flat cells that

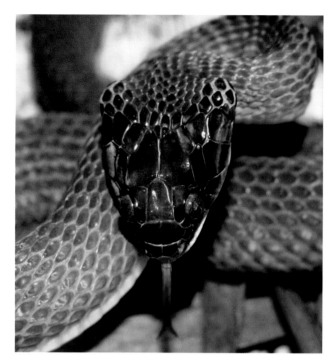

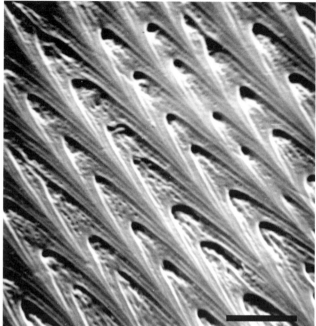

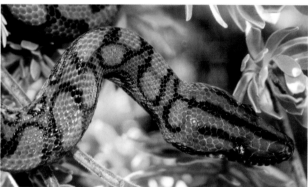

Figure 5.12. Photos of a Cross-barred Tree Snake (*Dipsadaboa flavida*) (**upper photo**) and a Rainbow Boa (*Epicrates cenchria*) (**lower photo**) illustrating iridescent scale colors attributable to structural features of the epidermal surfaces (not pigments). Note the blue and green colors on the edges of the scales and head plates, which are due to reflected light patterns dependent on the direction of lighting. Such structural colors are most vivid just after a snake has shed its skin. These are captive snakes owned by Ron Rozar and photographed by the author.

Figure 5.13. Microstructural projections on the surface of a ventral scute from the African Stripe-bellied Sand Snake, *Psammophis subtaeniatus*. The head-to-tail direction of the projections is from top to bottom in the photograph. The black scale bar at the bottom of the photograph equals 5 μm. Minute pores can be seen in the regions between the elevated projections running parallel with the length of the snake (arrows). Scanning electron micrograph by the author.

occur in the dermis, whereas epidermal melanophores (also called melanocytes) are thin, elongated cells that contribute pigment to regions of the epidermis. Once pigment is produced within melanocytes, it is "packaged" in a sense and transferred to epidermal cells (keratinocytes) that will produce keratin. Whether pigments are transferred between the dermis and epidermis is an entirely unresolved issue.

Pigment cells termed xanthophores contain oil-filled vesicles with suspended pigments called carotenes that are yellowish or orange in hue. The carotenes are taken up from the diet and are related to vitamin A. Pigment cells termed erythrophores contain oil with heterocyclic compounds called pteridines, and are reddish in color. Some consider the erythrophores to be a type of xanthophore that is reddish in color, in contrast to the other xanthophores that are yellow in color. Silvery chromatophores termed iridophores do not contain true pigments but contain crystals of guanine. Guanine is a purine that reflects light and imparts a noniridescent bluish or silvery white color. The color varies depending on the scattering of light and the surrounding pigments in the skin. They may also contain derivatives of other purines, and the combination of different crystals determines the variety of hues that are produced by diffraction, scattering, and reflection of light. The colors are structural and not attributable to true pigments. The different kinds of chromatophores may associate in the skin to produce various colors by virtue of their reflectance of light and their collective interference with reflected light.

In preserved snakes such as those in museum collections, the pigments contained in xanthophores and erythrophores are soluble in formalin or alcohol and thus slowly leach from the skin. Melanins are insoluble, so over time the colors of preserved snakes fade except for the patterns that are attributable to the distribution of melanins.

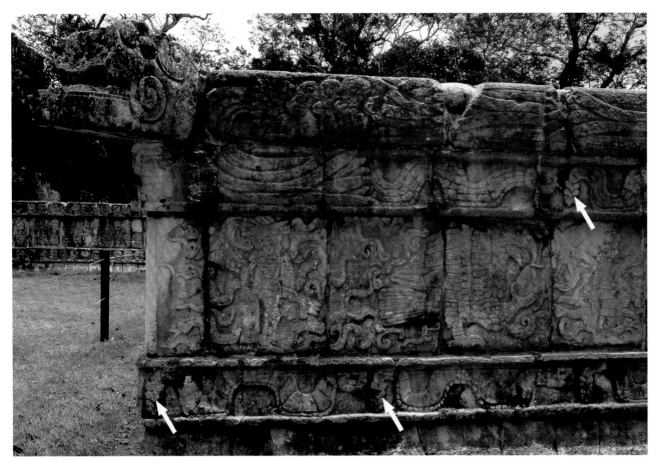

Figure 5.14. Part of the Mayan-Toltec ruins at Chichen Itza, Mexico. This wall is covered with iconography depicting many snakes, the larger one at the top representing the Mayan snake deity Kukulkan, or "Plumed Serpent." Feathers, or plumes, can be seen to decorate the stones at the top of the wall and just beneath it. Many of the other snakes represented in this stone structure clearly represent rattlesnakes. The white arrows point to some of the rattles at the tails of these stone serpents. Photograph by Ming-Chung Tu.

The Functions of Color Pattern

Anyone familiar with even a modest sampling of the diversity of snakes knows that they come in a variety of colors and patterns of color, which to the novice might not make much sense in terms of understanding reasons for the variation. Some snakes such as desert vipers appear quite well camouflaged against a background of sand (fig. 3.16), and thus we might suppose that diffuse, buff colors fit that purpose. Others seem brilliantly colored with amazing patterns of rings, bands, or blotches, and these are not necessarily *cryptic* (camouflaged). Still other snakes might appear dull when viewed from above, but the underside is a brilliant color that is obvious when presented by turning over or curling the tail (figs. 1.48, 1.50). Considering all that is known about these various color patterns reveals some generalizations regarding their function.

We begin by regarding color patterns to be phenotypic traits, which in some manner "fit" a snake to its environment. The contexts of "purpose" usually have to do with antipredator behaviors, social interactions, or the physical environment—for example, the relative heat absorption that influences body temperature. Investigations by Harvey Pough, James Jackson, and their coworkers suggest there is a correlation between the dorsal color pattern of snakes and the manner in which they respond to predators. Snakes with uniform colors or disruptive patterns of blotches, spots, or irregular crossbands tend to rely on crypsis, or concealment, to avoid being seen by potential predators. Some excellent examples are blotchy or speckled vipers that blend with their background when viewed upon rocky or course soils (fig. 1.25, 3.16); green or brown tree snakes that are concealed in green foliage or twigs and branches, respectively; and blotched or banded snakes when viewed among leaves (figs. 1.28, 1.29, 1.33, 3.16, 5.17). Many of these species also defend themselves with aggressive behaviors when the concealment fails. Thus, many viperid species will coil and strike when discovered by a human or other animal, rather than fleeing to escape. This behavior also tends to correlate with a lesser ability to crawl rapidly. These are generalizations, however, and there are many exceptions involving individuals or even species.

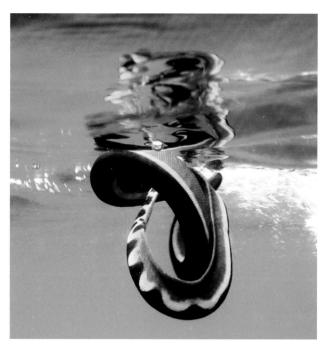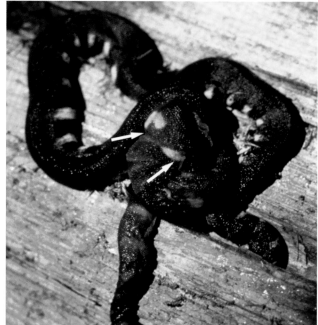

Figure 5.15. Left: Knotting behavior in a pelagic Yellow-bellied Sea Snake (*Pelamis platurus*) photographed in Costa Rica. The knotting behaviors of sea snakes are thought to be employed to remove debris and potentially settling ectoparasites (barnacles for example) as well as to remove old epidermis during skin shedding. The specimen shown in this photograph is not shedding its skin. **Right**: A Little File Snake (*Acrochordus granulatus*) photographed in the Philippines. The snake is outside of water to illustrate a "knot" that was being used to remove old epidermis during skin shedding. The arrows point to the location on the body where a tight coil (above arrowheads) is being used to push against part of the body where the old epidermis is sliding toward the tail and off the snake (below arrowheads). The old epidermis can also be seen as the wrinkled skin in the lower part of the photo. The greenish color is attributable to the presence of algae. The anterior part of the snake from which the skin has been removed is evident in the upper part of the photo. The photograph of *Pelamis* is by Joseph Pfaller, and that of the *Acrochordus* is by the author.

On the other hand, snakes that possess colors forming stripes or more uniform patterns than those discussed above tend to be more active and rely on rapid escape by fleeing away from potential predators. Herpetologist Edmund Brodie III found this to be true even within a species when he investigated color patterns of individuals of the Northwestern Garter Snake, *Thamnophis ordinoides*. Individuals of this species have colors that vary from distinct stripes to patterns of spots. When Brodie measured the tendencies of snakes to flee following provocation, he found that striped snakes tended to crawl away from the aggressor, whereas snakes with more blotched patterns were more likely to flee a short distance and then suddenly stop and assume a motionless position. Such behaviors are termed "reversals" and reflect a behavioral component of crypsis that is employed following the initial detection of an animal by a predator. It is a defensive tactic that does not rely greatly on speed. The behavior confuses a predator when a fleeing animal that is being followed rapidly and suddenly "disappears" (when it stops).

Optical illusions can be created by moving color patterns and their effects on visually foraging predators. Studies have found that the ability to perceive motion and the velocity of an object depends on the color pattern of the object and its surrounding field on which it moves. Striped snakes appear to be stationary when crawling slowly, and they can appear to be moving more slowly than they actually are. It is difficult for the eye of the predator to "fix" on a particular point on the fleeing snake and follow it, so the result can be that the stripe is seen momentarily but then suddenly the tail appears in a flash and the striped object vanishes! This optical illusion clearly has advantages for the escaping snake and suggests the striped pattern may be more effective in permitting escape than does some other color patterns when fleeing is involved. The striped pattern becomes more apparent with increasing size of garter snakes, and the tendency to flee from threats intensifies in older striped individuals of *Thamnophis ordinoides*.

Ed Brodie III also studied natural selection for combinations of color pattern and escape behavior in a population of *T. ordinoides*. Newborn snakes that were scored for behavior and color pattern in the laboratory were released into the wild, and their survival was followed by mark and recapture techniques. Snakes with the highest probability of survival performed uninterrupted flight if striped, but tended to flee evasively by performing reversals if they were

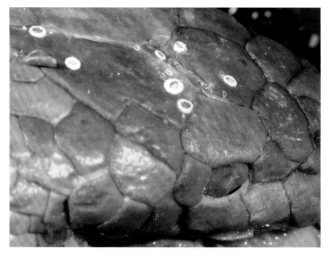

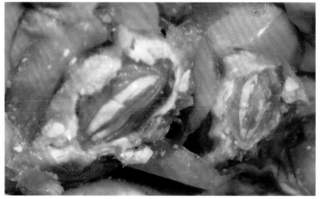

Figure 5.16. Barnacles encrusting into the skin atop the head of an Olive-headed Sea Snake, *Disteria major*. The lower photo shows a closer-up view of two such barnacles. Photographs by Sara E. Murphy.

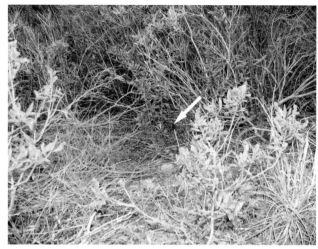

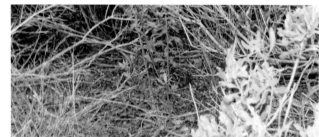

spotted or nonstriped. The covariation of color pattern and behavior help to explain the variation of color pattern that is seen in natural populations of this species.

Another important function of snake colors is that of a warning signal to predators. The warning function is termed *aposematism* and is probably best known in coral snakes of the genera *Micrurus* and *Micruroides*. These snakes are conspicuously colored with usually red, yellow, and black bands, which function as a warning signal to avian predators. Aposematic colors are most effective when they contrast strongly with that of the animal's background, and the warning colors tend to be avoided by would-be predators. Such contrasting colors have also been shown, or suspected, to be aposematic in other species of snakes including some sea snakes, other elapids, colubrids, and viperids (figs. 1.14, 1.41, 1.52 and below).

A very interesting example of an aposematic color pattern occurs in European Vipers, *Vipera berus*, which have a dorsal zigzag pattern that has been shown to be aposematic. The zigzag pattern of European vipers is not very conspicuous and could also have both a cryptic and aposematic

Figure 5.17. An Eastern Diamondback Rattlesnake (*Crotalus adamanteus*) resting on a sand dune at Sapelo Island, Georgia. From a distance (**upper photo**) the snake (arrow) is almost completely cryptic and difficult to see. At reasonably close range (**middle photo**) the snake remains cryptic. Only if the observer is right upon the snake does it become conspicuous (**lower photo**). Photographs by James Nifong.

function (fig. 1.25). The dorsal colors can reduce the detection by avian predators while the snake is coiled motionless, but change into a highly conspicuous and characteristic signal once the snake has been seen. Moreover, the pattern can create a "flicker-fusion" illusion during movement, which makes it difficult for a predator to focus on a moving snake and thereby increases the chances for escape. Many snakes are brightly banded, and during rapid crawling movement the bands create a similar effect, or they blur to produce a seemingly uniform color that also enhances escape by fleeing. A similar effect occurs in swimming sea snakes, many of which have banded coloration (figs. 1.43, 1.45).

Numerous venomous snakes possess potent venom and irritable defensive behaviors, but are cryptically colored and not conspicuously marked like the European vipers. The use of such weak color signals combined with strong defenses is a common phenomenon (see writings by John Endler). Many snakes are preyed upon largely by birds, and a number of these birds are specialists that feed primarily on snakes. If some predators avoid venomous snakes because of their coloration, while others do not, it makes sense to employ a color strategy that involves crypsis to avoid being seen by predators, while also having an aposematic function once an individual is seen.

Other examples of warning coloration include tail curling or exposure of ventral surfaces, which are brightly colored in various species of snakes (figs. 1.48, 1.50). The arboreal Red-tailed Rat Snake (*Gonyosoma oxycephalum*) of Southeast Asia presents blue colors to predators when it is in a defensive attitude, and similar defenses have also evolved in other arboreal species. The blue colors are sometimes revealed when body scales are spread apart by neck inflation, or when the mouth is opened or the tongue is flicked (fig. 5.18; see also fig. 6.19).

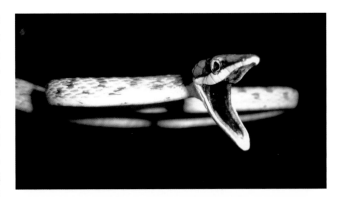

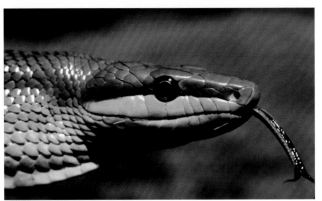

Figure 5.18. The **upper photo** shows the open mouth of a Brown (or Mexican) Vine Snake (*Oxybelis aeneus*) and reveals dark blue coloration that is displayed within. In the **lower photo** one sees the blue colors that decorate the tongue of a Red-tailed Rat Snake (*Gonyosoma oxycephalum*). This species also displays a dark blue spot on the inside of the mouth when it is opened in a threatening defensive display. The vine snake was photographed by Dan Dourson in Belize; the rat snake was photographed by the author.

Mimicry

The term *mimicry* refers to the phenomenon where organisms resemble one another in context of gaining an advantage in the avoidance of predators. Studies of coral snakes, in particular, have demonstrated the existence of mimicry systems in which harmless snakes resemble or "mimic" coral snakes in color pattern and thereby gain the benefit of signaling avoidance to avian predators (fig. 5.19; see also figs. 1.14, 1.52). Field studies by Ed Brodie III have provided direct evidence that avian predators avoid banded patterns of model snakes. Thus, there appears to be a generalized avoidance by free-ranging avian predators of ring patterns resembling those of coral snakes. Other plausible but less tested systems might involve mimicry of viperid body form and coloration by snakes such as American hognose snakes (*Heterodon* spp.; see fig. 1.49), or spreading the neck in a cobra-like fashion among various colubrid species of snakes. Many such displays occur in snakes that are not sympatric with an appropriate model species, however, and are likely to represent convergent evolution of defensive tactics (fig. 5.20).

Mimicry involving snakes might also extend to other kinds of organisms. For example, coloration of some tropical insects appears to mimic snakes, and the sophistication of the resemblance can be indeed remarkable (fig. 5.21). Tropical millipedes with ringed patterns might also gain some advantage in resembling ringed patterns of snakes, but this is simply speculation at present.

Melanism

Melanism refers to excessive pigmentation or blackening of the skin, usually determined by genetics and having evolutionary origin. In some cases, melanism is determined by recessive homozygotes at a single gene locus. The significance of melanism has attracted the attention of biologists since the 19th century. As in other reptiles, birds and mammals, melanism is quite common in snakes. In some circumstances, the melanism in individuals may be partial, and populations may reflect a mixture of melanistic and normally colored individuals representing either rare or well-established polymorphism. There are several plausible advantages for melanistic individuals, depending on the environment, ecology, and behavior of a species.

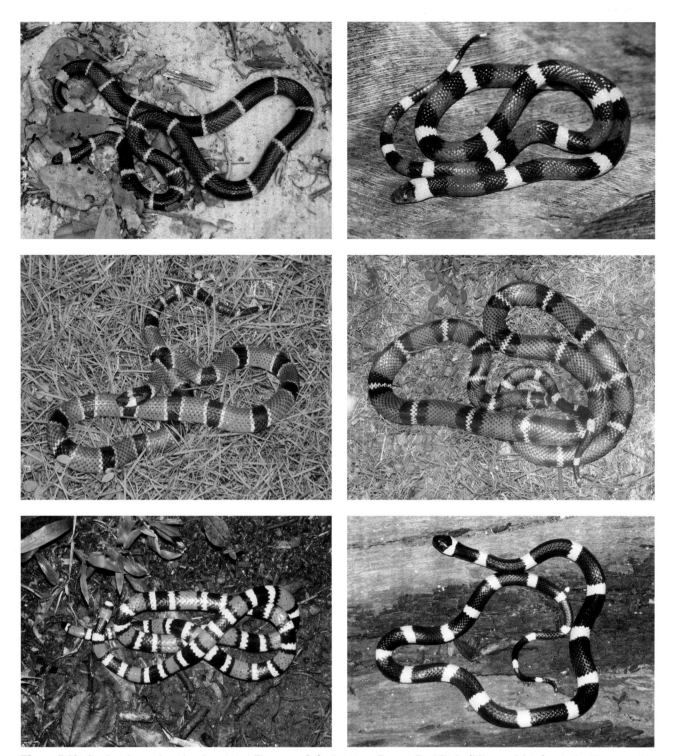

Figure 5.19. Coral snakes and coral snake mimics. The **upper left** photo is an Eastern Coral Snake (*Micrurus fulvius*), paired with a sympatric mimic (**upper right**), a Scarlet King Snake (*Lampropeltis elapsoides*). The **middle left** photo is a Central American Coral Snake (*Micrurus nigrocinctus*), paired with a sympatric mimic (**middle right**), a Black Milk Snake (*Lampropeltis triangulum gaigeae*). The **lower left** photo features a Brazilian Coral Snake (*Micrurus decoratus*), and the **lower right** photo features a Terrestrial Snail Sucker (*Tropidodipsas sartorii*) that is common throughout much of Central America. Note the variation of banding and ring patterns, all of which can have a generalized advantage of being avoided by avian predators. The *Micrurus fulvius* was photographed in Florida by Dan Dourson. The other snakes were photographed by the author: *Lampropeltis elapsoides* in south Florida; *Lampropeltis triangulum*, *Micrurus nigrocinctus*, and *Tropidodipsas* in Costa Rica; and *Micrurus decoratus* in Itatiaia National Park, Brazil.

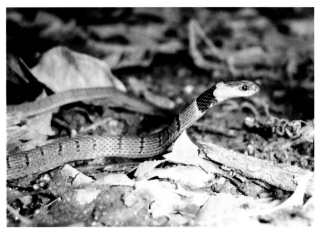

Figure 5.20. A Red Coffee Snake (*Nina sebae*) with threatening display. This snake is normally secretive and when uncovered it typically remains motionless (a behavior that has earned it the name "dormiloma," meaning "sleepyhead," in parts of Mexico). However, when startled or disturbed the snake may dorsoventrally flatten its neck and part of its body, crawl forward, and elevate its head. The snake also thrashes or moves its body jerkily to keep its red-colored back facing toward a potential predator. Such a head and neck display is relatively rare in snakes that are this small (maximum length 40 cm) and probably serves to make the snake look larger or more threatening. This snake was photographed in Belize by Dan Dourson.

One advantage clearly is cryptic in cases where black or very dark individuals match a dark background (figs. 5.22, 5.23). Examples are darkly colored specimens of the Southwestern Speckled Rattlesnake, *Crotalus mitchellii pyrrhus*, which occur on dark lava rock flows, as mentioned earlier, and the Arizona Black Rattlesnake, *C. cerberus*, which has a limited range in the vicinity of black lava outflows from an ancient volcano (fig. 5.22). Another context for crypsis is a match of dark skin color against charred backgrounds or objects that result from wildfires. From personal experience, I know that Southern Pacific Rattlesnakes (*C. oreganus helleri*, fig. 4.6) tend to be very dark in regions of Southern California that have had a history of frequent fires. Although wildfires are an ephemeral event, selection is very intense for perhaps one to three or four years afterward because of increased appearance of aerial predators that tend to forage in the open habitat. Moreover, charred stalks from shrubs tend to remain dark in color for many years, and the author has often confused these momentarily for snakes while walking through recently burned habitats.

Another adaptive context for melanism is a presumptive advantage for more rapid warming and thermoregulation in relatively cool environments. This has been shown to play an important role in a number of lizard species, as well as in garter snakes and melanistic color morphs of the European Adder, *Vipera berus*. Ralph Gibson, Bruce Falls, Tonya Bittner, and others have demonstrated that melanistic adult garter

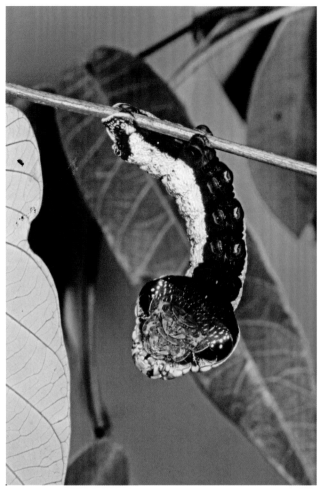

Figure 5.21. A Brazilian Hawkmoth caterpillar (*Hemeroplanes ornatus*, = *Leucorampha ornatus*) inflates itself to resemble a snake when it is frightened by a potential predator. The resemblance is amazing, and the caterpillar sways from side to side in effort to improve the resemblance. The would-be predator might even think the false snake is striking! Photograph by Lincoln Brower.

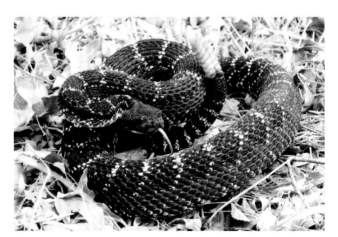

Figure 5.22. An Arizona Black Rattlesnake (*Crotalus cerberus*) illustrating the predominantly black color that renders this snake cryptic when seen against dark rocks that are part of an ancient lava flow associated with its range. Photograph by William B. Montgomery.

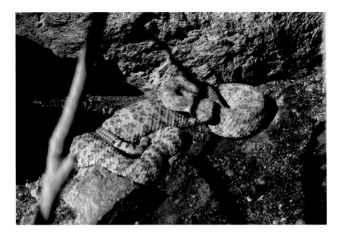

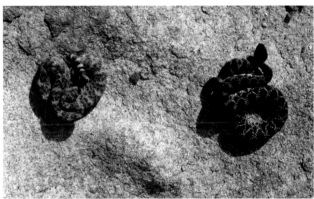

Figure 5.23. The **upper photo** features a Southwestern Speckled Rattlesnake (*Crotalus mitchellii pyrrhus*) that has emerged from a granite rock outcrop that was blackened by a recent wildfire. The charred rocks in this habitat are typically pinkish-orange in color, which matches the color of the snake. The **lower photo** illustrates the normal pink color of rocks in the vicinity (before the fire). The snake to the **left** is another Southwestern Speckled Rattlesnake (*C. m. pyrrhus*), and that to the **right** is a Southern Pacific Rattlesnake (*C. oreganus helleri*). This photograph was taken in the early morning, and shadows unintentionally exaggerate the dark colors. The speckled rattlesnake matches the rock more closely after it warms up and its colors lighten akin to the one in the upper photograph. The Southern Pacific Rattlesnake, on the other hand, is naturally quite black. It is an obvious mismatch of color with the pink rock, but it is relatively camouflaged on the blackened substrate following a fire. These snakes were photographed by the author in the southern Laguna Mountains of San Diego County, California.

snakes (*Thamnophis sirtalis*) maintain significantly higher body temperatures (by about 1.3°C) during the colder periods of the day when compared with normally colored morphs of this species. The higher body temperatures can influence rates of metabolism and growth of individuals, leading to increased reproductive success. Black morphs might also be active for somewhat longer periods of a year. However, melanistic individuals of a species may occur at particular locations, or at moderate to relatively low frequencies in a population, due to being conspicuous and subject to increased predation. The increased predation risk was demonstrated

for melanistic color morphs in an island population of *Vipera berus* by Claes Andrén and Göran Nilson.

Another function of dark pigmentation is protection of reproductive and other critical organs from harmful ultraviolet radiation. In various species, and particularly in those inhabiting open habitats with intense sunlight, dense layers of melanin can be found in the internal thin membranous tissues that surround the gut (called *peritoneum*), reproductive organs, and venom glands of venomous snakes. These internal melanins, in addition to those present in the skin, are thought to protect sensitive internal organs from the harmful effects of penetrating UV radiation. Changes in the amount of melanin and its dispersion throughout the skin significantly affect the amount of radiation that penetrates the body wall. Studies of color-labile desert lizards by Warren Porter and Kenneth Norris have demonstrated that lightening of the skin color doubles the amount of UV and visible radiation that penetrates the body wall to the peritoneum and is potentially mutagenic judged by effects on bacteria. Hence, the so-called "black peritoneum" is an important shield that guards against incoming radiation.

Changes of Color Pattern

The color patterns of snakes are generally fixed, and the lability (especially short-term variation) of color change in any individual is not as pronounced as what occurs in some other taxa such as frogs, lizards, and fishes. However, it is fairly common for snakes to exhibit significant change of color pattern during development, with juveniles exhibiting blotched or banded patterns that transform to uniformly colored or striped patterns in adults. In some cases, the changes in color pattern correspond with changes in behavior and appear to be related to crypsis or escape strategies. For example, juvenile Cottonmouths (*Agkistrodon piscivorus*) are orange or brownish in color with patterns of blotches and crossbands, whereas the adults are more uniformly colored brown or black (fig. 1.32 cf. fig. 2.28). The colors of the juveniles tend to provide crypsis related to a tendency of young snakes to spend more time immobile in situations where there are leaves or other ground vegetation in contrast to adults, which forage nocturnally in shallow water or muddy banks of ponds and streams. Put another way, the color pattern of juvenile cottonmouths resemble somewhat closely the color pattern of the related Copperhead (*Agkistrodon contortix*), which is very inconspicuous when coiled amid the leaf litter of a hardwood forest (fig. 1.32). Unfortunately, there are no quantitative data to confirm the tendency of juvenile cottonmouths to coil among leaf litter in comparison with the behaviors of adults.

Studies of the racer *Coluber constrictor* by Douglas Creer demonstrated that newborn and juvenile racers were more likely than adults to exhibit aggressive behavior in contrast to fleeing that is more characteristic of adults. The young snakes have a blotched color pattern in contrast with adults, which develop a more uniform color ranging from blue or brown to black. Generally, however, the significance of ontogenetic color changes in snakes is not well understood.

The changes of color that occur during ontogeny involve fixed pigment patterns that do not vary substantially from day to day, and the transformation from juvenile to adult patterns is an example of what is called *morphological color change*. These take place over the lifetime of an individual, or might describe evolutionary changes in which the color pattern of a species changes over relatively long periods of evolutionary time. On the other hand, shorter-term changes can occur over periods of minutes to hours in individuals experiencing hormonal or nervous stimulation of chromatophores, termed *physiological color change*. While common in some other animals, such changes are comparatively rare in snakes, but they do occur. The distinction is that physiological changes involve the movement of pigment (usually melanin) into or out of dermal melanophore processes (to cause darkening or lightening, respectively) whereas morphological color changes involve increases or decreases in the absolute numbers of melanophores that are present in the skin.

Physiological color change has been documented in several families of snakes including viperids, boids, tropidophiids, bolyeriids, and colubrids. In many cases it seems to be cyclical and related to activity or 24-hour light cycles. In other cases, colors may vary seasonally and might be difficult to detect by human visual systems. Scott Boback and Lynn Siefferman studied such phenomena in Boa Constrictors and suggested that physiological color changes can be related to underlying hormone cycles involving *melatonin* and *melanophore stimulating hormone* (or MSH). The patterns of color changes in snakes have probably evolved in relation to crypsis, thermoregulation, and sexual signaling in various species.

Some rattlesnakes tend to lighten with increased temperature or activity, and hormonal control of the relative state of melanin dispersion has been suggested to constitute the mechanism for controlling these changes. Early studies by Hermann Rahn revealed that high temperatures contracted melanophores in rattlesnakes, and the state of lightening resembled that seen in response to surgical removal of the pituitary gland, which eliminates the melanophore dispersing actions of pituitary hormones.

The Speckled Rattlesnake, *Crotalus mitchellii*, of the southwestern United States seems to be particularly labile in color pattern. Specimens that are captured on or near lava flows in the Mojave Desert appear nearly slate gray in color, whereas individuals captured on nearby areas of sand or light substrate can be a peppered whitish color in appearance. The author has also seen specimens of variable colors that generally match the predominant soils or rocks with which they associate, ranging from darker gray or bluish tones through lighter, usually pinkish colors. Moreover, these snakes appear capable of changing their dorsal color pattern to match not only the basic ground color but also the speckled appearance of granite rocks in their habitat. Nonetheless, the fundamental ground color of these snakes appears to become "fixed" sometime during early ontogeny (fig. 5.23).

Acquisition of Color Directly from Environment
Genetically based color patterns can also be affected by the adherence of dirt or mud particles that a snake contacts directly in its environment. Generally, the skin of snakes is kept exceptionally clean due, in part, to the hydrophobic nature of the microstructural properties of the epidermis. However, snakes that frequent muddy environments such as stream banks, or which occur in dry habitats with wind-blown dirt or sand, can accumulate a thin layer of debris that alters the normal skin color. One example is the adherence of mud to the skin of Cottonmouth snakes that crawl over muddy surfaces associated with stream banks or ponds (fig. 5.24).

Genetics of Snake Coloration
The genetics of skin color is not well studied in snakes, and much knowledge of genetic systems and expression related to coloration has been derived from investigations of other animals. Investigations of snake colors arise, however, in relation to two principal interests. First, evolutionary biologists interested in coloration, evolutionary principles, or natural selection recognize that snakes offer a diversity of fascinating color systems and are subject to selection pressures that provide useful experimental systems for understanding the underlying genetic mechanisms related to certain patterns or variation. Second, herpetoculturists are interested in breeding various mutant lines of color variants that have become popular in the pet trade. Various private and commercial breeding programs have yielded information about fundamental Mendelian genetics of color in various strains or subspecies of interest to buyers. Much of the knowledge related to these breeding programs has not been published in the scientific literature, but is available from various individuals who are involved (fig. 5.25).

Skin color in snakes and in other vertebrates can be subject to relatively rapid natural selection and expressed by

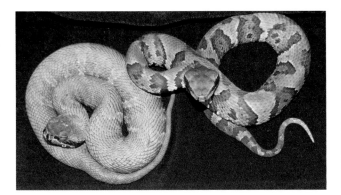

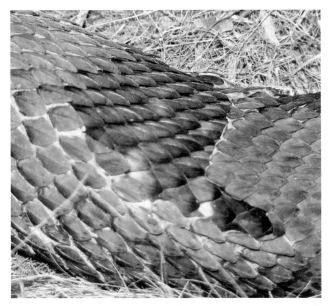

Figure 5.24. Florida Cottonmouths (*Agkistrodon piscivorus conanti*) with skin colored by a superficial layer of dried mud that occurs in the snake's natural habitat (Lower Suwannee National Wildlife Refuge). In the **upper photo**, two juvenile snakes are shown before (left) and after (right) shedding the skin. In the **lower photo**, an older individual from the same region is shown with part of the old epidermis removed just prior to skin shedding. The older, outer generation of epidermis is covered with a layer of dry mud from the animal's habitat, whereas the new skin revealed beneath is an entirely different color before it becomes covered with adhering mud particles. Photographs by the author.

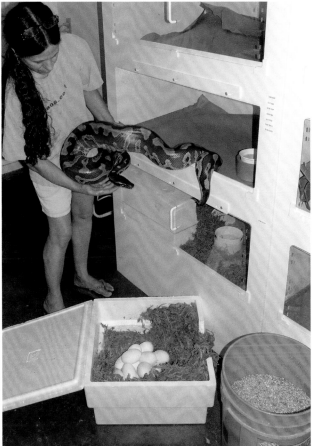

Figure 5.25. A working scene at Vida Preciosa International, Inc., better known as VPI. This is a commercial enterprise owned and operated by David and Tracy Barker near San Antonio, Texas. VPI is best known for its collection and captive breeding of pythons. Here Tracy is shown preparing eggs from the cage of a Red Blood Python (*Python brongersmai*) for artificial incubation. Successful captive breeding of various python species at VPI has produced numerous color variants, many of which are related to natural taxonomic and geographic variation. Photograph by David Barker.

comparatively simple genetic mechanisms. The production of melanin in snakes is controlled by a single pair of genes, which when recessive can result in albinism. Unlike mammals, however, an albino snake has normal amounts of red and yellow in the skin so the condition is more appropriately referred to as *amelanistic partial albinism*. Additionally, there are probably a number of genetic defects that are capable of producing amelanistic partial albinism. There is great variation in the quantity of black that is present in the skin, and the quantity can also be controlled by multiple alleles (alternate forms of a specific gene). There is a clear suggestion in some species that melanin related to color pattern is inherited differently from melanin that is scattered more diffusely throughout the skin.

A number of snake species become melanistic or variously darkened with age. Examples are the Northern Black Racer (*Coluber c. constrictor*), which is very black as an adult, the Eastern Hognose Snake (*Heterodon p. platyrhinos*), in which melanistic individuals are normal color variants, and insular Florida Cottonmouths (*Agkistrodon piscivorus conanti*), which darken to nearly uniform black color earlier in life than do conspecifics on the mainland (see color of the adult snake in the upper part of fig. 1.32). Some Eastern Garter Snakes (*Thamnophis s. sirtalis*) from nearshores of the Great Lakes are born jet black, and early breeding experiments suggested this to be attributable to a single pair of recessive genes. Subsequent work, however, has put this supposition into doubt. Richard Zweifel suggested that

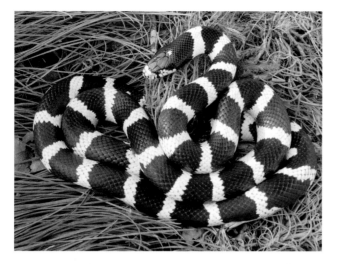

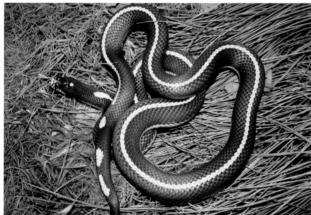

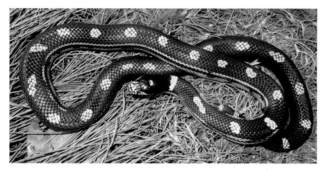

Figure 5.26. Three different color phases of the California King Snake (*Lampropeltis californiae*). The banded phase (**top**) is the more common form of this snake in the wild. The striped form (**center**) is less common but occurs somewhat commonly in the vicinity of San Diego. The spotted form (**bottom**) is quite rare but illustrates further variation of pattern in this species. These photos also illustrate variation of the ground color that ranges from brown to black. Photographs by the author.

melanism in this species may depend not only on genetic constitution but also on environmental influence, for example, cold temperature.

There is much normal variation in color pattern in species and populations of snakes, related to individual variation, ontogenetic changes, regional geographic differences,

and pattern dimorphism or polymorphism within a species. Color anomalies are noted by herpetologists from time to time in wild-caught snakes, and various abnormal patterns likely reflect genetic mutations or abnormal changes in genetic expression. A classical example of pattern dimorphism is seen in the California King Snake, *Lampropeltis californiae*. The usual color pattern consists of alternating black and white (or brown and yellow) bands, but an alternate pattern consists of a white stripe running lengthwise along the center of the back (fig. 5.26). The majority of snakes throughout the range of this species exhibit the banded pattern, but in the vicinity of San Diego about 40 percent of specimens exhibit the longitudinally striped pattern. Both patterns occur in snakes from the same litter and represent a natural dimorphism, the striped pattern having originated as a genetic mutation.

Finally, an interesting example of color polymorphism involves the Yellow-bellied Sea Snake (*Pelamis platurus*). This pelagic species has the largest range of any snake species and exhibits extensive variation of color and pattern. Most individuals have black or brown coloration largely restricted to the dorsal surface, mixed with spots, stripes, bands, or mottling of yellow, which predominates on the ventral surface (fig. 1.44). The tail is usually a mottled combination of black and yellow or white. All-yellow individuals have been reported from certain localities in Costa Rica and Panama. In particular, there appears to be a localized population of all-yellow individuals in the Golfo Dulce of southern Costa Rica (fig. 5.27). Alejandro Solórzano suggests that this population is relatively isolated within the gulf because of circulation patterns of surface currents within and outside the gulf. Preliminary evidence suggests that such isolation by currents might restrict gene flow between oceanic and gulf populations and contribute to what appears to be population differentiation.

Conclusions concerning Color Polymorphisms

The variability of snake coloration includes variation within populations and species, and this likely reflects, in large part, interactions with the environment and especially threats of predation. Snakes are very attractive prey to birds, and avian predation pressures can be very significant. To the extent that intraspecific color variation reflects polymorphisms, ecological and evolutionary consequences promote color "ecomorphs" involving coadapted complexes of genes. Recent comparative analysis of Australian squamates by Anders Forsman and Viktor Åberg demonstrates that species with variable color patterns have larger ranges, utilize a greater diversity of habitats, and are less likely to be threatened with extinction. These findings likely reflect theoretical predictions that variable color patterns, or *color polymorphisms*, enable a species to increase the efficiency

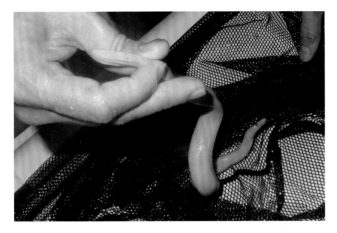

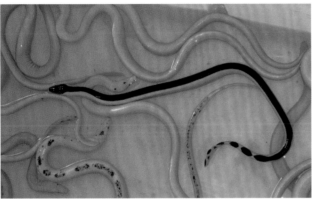

Figure 5.27. Yellow-bellied Sea Snakes (*pelamis platurus*) captured from a population of yellow color morphs at Golfo Dulce, Puntarenas, Costa Rica, and photographed by the author. Most of the snakes in this population are completely yellow, but a more "normal" bicolored snake is shown in the lower photograph for contrast with the yellow specimens as well as a snake that has diffuse black mottling on its dorsal surface.

with which it exploits resources of the environment through increased ability to utilize varied environments and to extend its range. Thus, snakes provide excellent model systems in which studies of coloration can reveal important principles related to population and evolutionary processes. On the other hand, snakes are fundamentally exquisitely colorful animals, and one does not need additional justification to enjoy the beauty that stimulates our raw emotions.

Additional Reading

Andrén, C., and G. Nilson. 1981. Reproductive success and risk of predation in normal and melanistic colour morphs of the adder, *Vipera berus*. *Biological Journal of the Linnean Society* 15:235–246.

Avolio, C., R. Shine, and A. J. Pyle. 2006. The adaptive significance of sexually dimorphic scale rugosity in sea snakes. *American Naturalist* 167:728–738.

Bechtel, H. B. 1995. *Reptile and Amphibian Variants: Colors, Patterns and Scales*. Malabar, FL: Krieger Publishing

Bittner, T. D., R. B. King, and J. M. Kerfin. 2002. Effects of body size and melanism on the thermal biology of garter snakes (*Thamnophis sirtalis*). *Copeia* 2002:477–482.

Boback, S. M., and L. M. Siefferman. 2010. Variation in color and color change in island and mainland boas (*Boa constrictor*). *Journal of Herpetology* 44:506–515.

Brodie, E. D., III. 1989. Genetic correlations between morphology and antipredator behavior in natural populations of the garter snake *Thamnophis ordinoides*. *Nature* 342:542–543.

Brodie, E.D., III. 1990. Genetics of the garter's getaway. *Natural History* 99:44–50.

Brodie, E. D., III. 1992. Correlational selection for color pattern and antipredator behavior in the garter snake *Thamnophis ordinoides*. *Evolution* 46:1284–1298.

Brodie, E. D., III. 1993. Differential avoidance of coral snake banded patterns by free-ranging avian predators in Costa Rica. *Evolution* 47:227–235.

Brodie, E. D., III, and F. J. Janzen. 1995. Experimental studies of coral snake mimicry: Generalized avoidance of ringed snake patterns by free-ranging avian predators. *Functional Ecology* 9:186–190.

Creer, D. A. 2005. Correlations between ontogenetic change in color pattern and antipredator behavior in the racer, *Coluber constrictor*. *Ethology* 111:287–300.

Endler, J. A., and J. Mappes. 2004. Predator mixes and the conspicuousness of aposematic signals. *American Naturalist* 163:532–547.

Forsman, A., and V. Åberg. 2008. Associations of variable coloration with niche breadth and conservation status among Australian reptiles. *Ecology* 89:1201–1207.

Gibson, A. R., and J. B. Falls. 1979. Thermal biology of the common garter snake *Thamnophis sirtalis* (L.). II. The effects of melanism. *Oecologia* 43:99–109.

Hedges, S. B., C. A. Hass, and T. K. Maugel. 1989. Physiological color change in snakes. *Journal of Herpetology* 23:450–455.

Hulse, A. C. 1971. Fluorescence in *Leptotyphlops humilis* (Serpentes: Leptotyphlopidae). *Southwestern Naturalist* 16:123–124.

Jackson, J. F., W. Ingram III, and H. W. Campbell. 1976. The dorsal pigmentation pattern of snakes as an antipredator strategy: A multivariate approach. *American Naturalist* 110:1029–1053.

Lillywhite, H. B. 2006. Water relations of tetrapod integument. *Journal of Experimental Biology* 209:202–226.

Lillywhite, H. B., and P. F. A. Maderson. 1982. Skin structure and permeability. In C. Gans and F. H. Pough (eds.), *Biology of the Reptilia*, vol. 12, *Physiology C, Physiological Ecology*. New York: Academic Press, pp. 379–442.

Maderson, P. F. A. 1965. Histological changes in the epidermis of snakes during the sloughing cycle. *Journal of Zoology* (London) 146:98–113.

Maderson, P. F. A. 1984. The squamate epidermis: New light has been shed. *Symposium of the Zoological Society of London* 52:111–126.

Maderson, P. F. A. 1985. Some developmental problems of the reptilian integument. In C. Gans, F. Billett, and P. F. A. Maderson (eds.), *Biology of the Reptilia*, vol. 14, *Development A*. New York: John Wiley & Sons, pp. 523–598.

Maderson, P. F. A., K. W. Chiu, and J. G. Phillips. 1070. Endocrine-epidermal relationships in squamate reptiles. *Memoirs of the Society for Endocrinology* 18:259–284.

Maderson, P. F. A., T. Rabinowitz, B. Tandler, and L. Alibardi. 1998. Ultrastructural contributions to an understanding of the cellular mechanisms in lizard skin shedding with comments on the function and evolution of a unique lepidosaurian phenomenon. *Journal of Morphology* 236:1–24.

Niskanen, M., and J. Mappes. 2005. Significance of the dorsal zig-zag pattern of *Vipera latastei gaditana* against avian predators. *Journal of Animal Ecology* 74:1091–1101.

Porter, W. P., and K. S. Norris. 1969. Lizard reflectivity change and its effect on light transmission through body wall. *Science* 163:482–484.

Pough, F. H. 1976. Multiple cryptic effects of cross-banded and ringed patterns of snakes. *Copeia* 1976:834–836.

Rahn, H. 1942. Effect of temperature on color change in the rattle-snake. *Copeia* 1942:178.

Sheehy, C. M., III, A. Solórzano, J. B. Pfaller, and H. B. Lillywhite. 2012. Preliminary insights into the phylogeography of the Yellow-bellied Sea Snake, *Pelamis platurus. Integrative and Comparative Biology* 52:321–330.

Solórzano, A. 2011. Variación de color de la serpiente marina *Pelamis platura* (Serpentes: Elapidae) en el Golfo Dulce, Puntarenas, Costa Rica. *Cuadernos de Investigación UNED* 3:89–96.

Tu, M.-C., H. B. Lillywhite, J. G. Menon, and G. K. Menon. 2002. Postnatal ecdysis establishes the permeability barrier in snake skin: New insights into lipid barrier structures. *Journal of Experimental Biology* 205:3019–3030.

Zweifel, R. G. 1998. Apparent non-Mendelian inheritance of melanism in the garter snake *Thamnophis sirtalis. Herpetologica* 54:83–87.

INTERNAL TRANSPORT

Circulation and Respiration

> As is well-known, snakes have a tendency to secrete themselves in very confining quarters and they are capable of passing through relatively small apertures and channels. It was noted earlier that the air sac reduces the changes in diameter necessary for ventilation. Possibly of greater importance in the present context is the fact that if one region of the body is entirely immobilized ventilation can be maintained by regions that are free. In attempting to record breathing movements by means of mechanical levers and cuff pneumographs it was found that most snakes are very sensitive to pressure on their ribs. Almost invariably the region in contact with the cuff ceases movement and ventilation is taken up elsewhere. It is reasonable to suppose that a similar reaction occurs in nature when a snake passes through a narrow passage.
>
> —*Harry S. McDonald, Herpetologica 15 (1959): 195*

The Need for Oxygen

Just like any other vertebrate, a snake requires oxygen in order to remain alive. Oxygen is required for cellular *respiration*, which in the strictest sense refers to the intracellular oxidation of organic substrates by molecular oxygen, coupled in turn to the generation of usable energy that becomes trapped in the molecular form of ATP. The organic substrates consist of macromolecules that are derived from the processes of digestion and absorption of the food that snakes eat. The well-known by-products of respiration are CO_2 and H_2O. The latter is called *metabolic water* and actually makes a small, but sometimes significant, contribution to the water input of an animal (see chapter 2). In more popular and lay usage, the term "respiration" is often used (inaccurately) as a name for the process of exchange of O_2 and CO_2 between the animal and its environment. The term *external respiration* is sometimes used in reference to breathing, which more accurately should be called *ventilation.*

Oxygen is acquired from the environment, while CO_2 escapes the body and dissipates to the environment. Both processes are fundamentally essential to life. Collectively, these are referred to as *gas exchange*, and any organ that evolves specifically for this task is called a *gas exchanger*. In the case of snakes, the gas exchanger is a lung, although some aquatic species can supplement pulmonary exchange (meaning "lung" exchange) with some intake of O_2 and losses of CO_2 across the skin. Internally, the oxygen is transported throughout the body by means of the blood circulation, which also transports CO_2 from the various body tissues back to the lung and skin (fig. 6.1).

Diffusion versus Convection: The Need for a Pump

The movement of gaseous molecules such as O_2 and CO_2 is by diffusion across the internal lung surfaces and from blood capillaries to the mitochondria of cells where the oxidation processes involving oxygen occur. The term *diffusion* refers to the movement of molecules by random motion that depends on the temperature and a gradient of concentration difference. The net movement occurs from higher to lower concentration (or, in the case of gases, partial pressure). Diffusion is a slow process, however, and in a moderate size snake—say, a boa that is 3 or 4 meters long—it would require literally a few years for oxygen to diffuse through tissues from the lung at the anterior quarter of the animal to the tissues in its tail! Thus, animals larger than a few centimeters in size, including all vertebrates, depend on the process of convection to speed the

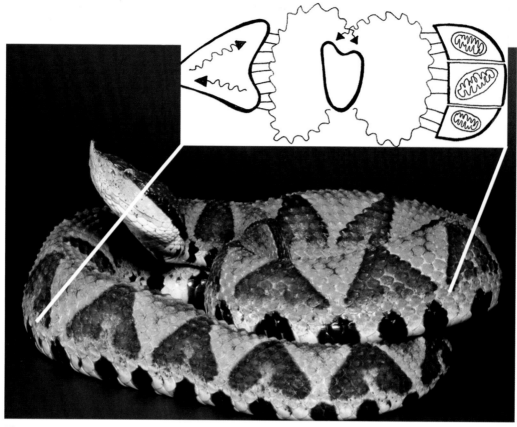

Figure 6.1. Schematic representation of lung ventilation, blood circulation, and transfer of respiratory gases (O_2 and CO_2) between the lung and blood and between the blood and tissues. The squiggly lines represent movement of gases by convection (or bulk flow transport), and the straight lines represent movement of gases by diffusion: oxygen from lung to blood (left part of schematic), and from blood to tissue and mitochondria (right part of schematic); CO_2 in the opposite directions. The circulation of blood is powered by muscular pumping of the heart (center of schematic). The snake to which the schematic arbitrarily applies is a *Deinagkistrodon acutus*, photographed in Taiwan by Ming-Chung Tu. The schematic representation of gas transport was drawn by Shauna Lillywhite.

movement of gaseous molecules as well as other substances around the body (fig. 6.1).

Convection refers to the bulk movement of something when it is carried in a medium such as air, water, or blood. Imagine you are outdoors and standing in front of your house. If the outside air was perfectly still and your neighbor across the street opened a perfume bottle outside, you would not smell it, and the movement of perfume molecules that happen to vaporize would be a slow process if it depended solely on diffusion from the source. However, if there is even a gentle breeze, you could smell the perfume if the vaporized molecules were carried by the air movements from the neighbor to you, assuming of course the wind is blowing in the right direction. Similarly, we could imagine the enhanced movement of a dye when a drop of it enters a body of water such as a pond or lake. The dye would not disperse very rapidly without movement of currents in the water (say by stirring) that would carry it from place to place. This is essentially the reason that circulatory systems evolved in animals. Indeed, some physiology books refer to

the blood circulation as a "transport system" because this is precisely how it functions in moving various things from place to place within the body. These include not only respiratory gases but also blood cells, various ions, nutrients, waste metabolites, hormones, water, and heat.

The circulatory system of a snake consists of a central muscular pump, the heart, and distributing vessels that move blood (the transport medium) around the body. The blood is red because of red blood cells that contain hemoglobin, which is a pigment that binds oxygen reversibly and permits the transport of much larger amounts of oxygen than would be possible otherwise (i.e., in simple solution). Thus, when the blood is oxygenated in the lung, the large majority of oxygen molecules is attached to hemoglobin and is transported within the red blood cells, which move freely while suspended in the blood plasma. The plasma is the liquid part of the blood and contains various dissolved substances—red blood cells, nutrients, and the like—and flows through the blood vessels. In the *capillaries*, which are the smallest blood vessels that service tissues, oxygen comes off the hemoglobin and diffuses into the cells that are oxidizing substrates in the process of respiration.

There are two fundamental circuits in the blood circulation of snakes and other terrestrial vertebrates. The *pulmonary circulation* consists of all the vessels that convey blood from the heart to the lung, where the blood is oxygenated in pulmonary capillaries before returning to the heart for pumping to all other body tissues. The *systemic circulation* consists of all the vessels that convey oxygenated blood from the heart to the body tissues where oxygen is exchanged for CO_2 in the systemic capillaries. Ideally, if the system operated as it does in a mammal, which has a four-chambered heart, all of the oxygenated blood from the lungs would be pumped to the systemic tissues, and all the relatively unoxygenated (termed deoxygenated) blood returning to the heart from the tissues would be pumped to the lungs for reoxygenation. In this system the blood flows from the systemic circuit through the heart to the lung, hence back to the heart for return to the tissues again, and so forth. The blood flows in series from the pulmonary vessels to the systemic vessels, then back to the pulmonary vessels, and so on, and the blood in the two respective circuits is kept separated. In vertebrates other than crocodilians, birds, and mammals, however, there is possibility for mixing of the two bloodstreams in the ventricle, which is not anatomically divided into two separate chambers.

The Heart: Central Pump and Controller of Shunts

The heart is a muscular pump and serves the important role of imparting motion to the blood that circulates throughout the system of interconnected blood vessels (fig. 6.2). Blood is returned to the heart in vessels called *veins*, which fill the heart with blood during its state of muscle relaxation. When the *cardiac* (heart) muscle contracts, much of the blood is ejected from the *ventricle* through outflow vessels that convey the blood to the various *arteries*. Before the blood enters the ventricle, it flows from the veins into two *atria* (individually termed *atrium*) that are capable of muscular contraction and positioned between the veins and the ventricle. It is the ventricle, however, that possesses stronger muscle and imparts the greatest force to the blood in order to produce movement throughout the system.

The heart of snakes is fundamentally similar to that of other squamates and turtles, but it differs substantially from that of crocodilians, birds, and mammals. The *sinus venosus* is the first heart chamber to receive venous blood from systemic veins, and it contains a "pacemaker" that initiates contraction and determines its timing. From here blood enters the right atrium. In comparison with "primitive" (basal) early vertebrates, the sinus venosus is reduced and the originally single atrium is divided into two distinct chambers. The muscular ventricle joins the two atria where each of two atrioventricular valves guards the entrances to the ventricular chambers. From the ventricle blood flows into three large arteries, and the base of these vessels is derived in evolutionary terms from the primitive *conus arteriosus*. The three arterial outflow vessels branch to form the pulmonary trunk and the right and left *aortic arches*, the latter vessels sending blood flow to the systemic tissues. There is a valved interaortic foramen that forms a tiny connection between the bases of the adjacent aortic arches. This opening allows possible shunting or movement of blood from one aortic arch to the other, but the functional significance of this connection has not been well studied in snakes. Contractile muscle tissue is dense near the base of the three outflow tracts and is especially important in controlling the resistance of the pulmonary trunk to the blood that is flowing to the lungs.

Figure 6.2. Heart of a Florida Cottonmouth (*Agkistrodon piscivorus conanti*). The snake weighed 656 g, and the heart shown weighed 1.6 g. At the **left**, the ventricle is shown in diastole, with the atria contracted while filling the ventricle with blood. The ventricle contracts in systole at the **right**, with the atria filling with new venous blood. Symbols are CA, *cavum arteriosum*; CP, *cavum pulmonale*; CV, *cavum venosum*; LAo, left aortic arch; RAo, right aortic arch; PA, pulmonary arch. The abbreviations CA, CP, and CV overlie the locations of the respective heart chambers, which are internal and cannot be seen. Note the coronary arteries that are visible as small vessels branching over the surface of the ventricle. Photographs by the author.

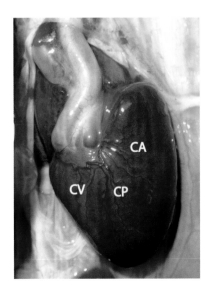
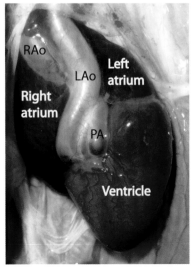

The right atrium receives deoxygenated blood returning from the systemic body tissues, and the left atrium receives oxygenated blood that is returning from the lungs. When the atria contract, their respective bloodstreams fill somewhat separated regions of the ventricle and are subsequently ejected into the appropriate outflow tracts: deoxygenated blood to the lungs via the pulmonary trunk and arteries, and oxygenated blood to the body via the aortic arches. The movement and separation of bloodstreams within the ventricle is complicated and subject to considerable variation depending on the prevailing physiological demands.

The ventricle is anatomically a single chamber and serves as a single pump to power the movement of blood into the major arterial branches leaving the heart. Internally and functionally, however, the ventricle is subdivided into three interconnected compartments (fig. 6.3). The *cavum arteriosum* receives oxygenated blood from the left atrium but has no direct connection to an outflow tract. Deoxygenated blood from the right atrium flows into a cavity called the *cavum venosum* and then across a muscular ridge to a third cavity called the *cavum pulmonale*. The muscular ridge is an incomplete muscular septum that partially divides the ventricle by separating the cavum pulmonale from the cavum arteriosum and cavum venosum. The latter two chambers are partially separated by a structure called the *vertical septum* and joined by an interventricular canal that communicates between the two. During filling of the ventricle, termed *diastole* (pronounced dye-ASS-toh-lee), the opened right atrioventricular valves lie across the opening to the interventricular canal and temporarily close it. Thus, oxygenated blood from the left atrium enters the cavum arteriosum and remains there during the period when the inter-ventricular canal is occluded by the valve structures. During contraction of the ventricle, termed *systole* (pronounced SIS-toh-lee), the atrioventricular valves close and prevent a reversed flow of blood back into the atria, also removing the physical occlusion of the interventricular canal. Hence, blood in the cavum arteriosum flows to the cavum venosum via the interventricular canal, and from this compartment it is expelled into the aortic arches. The contraction of the ventricle also compresses the muscular ridge against the opposite wall, which separates the cavum venosum from the cavum pulmonale. Deoxygenated blood residing in the cavum pulmonale exits the ventricle through the pulmonary trunk (hence pulmonary arteries) to the lung, but some of this blood may leak across the muscular ridge to enter the left aortic arch.

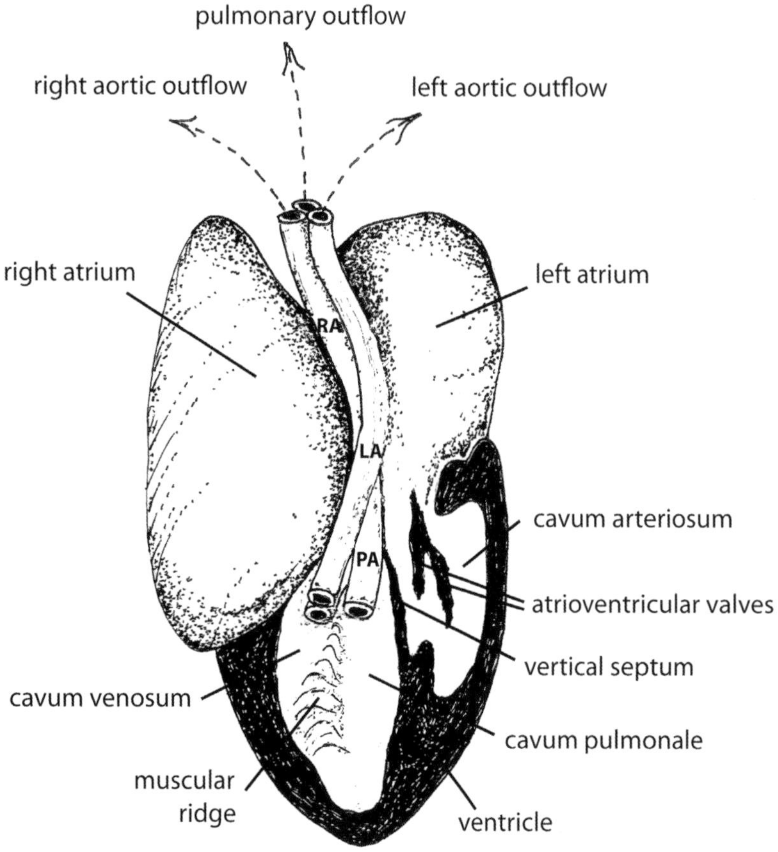

The contraction of ventricular muscle is not synchronous, and deoxygenated blood is propelled into the pulmonary arteries before oxygenated blood exits the ventricle. When the oxygenated blood is compressed by contraction of the adjacent ventricular walls, it encounters high resistance in the pulmonary trunk that is mostly filled with deoxygenated blood. Therefore, oxygenated blood enters the systemic arches partly because they offer less resistance.

A single ventricle such as that of a snake presents the potential for intracardiac shunting of blood from systemic to pulmonary streams, or vice versa. The term *shunt* basically refers to an alternate pathway. Thus, some of the blood that returns from the body tissues and is normally directed to the lungs might instead be "shunted" to the systemic circulation and thereby return to the body, whereas some of the oxygenated blood that returns from the lung

Figure 6.3. Schematic drawing of a generalized heart of a snake. This drawing illustrates the three chambers of the ventricle, which receive inflowing blood from the atria, and the connections to outflow vessels are shown. Label abbreviations are LA, left aortic arch; RA, right aortic arch; PA, pulmonary artery. See text for further explanation. Drawing by Dan Dourson and the author.

and is normally directed to the body might instead be "shunted" back to the lungs. These circumstances are termed intracardiac shunts and may result in either pulmonary bypass or systemic bypass (or both), involving some fraction of blood that is passing through the single ventricle.

Partial or complete pulmonary bypass is called a *right-to-left shunt* (R-L shunt), and partial or complete systemic bypass is called a *left-to-right shunt* (L-R shunt). The mechanisms controlling the magnitude and direction of shunting involve nervous control of the relative resistance or pressure differences in the pulmonary and systemic outflow tracts. For example, an increase in pulmonary vascular resistance will promote the translocation of a fraction of blood from the pulmonary to systemic circuit; that is, blood normally leaving the ventricle through the pulmonary trunk encounters increased resistance and instead is redirected to the systemic outflow tracts (R-L shunt). Such a mechanism has been termed *pressure shunting*. Alternatively, a passive mechanism for shunting can involve blood that is located within a space of the ventricle that is common to both pulmonary and systemic circulations at different phases of the heart cycle and is subsequently "washed" into the "wrong" circulation by inflowing or outflowing blood that is moving in the correct direction. This condition has been termed *washout shunting*. Both pressure and washout shunting probably occur under various conditions in most or all species of snakes, but the subject has not been well studied in reptiles other than turtles, crocodilians, and lizards. Furthermore, mixing in the ventricle can create both shunts simultaneously.

One of the more dramatic examples of pressure shunting in snakes occurs in the aquatic file snake, *Acrochordus granulatus*, investigated by myself and John Donald, who was a postdoctoral associate in my laboratory at the University of Florida. This snake is a resident of mangrove swamps and shallow tropical waters, where it remains submerged for periods up to several hours. During submergence when the snake is quiescent, blood flow completely bypasses the lung except for periodic moments when flow is directed to the lung briefly and at low flow rates. This pattern of intermittent shunting, attributable to increased resistance in the pulmonary artery, keeps the partial pressure of circulating oxygen low. This condition favors the uptake of oxygen across the skin (from a higher partial pressure in water) and inhibits the losses of oxygen to surrounding water under conditions where the ambient water is low in oxygen. In a crude sense, this has been likened to "metering" the oxygen stores in the lung and allowing the transfer of lung oxygen to circulating blood at low or minimal rates. Thus, the intracardiac shunt capabilities of ophidian hearts have advantages and would not be possible if the pulmonary and systemic flows of blood were completely separated, as in mammals.

High degrees of shunting have also been shown to occur in sea snakes, which dive to considerable depths (maximum recorded about 100 meters) and breathe intermittently at the surface of the ocean. Some species appear capable of remaining submerged for very long periods, however, by "cutaneous breathing" (uptake of oxygen diffusing across the skin, with release of CO_2 in the opposite direction).

Another important issue associated with diving is the prevention of decompression illness (also known as the "bends" or caisson disease). This occurs when nitrogen that diffuses into blood from the pulmonary air becomes pressurized at depth and "loads" the circulation. Then it forms bubbles when the blood is depressurized and the gas comes out of solution as the snake ascends to breathe air. Small bubbles that form in the blood circulation can block smaller blood vessels and thereby cause tissue damage, but this has not been evaluated well in snakes or other reptiles that might have vessel size and properties that are different from humans or other mammals in which decompression problems have been better studied. Roger Seymour and his colleagues have performed elegant studies that establish avoidance of decompression problems in sea snakes by virtue of a combination of shunting blood away from the lung (thus avoiding nitrogen loading from the compressed lung gas) and losses of blood nitrogen to the ambient water across the skin. All of the nitrogen that enters the blood in the lung is mixed with nitrogen-poor blood that has come from the skin. This goes out into the body, but the pressure of nitrogen never increases enough to cause the bends. So it is central shunting plus the ability to lose nitrogen through the skin that prevents the bends.

Blood Vessels and the Vascular Distribution System

The heart is connected to a marvelously complex system of vessels that distribute the blood throughout the body and return it for repeated pumping in a conventional manner that is fundamentally similar to what occurs in mammals. The vessels transporting blood away from the heart are termed arteries. As in mammals, they are characterized by having relatively thick walls with layers of smooth muscle and elastic tissue. The vessels that return blood from the tissues to the heart are called veins, and these are generally thinner than arteries but also contain muscle and elastic tissues. The veins are more "stretchy" than arteries and contain the major part of the circulating blood and thereby serve as a blood "reservoir." Capillaries are the smallest vessels of the circulatory system and collectively constitute the sites where respiratory gases, nutrients, ions, and other substances are exchanged with the interstitial fluid that surrounds cells of the various tissues. In the pulmonary circulation, the lung capillaries are where oxygen and CO_2 are exchanged between the blood and the air spaces within the lung (fig. 6.4). The smaller arteries leading blood to the capillaries are called *arterioles*, and the smaller veins leading blood away from the capillaries are called *venules*.

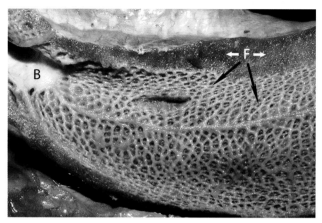

Figure 6.4. Respiratory, vascularized part of the lung of a Burmese Python (*Python molurus bivittatus*). The lung has been severed and laid open to reveal its internal anatomy (head end is to the left). The bronchial airway (B) opens into the lung where the internal air pockets (faveoli) are seen. Three-dimensionally, the faveoli (F) form a thickness of highly vascular red tissue comprising the wall of the lung. The density of blood capillaries in this tissue gives rise to its intense red color. Oxygen and CO_2 are exchanged between the blood capillaries of the faveoli and the lung air within the faveoli, derived from the pulmonary air that is ventilated in and out of the lung. Photograph by John Roberts.

The arterial outflow tracts from the ventricle include the right and left aortic arches, which typically leave the ventricle ventromedially and arch around the esophagus to run toward the tail. Not far from the heart these two arches merge in the dorsal midline to form the *dorsal aorta* (fig. 6.5). The *carotid arteries* leave the right aortic arch near the cranial ends of the atria and carry blood to the head and brain. The left carotid artery is usually the dominant vessel and typically about the same diameter as the right aortic arch. The right carotid artery is smaller in diameter and may be absent or vestigial in some taxa of more advanced snakes (Caenophidia). A *vertebral artery* arises from the right aortic arch near where it curves to run in a posterior direction. The anterior vertebral artery courses toward the head for variable distances and then disappears in the musculature between the vertebrae. Branches of this vessel perfuse the muscles of the body wall, skin, esophagus, lung fascia, and head. Progressing in the opposite direction toward the tail, a series of vertebral vessels originates from the dorsal aorta in addition to prominent branches to the principal organs of the body cavity. The caudal segment of the aorta terminates within the tail.

The third arterial outflow tract from the ventricle gives rise to the pulmonary artery (fig. 6.5). The pulmonary trunk originates from the ventricle immediately adjacent to the aortic arches, and all three vessels emerge from the ventricle to course for a short distance as a *truncus arteriosus*,

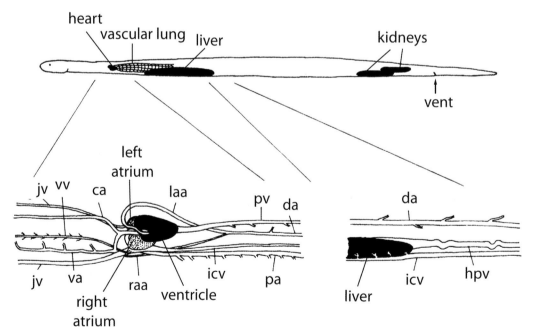

Figure 6.5. A schematic diagram of a snake showing the major blood vessels in two regions of the body. The arrangement of internal anatomy is based on that of a rat snake (*Elaphe* or *Pantherophis* spp.), which has a relatively anterior position of the heart. The ventricle, liver, and kidneys are shown in black; the atria are stippled; and the vascular lung is crosshatched. The blood vessel abbreviations are **ca**, carotid artery; **da**, dorsal aorta; **icv**, inferior caval vein; **jv**, jugular vein; **hpv**, hepatic portal vein; **laa**, left aortic arch; **pa**, pulmonary artery; **pv**, pulmonary vein; **raa**, right aortic arch; **va**, vertebral artery; **vv**, vertebral vein. Redrawn by the author after fig. 1 in J. A. Donald and H. B. Lillywhite, Adrenergic innervation of the large arteries and veins of the semiarboreal rat snake *Elaphe obsoleta*, *Journal of Morphology* 198:25–31, 1988.

Figure 6.6. Corkscrew structure of the portal vein in a Florida Cottonmouth (*Agkistrodon piscivorus*). The corkscrew turns of this segment of portal vein can be seen in the central part of the photograph, adjacent to the posterior aspect of the liver. The posterior direction (toward the tail) is to the right in the illustration, indicated by the arrow in the **inset**. The inset is a schematic illustration of how "damming" of blood movement can occur hypothetically if there is retrograde (reversed and wrong direction) flow in the vein, e.g., through a gravitational surge of blood. The damming effect is seen in the lower part of the inset where blood (dark stippling) collects at one of the turns of the "corkscrew," which collapses on itself because of pressure of the surging blood. The direction of normal blood flow, returning to the heart, is from right to left. Photograph and drawing by the author.

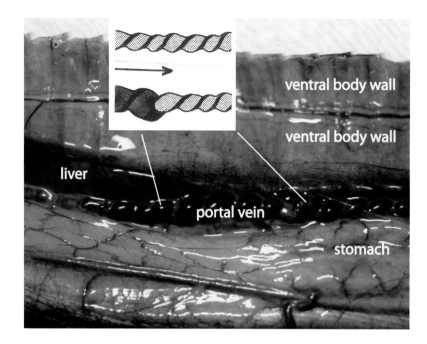

bound together by common elements of fibrous fascia. Eventually the pulmonary artery divides in variable patterns in different taxa, but there is usually a single prominent branch, or two branches that course in opposite directions away from the heart. In most species the anterior branch is the predominant and longest pulmonary vessel, which services a vascular lung that is near the heart (see below).

Blood from the lung is returned to the heart in one or more pulmonary veins, and the pulmonary drainage parallels the pulmonary arterial system. Pulmonary venous blood returns from the lung to the left atrium. Anterior drainage from tissues other than the lung returns to the heart in usually two jugular veins, one being dominant (the right) or the two joining to form a superior caval vein that conveys blood to the right atrium (fig. 6.5). The inferior caval vein originates from two renal veins in addition to a hepatic portal vein and numerous parietal veins, returning blood to the heart from the posterior body cavity. The portal vein branches profusely within the liver but also conveys blood directly to the inferior caval vein. Variable portions of the portal vein may show a "corkscrew" configuration at the level of the liver and immediately posterior to it in terrestrial taxa of snakes (fig. 6.6). This structure conceivably acts as a bidirectional valve and prevents gravitational surges of large volumes of blood that is associated with the liver and vessel lumen. The inferior caval vein and the hepatic portal vein run parallel in close proximity posterior to the liver.

Snakes have an extensive system of lymphatic vessels, which often parallel the blood vessels as perivascular lymphatics. Major arteries, for example, might be surrounded by a sleeve of fluid that flows in the lymphatic vessel surrounding the artery. The *lymphatic fluid* (also called *lymph*) that fills these vessels resembles blood plasma and is derived from excess filtration of fluid at the capillaries. This fluid eventually merges with the venous system, where it is returned to the heart and recirculated in blood. The lymphatic vessels of snakes are fascinating in their structural complexity but have not been well studied.

Properties of Blood

Blood Volume

The volume of blood contained in the circulation is an important parameter that is, of course, essential for adequate pressure and flow in the vascular distribution system. Circulating blood volumes have been measured in a few species of snakes and generally correspond to about 6 percent of the body mass. File snakes (*Acrochordus* spp.) may have blood volumes about twice this amount, and the extra volume is thought to improve the storage of oxygen and thereby prolong the diving times in tropical waters where this species lives (see below). Measurements of fluid movements between blood vessels and the surrounding interstitial fluids have been evaluated in some snakes and suggest that capillary permeability is relatively great. Therefore, plasma can move relatively freely across capillary walls, and the blood volume is potentially labile. For example, interstitial fluid moves into the blood compartment when there are losses of blood due to hemorrhage, whereas activity such as locomotion may filter blood in the opposite direction and transiently reduce the blood volume (as much as 17 to 22 percent in some rattlesnakes).

Although the circulating blood volume may be subject to transient disturbance, this important parameter is, in fact, well regulated over time. The lymphatic system may also provide an important reservoir of fluid that might contribute to the regulation of blood volume, as is the case in amphibians.

Blood Oxygen Capacity

The amount of oxygen that is present in the blood is related to the absolute volume of blood, and to the amount of circulating red blood cells with their characteristic content of hemoglobin. Considering somewhat sparse data that are available for snakes, the amounts of red blood cells and oxygen that are present in the blood are generally similar to that in other reptiles. *Hematocrit* values, which represent the volume of red cells per unit of blood volume, generally range between 20 and 30 percent with marine species representing the higher values. Exceptionally high values (around 50 percent) have been reported in marine file snakes. Maximum oxygen capacity is around 10 vol% (which indicates the volume of oxygen per unit volume of whole blood, expressed as a percentage). Again, file snakes (*Acrochordus*) exhibit higher values that are thought to be important for the storage of oxygen in relation to diving.

The molecular properties of hemoglobin are also important and determine its affinity for oxygen at a given pressure of oxygen to which the blood is exposed. Typically, hemoglobin binds oxygen in adequate amounts to saturate its binding sites at normal atmospheric pressures of oxygen in the air that is breathed into the lungs by snakes and other air-breathing vertebrates. Diving aquatic snakes may have hemoglobin with slightly greater oxygen affinity because of the requirement for extracting oxygen from lung air that becomes relatively depleted of oxygen (which reduces the oxygen pressure proportionately) during the time underwater when the snake is not breathing atmospheric air and the lung becomes essentially a "closed system." Differences in oxygen affinity of hemoglobin might also be related to differences in levels of behavioral activities, or other factors that are not yet well studied.

The blood properties of snakes can vary substantially with temperature, ontogeny, nutrition, and activity. The amount of data is limited for snakes, and the significance of all the variation that has been observed has not been fully evaluated. We may conclude however—with some measure of caution—that the transport of respiratory gases is maximal or "optimal" in supporting activities at preferred body temperatures in characteristic environments in which a given species has evolved. This appears to be generally true in a variety of ectothermic vertebrates.

Hemodynamics: The Physics of Flow in the Vascular Fluid System

The transport function of the blood circulation requires that fluid moves at appropriate rates throughout the body, and this depends on the pumping action of the heart and the nature of the vessels that distribute blood from the arteries to capillaries. There must also be sufficient flow in the venous system so that blood returns to the heart for further pumping. The distributing vessel system, especially the smaller arterioles and capillaries, presents a certain resistance to the flow of the blood, and the quantitative expression of this resistance is called *peripheral resistance*. The resistance depends on the geometry of the vascular system, especially the diameter of the distributing vessels. Smaller diameter vessels present a greater resistance to flow than do larger diameter vessels. Thus, most of the resistance to blood flow occurs in the *microvasculature*, which includes the smaller arterioles and capillaries.

The viscosity of the blood is another parameter influencing the resistance to blood flow. In essence, this refers to the interaction of the vascular geometry with the viscosity of the flowing fluid that determines how well the blood moves. Frictional interactions between concentric layers of blood moving past each other vary with the velocity of movement and the size and length of the vessels. The nature of the blood also is important. The viscosity of blood is greatly increased over that of water by the presence of red blood cells, which also have frictional interactions with the surrounding blood plasma and especially suspended proteins that have "sticky" qualities when contacting the outer walls or membranes of the red blood cells. The greater the number of red blood cells the greater the viscosity of the blood relative to water.

The muscular contraction of the heart's ventricle creates pressure in the blood that is contained within it. This pressure adds energy to the blood, which imparts motion and powers its circulation. Because of the heart's pumping action, the energy content of blood is highest in the arterial outflow tracts and is dissipated during flow in overcoming the peripheral resistance. Thus, there is a gradient of energy from the heart to the capillaries, and on to the veins, which induces flow. Blood pressures in the veins are very low, nearly zero, and the heart reenergizes the blood to produce continued flow into the arteries. This system is somewhat analogous to the continuous movement of water through a fountain, as example one that sprays water in an upward stream that falls into a quiet pool below. The spout of water flow at the fountain is powered by a pump that pressurizes the water. The water in the pool is relatively still and flows at low energy level back to the pump where it is again pressurized and sprayed into the air against gravity.

The parameter of foremost physiological importance in the snake's circulatory system is the actual *flow* of blood, which is of course necessary for the transport of materials around the body. The related parameter that energizes the flow is the blood *pressure*, and this is what a physician usually measures as an indicator of the overall health and well-being of a person's blood circulation. The pumping action of the heart produces repetitive "pulses" of arterial pressure that vary from a systolic high (related to ventricular contraction) to a diastolic low (when the ventricular muscle is relaxed and the heart chambers are refilling with blood). Thus, in a human, the arterial systolic pressure is around 120 mm Hg and the diastolic pressure is around 80 mm Hg, giving a geometric mean of about 100 mm Hg. The mean value and the difference between systolic and diastolic pressures are related to the *heart rate* (frequency of heart contractions) and the level of peripheral resistance in the blood vessels. Mean levels of systemic arterial blood pressure in snakes typically vary from lows of 20–30 mm Hg to highs of 50–80 mm Hg in various species. Pulmonary arterial pressures run lower at about 15–30 mm Hg (see below). Venous blood pressures in both systemic and pulmonary circuits are very low, approaching zero, except when the vessels are compressed by the body during activities such as locomotion, climbing, constricting prey, and so on. External compression of the veins produces transient increases of pressure independent of the action of the heart and the levels of blood pressure in the arteries.

Although there are mechanisms that ensure that regional or local blood flow rates are adequate for the needs of the tissue, the overall ability of the central circulation to provision these collective flows is related to the regulation of the central arterial blood pressure. The principal determinants of the arterial blood pressure are the ventricular outflow of blood (called *cardiac output*) and the level of peripheral resistance. Both of these parameters are regulated principally by the nervous system, with lesser but important controls exerted by circulating hormones and the influence of tissue metabolites and chemicals that act locally on the smooth muscle of the blood vessels.

The cardiac output is determined by the rate and strength of the heart contractions, which are driven primarily by the influence of chemicals called *catecholamines*. These are released from nerve endings (as "neurotransmitters") at the heart muscle and may also be circulating as hormones derived from the medullary (deeper, internal) portion of the adrenal glands. The familiar catecholamines are known as *epinephrine* and *norepinephrine*, which are chemically very similar both in structure and actions. These same catecholamines also act at nerve endings in the walls of the blood vessels, especially arterioles, to influence the state of constriction of the smooth muscle. Circulating catecholamines have similar effects, and mostly these cause constriction of the smooth muscle (called *vasoconstriction*), but they may also cause dilation or relaxation of the smooth muscle (called *vasodilation*) in certain parts of the vasculature. *Acetylcholine* is another chemical that is released from nerve endings at the heart and causes slowing of the heart rate. Generally, the heart rate is determined by a balance or a "push-pull" action between acetylcholine and catecholamines.

How do the nerve endings and adrenal medulla know when and how much of these regulatory substances to secrete? Regulation is accomplished by a feedback system of information involving sensitive structures called *baroreceptors* that monitor the moment-to-moment changes in arterial blood pressure. The baroreceptors are actually a discrete collection of nerve endings located in the walls of central arterial outflow vessels, especially the base of the pulmonary artery and possibly the carotid artery. These are sensitive to stretch, which indirectly monitors the blood pressure. Increasing pressure tends to stretch the vessel wall slightly, and a decrease in pressure has the opposite effect. Information from these nerve endings is sent via nerve signals ("impulses" or "action potentials") to the central nervous system and interacts with other nerves in the brain to direct an outflow of nerve signals to modify the release of chemicals from nerve endings at the heart, peripheral blood vessels, and the adrenal medulla. So, as an example, a decrease in blood pressure reduces the stretch of baroreceptors, which then send signals to the brain, where integration results in increased signaling from the nerves that release catecholamines at the heart, blood vessels, and adrenal medulla. Simultaneously, the integration also decreases the release of acetylcholine from other nerve endings that are acting on the heart. The result is an increase in the rate and strength of the heartbeat, which increases the cardiac output, and a simultaneous increase in peripheral resistance due to vasoconstriction of peripheral vessels. These actions collectively tend to restore (increase) the arterial pressure. Alternatively, any transient increase of arterial pressure (above normal) produces the opposite effects.

There are undoubtedly multiple baroreceptors associated with the central blood vessels near the heart. In mammals, stretch-sensitive receptors are located in the aortic arch, the carotid artery, heart muscle, and major veins. Many of the blood vessels, including veins, can be to some degree stretch-sensitive in relation to the monitoring of blood pressure. The situation is probably similar in snakes, but these various receptors involved in the regulation of blood pressure have not been well studied in this group of vertebrates.

Gravity and Blood Circulation: Putting It All Together

Gravity's Challenge

Gravity has an important influence on blood circulation that is potentially expressed in animals that are especially long or tall with upright posture. According to the third "law of Pascal," fluid pressure increases with depth in any fluid column (fig. 6.7). Such pressure is independent of any other force, such as heart pumping that pressurizes the fluid, and is called *gravitational pressure* or, more commonly, *hydrostatic pressure*. It also follows that the pressure increase at the bottom of a fluid column depends on the height of the column, and therefore the gradient of pressure (attributable to gravity) from top to bottom of a column depends on its height. The pressure also increases from top to bottom of a fluid column that is tilted at an angle and not necessarily fully vertical. The increased pressure at the bottom of the column depends on both the length of the fluid column and its angle of tilt. More specifically, the increased pressure at the

bottom of any fluid column is dependent on the absolute height of the column. If a fluid column such as a blood vessel is turned from horizontal to vertical, the pressure decreases at the top of the column and increases at the bottom. There is a point or level near the center of the fluid column where the pressure necessarily does not change, and this is called the *hydrostatic indifferent point*. Importantly, these changes in pressure within a fluid column attributable to gravity occur whether the fluid is stagnant or is circulating, as in the blood vessels of a living animal.

Snakes are excellent model animals for studies of gravitational effects on blood circulation owing to their elongate body form and diversity of behaviors and habitats. At one extreme, arboreal or scansorial (climbing) species of snakes at times adopt fully upright postures when the blood vessels become long fluid columns with gradients of gravitational pressures related to the absolute height of the blood column. The ambient pressure is atmospheric, or by conventional reference zero, so the fluid pressures in vessels push outward on the vessel walls and tend to distend them.

At another extreme, fully aquatic snakes exist in a fluid medium in which vertical gradients of gravitational pressure in water counteract the nearly identical gradients in a snake's blood circulation owing to the near match of fluid density between blood and water. Thus, gravitational fluid pressures in the blood vessels are almost exactly counterbalanced by the external water pressures (which act across the body tissues) and there is no tendency for the gravitational blood pressures to distend vessels (fig. 6.7). Consequently, selection pressures for cardiovascular adaptations to counteract gravity are effectively not present in the aquatic medium in which fully aquatic forms have spent much of their evolutionary history (fig. 6.8).

Gravity challenges the circulation primarily in two ways. First, when the body is upright, the heart must pump against the pressure at the base of the arterial column between the heart and head. In animals like giraffes, long snakes, and perhaps certain longer-necked prehistoric dinosaurs this pressure can be considerable. More specifically, the ventricle must produce a pressure that exceeds the pressure at the point of outflow into the

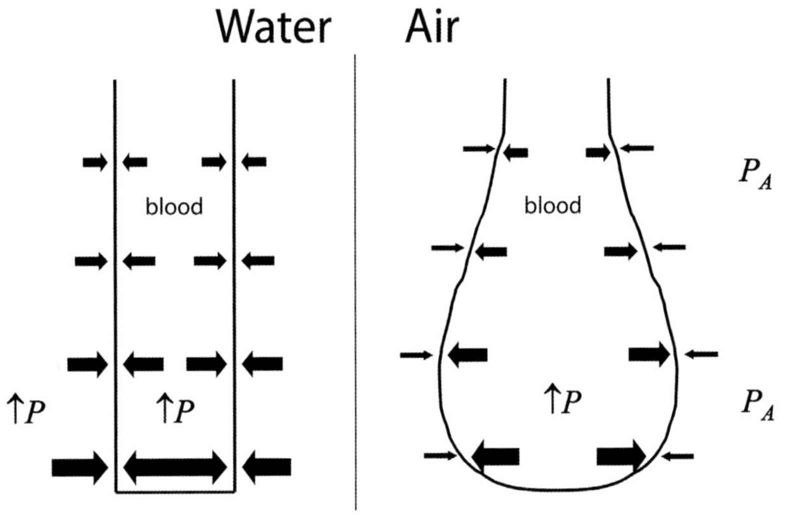

Figure 6.7. Schematic drawing to illustrate the effects of pressure on a liquid such as blood that is held within a vessel, for example, a vein. The magnitude of pressure is indicated by the width of the arrows. Pressure increases with depth in any column of liquid. If the vessel containing liquid is in water, the external pressure is nearly equal to that of the blood within the vessel at any point of depth in the liquid column, so the pressures (P) acting on opposite sides of the wall of the vessel are essentially equal and cancel each other (**left-hand** figure). If the vessel is in air, however, the ambient pressure outside the vessel is everywhere atmospheric (zero by convention), whereas the pressure in the blood inside the vessel increases with depth according to the Law of Pascal. (Pressure also increases with depth in a column of air, but the effect is negligible at this scale because of the lesser density of air compared with water.) Therefore, in the case of a vessel in air (**right-hand** figure), the net pressure acting across the wall of the vessel (inside to outside) increases with depth in the vessel. This net increase in transmural (across the wall) pressure causes the vessel to distend in its lower part and creates a condition called "blood pooling." See text for further explanation. Drawing by the author.

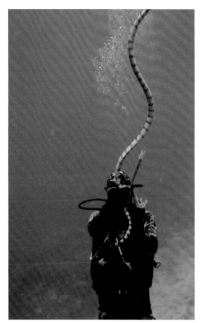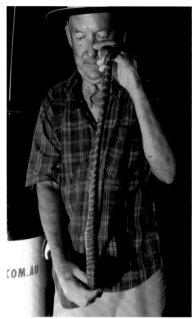

Figure 6.8. Views of two aquatic snakes illustrating the effects of gravity on internal body fluids. In the photo on the **left**, Arne Rasmussen holds a sea krait (*Laticauda colubrina*) vertically in seawater, and there is no evidence for blood pooling in this individual. In the photo at the **right**, Warren Watkins holds an aquatic file snake (*Acrochordus granulatus*) vertically outside of water. One can easily see the distension of the lower body, which is due to body fluids— especially blood—"pooling" in response to gravity. A part of the distension is probably attributable also to sagging of viscera. Compare these photographs with the illustration in fig. 6.7. The photo at the left was taken by Erik Frausing in Sulawesi. The photo at the right was taken by the author on the Embley River, Cape York Peninsula, Australia.

arterial column above the heart in order to promote flow. Such pressure should exceed the gravitational pressure by a considerable factor if there is to be sufficient pressure at the head to perfuse the cranial blood vessels. Moreover, these pressures should be positive because if the blood pressure falls to zero or becomes negative anywhere along the arterial branches, the vessel will collapse because of greater external pressure acting on the vessel wall. Again, there would be no flow of blood in this circumstance. Therefore, blood flow into the head and brain becomes a challenge for long snakes that climb with the head up.

The second challenge to blood circulation from gravity is the tendency for pressures to increase in blood vessels below the heart, especially at the feet and lower legs of terrestrial tetrapods and near the tail or caudal end of an elongate snake. These pressures can cause excess filtration of blood plasma at capillaries, thereby producing edema and swelling in tissues, and may also cause blood to "pool" in vessels that are especially distensible or compliant, particularly veins (fig. 6.7). The tendency for blood to pool in these lower vessels reduces the rate at which venous blood returns to the heart, which in turn diminishes ventricular filling and cardiac output. Under this scenario, severe or even moderate blood pooling can reduce the cardiac output sufficiently to lower the arterial pressure.

Snakes, Posture, and Gravity

Gravity clearly poses a challenge to three-dimensional uses of terrestrial habitats by long snakes. The problem is diminished or goes away in two circumstances. First, completely aquatic snakes are immune to the gravitational disturbance of blood circulation because of the stabilizing effects of external hydrostatic pressures that match the intravascular gradients of gravitational pressure during postural changes (see above). Second, relatively short species of snakes (< about one meter) experience little problem during vertical postures because of the limited length of blood columns and, therefore, limited gradients of gravitational pressure. However, for many terrestrial species of snake that utilize vertical dimensions of habitat, gravity potentially challenges the capacities of snakes to regulate arterial blood pressure and to maintain adequate blood flow to the head and other critical organs.

Many terrestrial species of snakes, and especially those that climb, have evolved marvelous defenses that guard against gravity's effect on blood circulation. Semiarboreal colubrid (especially rat snakes, genus *Elaphe* or *Pantherophis*) and elapid snakes have demonstrated abilities to regulate arterial blood pressure and to maintain adequate blood flow to the head during head-up postures. In some individuals, the precision of such regulation is excellent, and carotid blood flow remains at usual levels even when the body is fully vertical. Note that the carotid artery is the principal route of blood flow to the head of snakes. The cardiovascular "performance" of various scansorial species is consistent with a suite of physiological and morphological characteristics that evidently coevolved to counteract gravitational forces acting on the circulation, and these are quite similar to comparable adaptations that have been studied in humans and other mammals.

The arsenal of adaptive traits that counteract gravity's effect on blood circulation include morphological, physiological, and behavioral attributes (fig. 6.9). Morphological traits include anterior location of the heart, which can be as close as 11–12 percent of body length to the head, and relatively "tight" tissues that surround blood vessels and counteract the tendencies to blood pooling, especially in lower body veins. The tight nature of the tissues includes properties of the skin and body wall as well as the tissue spaces immediately surrounding certain vessels (for example, in the tail). The position of the heart close to the head shortens the gravitational column (pressure) against which the heart must work during head-up posture and tends to ensure adequate perfusion of head and brain tissues at all angles of body attitude. Such heart position, of course, increases the problem when the snake is in a head-down position. However, perfusion of the tail and lower body is less important than is the adequate and uninterrupted perfusion of the brain. It is interesting to think about the evolutionary migration of the heart in different taxa of snakes, which might not be possible in some other tetrapods in which the heart is constrained to a thoracic cavity that is surrounded by rigid vertebrae and ribs.

In contrast with scansorial terrestrial species of snakes, fully aquatic species such as file snakes and sea snakes exhibit generally looser tissues surrounding blood vessels and a more central position of the heart (generally 30–45 percent of total body length from the head). Other things equal, a central heart location is energetically more efficient with respect to pumping of blood throughout the entire elongated animal. Thus, natural selection probably favors a central location in circumstances where gravity's influence is reduced. The variation in heart position among species of snakes is quite likely related to the extent of time that ancestral species have been subjected to selection forces associated with particular habitats. Of course, other factors such as the size of prey and feeding habits might also influence heart position in snakes.

Roger Seymour and I demonstrated that the mean (resting) arterial blood pressure ranges from higher (50 to 70 mm Hg) to lower (20 to 30 mm Hg) in species of snakes ranging from

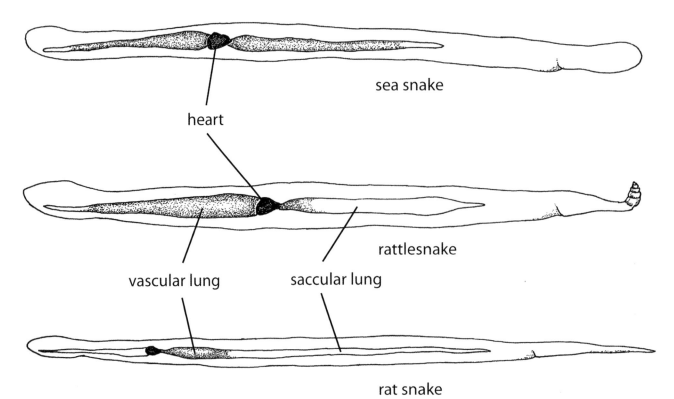

Figure 6.9. Schematic features of snakes that counteract gravity disturbance to blood circulation. **Upper drawing** features a sea snake that is characterized by an elongate *vascular lung* and a relatively short *saccular lung* segment. The **middle drawing** features a ground-dwelling rattlesnake that has a comparatively central heart position (with respect to length) and an elongate *tracheal lung*. The saccular segment of lung is relatively short, but less so than in the sea snake. The **lower drawing** features a semiarboreal rat snake that has a relatively anterior heart and a very short vascular lung that is located near the heart. The saccular lung comprises a relatively elongate segment of the lung structure. The rat snake is relatively more slender than the other snakes and has comparatively "tight" tissues surrounding blood vessels, in addition to superior nervous control of vessel constriction compared with the other snakes (these features not shown). Drawing by Dan Dourson, after fig. 6 in H. B. Lillywhite, Circulatory adaptations of snakes to gravity, *American Zoologist* 27:81–95, 1987.

scansorial to aquatic in behaviors. Also, regulation of arterial pressure is much tighter in the arboreal/scansorial species. Finally, mean arterial pressures in terrestrial snakes increases in exact proportion to the distance between the heart and head.

Structure and Function of the Ophidian Lung

Like other vertebrates, snakes possess a lung that is used for exchange of respiratory gases between the animal's blood circulation and the outside aerial atmosphere. Air is breathed in and out of the system by means of nostrils, or nasal openings, which are paired and referred to as external *nares* (singular is *naris*). Some species such as sea snakes possess nasal valves in the nostril consisting of erectile tissue (fig. 6.10). The nasal passages communicate with the roof of the pharynx, from whence air passes into the trachea via the glottis when the jaws are normally closed. (A glottis with the mouth open can be seen in fig. 8.5.) The trachea communicates with the bronchial airway and remainder of the lung as a tubular air-conducting system (see bronchial airway in fig. 6.4).

The lung proper is shaped somewhat like a spindle and has a voluminous central space (lumen) that is free of tissue (fig. 6.11). The inner surfaces are lined by a very thin layer of tissue, or *parenchyma*, that is typically less than 3 or 4 mm in thickness. Fundamentally, the lung can be divided into two functionally different regions: the "respiratory" segment consists of highly vascularized exchange tissue, hereafter referred to as *vascular lung*, and in most cases there is also a simple extension of flat, thin epithelium known as the *saccular lung*. The vascular lung, including sometimes tracheal segments, is the region of the lung that functions in respiratory gas exchange (O_2 and CO_2), whereas the

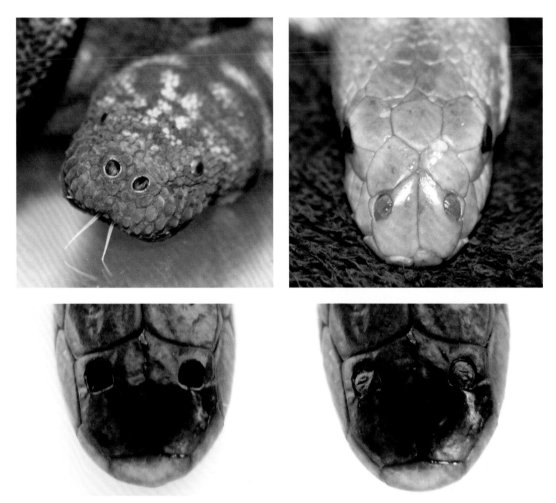

Figure 6.10. Views looking down on the snout of sea snakes, illustrating narial valves just inside the nostrils. The **upper left** photograph shows the narial valves in a Little File Snake (*Acrochordus granulatus*) photographed by the author in Queensland, Australia. Note the fleshy valves come together in a vertical plane. The **upper right** photograph shows the closed fleshy valves in a Shaw's Sea Snake (*Lapemis curtus*) photographed by the author in Queensland, Australia. The **lower** photographs illustrate a Yellow-bellied Sea Snake (*Pelamis platurus*) breathing naturally outside water. The photos capture the narial valves open (left) during inhalation of air and closed (right) during pauses between breaths. This specimen was photographed in Costa Rica by Coleman M. Sheehy III.

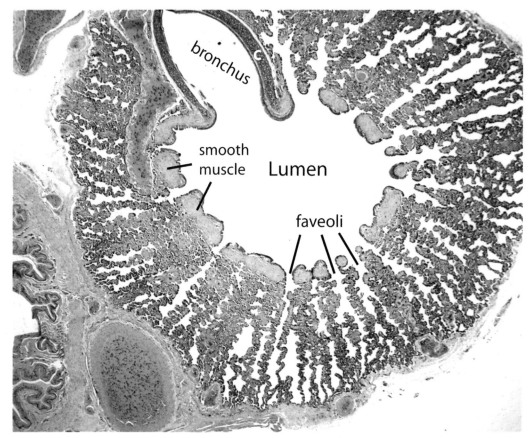

Figure 6.11. Histological cross-section through the lung of a king snake (*Lampropeltis getula*). The bronchial conducting airway is continuous with the central lumen, which opens into numerous faveoli. The bronchial airway has walls that are stiffer than the other lung structure, and comprised of cartilage (dense blue tissue, c). Adjacent faveoli are separated by a connective tissue septum, and the luminal end of each septum contains a bundle of smooth muscle. The histological stain is H & E. Microphotograph by Elliott Jacobson.

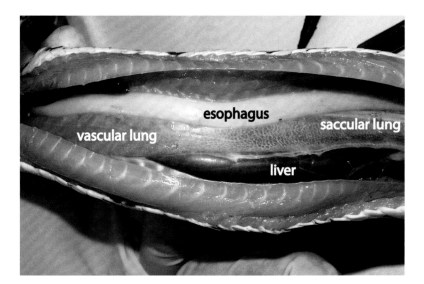

Figure 6.12. Ventral view of the anterior coelomic cavity featuring segments of the right (dominant) lung in a Diamond Python (*Morelia spilota spilota*). The respiratory segment of the lung, termed the *vascular lung*, is adjacent to the esophagus and near the liver. The vascular lung is red because of the numerous blood capillaries involved in gas exchange. Note that the vascular lung gradually transitions to the *saccular lung*, in which three-dimensional *faveoli* are lacking and there are no blood vessels involved in gas exchange. Individual and increasingly shallow faveoli are seen in the region of transition in the center of the photograph. The head and the heart of this snake are to the left in the illustration. Photograph by Elliott Jacobson.

saccular lung receives only a nutritive blood supply and does not function in gas exchange (figs. 6.9, 6.12).

Of the internal viscera of snakes, the lung is perhaps the most variable in size and complexity. Unlike other vertebrates having symmetrically paired lungs, the left lung is greatly reduced or vestigial in most species of snakes, and the right lung becomes elongated as the prominent single functional lung that is evident to the observer. In various species, including both primitive and advanced taxa, the left lung has been lost entirely. When present, the length of

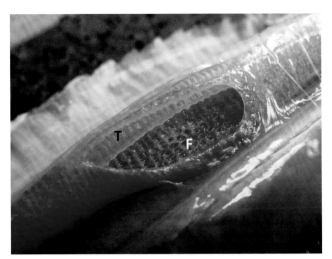

Figure 6.13. Ventral view of the tracheal lung of a Florida Cottonmouth (*Agkistrodon piscivorus conanti*). A cut in the lung reveals the inner aspect featuring partly collapsed *faveoli* (F) and the cartilaginous *trachea* (T) above. The lumen of the trachea and the lung are continuous, and the vascular lung shown here expands outward during normal breathing by the snake. Photographed in Florida by the author.

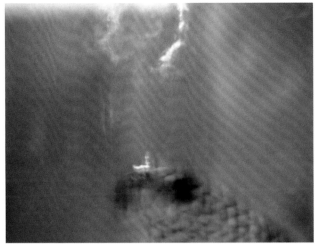

Figure 6.14. Streams of air bubbles can be seen rising from the nostrils of a Chinese Sea Krait (*Laticauda semifasciata*). This snake is adjusting its buoyancy by exhaling air after it submerged in a tank of seawater. Photographed by the author in Taiwan.

the left lung varies from 1 to 31 percent of snout-vent length, whereas the length of the right lung varies from 8 to 82 percent of snout-vent length. Only in some primitive snakes (e.g., xenopeltids and boids) do the lungs function as paired structures. A nice summary of quantitative measurements of ophidian lungs has been published by Van Wallach in the *Biology of the Reptilia* series.

With the exception of certain aquatic snakes (see below), the vascular lung in the majority of species is best developed near the heart, often beginning at or just anterior to the heart or ventricle, and extending for variable distances in a posterior direction. Additionally, members of about half of living snake families possesses a *tracheal lung*, which functions as the principal gas exchange organ in the region anterior to the lung. This is especially prominent in viperid species of snakes (figs. 6.9, 6.13).

The lungs of snakes are generally cigar-shaped (fusiform) and have an elongated central lumen that is arranged as a single longitudinal unit. One exception to this structure is the lung of the aquatic file snakes, *Acrochordus* spp., which consists of either two or four longitudinal lungs that are fused into a single organ having two or four corresponding air chambers in transverse sections. In all snakes the entire lung is attached to the body wall or associated membranes and is surrounded by other viscera. The internal surfaces are lined with a thin layer or vascularized tissue (vascular segment) and thin, membranous tissue (saccular segment). The total length of the lung can be somewhat short (e.g., 16 percent of total body length in *Uropeltis*), or extremely long (94 percent of total body length in *Acrochordus granulatus*).

The lung volume can be very large and represents from 30–53 percent of the body volume in some European vipers. When snakes are engaged in defensive displays with the lung fully inflated, these percentages are no doubt even larger but have not been measured. Obviously, the lung volume at any time varies considerably with the ventilatory status of the snake, and aquatic species adjust the volume to regulate buoyancy at various depths (fig. 6.14).

Respiratory gases are exchanged between the pulmonary blood and ventilated air across the thin, vascularized parenchyma of the vascular lung. The parenchyma is variously sculptured in different species to increase the area of exchange surfaces. The structural elaboration of parenchymal surfaces varies from a single layer of low relief trabeculae, or pockets, that lie in a polygonal pattern on the lung wall to a multilayered honeycomb-appearing structure consisting of raised walls or septa that form cubicles or compartments that may be deeper than wide (figs. 6.4, 6.11, 6.13). These structures are somewhat similar to the alveoli present in mammalian lungs, except the parenchymal units in snakes are not homologous structures and are termed *faveoli* (singular *faveolus*) because they resemble a honeycomb. The faveolar parenchyma of snakes is highly variable and may exhibit up to four levels of subdividing walls or septa (figs. 6.4, 6.11). The septa separating individual faveoli contain capillaries on both sides and are supported by connective tissue with collagen and elastin fibers. The diameters of individual faveoli typically vary from a fraction of a millimeter to several mm (e.g., 7 mm in the viperids *Atheris* and *Causus*). The faveolar parenchyma of the vascular lung is variable within individuals as well as among species. It is most deeply partitioned near the heart and more sparsely partitioned with increasingly shallow depressions or pockets posteriorly where the vascular lung transitions to saccular lung (fig. 6.12).

Lung Ventilation: How Do Snakes Breathe?

The lungs of reptiles, including snakes, are filled by a mechanism that involves aspiration of air into the lungs. The lungs are expanded by muscular effort, and this creates a negative pressure with respect to atmospheric pressure around the animal. Thus, air moves in response to a pressure gradient from outside to inside during the inflow phase of the breathing cycle, called *inspiration*. The opposite outflow of air, or *expiration*, is attributable to passive elastic recoil of the stretched lung and surrounding tissues, in addition to ventilatory muscles that help to squeeze the lung and thereby assist the expulsion of air. Gravity may also assist the passive component of expiration by creating a downward force on the expanded ribs and elevated body. Paired ribs surround the internal organs, including the lung, and run the length of the body cavity in snakes. Intercostal muscles between adjacent ribs act to move the ribs forward and outward, thereby expanding the lung and body wall during inflation, while other sets of muscles pull the ribs inward to compress the lung space during expiration.

Breathing is intermittent, and the air that is inspired into the lung typically is held there for variable periods (called *apnea*) before the air is expired. Only a fraction of the lung air is inspired or expired in a given breath, and several cycles of breathing are usually required to "turn over" the lung air completely. The glottis is open during inspiration, allowing air to flow into the lung when its internal space expands. Following the active inspiration of air, the inspiratory muscles relax and the glottis is closed. Elastic recoil of the lung causes the lung space to compress slightly, but the lungs are maintained in a partly inflated state during the period of apnea. After some while consisting of fractions of a minute or longer, the glottis is opened and air is expired from the lung, which empties partially and then expands immediately for the next cycle of inflation. Terrestrial snakes usually take a single breath at a time, spaced apart by variable apneic periods depending on the need. Aquatic snakes, however, typically have long apneic periods, or breath-hold, while they are submerged. When these snakes surface to breathe, several or more breaths are exchanged before the animal dives once again.

Respiratory Properties and Functions of Blood

The blood of snakes serves to transport oxygen from lungs to body tissues, and carbon dioxide from body tissues to lung. These gases diffuse freely across the thin barrier between the blood and lumen of the lung, and across the thin barrier between blood and cells of the various body tissues (fig. 6.1). The exchanges occur within capillaries, which have thin and very permeable walls that are designed for such exchange.

The amount of respiratory gases that might dissolve freely in the blood plasma would not be sufficient to meet the transport needs of an active vertebrate animal such as a snake. Therefore, the role of hemoglobin—carried within red blood cells—is very important. Once oxygen diffuses into the blood plasma across the capillary wall, it diffuses very rapidly to hemoglobin, where it attaches to specific sites. Each "molecule" of hemoglobin has four subunits, each with a *heme* group containing iron. Once oxygen attaches to one of the heme sites, the probability increases that the other sites will bind other oxygen molecules. When all the sites are bound on all the hemoglobin molecules, the blood is said to be "saturated" with oxygen and exhibits its maximum transport capacity. The maximum transport of oxygen by hemoglobin is, very roughly, about 20 to 40 times greater than the amount that might be carried in simple physical solution (plasma) without hemoglobin.

There are two important features of the physical environment of hemoglobin that determine how much oxygen it carries and can provide for respiration. First, the tendency for oxygen molecules to bind with hemoglobin depends on the partial pressure of oxygen in the blood. Typically, oxygen binds to hemoglobin at pressures that occur within the ventilated lung, and the pulmonary blood saturates with oxygen during its passage through the vascular lung parenchyma. Second, the physical diffusion of oxygen either from the lung air into pulmonary capillaries, or from systemic capillaries into respiring tissues, depends on the gradient of oxygen pressure. That is, there must be a difference of oxygen partial pressure in order for oxygen to diffuse, and it will move from a region of higher to lower pressure. This is why lung ventilation is important, because it maintains the oxygen pressure closer to the ambient atmospheric value and thereby maximizes the pressure that drives diffusion into the lung capillaries. Because some of the oxygen is removed from the blood during its passage through systemic capillaries, the relatively oxygen-deficient blood that is returned to the heart from tissues and sent to the lung for reoxygenation is at an oxygen pressure lower than that of the pulmonary air within the lung lumen. Therefore, oxygen diffuses from the lung air into the capillaries within the lung. At the other end—systemic tissues—the removal of oxygen by respiring mitochondria within cells lowers the oxygen pressure well below that of the systemic blood, so now the oxygen diffuses from the pressure in the blood (equilibrated to atmospheric air within the lung) to the much lower pressure in tissues that act as the "sink" for the oxygen.

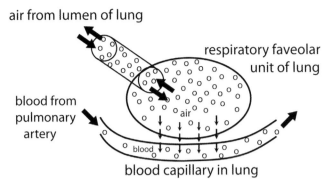

air from lumen of lung

respiratory faveolar unit of lung

blood from pulmonary artery

air

blood

blood capillary in lung

Figure 6.15. Schematic representation of oxygen transfer by diffusion from lung air into blood of a pulmonary capillary. The density of bubbles in the illustration represents the concentration and pressure of oxygen molecules, which are greatest where the air is ventilated in and out of the faveolar exchange unit (upper and left part of figure) and becomes relatively depleted where oxygen diffuses into the blood capillary. The blood capillary carries relatively oxygen-deficient blood returning from the body tissues (entry at left), and this blood becomes relatively more oxygenated as it passes through the lung faveolar exchange unit (center to right). Drawing by the author.

Thus, there are two competing processes that occur in the lung with respect to oxygen: diffusion into blood tends to lower the oxygen pressure, and renewal of oxygen by ventilation tends to elevate the oxygen pressure. The actual oxygen pressure in the lumen of the lung at any given time depends on the balance between these two opposing processes (fig. 6.15).

It is important to realize that the oxygen that binds to sites on hemoglobin does not contribute to the blood levels of oxygen pressure. Thus, the oxygen pressure is determined by the amount of free oxygen in the blood plasma immediately surrounding the hemoglobin. At any given level of this pressure, the hemoglobin saturates to the extent determined by its binding properties in relation to the oxygen pressure.

Like other vertebrates, the hemoglobins of various species of snakes are adapted to load and deliver oxygen according to evolved properties that are appropriate for the gaseous environment, rate of metabolism, and the activity regimen of the animal, but these have been studied in but a few species of snakes. The blood of file snakes (*Acrochordus* spp.) is unusual because of their generally sluggish behavior, comparatively low rates of metabolism, and especially their tendency to be reclusive—probably to avoid possible predators. These snakes have a comparatively large volume of blood, a high ratio of red blood cells (and thus hemoglobin) to plasma, and possession of hemoglobin that has an unusually high affinity for oxygen and is capable of binding oxygen at relatively low oxygen pressures. These aquatic snakes exchange a portion of their respiratory gases across the skin (8–24 percent of O_2; 33–76 percent of CO_2), so it is important that the hemoglobin not release its oxygen at

low pressures that might prevail in water. The high affinity of the hemoglobin ensures that oxygen will be attracted from the aqueous environment that is near to the skin capillaries as well from lung air, and that diffusion losses to water that might be deficient in oxygen are minimized. In addition to this feature of acrochordid hemoglobin, the skin capillaries are associated with arterial vessels that can shunt blood toward or away from the skin.

In the case of Little File Snakes (*Acrochordus granulatus*) that live in the Philippines, I have measured nearly zero oxygen in water within mud burrows where these snakes occur at the bottom of mangrove habitats. Presumably in these situations blood is shunted *away* from the skin to avoid cutaneous losses of oxygen due to diffusion from blood to water. On the other hand, high levels of oxygen pressure occur in the open waters of these mangroves especially at certain times of the day. During these times blood flow is presumably shunted *to* the skin in order to capture oxygen from the ambient water as well as diffuse away CO_2. These comments are speculations, and the phenomena associated with blood flow patterns to skin require much further investigation. Sea snakes, incidentally, exchange higher proportions of respiratory gases across the skin, and they are probably subjected to higher environmental pressure of oxygen than are file snakes living in mangroves.

Here we need to mention that the gaseous by-product of respiration, CO_2, is transported in the blood with a reversal of features that have been described for oxygen. Thus, CO_2 diffuses from respiring cells into systemic blood capillaries and then flows to the lung, where it diffuses across the vascularized pulmonary parenchyma into the air of the lumen, from where it is ultimately ventilated away to the atmosphere. Some of the CO_2 forms an attachment with hemoglobin, but in a way that is different from oxygen and in far lesser amounts. The majority of the gas becomes hydrated and is transported in plasma in the form of bicarbonate ion (HCO_3^-). Carbon dioxide is highly soluble in water, and relatively little is transported as a gas in physical solution. Hemoglobin also plays an important role in buffering the pH of the blood, for acid is formed when CO_2 combines with water to form H^+ and HCO_3^-.

The control of breathing and transport of blood gases is driven by the need to eliminate CO_2 as much as the need to acquire oxygen. Also, the need to eliminate CO_2 is coupled to the requirement for regulating the pH of blood and other body tissues. Because the hydration reaction of CO_2 to form bicarbonate (HCO_3^-) also produces acid (H^+), respiration tends to acidify the blood unless the H^+ is buffered and/or removed from the body. Both processes occur. Hemoglobin and other components of the blood tend to buffer the H^+, but over time the CO_2 being produced from metabolism must be eliminated or the pH will ultimately decrease to lethal levels. Decreases in blood pH and increases in blood CO_2 tend to provide the more important respiratory signals controlling ventilation in tetrapod vertebrates, although diminishing levels of blood oxygen also participate.

Nonrespiratory Functions of the Lung

The saccular segment of lung—simply called "air sac" in earlier literature—functions as a "bellow" because the volume expansion of the entire lung pulls air into the "sac" and this same air exits the lung when it is expired. Hence, the relatively large volume of the saccular region of the lung helps to ventilate the vascular lung, in essence alternately "pulling and pushing" air across it. The saccular region also allows storage of air, in addition to that which is within the vascular lung. This means there is added storage of oxygen, which can be moved to the faveolar surfaces either by diffusion or, more effectively, by convection due to body movements or active contractions of smooth muscle that occurs in the lung wall. The bellows and storage functions of the saccular lung are, of course, indirectly related to respiration.

The storage function might be particularly important in aquatic or semiaquatic species of snakes because it increases the time that a snake might remain submerged without needing to surface for breathing air. In sea snakes the terminal saccular segment of the lung is exceptionally thick and muscular (fig. 6.16), presumably important for storage but with capability to "inject" by muscular contraction the pressurized air into the respiratory parenchyma at periodic intervals. No one knows if, or how, this feature is actually used by sea snakes.

Inflation of the total lung increases the body size of a snake, and extreme inflation is typically used in many pit vipers to enlarge the appearance of the body during defensive displays. Irritated rattlesnakes, for example, characteristically coil with an inflated body while rattling (fig. 6.17). Also in connection with defense, this inhaled air can be expelled to produce loud hissing sounds in a variety of species (see chapter 8). More about inflation displays is explained in the next section.

Bayard Brattstrom is one of the first of many herpetologists to have suggested there are various other functions of the saccular lung that are related to physiology. When snakes become overheated, they may begin to pant, as do lizards and other terrestrial vertebrates. Panting consists of rapid, shallow breathing that exchanges air across the moist membranes of the lung and its associated airways. This convection removes water by evaporation, and in the process heat is also removed from the evaporating surfaces. This is called *evaporative cooling* and is a mechanism employed to cool the body, or at least slow the rate of warming toward a lethal temperature. If the body has been warmed through accumulation of heat from solar radiation or contact with a warm substrate, it likely will be warmer than the surrounding air. Therefore, air that is moving in and out of the lung will remove heat by internal conduction and radiation from the body surrounding the lung as well as from evaporative cooling of the lung parenchyma (largely in the anterior part of the lung and associated airways such as the trachea). Of these phenomena, evaporative cooling is likely to be most significant (see fig. 4.13; also chapter 4).

The saccular lung might also play some role in reducing the temperature of the testes in male snakes. Sperm development is sensitive to temperature, and heat-induced sterility is the probable reason for the descent of the testes in mammals, which keeps the testes generally at temperatures that are lower than the core body temperature. Cooler air

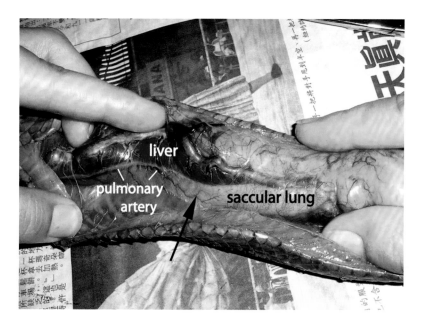

Figure 6.16. Muscular termination of the *saccular lung* of a Chinese Sea Krait (*Laticauda semifasciata*). The white, opaque, and thick appearance of this organ reflects its function for storage, having lots of muscle and thick tissue that is not well vascularized for gas exchange. The arrow points to the termination of the *vascular lung* that is functional with respect to gas exchange. The red lung tissue to the left of the arrow is the posterior aspect of the vascular lung, the arrow indicating its transition to saccular lung near the termination of the pulmonary artery. Above the lung structure an engorged portal vein can be seen returning systemic blood to the heart through the liver. Photograph by Coleman Sheehy III.

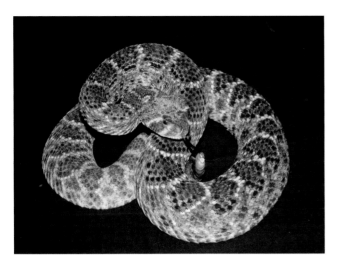

Figure 6.17. A Western Diamond-backed Rattlesnake (*Crotalus atrox*) in a defensive posture. The lung is abnormally inflated by the snake to increase its apparent size, which accounts for the spreading of scales to reveal the interscale tissue—most notably visible in the lower front of the figure. This snake was photographed in Texas by the author.

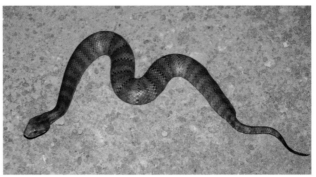

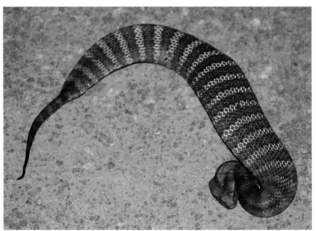

Figure 6.18. Defensive posture being displayed by a Hill Death Adder (*Acanthophis rugosus*) in northern Queensland. The **upper photo** shows the snake's normal body form before flattening. The **lower photo** shows the snake while it is flattened in defensive posture. Note the body is extremely flattened, likely in attempt to look larger to a potential predator. The color of this snake matches that of "red" soils characteristic of the region in which it was photographed. Photographs by Lauren Dibben.

that is ventilated in the posterior saccular lung might play some role in the regulation of testes temperatures in snakes.

The entire lung including the extensive saccular segment in terrestrial species appears to be important in assisting support of the body, given that ribs are free ventrally except for attachment to skin and there is no sternum. When air is withdrawn entirely from the lung, terrestrial snakes can become extremely flattened when fully extended on a flat surface (fig. 6.18). Adjustments of the total lung volume also are important for the ability of sea snakes to control buoyancy and orientation. Diving marine snakes have been observed to vent excess air after arriving at a particular place in a water column (sea snakes, fig. 6.14, and *Acrochordus*), or to adjust their vertical location (Yellow-bellied Sea Snake, *Pelamis platurus*) soon after submerging from a bout of air-breathing at the water surface. Presumably, these snakes are adjusting buoyancy to a neutral condition that is appropriate for the particular depth at which they choose to remain or be active.

Structure and Function of Tracheal Air Sacs

More than 30 species of Asian snakes possess *tracheal air sacs*, which are nonpulmonary, saccular extensions of the trachea and have been called various names including *tracheal diverticula*, *neck sacs*, and *tracheal chambers*. These are present in numerous colubrid snakes, especially arboreal species, and the King Cobra, *Ophiophagus hannah*. All of the genera, and probably all of the species, that possess these structures engage in some form of extended neck display, and all are restricted to central and southern Asia.

The tracheal air sacs of the Asian Red-tailed Rat Snake, *Gonyosoma oxycephalum*, are representative and illustrated in figure 6.19. These structures are located in the ventral body cavity immediately below the trachea. They are derived from the tracheal airway, but are secondary and accessory parts of the pulmonary system. The air sacs are thin, fragile, translucent, and poorly vascularized membranes. They do not receive blood from the pulmonary artery and cannot have any direct significant role in respiratory gas exchange. Each individual air sac is separated from adjoining neighbors by a transverse septum, and there are 11–15 separate sacs associated with the trachea and collectively extending from the head to the heart (about 16 percent of total body length). The air within each air sac communicates with tracheal air by means of a foramen (hole) in the tracheal membrane, just above the tips of the cartilaginous tracheal rings (fig. 6.19). There is a single foramen associated with each individual air sac.

The air sacs might be inflated by one or a combination of two mechanisms. Ventral expansion of the neck might

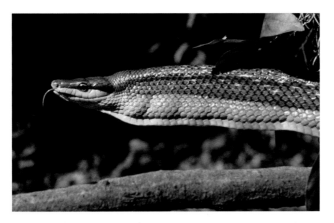

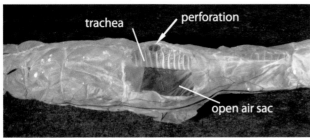

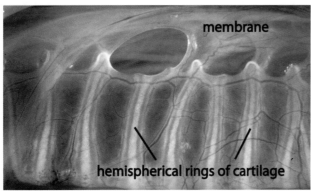

Figure 6.19. Inflation of the neck by tracheal air sacs in the arboreal Red-tailed Rat Snake (*Gonyosoma oxycephalum*). The **upper photo** shows a snake with its neck inflated in a defensive display, and the individual air sacs can be seen as distinct bulges at the anterior aspect of the neck. The **middle photo** illustrates a dried cast of several air sacs with one unit cut open to reveal the open space inside and its communication with an individual foramen (arrow) that perforates the tracheal airway. In the **lower photo** the foramen and cartilaginous tracheal rings are seen with more detail in fresh tissue. The foramen or aperture opens in the tracheal membrane and is about 3 mm in diameter. Photographs by the author.

enlarge the air sacs and draw air into them under negative pressure. Or air might be forced into the air sacs from the trachea and lung, which would be a positive pressure mechanism. Because the air sacs can be seen to bulge during defensive displays (fig. 6.19), it seems likely that a positive mechanism is active at least in some circumstances. Also, the membranous air sacs are overlain by muscle, so there is some likelihood that contractile activity of these muscles exerts forces directly on the saccular

membranes, in addition to control by adjoining lung pressures or movements of the body wall.

There are two plausible functions of the tracheal air sacs of snakes. First, Bruce Young has shown experimentally that these saccular structures can act as resonating chambers that modify the acoustic properties of hissing sounds, especially in the King Cobra (see also chapter 8). Second, the air sacs greatly enlarge the neck in a vertical dimension during defensive neck displays. In the Red-tailed Rat Snake, neck displays are easily evoked when snakes are disturbed, and the air sacs become prominent by extreme inflation during a display (fig. 6.19). Both of these functions—sound modification and neck inflation—are related to defense.

Concluding Remark

Few persons probably give much thought to how the blood circulates within a snake and how the lung functions to assist in the delivery of oxygen. Yet these are absolutely critical needs in the life of a snake, and both circulatory and pulmonary functions depart from the ordinary because of the elongate body of a snake, how it feeds, and how it moves. Understanding the physics of blood circulation, for example, can open one's eyes to understanding some of the environmental constraint that influences the behaviors of snakes, and how evolutionary adaptation can be so very different in aquatic and terrestrial environments. Hopefully, the subjects discussed in this chapter will help to stimulate one to ponder more deeply, and to contemplate new questions, regarding the structure and function of these fascinating reptiles.

Additional Reading

Brattstrom, B. H. 1959. The function of the air sac in snakes. *Herpetologica* 15:103–104.

Brischoux, F., G. E. A. Gartner, T. Garland Jr., and X. Bonnet. 2011. Is aquatic life correlated with an increased hematocrit in snakes? PLoS ONE 6(2): e17077. doi:10.1371/journal.pone.0017077.

Burggren, W., A. Farrell, and H. Lillywhite. 1997. Vertebrate cardiovascular systems. In W.H. Dantzler (ed.), Handbook of Physiology, Section 13: Comparative Physiology, Vol. I. Oxford University Press: New York, pp. 215–308.

Conklin, D. J., H. B. Lillywhite, B. Bishop, A. R. Hargens, and K. R. Olson. 2008. Rhythmic contractility in the hepatic portal "corkscrew" vein of the rat snake. *Comparative Biochemistry and Physiology*, Part A, 152:389–397.

Frenkel, G., and E. Kochva. 1970. Visceral anatomy of *Vipera palaestinae*: An illustrated presentation. *Israel Journal of Zoology* 19:145–163.

Graham, J. B., J. H. Gee, J. Motta, and I. Rubinoff. 1987. Subsurface buoyancy regulation by the sea snake *Pelamis platurus*. *Physiological Zoology* 60:251–261.

Jensen, B., A. S. Abe, D. V. Andrade, J. R. Nyengaard, and T. Wang. 2010. The heart of the South American Rattlesnake, *Crotalus durissus*. *Journal of Morphology* 271:1066–1077.

Jensen, B., J. M. Nielsen, M. Axelsson, M. Pedersen, C. Löfman, and T. Wang. 2010. How the python heart separates pulmonary and systemic blood pressures and blood flows. *Journal of Biology* 213:1611–1617.

Jensen, B., J. R. Nyengaard, M. Pedersen, and T. Wang. 2010. Anatomy of the python heart. *Anatomical Science International* 85:194–203.

Lillywhite, H. B. 1985. Postural edema and blood pooling in snakes. *Physiological Zoology* 58:759–766.

Lillywhite, H. B. 1987. Circulatory adaptations of snakes to gravity. *American Zoologist* 27:81–95.

Lillywhite, H. B. 1995. Evolution of cardiovascular adaptation to gravity. *Journal of Gravitational Physiology* 2:P1–P4.

Lillywhite, H. B. 2005. Cardiovascular adaptations to gravity: Lessons from comparative studies of snakes. In A. Hargens, N. Takeda, and P. K. Singal (eds.), *Adaptation Biology and Medicine*, vol. 4, *Current Concepts*. New Delhi, India: Narosa Publishing House, pp. 68–81.

Lillywhite, H. B., J. S. Albert, C. M. Sheehy III and R. S. Seymour. 2012. Gravity and the evolution of cardiopulmonary morphology in snakes. *Comparative Biochemistry and Physiology* Part A 161:230–242.

Lillywhite, H. B., and T. M. Ellis. 1998. Structure and function of tracheal air sacs in the Asian snake *Gonyosoma oxycephalum*. *Hamadryad* 23:121–126.

Pough, F. H., and H. B. Lillywhite. 1984. Blood volume and blood oxygen capacity of sea snakes. *Physiological Zoology* 57:32–39.

Rosenberg, H. I. 1973. Functional anatomy of pulmonary ventilation in the garter snake, *Thamnophis elegans*. *Journal of Morphology* 140:171–184.

Seymour, R. S. 1974. How sea snakes avoid the bends. *Nature* 250:489–490.

Seymour, R. S. 1982. Physiological adaptations to aquatic life. In C. Gans and F. H. Pough (eds.), *Biology of the Reptilia*, vol. 13, *Physiological Ecology*. New York: Academic Press, pp. 1–51.

Seymour, R. S. 1987. Scaling of cardiovascular physiology in snakes. *American Zoologist* 27:97–109.

Seymour, R. S., and J. O. Arndt. 2004. Independent effects of heart-head distance and caudal blood pooling on blood pressure regulation in aquatic and terrestrial snakes. *Journal of Experimental Biology* 207:1305–1311.

Seymour, R. S., and H. B. Lillywhite. 1976. Blood pressure in snakes from different habitats. *Nature* 264:664–666.

Wallach, V. 1998. The lungs of snakes. In C. Gans and A. S. Gaunt (eds.), *Biology of the Reptilia*, vol. 19. Ithaca, NY: Society for the Study of Amphibians and Reptiles, pp. 93–295.

Young, B. A. 1991. Morphological basis of "growling" in the King Cobra, *Ophiophagus hannah*. *Journal of Experimental Zoology* 260:275–287.

Young, B. A. 1992. Tracheal diverticula in snakes: Possible functions and evolution. *Journal of Zoology* (London) 227:567–583.

7

PERCEIVING THE SNAKE'S WORLD

Structure and Function of Sense Organs

As one approaches a snake in the wild, the first evidence that the presence of an intruder has been recognized is likely to be given by the tongue. The eyes are without the possibility of expression or winking; there are no ears to cock forward. Instinctively endeavoring to remain undiscovered through its blending coloration, the snake will seldom move until it seems to detect that it has been noticed by the trespasser. And so the flicking tongue is being employed in some way to investigate the stranger; to give some indication of his character and intentions. Until quite recently, the nature of the impression conveyed by the tongue and the course of its transmission to the snake's consciousness were unknown. Now the tongue is believed to be an adjunct to the sense of smell, although not the sole vehicle of that sense.

—*Lawrence M. Klauber,* Rattlesnakes. Their Habits, Life Histories, and Influence on Mankind *(1956), 396–97*

The Need for Information

Try to imagine how a snake perceives its world as it slithers through grass, makes its way through tropical vegetation high in a canopy forest, or swims through the ocean across a coral reef. Behind your head is a long, thin body. You have no external ears, but your eyes are large, your tongue flicks regularly, and your long body pushes against fluid or objects in the physical environment. We know that snakes have marvelous senses, including ways of perceiving their world in some ways that we cannot. Some senses have been well studied, while others have been neglected relative to what is known in other animals. What is certain is the brain of a snake receives a rich variety of information about its external world, and this information is important to the survival and success of snakes as a group.

During the evolution of vertebrates, increases in body size and specializations for living in many different habitats occurred only with an increase in capacity for constant surveillance of the environment. Animals acquired increasing sensory capabilities for acquiring information, as well as development of the central nervous system for processing and using the information. Animals had to know what was in their environment and how to respond appropriately. Because the head end of bilaterally symmetric animals meets the environment first, sensory structures tend to be concentrated at, or near, the head. This is true for snakes, although the body is also rich in having numerous sensory structures and responses to the environment. In this chapter we shall explore the sensory world of snakes, considering what is known about the various senses and the organs that acquire information in various modalities.

The term *modality* refers to the qualitative nature of a *stimulus*—whether it is light, sound, vibration, and so on. A stimulus refers to any form of energy that excites a *receptor*, and a receptor in turn is defined as a structure that is excited by, and transduces, a stimulus. Receptors are typically specialized nerve endings or sometimes other cells that are modified to receive a particular stimulus and are themselves coupled to specialized nerve endings. The rods and cones of the eye are examples. A *transducer* is any device (biological or not) that changes energy from one form to another. So, continuing with the eye as an example, the rods and cones transduce captured light energy that falls upon them into the bioelectric signals that travel along nerve membranes. It is amazing to think that, regardless of the modality of stimulus—light, heat, sound, and so on—all stimuli are transduced into the same form of energy that travels as nerve impulses to the brain. The specificity of the nerve pathway and the area of the brain receiving signals determine the sensation that the animal perceives, such as light or sound.

Vision: What the Eyes See

Snakes generally have good vision, but it is better developed in arboreal snakes than in many others, and is poorly developed in burrowing and possibly some aquatic species living in turbid waters. Fundamentally, the eye of a snake is quite similar in physical features to the eyes of other vertebrates, including humans (fig. 7.1). It is shaped like a cup. There is a bilaterally symmetric pair on the head, and the "eyeball" is spherical. Light entering the eye passes through a transparent layer of tissue called the *cornea*, which is continuous with connective tissue termed the *sclera*. The latter forms what is called the "white" of the eye in humans. The sclera of snakes does not possess a densely fibrous, cartilaginous, or bony ring that is present in some other vertebrates, however. The entering light next passes through fluid within the eye chamber and is absorbed by the *retina*, which is a tissue layer containing the visual receptors, termed rods and cones. Just behind the cornea are the *iris* and *lens*. The iris consists of pigmented smooth muscle surrounding an opening called the *pupil*. The iris can constrict or dilate and thereby controls the aperture of the pupil, allowing more or less light to enter. In dim light the iris dilates, the pupil enlarges, and more light is allowed into the eye (fig. 7.2).

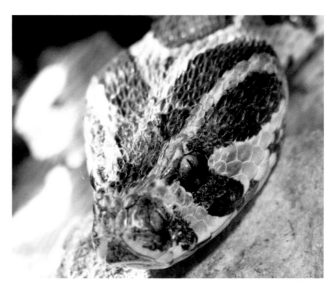

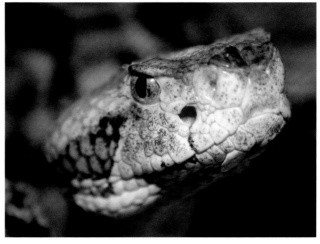

Figure 7.2. Photographs of two viperid snakes illustrating differences in pupil dilation. The **upper photo** is a Palestine Viper (*Daboia palaestinae*) that was photographed in bright light. The **lower photo** features a Timber Rattlesnake (*Crotalus horridus*) that was photographed in dim light. Both species have a vertically elliptical pupil, but the pupil in the upper photograph is relatively more contracted to admit less light under the brighter condition. Both snakes were captive specimens at the University of Texas at Arlington and were photographed by the author with permission of Carl Franklin.

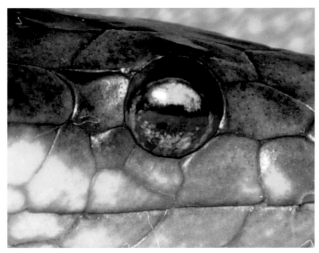

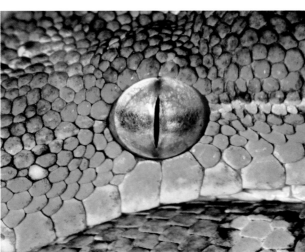

Figure 7.1. The eye of a Yellow-bellied Sea Snake (*Pelamis platurus*) (**upper photo**) and a GreenTree Python (*Morelia viridis*) (**lower photo**). Notice the diffuse pigments in the eye of the sea snake and the vertically elliptical pupil of the tree python. The upper photograph is by Coleman Sheehy III, and lower photograph is by Nicholas Millichamp.

In species having a so-called "slit pupil" (figs. 7.1, 7.2, 7.4. 7.5) the arrangement of muscles around the "slit" makes it easier to control the amount of light entering the eye with minimum muscular contraction. Slit pupils can open to a fully round pupil in dim light, and the slit is not required for nocturnal vision. A number of nocturnal species do not have a slit pupil and are well able to see under conditions of dim light. The slit simply affords finer control over light entry in nocturnal or crepuscular species having retinas that are adapted for dim light conditions, but might also be exposed to bright light conditions.

The lens is behind the iris and bends the light rays toward each other as light passes through this structure. The bending of light in this way is called *refraction*, and the degree of refraction depends on the curvature of the lens. The cornea also refracts light, and the further refraction afforded by the lens is simply "fine-tuning" of the process. The point at which the light rays converge after passing through the cornea and lens is called the "focal point." In

order to produce a clear image, the light must converge at a focal point that is on the retina (fig. 7.3). This is accomplished in snakes by moving the entire lens in relation to the retina using muscles within the iris. Enlarged muscles of the iris apply pressure to the vitreous fluid, which forces the rigid, spherical lens forward. The lens moves back passively when these muscles are relaxed. Such a means of so-called *accommodation* is a principal difference from other vertebrates in which the eye is focused by changing the curvature of the lens by means of ciliary muscles (also called "ciliary bodies") that were conceivably lost in the ancestors of snakes. The peculiar mechanism for focusing the eyes of modern snakes is presumably derived independently from other vertebrates, and likely represents the evolutionary "use" of the degenerated ancestral eye parts.

Snakes lack eyelids, and what is called a *spectacle* consists of fused corneal and scleral tissue with epidermis. The spectacle is protective and serves the same function as eyelids. In addition, the spectacle has been shown to contribute to

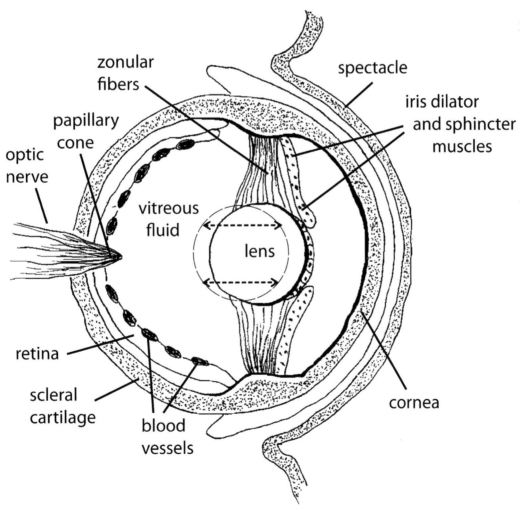

Figure 7.3. Schematic illustration of a generalized eye of a snake. Light passes through the lens and activates photoreceptors that are arrayed on the retina. Snakes focus the light by means of contracting iris muscles that increase pressure on the vitreous fluid and thereby move the lens forward. The dashed lines indicate such movement of the lens. Drawing by Dan Dourson.

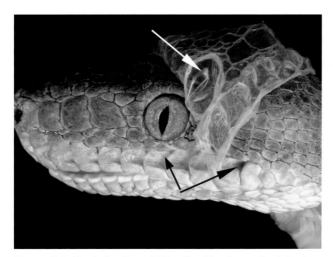

Figure 7.4. Head of an Emerald Tree Boa (*Corallus caninus*) that is beginning to shed its outer generation of epidermis. The shed *spectacle* that previously covered the eye can be seen immediately behind the eye (white arrow). Note also a series of *labial pits* running lengthwise along the series of upper labial scales (black arrows). The external nostril is at the front of the head to the left in the photo. Photograph by Elliott Jacobson.

Figure 7.5. Head view of an arboreal Oriental Whipsnake (*Ahaetulla prasina*) featuring the keyhole eye and lateral depression along the side of the head, extending from the eye to the snout. The **inset** illustrates binocular vision and overlap of the visual field in this species, related to the narrowed snout and the relative position of the eyes. Note the extended tongue with tines together. Photograph by the author.

the refractive properties of the eye. The spectacle is renewed when the epidermis is shed at each skin-shedding cycle (fig. 7.4). Because of the lack of eyelids, snakes will never wink at you in spite of what they might be thinking.

Most snakes, as well as most vertebrates, have two overlapping visual systems within the retina. One contains *rods*, which are sensitive to dim light and are responsible for night vision, and the other contains *cones*, which provide color vision under conditions of bright light. Rods and cones are light-sensitive cells that are characterized by possession of different visual pigments called "opsins." These are proteins that are conjugated with a light-absorbing derivative of vitamin A. Eyes that possess both rods and cones are said to have "duplex retinas."

Gordon Walls, who was a research associate in ophthalmology at Wayne University College of Medicine, wrote an early treatise on the adaptive diversity of vertebrate eyes and pointed out that the eyes of snakes exhibit a wide range of ratios of rods to cones. Many snakes are considered to have color vision, except for burrowing forms in which the eyes are degenerated to varying degrees. Diurnal snakes—especially many terrestrial colubrids and elapids—have a round pupil and a retina that is characterized by a high ratio of cones to rods. The various types of cones contain pigments that are sensitive to different colors, although color vision can be restricted depending on the degree of spectral overlap of the pigments. Some diurnal elapids and colubrids (e.g., garter snakes, *Thamnophis sirtalis*) have been shown to have a retina that contains strictly cones, and there are four distinct cell types expressing different visual pigments.

Depending on the pigments that are present, diurnal snakes possess dichromatic or trichromatic color vision. Under certain conditions of moderate lighting, rod pigments may also be active and contribute to what some have called a "conditional" form of color vision.

On the other hand, crepuscular, nocturnal, or burrowing species of snakes often have a slit pupil and a retina that has exclusively or mostly rods. Only very recently have the molecular properties of visual pigments been studied in snakes. Certain henophidian snakes that are partly nocturnal (Ball Python, *Python regius*) or nocturnal and semifossorial (Sunbeam Snake, *Xenopeltis unicolor*) were shown to possess duplex retinas, although rods accounted for more than 90 percent of the total photoreceptors. Although these snakes are phylogenetically basal, their cones express two of the four classes of ancestral vertebrate cone pigments and provide these species with dichromatic color vision. In strictly fossorial species, however, there is no need for color vision, which is likely to be totally lacking in many such snakes.

Yang Liu and collaborators have investigated the variation of the size of eyes and how this correlates with behavior and habitat among colubrid species of snakes. The diameter of the eye is larger in diurnal than nocturnal species, both in absolute and relative terms. Furthermore, arboreal species have larger eye diameters than do terrestrial and aquatic species. The eye diameters of terrestrial species are similar to those of semiaquatic species, but larger than those of fossorial species. The findings suggest that variation of eye size reflects adaptation to specific habitats, foraging, and other behaviors.

The pair of eyes that occur on the head of snakes occupy a considerable variation of position, usually on the sides but having varying distances from the snout and sometimes positioned higher on the head. Probably most snakes have a wide field of vision, ranging from a little over 100° to more than 160° in various species. Snakes also have *binocular vision*, which refers to the overlapping visual fields of the two eyes (fig. 7.5). Images are focused on each of the two retinas simultaneously, and this aids in the perception of depth and distance. Binocular vision is especially well developed in species of arboreal snakes, which must judge distances and slight movements during prey capture. In the Asian colubrid *Ahaetulla prasina* (an arboreal species), the range of binocular

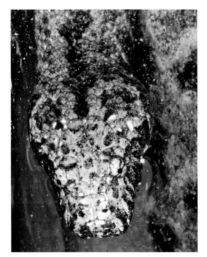 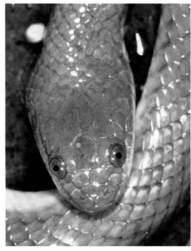

Figure 7.6. Dorsally positioned eyes in two highly aquatic homalopsid snakes, Jagor's Water Snake (*Enhydris jagorii*) (**left**) and the Rice Paddy Snake (*Enhydris plumbea*) (**right**). Snakes were photographed in Thailand by John C. Murphy.

vision is about 45° compared with 20° to 30° in some other species. In this and some other arboreal colubrids, the snout is pointed and there is a depression on each side of the head that minimizes the nasal area and thereby increases the range of visual overlap for the two eyes (fig. 7.5). Snout attenuation is characteristic of many species of arboreal snakes, likely as an aid for enhancing binocular vision. Also, when these snakes orient to a prey, the tongue is extended with the tines together, almost as if it acted as a "pointer."

Perhaps a dozen or more arboreal colubrid snakes in Asia and Africa (e.g., *Dryophis*, *Ahaetulla*, *Thelotornis*) have horizontal pupils that provide "wraparound" vision while enlarging the forward binocular field. The shape of the pupil in some species also resembles a "keyhole" that is centered over the lens (fig. 7.5). These snakes are considered to have very acute vision and comparatively keen abilities to detect movement and to judge distance. They also possess a *fovea centralis*, which is a depression on the retina where there is a relatively high density of cones and therefore maximal visual acuity.

Some aquatic or semiaquatic species that spend time with the head at the surface of water have eyes that are positioned higher up on the head (fig. 7.6; see also figs. 1.23, 4.8). This enlarges and shifts the binocular field of vision so that these snakes can better see what is above them, whether in water or at its surface. Examples are the file snakes (*Acrochordus* spp.) and some homalopsid species (e.g., *Cerberus rhynchops*). Many bottom-dwelling fishes also have dorsal binocular fields. Moreover, the higher the eyes, the lesser amount of head that needs to protrude above the water when the snake is at the surface, which might render snakes less conspicuous to visually oriented predators. The eyes are also dorsally displaced in

some burrowing or desert snakes that spend time cratered into sand with just the eyes protruding (figs. 1.20, 3.16).

The coloration of the eyes of snakes shows much variation, often related to rendering the eye inconspicuous. Eye stripes and other forms of head coloration also serve to render the eyes cryptic (see figs. 1.29, 1.32, 1.36, 1.43, 1.48, 7.8). However, in many snakes the eyes are also very conspicuous, perhaps the inadvertent result of its necessary prominence as a sensory organ. To be quite honest, we do not know why the eyes of many snakes are colored the way they are, nor need we always assume that these colors have some functional or adaptive value (see fig. 1.53).

Many snakes that are diurnal predators depend highly on vision for orientation to objects. They can maintain visual contact with potential prey items and respond to subtle cues such as respiratory movements of lizards and the movement of antennae of insects. Visual information about the position and prominence of an object is increased by viewing it from more than one angle simultaneously, conferred by binocular vision, or in rapid succession invoked by movements of the head. Head swaying occurs in a number of snakes in contexts related to prey capture.

Hearing, Vibrational, and Equilibrium Sense: Function of the Ears

Hearing and Vibration Sense

Snakes do not have external ears such as the elaborate structures characteristic of terrestrial mammals that function to collect and focus sound energy onto a tympanic membrane. Nor do snakes have a tympanic membrane or any external opening or canal that conducts sound energy to the inner ear, which is the organ of hearing. In other words, snakes have (secondarily) lost a tympanum and middle ear, which previously evolved independently in all major lineages of tetrapods. Because snakes are anatomically peculiar in this way—possibly a reflection of fossorial or aquatic ancestry—it was thought for many years during the history of herpetology that snakes cannot hear. The inner ear is well developed, however, so many herpetologists assumed that it responds to vibrational stimuli that are first transmitted from the ground through the head tissues, and ultimately to the sensitive receptors that are responsible for hearing in other vertebrates. Since the 1970s it has been learned from both physiological and behavioral studies that snakes indeed respond to vibrational stimuli that occur on the ground, in air, or even water. Therefore, the popular notion that snakes are deaf is not true, although hearing is restricted to a limited range of sound frequencies, from approximately 50 to 1000 Hz (= cycles per second). By comparison, humans can sense airborne vibrations in the range from 20 to 20,000 Hz. By definition, hearing refers to the sensory detection of airborne vibrations by the inner ear, as distinct from very low-frequency vibrational stimuli transmitted by the ground or by solid objects that might be in contact with an animal.

Snakes lack a tympanic membrane, or eardrum, and the element responsible for transmitting vibrational stimuli to the inner ear consists of a single thin bone called a *columella*. The columella is equivalent to what is termed the stapes in mammals. The columella is attached by means of a short ligament, and sometimes cartilaginous structures, to the quadrate bone, which is the posterior element of the upper jaw and articulates with the lower jaw at the rear angle of the head (see fig. 7.7; also figs. 2.5, 2.6). Thus, either airborne sound pressures or vibrations from the ground affecting the body of a snake are transmitted through tissues surrounding the jaws, the bones and joints of the jaw, the long axis of the columella, and finally to fluid of the inner ear on which the other end (footplate) of the columella is attached. The space that accommodates the columella is extremely reduced and immediately surrounds this structure, or is lost entirely.

The inner ear of snakes is fundamentally similar to that of other vertebrates (fig. 7.7). It consists of a bony structure that encloses a labyrinth of liquid contained within saccular structures, semicircular canals, and a cochlear duct or canal. The latter is an outgrowth of the saccular structure and becomes elongated and coiled to form the cochlea of mammals. The structure is not elongated in snakes or other reptiles, but like the cochlea of mammals contains sensitive *hair cells* that are arrayed on a vibration-sensitive membrane called the *basilar membrane*. This is the region of the inner ear that is sensitive to vibrational stimuli or sound and provides the sense of hearing. Energy in the vibrational movement of the columella moves the *oval window*, a membrane that moves to create vibrational waves in the liquid of the cochlear canal. These movements in liquid cause motion of the basilar membrane, which in turn creates shearing movements of the hair cells. The cellular membranes of the "stimulated" hair cells create the bioelectric potentials that are ultimately expressed as nerve signals that travel through the auditory nerves to the brain where the "sound" is interpreted.

Christian Christensen and colleagues recently demonstrated that Ball Pythons (*Python regius*) are sensitive to sound-induced vibrations, but they have lost the sensitivity to airborne sound pressure that is sensed by the tympanic membrane of other tetrapods. Both aerial sound and substrate vibrations that are incident on a snake's body are transmitted to the inner ear by a mechanical pathway through the tissues of the head. The ear transduces the tissue-borne vibrations into a neural response that travels to the brain via the auditory nerve. The original stimulus of sound or vibration can elicit a response regardless of where it impinges on the snake (head, tail, trunk, or tail).

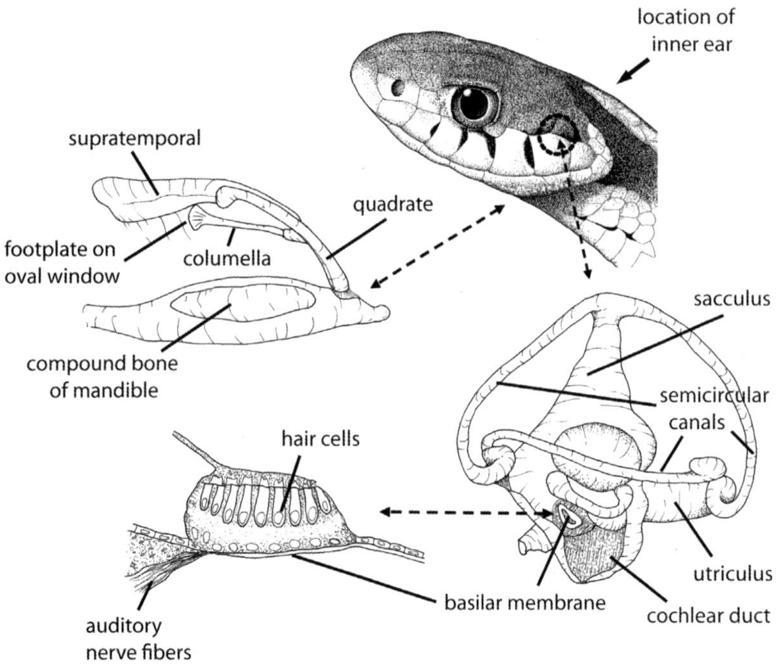

Figure 7.7. Schematic illustration of the hearing apparatus of a snake. The individual elements of artwork were drawn by Dan Dourson and based, in part, on figs. 20-12, 20-16, and 20-21 in E. G. Wever, *The Reptile Ear* (Princeton, NJ: Princeton University Press, 1978).

It is not clear why the hearing of snakes is restricted to such a narrow band of frequencies. This could be related to several factors, including (1) the pathway of tissues through which a sound stimulus must be conducted before reaching the basilar membrane, (2) dampening of vibrational stimuli by inner ear fluids that dissipate the pressure waves differently than in mammals, and (3) properties of the auditory neurons that behave somewhat differently than those of other terrestrial vertebrates. Regardless of the frequency limitations, the sensitivity of snakes to vibration and sound is remarkably good. The populations of neurons that respond to airborne sounds or ground vibrations are thought to largely overlap and could, in fact, be essentially the same.

Given the repertoire of senses that snakes possess, one might question whether hearing or vibrational sense is actually useful to snakes and whether acquired acoustic information is used adaptively. It is definitely clear that this is the case. An excellent example is the auditory localization of ground-borne vibrations in Desert Horned Vipers, *Cerastes cerastes*. Bruce Young and Malinda Morain demonstrated in laboratory studies that these snakes can localize and strike live mice using only vibrational cues. The footsteps of a mouse cause the propagation of surface waves in sand, and these are detected by the snake when it rests with its lower jaw on the sand. The incoming surface wave sets the two independent sides of the lower jaw in motion, and these vibrational stimuli are then relayed through the quadrate and columella to the inner ear. There are, of course, two receivers in the form of each inner ear. Because each side of the jaw can move independently of the other, a vibrational wave originating in sand from the right side will stimulate the right side of the lower jaw slightly earlier than the left, and vice versa. A very small difference in the arrival time of the wave stimulus at the right and the left ear is sufficient for the snake's brain to discriminate the direction of the vibration source.

It has also been shown experimentally that the midbrain of sea snakes (*Lapemis curtus*) responds with electric potentials to vibrating motions and pressure fluctuations in water. The sensitivity is low but probably sufficient for the detection of fish-generated motions in water. Both file snakes (*Acrochordus granulatus*) and sea snakes (*Pelamis platurus*) are sensitive to motions caused by swimming fish. Some sea snakes have been observed to approach and eventually bite into a vibrating object. Bruce Young has also demonstrated that swimming anacondas will attack underwater speakers playing the sounds that are made by swimming rats.

Vestibular System and the Sense of Equilibrium

As in other vertebrates, snakes possess what is called a *vestibular system* consisting of patches of hair cells in the saccular structures (*sacculus, utriculus*) and *semicircular canals* of the inner ear. These hair cells are sheared by movements of fluid and solid structures that might be affixed to the tips of the hair cells when the animal changes position in space. As with auditory neurons, nerve endings associated with the vestibular hair cells relay messages on to the brain and provide a sense of movement and orientation. Very little neurobehavioral research has been conducted with the vestibular system of snakes, which is assumed to function similarly to that of other vertebrates. Movement and orientation also depend on appropriate inputs from *proprioceptors* in muscles, tendons, and joints. These provide the sense of position and relative motion of body parts.

Interestingly, rat snakes (*Elaphe quadrivirgata*) have been subjected briefly to microgravity that is induced momentarily by parabolic flights using special research aircraft. Apparently, the loss of surface contact and normal proprioceptive stimuli from muscles and joints caused these snakes to become aggressive and to strike their own body when they lost orientation momentarily during free fall that produced microgravity during the parabolic flights on the aircraft.

Chemoreception: Flicking Tongues and Sniffing Noses

Anyone familiar with snakes has noted their tendency to protrude the tongue and flick it toward objects (fig. 7.8). In folklore the serpent's tongue has been regarded as a stinger, which surely brings death from a venomous species such as the adder. The tongue has also been regarded as a cleaning device and as a tactile structure providing a sense of fine touch. Today, however, most herpetologists regard the snake's tongue to be a sensory aid that during flicking acquires volatile chemical molecules from the environment and helps to guide the animal's behavior. Scientists working in the 1920s and 1930s demonstrated an important connection between tongue-flicking and the chemical senses: molecules acquired by the tongue stimulate chemosensory structures above the palate, which are called *vomeronasal organs* or Jacobson's organ. Although much attention has been given to the role of the tongue in chemoreception, it is only an accessory contribution to the rich fabric of chemical senses that help make up a snake's world. Functional distinctions of the chemical senses are difficult because of the interplay with other senses and a requirement for very carefully controlled experiments involving invasive techniques.

Smell and the Olfactory Epithelium of the Nasal Cavity

The nasal cavity of snakes bears a rich sensory epithelium that is sensitive to airborne molecules and allows the detection of

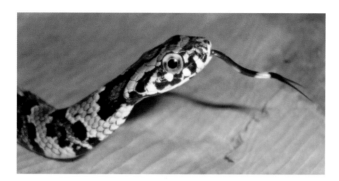

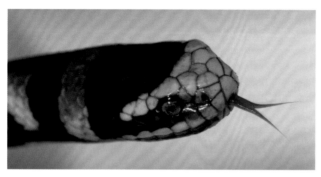

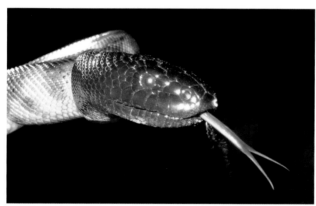

Figure 7.8. Upper photo: Tongue flick of a False Fer-de-Lance (*Xenodon rabdocephalus*) photographed in Belize by Dan Dourson. **Center photo:** Tongue flick of a Yellow-lipped Sea Krait (*Laticauda colubrina*) photographed in Sulawesi by Arne Rasmussen. Note the extent of tongue protrusion is different in the two species and is exceptionally long in *Xenodon*. The extent of protrusion in marine snakes is typically less than in terrestrial snakes. **Lower photo:** Tongue flick of a Black-headed Python (*Aspidites melanocephalus*) photographed in northern Queensland, Australia, by the author. Note the tines are separated in all photographs.

volatile chemicals (fig. 7.9). There has been a popular notion that the olfactory sense originating from activation of these nasal receptors triggers tongue-flicking and is of secondary importance to the vomeronasal system. However, there are behavioral circumstances in which olfaction appears to be dominant, and the olfactory regions of the brain are relatively large. Moreover, some studies have found the olfactory epithelium to be more sensitive than the vomeronasal epithelium to chemical stimuli. The principal conclusion here is that snakes can smell using their nasal passageways to sample

volatile odors. How useful this information is in relation to other sensory inputs is not entirely clear, and there is much more scientific work that needs to be accomplished before we will have a better understanding of this subject. Clearly in snakes as in many other vertebrates, odorous molecules are delivered to the olfactory mucosa by inhaling or sniffing with the nose. Stimulating molecules must be both volatile and adsorbed by the olfactory mucosa.

I once kept a Gaboon Adder (*Bitis gabonica*, fig. 1.28) for some while and was impressed at how consistent was its feeding behavior. Typically, it would lie within a box inside its cage with its head protruding about half its length from an opening in the box at the level of the cage floor. Whenever I put a live mouse or rat inside the cage, the snake remained perfectly still except for two changes that told me it was alert to the presence of the mouse. First, there was a brief and rapid eye movement. Second, body movements indicated the snake was breathing more rapidly and shallowly, but the tongue was not protruded in flicking that is characteristic of many other species when they are presented with food. The snake waited until the mouse came within a critical distance of its head before striking and holding the mouse, which was impaled by the snake's fangs. This strike distance was surprisingly short—about two mouse lengths—but the snake always succeeded in capturing and paralyzing the mouse quickly. One could suppose that the lack of tongue-flicking was part of the furtive behavior of the snake while it was waiting to ambush the mouse. It further seems likely that the rapid but shallow ventilation enabled the snake to increase the rate of sampling of airborne odors emanating from the mouse. Thus, in this circumstance the chemosensory input from the mouse to snake did not involve the vomeronasal system, but rather the olfactory epithelium.

Recently, two investigators from Kyoto University, led by Takushi Kishida, demonstrated that genes related to olfactory receptors are greatly reduced in completely aquatic sea snakes (hydrophiines) but are still maintained in semiterrestrial laticaudine sea kraits (Laticaudini). Relatively large-scale degeneration of these genes in the hydrophiine sea snakes following separation from their terrestrial relatives supports the hypothesis that olfactory receptors have little use in the aquatic environment.

Chemical Sense and the Vomeronasal System

The vomeronasal system appears to provide highly important sensory input to snakes and influences many of their behaviors. The vomeronasal organ consists of paired structures located near the nasal cavity from which it originates (fig. 7.9). However, during development it becomes isolated from the nasal passages to form two spherical structures, each bearing sensory epithelia on the inner surface. These open and communicate with the roof of the mouth through

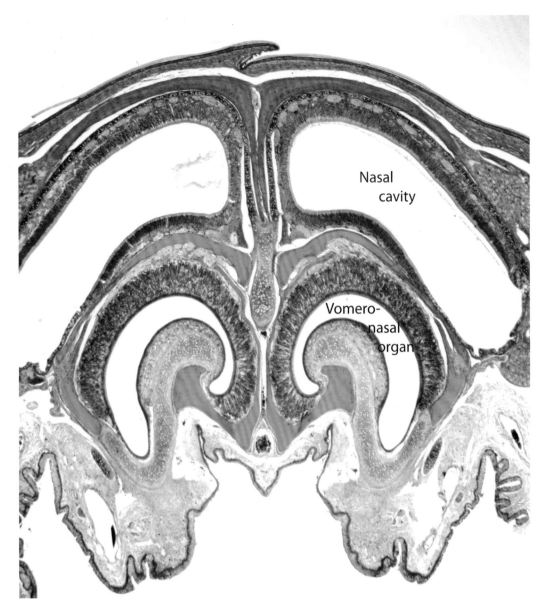

Figure 7.9. Photomicrograph of a cross-section through the anterior head region of an Eastern Corn Snake (*Pantherophis guttatus guttatus*). The *nasal cavity* and *vomeronasal organ* both have paired chambers lined with sensory epithelium. The tissues have been stained with a standard histological stain, H & E. Photomicrograph by Elliott Jacobson.

two small respective orifices in the palate. Sensory cells comprising the vomeronasal epithelium contact and react to molecules that are brought into the mouth by means of the tongue, and the activated cells send nervous signals to the accessory olfactory bulb in the brain via the vomeronasal nerve. This nervous pathway is separate and different from that associated with the nasal olfactory epithelium.

The stimulus molecules are delivered to the vomeronasal openings either by direct contact with the tongue or by contact with ridges or pads on the floor of the mouth immediately anterior to the tongue sheath. Thus, in the latter case, stimulus molecules are first wiped from the tongue onto tissues in front of the tongue sheath before being transferred

to the vomeronasal openings. Early evidence that the tongue was involved in delivery of particles to the vomeronasal organ came from experiments published in 1932 by H. Kahmann in which snakes that tongue-flicked a piece of carbon and were sacrificed shortly thereafter had sooty particles in the lumen of the vomeronasal organ. Similarly, snakes that have tongue-flicked cotton swabs soaked in prey extracts mixed with tritiated proline were shown by subsequent sacrifice and autoradiography to have radioactive material in the vomeronasal organ but not on the olfactory epithelium.

Generally, it is not clear to what extent snakes apply the tongue tips to the vomeronasal openings, or simply wipe the adjacent tissues. In many snakes, the tongue tips appear to be too blunt to actually enter the vomeronasal canal orifices. Also, some species are observed to completely retract the tongue into the tongue sheath before the mouth is closed following tongue protrusion. Experiments using X-ray cinematography and pythons have shown that the tongue does not enter the lumen of the vomeronasal organ during multiple investigative tongue-flicks.

The tongue of snakes possesses morphological specializations that appear to enhance its ability to collect and transport odorants from the environment during tongue-flicking. Histological and electron microscopic studies show there are minute papilla-like processes and shallow depressions of various sizes on the tongue's surface, and the forked regions of some colubrids have modified epithelial cells that bear numerous microscopic projections, termed "microfacets," while some other species exhibit ridges made up of projections resembling microvilli and small pores. These are thought to aid in the collection and retention of odorant particles. Moreover, tissues on the floor of the mouth beneath the openings to the vomeronasal organs exhibit a surface anatomy of folds and pores. These oral tissues also contain mucous glands that provide lubrication and enhance the adherence of substances. It has been postulated that oral secretions pool in this region, and these fluids conceivably absorb the odorant molecules and transport them into the vomeronasal organ.

Thus, the snake's tongue is used in flicking to sample odors in the environment and thereby assists with the detection of chemicals. When the tongue is protruded from the mouth, the tines are usually spread and are swept through the air or touched upon the substrate or other objects in front of the animal and, in so doing, collect a sample of chemicals from the environment (fig. 7.10; see also figs. 5.8, 5.12). The tongue is retracted into the mouth and transfers the chemical stimuli to the vomeronasal organ via the small ducts that lead to each organ. The odorant molecules then bind to receptor cells on the sensory epithelia in the lumen of each vomeronasal organ. Axons of the receptor cells are bundled together and form the nerve that communicates signals onward (via other higher-order nerve cells) to the brain.

The signals from each vomeronasal organ appear to be processed separately within the brain, so that the animal is able to discriminate stimuli from each tine of the tongue. Theoretically, this provides a snake with the ability to discriminate between paired stimuli from the two separate tines and therefore to detect directional differences of odorant molecules in the snake's environment. Many snakes (but not all) separate the tines of the tongue widely during flicking, which increases the distance between sampling points when odor molecules are being sampled and retrieved (figs. 5.12, 7.8, 7.10). The greater the distance between sampling points, the greater the likelihood that a chemical gradient can be detected during a single flick.

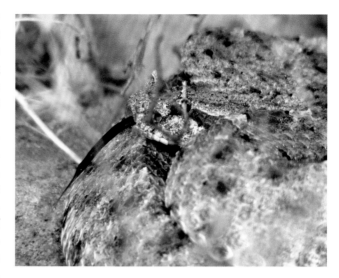
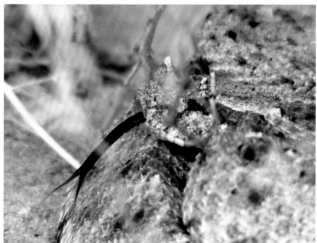
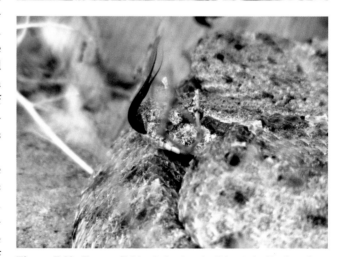

Figure 7.10. Tongue-flicking behavior of a Sidewinder Rattlesnake (*Crotalus cerastes*) photographed by the author in the Anza-Borrego Desert of California. The tines are sometimes together (**upper photo**) but usually spread widely as the tongue is waved in a vertical arc while protruded for several seconds at a time (**middle and lower photos**). The change of tine separation reflects the active muscular control of the tongue. This snake was in a defensive posture during this series of photographs. When investigating an object more directly, the tongue is protruded toward the object without the wide vertical swing that is seen here.

Laboratory experiments have demonstrated, however, that there is no change in the trailing ability of certain rattlesnakes (*Crotalus oreganus*) when a vomeronasal nerve is unilaterally severed. In other contexts, the tongue may be extended with the tines held together (e.g., fig. 7.5).

Snakes are well known to use their vomeronasal system to detect prey odors, and many investigators consider this system important for behaviors related to courtship, mating, feeding, and aggregation. At least in the more advanced snakes (viperids and colubrids) behavioral performance in these contexts falls off if the brain is deprived of input from the vomeronasal receptors. An interesting example is the well-studied predatory behaviors of rattlesnakes (*Crotalus* spp.). The brain of the rattlesnake receives input from receptors related to both chemosensory systems, vision, and infrared stimuli from the facial pits (see below). All this information is integrated within the central nervous system to produce the appropriate motor response, for example, striking to capture prey. There is convergence in the chemosensory systems, which means that neurons conveying information from separate olfactory and vomeronasal receptors act to influence the same cells to which they transfer stimulation within the central nervous system. However, when the brain is deprived of vomeronasal input, strike performance decreases and trailing behavior following a strike is lost entirely. So the olfactory input does not compensate for the loss of vomeronasal input, in spite of convergence in these two systems. Further, when snakes are deprived of chemosensory input to the brain, the sensory information from vision and radiation does not compensate and predatory performance also declines. Thus, chemosensory information (especially that of the vomeronasal system) seems to be very important in the multimodal sensory systems involved with such complex behaviors as hunting and procuring prey.

Do Snakes Have Taste Buds?

There are numerous sources of information about snakes that state categorically that these reptiles cannot taste and they have no taste buds. Usually these statements are followed by descriptions of the vomeronasal system and its importance in the chemosensory abilities of snakes. Generally, there has been a tendency to downplay, or even ignore, the sense of taste in snakes—probably in large part due to the obvious behavior of tongue-flicking and the intense interest in its significance. The scientific literature on taste in snakes has been limited as well as contradictory.

Recently, taste buds have been reported to be present on the soft tissues inside the mouths of advanced snakes (*Crotalus*) and in some basal scolecophidians. These structures are similar in appearance in the two disparate groups and resemble taste organs that have been described in other reptiles. The number of taste buds is relatively few in any given animal, and these are restricted to the mucosa of the palate adjacent to the vomeronasal organ.

Sensory papillae considered to be taste buds also have been described in sea snakes and also a colubrid snake (*Elaphe quadrivirgata*), wherein these were demonstrated to be present along the tooth rows. Each sensory papilla is comprised of a single taste bud and free nerve endings in the epithelium, and there are corpuscle-like structures in associated connective tissue beneath. These are regarded to represent a compound sensory system that may receive both chemical and mechanical information from prey.

It remains equivocal whether taste buds on the tongue are functionally important, for their presence has been reported as well as refuted in different species. I have observed behaviors of snakes that involve actions elicited from tongue protrusion before the tongue is withdrawn back into the mouth, thus suggesting that the tongue itself is sensory. Considering all the information available, there seems to be little doubt that snakes possess sensory receptors within the mouth that probably respond to multiple stimuli including chemical, mechanical, and (possibly) thermal characteristics of prey. Indeed, they may well possess some of the more specialized and useful chemosensory systems that are known among vertebrates.

Sensing Thermal and Infrared Radiation

Cutaneous Receptors and Temperature Sense

Like other vertebrates, snakes are able to sense temperature and respond to gradients of temperature and sources of heat in their environment. As ectotherms, snakes thermoregulate most generally by basking at sources of heat that is absorbed either by radiation or by conduction from the substrate (see chapter 4). To function effectively and efficiently in its thermal environment, snakes therefore must have a good temperature or heat sense. Like other animals much of the sensory information related to heat and temperature is probably sensed by free nerve endings in the skin. Therefore, it seems likely that a snake can sense the distribution of temperature along its body, as well as sense the nature of heat fluxes from the environment in relation to the length of the body. Much is known about the properties of thermoreceptors in animals, but there is a paucity of such information as it applies directly to snakes. Instead, most attention to ophidian heat-sensing has been directed to understanding specialized infrared receptors in boas, pythons, and pit vipers.

Facial Pits and Sensing of Infrared Radiation in Snakes

The ability to sense infrared, or "thermal," radiation has evolved independently in crotaline pit vipers and in several taxa of boas and pythons. Anatomically, the facial pits of pit vipers (from which they get the name) occur as a pair of individually prominent pit organs, one on each side of the head, each located generally between the eye and the nostril (fig. 7.11). These are sometimes termed *loreal pits* as well as *facial pits* or *pit organs*. In some boas and pythons there are multiple, comparatively smaller pit structures that are aligned along variable lengths of the upper and sometimes lower lip, in or between the scales (figs. 7.4; see also figs. 1.17, 1.22). These are termed *labial pits* in contrast to the loreal pits of pit vipers. The facial pits of pit vipers are considered to be more advanced, and they differ in some structural details from those of boas and pythons. In both cases, however, pit organs enable snakes to detect thermal contrast (fig. 4.13) and to form spatial images related to radiation from the environment within the infrared regions of the electromagnetic spectrum. The infrared imaging system provides a spatial image of the thermal environment and thus complements the snake's visual system.

The individual pit organ of pit vipers consists of a deep, saccular pocket having a thin membrane stretched across it. There is an air-filled chamber behind the membrane, so each side of the membrane contacts air. The membrane is highly vascular and innervated with many heat-sensitive receptors, which are formed at the terminal endings of the trigeminal nerve. That is, each receptor is part of the trigeminal nerve and not a separately modified sensory cell. The pit organs of boas and pythons are similar except the membrane is not suspended and instead lines the inner reaches of the recessed pocket. Like the crotaline membrane, the membrane of boas and pythons is richly innervated and vascularized, but it differs in not having an underlying cavity. Probably for this reason, infrared detection in pit vipers has been shown to be more sensitive than that for pythons both in electrophysiological studies of neural responses and in investigations of behavioral responses. The distance at which snakes can detect an infrared stimulus also differs in the two groups of snakes: about 100 cm in pit vipers and about 30 cm in boids.

Research using scanning electron microscopy (SEM) and other imaging techniques has revealed that the stratum corneum of the pit organ is covered with microscopic pores or indentations termed *micropits* or *nanopits*. These vary from 1–2 µm in diameter to smaller than 0.5 µm diameters in both boid and crotaline snakes. The average spacing of nanopit arrays on the pit epidermis has been determined to be from 520 to 808 nm, which is close to a structural spacing required for efficient reflection of ultraviolet and visible radiation (characteristic of sunlight) without affecting the absorption of infrared radiation. Thus, it has been suggested that the "ultramicrostructural" (nanostructural) features of the surface stratum corneum of pit organs protects the infrared imaging sensors from high-energy flux of photons in ambient light and selectively absorbs infrared radiation, thereby enhancing the resolution of infrared images. The

spacing of nanopits on epidermis outside the receptor organ areas is different (330 nm). It is not clear, however, exactly where the epidermis from these pit organs was sampled, so the functional significance remains uncertain.

In summary, scale surface and pit organ morphologies have been examined with high-resolution techniques that have revealed three-dimensional details of nanostructures on these surfaces. The dimensions of micropits are shown to vary depending on their location on the snake's body, and the surface of the pit organ is distinct from other scale surfaces that bear

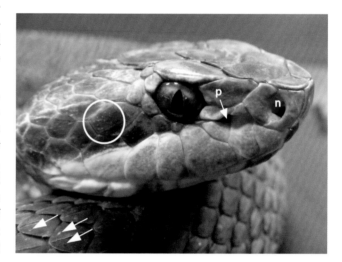

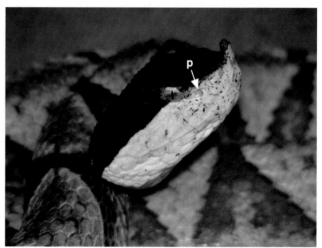

Figure 7.11. Pit organs of pit vipers. The **upper photo** illustrates sensory structures on the head and scales of the Florida Cottonmouth (*Agkistrodon piscivorus conanti*). The external *naris* (n) and *pit organ* (p) are prominent on the head anterior to the eye. Paired *apical pits* are visible on some of the body scales just to the left of the arrows. The white circle surrounds tiny projections on a head scale that are probably sensory (although this is speculation on the part of the author). The **lower photo** illustrates the pit organ (p) just below the arrow on the head of a Chinese Moccasin (*Deinagkistrodon acutus*). The membrane of the pit organ can be seen within the pocket of the structure. The cottonmouth was photographed in Florida, and the Chinese Moccasin was photographed in Taiwan, by the author.

these same structures. The dimensions, spacing, and size distribution of micropits depend on the scale type, and those that are associated with pit organs appear to enhance the absorption of infrared radiation while scattering ultraviolet and visible light in comparison with other body surfaces. One other possible advantage of the nanostructural features of pit organ membranes is to lower the surface thermal conductivity, which might enhance the detection of thermal contrasts related to patterns of radiation impinging on the pit membrane.

In pit vipers there are roughly 1,600 sensory cells arrayed on the membrane, which has a field of view of about 100 degrees. The open entry to the pit is relatively large compared to the membrane, and radiation entering the pit strikes many points on the membrane. If the radiation intensity striking the membrane is larger than the emitted thermal radiation of the membrane itself, the membrane will heat up at that location. The nerve fibers in the membrane are constantly firing (action potentials, or nervous "impulses") at a low rate determined by the average thermal radiation of all objects in the receptive field of the pit organ. When a localized stimulus (fig. 4.13) raises the temperature of nerve fibers above "background," the nerves are stimulated to increase their firing rate, which increases the rate of signal traffic going to the part of brain connected to those particular fibers. These nerve fibers are estimated to be sensitive to temperature changes of at least 0.001°C! All of the nerve signals from the pit organs arrive ultimately at the optic tectum of the brain, which also receives information from the visual, motor, and auditory systems. Some of the neurons in the optic tectum respond to combined infrared and visual stimulation, which produce overlapping maps that are relayed to the forebrain. Thus, the infrared and visual information, along with other sensory inputs, merges to form imagery of the external world in a manner that we cannot well imagine.

The spatial heat distribution in the environment produces a heat image on the pit membrane, but it is blurred to a large extent. In the brain, however, the superposition of information enables a reconstruction of the blurred image on the membrane so that what the snake "sees" in infrared is conceivably clear and three-dimensional. This provides a remarkable sense that can detect the difference in temperature between a moving prey, such as a mouse, and its surroundings on the scale of thousandths of degrees Celsius!

Given the means by which the infrared-sensitive neurons in the pit organ respond to a stimulus, scientists have been interested in the observation that localized blood flow in the rich vasculature of the pit membrane changes in response to the heating of the receptors that are subjected to an infrared stimulus. In response to heating, the smooth muscle elements of the pit organ blood vessels act locally and directly to increase blood flow in response to localized heating by a focused laser stimulus. Thus, it is believed that the rich vasculature and blood flow associated with pit organs constitute a cooling system (by carrying heat away) that enhances, or fine-tunes, the resolution of images.

Numerous studies have demonstrated the abilities of boid and crotaline snakes to utilize pit organs to image and target prey (see fig. 4.13), and these are the only animals known to form images of infrared radiation and to use this information adaptively. Rattlesnakes that are blinded experimentally, or are born blind, can target and strike prey accurately. Similarly, in boid snakes normal vision is not required for accurate prey targeting, although it is interesting that Burmese Pythons (*Python molurus*) born with a single eye preferentially target prey on the sighted side. On the other hand, experimental occlusion of the pit organs does not eliminate the ability of a rattlesnake to target prey accurately, although the targeting distance is decreased. Boid and crotaline snakes are further unique among animals in using information from two distinct parts of the electromagnetic spectrum (infrared plus vision) to form spatial representations of their environments in the brain. Both infrared information and visual information are likely to be normally involved in capturing prey. As with eyes and vision, pit organs are often directed forward in such a manner as to provide overlapping fields of environmental stimulus, analogous to binocular vision (fig. 7.12).

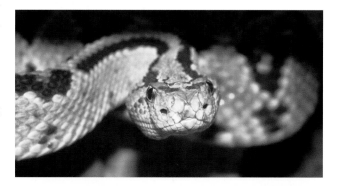

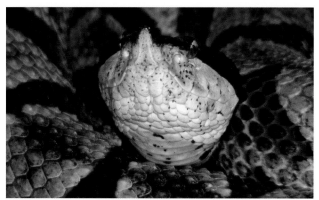

Figure 7.12. Paired facial pit organs of a South American Rattlesnake (*Crotalus durissus*) and a Chinese Moccasin (*Deinagkistrodon acutus*). The forward-projecting and overlapping sensory fields of the bilaterally paired pit organs and also the eyes of these snakes are evident in these views. Photographs by the author.

The majority of behavioral research on the use of infra-red radiation has related to the targeting and capturing of endothermic prey such as rodents. However, it seems also obvious that pit organs can be used to survey all of the spatial variation of the thermal environment, and this information might be used for judging movements related to thermoregulation, as well as capturing prey. Indeed, experiments have demonstrated that rattlesnakes use their facial pits to guide thermoregulatory behaviors. In one series of interesting tests reported by Aaron Krochmal and George Bakken, Western Diamond-backed Rattlesnakes (*Crotalus atrox*) selected a relatively cool refuge when given choices of retreat sites that simulated natural conditions of hot desert habitat. The snakes detected the appropriate artificial burrow from a distance of about 1 meter. However, when a snake's facial pits were blocked with insulating polystyrene and covered with a piece of aluminum to reflect thermal radiation, it could not locate the cooler burrow as before. When the foil and polystyrene were removed, the snakes quickly found the cooler burrows once again. These snakes clearly were using their facial pits to seek refuge from heat when placed in a hot environment.

Pit organs are probably used to survey the environment in a general way, and the infrared imagery that is integrated with visual and other sensory inputs likely guides a variety of behaviors. Both prey capture and thermoregulation are now accepted by scientists to be documented functions of crotaline facial pits. Some infrared pit organs also respond to touch, however, and the temperature sensitive neurons can also function as touch neurons. The evolutionary origin of these exquisite sensory organs remains an unresolved mystery.

Supranasal Sacs of Vipers

The pit organs of boas, pythons, and pit vipers are externally obvious structures, and it is only natural that they have attracted early attention and study. Less obvious structures in some other snakes might serve similar functions, however. Many of the Old World vipers (Viperinae) and night adders (Causinae) possess a *supranasal sac*, which is a recess located beneath the supranasal or internasal scale and the nasal scale. The sac has an inconspicuous slit-like opening and is innervated by nerve endings much like those of the labial pits of boas and pythons. The inner recess of the sac bears ciliated epithelium and secretory tubules that evidently deliver mucus that forms a think covering over the epithelium.

The supranasal sacs of viperine snakes are rarely mentioned, but some researchers have suggested that they might function as heat detectors similarly to the more familiar pit organs of boids and pit vipers. Behavioral studies have shown that Puff Adders (*Bitis arietans*) and Russell's

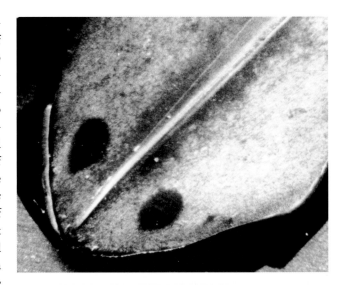

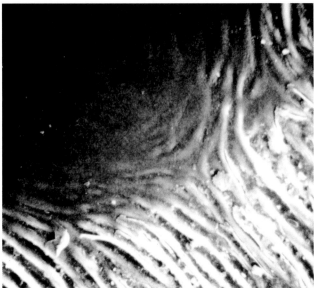

Figure 7.13. Scanning electron micrographs of the apical pits on an individual scale of a Florida Cottonmouth (*Agkistrodon piscivorus conanti*). The **upper photo** illustrates paired pits near the caudal (rear) end of a body scale. The **lower photo** is magnified another 25-fold and illustrates the transition of scale topography from the normal sculptured surface (lower aspect of photo) to the flat and smooth depression of the apical pit (upper left aspect of photo). Photographs by the author.

Vipers (*Daboia russelli*) preferentially strike at warm objects in the laboratory. Further research will shed more light on the structure and function of these putative sense organs, and perhaps other similar structures are yet to be discovered in the facial anatomy of other taxa of snakes.

A small pit has been described within each nostril of some species of *Trimeresurus* and in some other pit vipers. These consist of a minute pore lying on the inner posterior wall of the nostril, without any grooved connection with the main nasal cavity. These structures have been termed "nasal pores," but their function has not been investigated.

Sensory Organs in Skin

Imagine again you are a snake, and you have a very long body without limbs. It seems a most justifiable conclusion that sensory input along the length of the body is an important requirement for survival. Note also your body is covered with scales, and there are cornified folds in the epidermal layers between scales that allow bending and mobility. Not surprisingly, the scales of snakes have sensory structures that provide important information about the environment and a snake's sense of where it is and how it should move in response to the environment. Cutaneous sensory structures have been known for a long time, yet we know comparatively little about the details of their function.

Free nerve endings in the skin are capable of transmitting information about temperature and mechanical stimuli to the central nervous system, and these are probably important to the sensory world of a snake. Other structures appear more prominent and specialized, with attached nerves suggesting these to be sensory in function. File snakes (*Acrochordus* spp.) have prominent epidermal spines on each scale, and these are associated with a rich blood supply and connections with nerves. They are speculated to be mechanoreceptors important for detecting water displacements. Little File Snakes, *Acrochordus granulatus*, are very sensitive to mechanical stimuli in water, and they respond very rapidly to certain movements that are made by nearby fishes. These snakes enwrap fish with body or tail coils with extreme rapidity in response to these movements. Thus, it appears the innervated spines are used effectively in prey capture. Some sea snakes are sensitive to low-amplitude water motions, and the inner ear cells as well as scale structures may be involved in the detection of hydrodynamic stimuli. Behavioral studies also indicate that some sea snakes (*Pelamis platurus*) are sensitive to water motions caused by swimming fish. Small spines are sometimes seen on the scales of this species and are probably sensory (fig. 5.9). Physiological investigations have demonstrated nerve responses originating from both mechanoreceptors and separate temperature receptors in the skin of snakes, but the precise nature and identity of these receptors is unknown. Some mechanoreceptors of snakes (which respond to vibrations) resemble somewhat the Pacinican corpuscles of mammals. They possess layers of lamellar cells, but they lack the corpuscular end-organs that are characteristic in mammals.

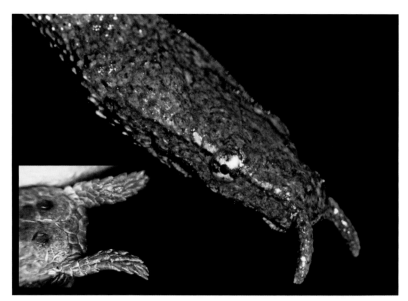

Figure 7.14. Head of the Tentacled Snake (*Erpeton tentaculatum*, an aquatic homalopsid) illustrating the paired mechanosensory appendages ("tentacles") protruding from the snout. These structures sense vibrational stimuli in water and are useful, for example, in capturing fish (see chapter 2). The **inset** shows the epidermal and scaled nature of the tentacles in closer detail, and also illustrates the closed mode of the narial valves. Photographs by John C. Murphy.

The scales of all snakes have various microstructural features on their surfaces (see chapter 5), and these include hair-like projections, pits, spinules, and what appear to be microscopic holes. Some of these features might act as collection or transducing receivers of information from the environment, but this has not yet been the subject of definitive research. Some scientists have even suggested that innervated scale structures might be used for the detection of weak electric fields, as is known in some other aquatic animals.

Many snakes (but not all taxa) exhibit structures near the posterior tip of the dorsal scales termed *apical pits*. These are typically paired (symmetrically to either side of the scale midline) sense organs recessed in a small depression having a smooth surface and visible to the naked eye in many species (figs. 7.11, 7.13). They occur on scales over the body and the tail. Similar structures having variable appearances and distribution occur on the head scales of snakes, and are known as *head pits* or *parietal pits*. These may have an elaborate three-dimensional structure within the skin and appear to be possible sense organs. The function of all these superficially positioned "pits" is completely unknown, however.

Harold Heatwole has noted that the tails of certain sea snakes are sensitive to light, and he postulates there are diffuse light receptors on the skin of the paddle-shaped tail. Olive Sea Snakes (*Aipysurus laevis*) tend to rest at night with their bodies inside crevices of coral, but the tail remains exposed and extends upward outside the coral. When light is shown on the tail, the snake is disturbed, suggesting a behavioral response to the stimulation of the cutaneous light receptors.

Finally, I mention the unique pair of scaled appendages that protrude from the rostral margins of the head of the aquatic Tentacled Snake (*Erpeton tentaculatum*) (fig. 7.14). These tentacles are very sensitive mechanoreceptors that respond to vibrational movements in water. They are densely innervated and are used to detect the position of fish that comprise their prey. Strikes at prey (see chapter 2) can be guided by either visual or mechanical cues, but normally the position of fish is signaled by integration of both visual and mechanosensory cues that are integrated in the brain. Tentacled Snakes are completely aquatic and feed almost exclusively on fish. The tentacle appendages are perhaps most useful when snakes are in turbid water or feeding at night when visual cues are less useful to localize prey.

Concluding Remarks

As with we humans, so it is with snakes: our sense organs enable us to perceive the world around us, and they determine how we view it. The amazing thing is that all the sensory input of stimuli—light, heat, sound, and so on—becomes transduced into the same form of signals that move almost instantaneously (along nerve pathways) to our brain as action potentials, where they are interpreted. How a snake "views" its world might be quite different from how we humans view ours. Consider, for example, what it might be like to view the world around us as thermal images that are constructed in the brain from signaling that originates in pit organs. On the other hand, perhaps our perception of the world around us is not really that different from that of a snake. Think about this.

Additional Reading

Amemiya, F., R. C. Goris, Y. Masuda, R. Kishida, Y. Atobe, N. Ishii, and T. Kusunoki. 1995. The surface architecture of snake infrared receptor organs. *Biomedical Research* (Tokyo) 16:411–421.

Bakken, G. S., and A. R. Krochmal. 2007. The imaging properties and sensitivity of the facial pits of pitvipers as determined by optical and heat-transfer analysis. *Journal of Experimental Biology* 210:2801–2810.

Berman, D. S., and P. Regal. 1967. The loss of the ophidian middle ear. *Evolution* 21:641–643.

Bulloch, T. H., and R. B. Cowles. 1952. Physiology of an infrared receptor: The facial pit of pit vipers. *Science* 115:541–543.

Burghardt, G. M. 1970. Chemical perception in reptiles. In J. W. Johnston Jr., D. G. Moulton, and A. Turk (eds.), *Advances in Chemoreception*, vol. 1, *Communication by Chemical Signals*. New York: Appleton-Century-Crofts, pp. 241–308.

Burns, B. 1969. Oral sensory papillae in sea snakes. *Copeia* 1969:617–619.

Campbell, A. L., T. J. Bunning, M. O. Stone, D. Church, and M. S. Grace. 1999. Surface ultrastructure of pit organ, spectacle, and non pit organ epidermis of infrared imaging boid snakes: A scanning probe and scanning electron microscopy study. *Journal of Structural Biology* 126:105–120.

Caprette, C. L., M. S. Y. Lee, R. Shine, A. Mokany, and J. F. Downhower. 2004. The origin of snakes (Serpentes) as seen through eye anatomy. *Biological Journal of the Linnean Society* 81: 469–482.

Catania, K. C., D. B. Leitch and D. Gauthier. 2010. Function of the appendages in tentacled snakes (*Erpeton tentaculatus*). *Journal of Experimental Biology* 213:359–367.

Chiszar, D., C. Andren, G. Nilson, B. O'Connell, J. S. Mestas Jr., H. M. Smith, and C. W. Radcliffe. 1982. Strike-induced chemosensory searching in Old World and New World pit vipers. *Animal Learning and Behavior* 10:121–125.

Christensen, C. B., J. Christensen-Dalsgaard, C. Brandt, and P. T. Madsen. 2012. Hearing with an atympanic ear: Good vibration and poor sound-pressure detection in the royal rython, *Python regius*. *Journal of Experimental Biology* 215:331–342.

De Cock Buning, T., S.-I. Terashima and R. C. Goris. 1981. Python pit organs analyzed as warm receptors. *Cellular and Molecular Neurobiology* 1:271–278.

De Haan, C. C. 2003. Sense-organ-like parietal pits found in Psammophiini (Serpentes, Colubridae). *Comptes Rendus Biologies* 326:287–293.

Ebert, J., S. Müller, and G. Westhoff. 2007. Behavioural examination of the infrared sensitivity of ball pythons. *Journal of Zoology* 272:340–347.

Fuchigami, N., J. Hazel, V. V. Gorbunov, M. Stone, M. Grace, and V. V. Tsukruk. 2001. Biological thermal detection in infrared imaging snakes. 1. Ultramicrostructure of pit receptor organs. *Biomacromolecules* 2:757–764.

Goris, R. C., Y. Atobe, M. Nakano, K. Funakoshi, and K. Terada. 2007. Blood flow in snake infrared organs: response-induced changes in individual vessels. *Microcirculation* 14:99–110.

Grace, M. S., W. M. Woodward, D. R. Church, and G. Calisch. 2001. Prey targeting by the infrared-imaging snake *Python*: Effects of experimental and congenital visual deprivation. *Behavioural Brain Research* 119:23–31.

Hartline, P. H. 1971. Physiological basis for detection of sound and vibration in snakes. *Journal of Experimental Biology* 54:349–371.

Hartline, P. H., and H. W. Campbell. 1969. Auditory and vibratory responses in the midbrain of snakes. *Science* 163:1221–1223.

Hartline, P. H., and E. A. Newman. 1981. Integration of visual and infrared information in bimodal neurons of the rattlesnake optic tectum. *Science* 213:789–791.

Jackson, M. K., and G. S. Doetsch. 1977. Functional properties of nerve fibers innervating cutaneous corpuscles within cephalic skin of the Texas rat snake. *Experimental Neurology* 56:63–77.

Jackson, M. K., and G. S. Doetsch. 1977. Response properties of mechanosensitive skin nerve fibers innervating cehalic skin of the Texas rat snake. *Experimental Neurology* 56:77–90.

Kahmann, H. 1932. Sinnesphysiologische studien an reptilien: 1. Experimentelle untersuchungen über das Jakobsonische organ der eideschen und schlangen. *Zoologische Jahrbücher Abteilung für allgemeine Zoologie ünd Physiologie der Tiere. Jena.* 51:173–238.

Kardong, K. V., and H. Berkhoudt. 1999. Rattlesnake hunting behavior: Correlations between plasticity of predatory performance and neuroanatomy. *Brain Behavior and Evolution* 53:20–28.

Kardong, K. V., and S. P. Mackessey. 1991. The strike behavior of a congenitally blind rattlesnake. *Journal of Herpetology* 25:208–211.

Kishida, T., and T. Hikida. 2010. Degeneration patterns of olfactory receptor genes in sea snakes. *Journal of Evolutionary Biology* 23:302–310.

Krochmal, A. R., and G. S. Bakken. 2003. Thermoregulation is the pits: Use of thermal radiation for retreat site selection by rattlesnakes. *Journal of Experimental Biology* 206:2539–2545.

Krochmal, A. R., G. S. Bakken, and T. J. LaDuc. 2004. Heat in evolution's kitchen: Evolutionary perspectives on the functions and origin of the facial pit of pitvipers (Viperidae: Crotalinae). *Journal of Experimental Biology* 207:4231–4238.

Liu, Y., L. Ding, J. Lei, E. Zhao, and Y. Tang. 2012. Eye size variation reflects habitat and daily activity patterns in colubrid snakes. *Journal of Morphology* 273:883–893.

Molenaar, G. J. 1992. Anatomy and physiology of infrared sensitivity of snakes. In C. Gans and P. S. Ulinski (eds.), *Biology of the Reptilia*, vol. 17. Chicago: University of Chicago Press, pp. 367–453.

Newman, E. A., and P. H. Hartline. 1982. The infrared "vision" of snakes. *Scientific American* 246:98–107.

Nishida, Y., S. Yoshie, and T. Fujita. 2000. Oral sensory papillae, chemo- and mechano-receptors, in the snake, *Elaphe quadrivirgata*: A light and electron microscopic study. *Archives of Histology and Cytology* 63:55–70.

Parker, M. R., B. A. Young, and K. V. Kardong. 2008. The forked tongue and edge detection in snakes (*Crotalus oreganus*): An experimental test. *Journal of Comparative Psychology* 122:35–40.

Povel, D., and J. van der Kooij. 1997. Scale sensillae of the file snake (Serpentes: Acrochordidae) and some other aquatic and burrowing snakes. *Netherlands Journal of Zoology* 47:443–456.

Schwenk, K. 1994. Why snakes have forked tongues. *Science* 263:1573–1577.

Schwenk, K. 1995. Of tongues and noses: Chemoreception in lizards and snakes. *Trends in Ecology and Evolution* 10:7–12.

Sivak, J. G. 1977. The role of the spectacle in the visual optics of the snake eye. *Vision Research* 17:293–298.

Walls, G. L. 1967. *The Vertebrate Eye and Its Adaptive Radiation*. New York: Hafner Publishing. Facsimile of 1942 edition.

Westhoff, G., B. G. Fry, and H. Bleckmann. 2005. Sea snakes (*Lapemis curtus*) are sensitive to low-amplitude water motions. *Zoology* 108:195–200.

Wever, E. G. 1978. *The Reptile Ear*. Princeton, NJ: Princeton University Press.

York, D. S., T. M. Silver, and A. A. Smith. 1998. Innervation of the supranasal sac of the puff adder. *Anatomical Record* 251:221–225.

Young, B. A. 1990. Is there a direct link between the ophidian tongue and Jacobson's organ? *Amphibia-Reptilia* 11:263–276.

Young, B. A. 1993. Evaluating hypotheses for the transfer of stimulus particles to Jacobson's organ in snakes. *Brain, Behavior and Evolution* 41:203–209.

Young, B. A. 2003. Snake bioacoustics: Toward a richer understanding of the behavioral ecology of snakes. *Quarterly Review of Biology* 78:303–325.

Young, B. A., and A. Aguiar. 2002. Response of western diamondback rattlesnakes *Crotalus atrox* to airborne sounds. *Journal of Experimental Biology* 205: 3087–3092.

Young, B. A., J. Marvin, and K. Marosi. 2000. The potential significance of ground-borne vibration to predator-prey relationships in snakes. *Hamadryad* 25:164–174.

Young, B. A., and M. Morain. 2002. The use of ground-borne vibrations for prey localization in the Saharan sand vipers (*Cerastes*). *Journal of Experimental Biology* 205:661–665.

8

SOUND PRODUCTION

A cornered gopher or bull snake is the picture of a vindictive and dangerous creature. It coils and vibrates its tail, and lunges repeatedly at any intruder. It hisses violently, having a peculiar construction of the epiglottis that accentuates the sound. This frightening pose will quite convince an observer that so ferocious an animal had best be let alone, which is exactly its purpose.

—*Lawrence M. Klauber,* Rattlesnakes *(1956), vol. 1, p. 22*

Most people probably consider snakes to be generally silent creatures, making little noise during chance encounters, or when being seen at a zoo or filmed for a television documentary. Limited knowledge also suggests to most people that snakes cannot hear, or at least cannot hear well. This view is strengthened by considering that snakes do not have external ears, and many older writings have stated or implied that snakes cannot hear, although they are sensitive to ground-borne vibrations. Although snakes may not hear well, those that hiss or rattle can make loud enough sounds to alarm persons who might encounter them.

Sound in the Environment
What we call "sound" refers to fluid-borne vibrations (usually in air) that impinge on a sensory structure (the ear) where the energy of the vibrations is transduced into nerve signals (see chapter 7). The nerve signals travel to the central nervous system, where they are interpreted by the appropriate (auditory) region of the brain. If the vibrational stimuli fall within the frequency range that is perceived by human ears and brain, the stimuli are called sound. The human ear can detect airborne vibrations in the range of frequencies from roughly 20 to 20,000 Hz (Hertz, = cycles per second).

A similar phenomenon would be expected to occur in snakes, except that the animals lack an external ear and ear canal. Therefore, one might suppose that snakes cannot hear at all, but this is not true. There are many animals that lack externally obvious ears, yet they can "hear" vibrational stimuli that are transduced through the tissues of the head, internal bony structures, or other mechanisms such as the vibrations of air sacs in fishes. In snakes, vibrations are conducted through the tissues of the head (including the columella) to stimulate the inner ear, as described in chapter 7.

At lower frequencies, even for humans, there is some overlap (and fuzzy distinction) between what we might call a "vibration sense" and hearing. This may be especially true for snakes, given they respond to vibrational stimuli largely within the range of several dozens of Hz to about 600 Hz, with little or no ability to detect stimuli in excess of about 1,000 Hz. Both the inner ear and the tissues of the body surrounding it are capable of responding to both ground-borne vibrations and airborne sounds (see chapter 7). So we know that snakes can sense at least many of the noises that they themselves produce. How they use this information in relation to various behaviors is a subject that is in need of much further study.

Externally Produced Sounds
Many snakes use the external body surfaces to produce sound, and various sounds are also made unintentionally by moving snakes in many circumstances. Thus, the "swishing" sounds made by racers or other large snakes crawling through dry grasses, the "humming" sounds of snakes moving over damp sand (as on a beach), and the "scraping" sounds of larger snakes that crawl among or over rocks all provide detectable auditory stimuli that alert other animals to a snake's presence and potentially inform the snake about its movements. Other sounds are made in specific contexts related to defense, sometimes using specialized features of a snake's morphology.

Rubbing of Scales

The scales on the body of snakes are fortified at their outer surfaces by numerous layers of keratin (see chapter 5). This material is derived from living cells and consists of dead interlocking elements of protein. Keeled scales have the outermost layers elevated into ridges or other protuberances on the scale surfaces, usually along the midlines (figs. 5.8–5.10). These scales can create sounds when they are rubbed against objects or against each other.

In certain snakes, the scales are deliberately rubbed together by precisely orchestrated body movements to produce sounds that are assumed to be defensive. The behavior is notable in snakes of the genera *Echis* (Saw-scaled Vipers), *Dasypeltis* (egg-eating snakes), and *Aspis* (some adders). The rubbing sound is especially pronounced in Saw-scaled Vipers, hence the common name. The lateral body scales are prominently keeled (fig. 8.1), and they rub against each other when segments of the body trunk make contact and slide in opposite directions while the snake is in a loose, but writhing, coil. The mutual abrasion of opposite-facing scales produces a "raspy" sound, which has not been analyzed in detail.

Two other observations are noteworthy. First, the lateral location of the relatively more prominent scale ridges (where the rubbing contact occurs) suggests these are a specific adaptation that has evolved in relation to the scale-rubbing behavior. Second, the rubbing of scales occurs only in circumstances that suggest that the function of this behavior is defensive.

Tail Vibration and Rattling

Many snakes, both venomous and nonvenomous, vibrate or shake their tails when they are disturbed or threatened. Such tail vibrations produce audible sounds depending on the substrate that contacts the tail, the speed of shaking,

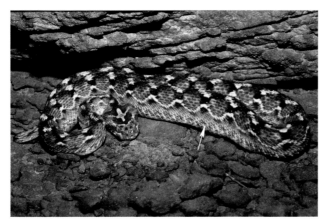

Figure 8.1. A Saw-scaled Viper (*Echis carinatus*) in south India, illustrating the highly keeled condition of lateral body scales (arrow) that are rubbed together to produce a defensive rasping sound. Photograph by Indraneil Das.

and the mass and nature of the tail. A vibrating tail of, say, a Bullsnake or Gopher Snake (*Pituophis catenifer*) will produce a startling sound when it shakes among dry leaves, but the sound would be very different and muted if the tail was shaken upon sand or in damp grass. The ability of the tail to produce sound also might depend on projections or appendages that are present at the tip of the tail in some species (rattlesnakes). In another context, I have observed that shaking the tail may serve to disperse musk in presumably chemical defensive responses (e.g., Cottonmouths, *Agkistrodon piscivorus*).

The most obvious example of enhanced acoustic signals in tail shaking is that associated with the rattles of rattlesnakes (genera *Crotalus* and *Sistrurus*). The rattle is similar in all species with respect to its fundamental structure, except for size. It can be considered an epidermal appendage, having evolved from proliferated horny tissue that is derived from the outermost *stratum corneum* at the tip of the tail (see chapter 5). The rattle consists of interlocking segments of keratin, each fitting loosely within another, and a new segment is added at each cycle of ecdysis (fig. 8.2). A prerattle segment on the tip of the tail, called a *prebutton*, is present at birth but is lost at the first ecdysis. The first permanent and distal segment on the rattle is called the *button* (fig. 8.3). Only after the second ecdysis does the rattle consist of two interlocking segments that can make sound. Each added segment increases in size as the snake grows larger, becoming more uniform as growth slows in adulthood (fig. 8.3). The rattle appendage, when shaken vigorously by its owner, produces the buzzing or hissing-like noise (similar to escaping steam or pressurized air) that results from the interlocking segments of the rattle striking against each other when the tail is shaken vigorously by tail muscles that are specialized for "rattling." The sound of such a rattle is weak when there are only a few segments, but increases with the addition of more segments as the snake grows in size.

People generally find rattlesnakes to be "noisy" animals, but many folks do not appreciate the elegant qualities of the rattle and the tail that shakes it. The rattling of a rattlesnake rattle is one of the faster movements made by vertebrates, and the so-called *shaker muscles* in the tails of rattlesnakes are among the faster muscles that are known in nature. These muscles can sustain contraction frequencies of 20–100 Hz for as long as several hours! The contraction frequency, and hence the oscillation frequency of the rattle, is dependent on temperature. In adult Western Diamondbacked Rattlesnakes, *Crotalus atrox*, the contraction frequency is 15 Hz at a temperature of 10°C, whereas the contraction frequency increases to 85 Hz at 35°C. The shaker muscles have large deposits of glycogen and are quite resistant to fatigue. Numerous mitochondria and blood capillaries are present in the muscle, which has comparatively small contractile elements and much noncontractile tissue. Consequently, the muscle is weak, albeit very effective in moving the lightweight rattle segments very rapidly to produce the characteristic rattling sounds.

There are three large shaker muscles on each side of the tail in *C. atrox*. (These correspond to the *M. longissimus dorsi*, *M. iliocostalis*, and *M. supracostalis lateralis* in the body of the snake.) Each muscle appears to be a single motor unit with fibers that contract synchronously. The individual contractions (called *twitches*) are "all-or-none" and involve all of the contractile elements. Brad Moon at the University of Louisiana, Lafayette, has shown that the muscle forces exerted on the rattle segments produce two motions: lateral displacement and torsion (fig. 8.4). The twisting motion enhances sound output, and particularly helps maintain sound output in long rattles, which have heavily dampened lateral displacements.

Recent investigations by Bruce Young, Ilonna Brown, Patrick Cook, and their colleagues have modeled the rattle as a multidimensional oscillator, and the acoustic profile of the rattling sound can be predicted by measuring the size of the rattle or even just the basal segment of the rattle. The rattle can be considered a kinetic chain, producing sound as interlocking adjacent segments of the rattle are shaken against each other, generally back and forth from side to side (the "oscillator") (fig. 8.4). Lateral displacement of the rattle segments during rattling oscillations is greatest at the tip and diminishes toward the base. In snakes having a large number of rattle segments, the segments near the base of the tail show little variation in size (fig. 8.3). This consistency in size produces a corresponding consistency in the frequency of sound that is produced during rattling. A

"typical" rattling sound can be described as broad-band noise spanning from roughly 2,500 to 19,000 Hz with a dominant frequency near 9,000 Hz. Note that this range does not overlap with that of rattlesnake hearing (see chapter 7). There is no frequency or temporal modulation of the sound at constant temperature and uninterrupted rattling. In some rattlesnakes not especially prone to rattle vigorously, the tail may twitch periodically or rattle for brief periods with resting pauses in between.

As temperature increases the frequency of rattling, the frequency of muscle twitches that power the rattling movements increase and the movements of the rattle segments require higher forces and accelerations. Yet the energy cost per twitch of rattling has been found to be independent of the twitch frequency. Recordings of the joint motions (between segments) and associated forces by Brad Moon, Kevin Conley, and Stan Lindstedt indicate that the increasing force of a twitch is offset by a shorter duration of each twitch, which keeps the energetic cost per twitch cycle nearly constant over a wide range of temperatures and twitch frequencies. Also, as the twitch frequency increases, the lateral displacement of the rattle decreases. Therefore, the increasing forces that are acting on the rattle segments are offset by reductions in the lateral displacement of the rattle, thereby keeping the mechanical work and force required to shake the rattle low. At higher frequencies of rattling (tail shaking), the decrease in lateral displacement of the rattle is a major factor in keeping the work and energy demand from increasing as much as it would if lateral displacement remained constant as the frequency increased. Fundamentally, the cost of any muscle contraction is proportional to the force and duration of the contraction. In the rattlesnake shaker muscles, there is a trade-off between

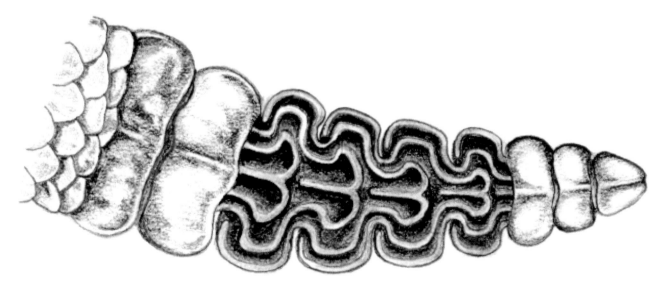

Figure 8.2. Drawing of a rattlesnake rattle illustrating the interlocking of individual segments in the central part of the rattle. Drawing by Amanda Ropp.

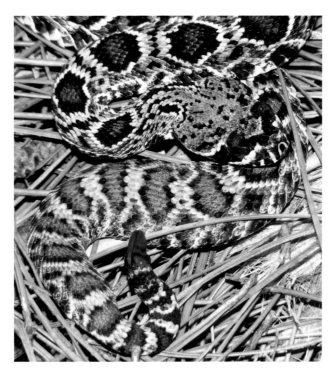

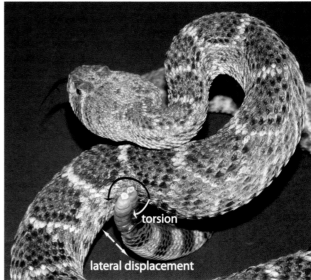

Figure 8.4. The rattle of a Western Diamond-backed Rattlesnake (*Crotalus atrox*) illustrating the forces that are involved in movements of the rattle (arrows) during shaking by the shaker muscles. Photograph by the author.

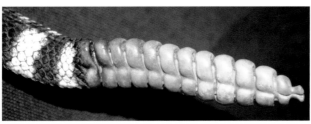

Figure 8.3. The **upper photo** illustrates the button at the tip of the tail of a baby Eastern Diamondback Rattlesnake (*Crotalus adamanteus*). This will become the terminal segment of the rattle as the snake grows and adds rattle segments. The **lower photo** shows the rattle of an adult Western Diamond-backed Rattlesnake (*Crotalus atrox*). The terminal button has been lost to wear in this individual. Both photographs are of living snakes and taken by the author.

the force and duration of twitches with changing frequency, which keeps the energetic cost per twitch constant. Thus, as temperature increases, higher muscle forces accelerate the rattle faster, but for shorter periods and over smaller lateral excursions. The diminished lateral displacement allows rattle motion and sound production to be sustained for very little work.

Prolonged rattling of the shaker muscle necessitates considerable blood flow, which supplies oxygen and removes waste metabolites associated with the muscle activity (especially lactate). William Kemper, Stan Lindstedt, and their colleagues demonstrated that the sustained rate of blood flow through the rattlesnake shaker muscles (> 450 ml · min^{-1} · 100 g $^{-1}$ muscle) is among the higher levels reported and exceeds that of the skeletal and heart muscles in exercising racehorses! During rattling, the increases in blood flow, extraction of

oxygen from blood flowing through the shaker muscles, and high rates of lactate removal by the circulation all contribute to the avoidance of fatiguing muscle during rattling at high frequencies. The unusually high glycolytic flux of lactate, and the supply of ATP related to it, help to meet a substantial fraction of the ATP energy demand of continuous shaker muscle contractions. Lactate results from the production of ATP energy in metabolic pathways (glycolysis inside muscle) that do not require oxygen. With respect to the energetics of the rattlesnake shaker muscles, their mechanical efficiency is comparable to other muscles that operate at very high frequencies, for example the flight muscles of insects.

According to the early thoughts of Lawrence Klauber, published in 1956, "The rattle is used as a warning signal; upon this, experience permits no argument: if it has alternative purposes . . . they are not matters of daily observation." Although other hypotheses and theories have been proposed by various persons, it seems to be generally accepted that certainly the dominant, if not sole use of the rattle, is in defense against potentially dangerous animals, such as predators or large animals that could trample a snake. Some imagined uses of the rattlesnake rattle are amusing, including ideas that rattlesnakes always warn an intruder by rattling in advance of a strike. Some folks living during the 1700s and 1800s believed that a snake always rattles three times before striking! Some Brazilian peoples believe that venomous snakes, including rattlesnakes, decoy small birds and mammals by imitating their calls. However, rattlesnakes rattle only in defensive contexts, and not always before the snake strikes.

The complex structure of the rattlesnake rattle is remarkably similar across all species, suggesting to most herpetologists that this structure evolved only once during rattlesnake evolution. Based on the dating of fossil rattlesnakes, rattles have been in existence for at least 5 million years. How rattles evolved is still unknown and basically a matter of speculation and debate.

Internally Produced Sounds

Hissing is the most common means by which snakes produce sounds. Surprisingly, however, there is another novel means by which sounds are produced, involving the opposite end of the animal. In all cases, the production of sound involves compressive forces that act to dispel air from internal storage sites.

Hissing and Related Sounds

I recall as a young boy the very first rattlesnake that I captured, together with a person who was my best friend at the time. This dramatic occasion occurred during December in Southern California, at a site consisting of rocky caverns and outcroppings on the Irvine Ranch (today very near the University of California at Irvine campus). We were exploring the region, as we often did for pure outdoor fun. Insofar as the seasonal weather was quite cool we were not even thinking about collecting snakes. However, we discovered a very large Red Diamond Rattlesnake (*Crotalus ruber*) visible within a rock crevice, so we pulled it out with a stick and set it in the open where we could check it out—with what I must say was great excitement! The snake slowly drew itself into a coil but did not rattle. I do not recall the temperature, but I suspect the shaker muscles of the tail might have been too cold to rattle effectively, so the defensive behavior was different from what we had anticipated. The snake slowly, over many seconds, inflated itself to a girth that appeared more than twice its normal size. Then, just as slowly, it gradually released the air during one, long, drawn-out, extraordinary hiss. The defensive effect was quite dramatic and twofold in purpose. First, the snake appeared larger, and for two boys messing with their first venomous snake, the perception of size had a chilling effect. Second, the sound of the hiss clearly impressed on us the danger that was before us in the form of this large snake. To conclude the story, we captured the rattlesnake, took it home, and held it for a week in captivity, then released it back to the wild on the following weekend.

This story helps to emphasize an important concept. As discussed in chapter 6, the elongated lung of snakes bestows numerous functions in addition to its primary job of exchanging respiratory gases, oxygen and carbon dioxide. In the case of the Red Diamond Rattlesnake, the lung volume was maximized by the prolonged inhalation, and the large storage of air permitted a prolonged hiss and thereby exaggerated the effect of instilling caution (and, at best, fear) on the part of any would-be predator.

Hissing

Hissing is an important defensive action in snakes, which otherwise have no "voice" to startle or alarm an approaching predator. The most important function of the hiss is probably to alarm an approaching animal and thereby either scare it away or, at least, instill caution on the part of an advancing predator and slow its advance toward the snake. This delay gives the snake more time either to escape or to optimize the position from which it can launch a strike or other defensive action, if necessary.

The hiss of a snake is clearly audible to humans. The sounds vary from low, guttural noises to sharper sounds resembling escaping steam or noisy gusts of air escaping through a tube. However, the hissing sounds of snakes are thought to have a very low potential for encoding information and can be generally regarded as a simple defensive warning. There is a remarkable acoustic similarity among hisses from many species of snakes, and the simplicity of the sounds has been said to approach the levels determined for "white noise." Most hisses are essentially high intensity, unmodulated, dynamic flows of ventilatory air. These are characterized by a generally simple acoustic structure with little frequency or amplitude modulation and little or no temporal patterning.

The mechanism of the hiss in most snakes involves several elements. First, the energy that "drives" the production of sound is attributable to the movement of air within the lung and through the opening of the trachea or larynx. The release of air during exhalation that is associated with a hiss is due either to passive recoil of the inflated lung and stretched body wall, or to active compression of the body and lung by surrounding muscles, or both. Second, the production of sound as a result of escaping air involves an interaction involving the dynamic flow of the air, the length of the tracheal airway, and the aperture (*glottis*) of the trachea (fig. 8.5). The frequency of the hissing sound depends on the length and diameter relationships of the trachea and/or larynx. The trachea is essentially a long tube with one end that can be opened or closed by muscular actions of the glottis. Exhalation of air from the trachea through the glottis induces vibration of air within the trachea. The frequency of such vibration, and thus the sound that is produced, is directly related to the length of the tube. Of course, the trachea is not a solid tube (of cartilage) but contains a flexible membrane for part of its circumference (figs. 6.13, 6.19). Thus, vibrations of the tracheal membrane can also influence the sound that is produced. Vibrations of the tracheal membrane are dependent on the vibrations of the

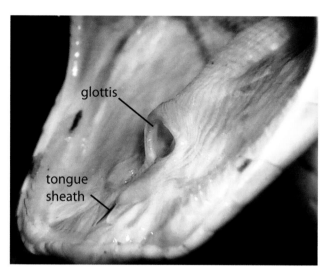

Figure 8.5. Lower mouth of a Neotropical Bird Snake (also called Puffing Snake) (*Pseustes poecilonotus*) showing the open glottis with tongue sheath beneath. Photograph by Dan Dourson.

air within the trachea, and the tensioning of the tracheal membrane. Finally, hissing sounds can be produced during both inhalation and exhalation of pulmonary air.

Dr. Bruce Young, currently at the University of Massachusetts, Lowell, has focused much of his research program on evaluating the sound production and sound-producing mechanisms of snakes. He has suggested a good analogy for understanding the hissing noises of snakes, and this is the musical instrument that we call a flute. Flutes are classified according to their length, and the longer the flute the lower the frequency it is able to produce. For a given flute, the finger holes (allowing escape of exhaled air by the player) farthest from the air source produce the sounds of lowest frequency, whereas those adjacent to the air source produce the sounds having highest frequency. These features are analogous to the length of the trachea and the relative position of the opening (see also the section on "growling" below).

Ventilatory air flow in snakes is produced by localized movements of the ribs, and such actions have been referred to by Herb Rosenberg as the "costal pump." In some snakes the defensive hisses exhibit a quadriphasic temporal pattern characterized by (1) an initial exhalatory hiss, followed by (2) a brief transitional pause; (3) an inhalatory hiss; and then (4) a second pause or period of rest. The costal pump is responsible for generating this pattern, and the role of the pulmonary tract is generally passive. *Abduction* of the ribs (movement away from the central axis) produces negative pressure in the lungs and powers inhalation, sometimes resulting in an inhalation hiss. *Adduction* of the ribs (movement toward the central axis) does the opposite, increasing pressure within the lung and powering exhalation with associated hissing. Expansion of the body (on inhalation) is a common feature of defensive displays of snakes, and the

exchange of air between the trachea, lung, and environment is often accompanied by hissing sounds.

The noise of a hiss is a broad spectrum of sound, spanning frequencies from roughly 3,000 to 13,000 Hz. There is a dominant frequency at around 7,500 Hz, with little variation related to species or body size. While some herpetologists have suggested that snakes have the capability to modulate the amplitude and temporal properties of the hiss (changes through time), there is no convincing evidence for such modulation. Snakes have two muscles that can act to alter the diameter of the glottal opening, which could change the nature of the hiss by altering the velocity of the air flow. Such active modulation of the glottal opening could possibly be employed to modulate the hiss, but no one has yet confirmed that this actually occurs in any of the species that have been studied. Moreover, studies of artificial hissing in Puff Adders (*Bitis arietans*) by Bruce Young suggest it would be nearly impossible for the snake to produce an acoustically complex hiss, and the trachea of this species imparts no distinct acoustic signature to the exhaled airstream. The larynx is simply not able to modulate frequency of the exhaled airstream even if the glottis is forcibly occluded against the flow of air by electrical stimulation of the *Constrictor laryngis* muscle.

The hiss of the colubrid snakes *Pituophis melanoleucus* and *P. catenifer* is especially noteworthy. These species are called Pine, Bull, or Gopher Snake depending on the subspecies and region of occurrence. The defensive hisses of these snakes can be very loud and have what has been described as a "raspy" texture. Unlike most other species of snakes, the frequency range of the hiss of *P. melanoleucus* spans the range from 500 to 9,500 Hz.

The larynx of *Pituophis* is unusual in having two morphological specializations: (1) a dorsal extension of the cricoid cartilage that is sometimes referred to as an "epiglottal keel"; and (2) a flexible, horizontal shelf of tissue called the "laryngeal septum" that divides the anterior portion of the larynx. The laryngeal septum can be regarded as the first described "vocal cord" of a snake. It is a uniquely unpaired structure compared with the paired vocal cords of other vertebrates, and it has not been found in species of snakes other than *P. melanoleucus*. Bruce Young and his coworkers have studied sound production in this species and were able to demonstrate that the laryngeal septum vibrates and contributes harmonic elements in the defensive hisses of *Pituophis*, whereas the epiglottal keel has little influence on the quality of these hissing sounds. A *harmonic* is an overtone—present in the calls of some frogs, bats, and other animals—whose frequency is a whole-number multiple of a fundamental frequency. Vibration of the laryngeal septum of *Pituophis* produces harmonics that have a fundamental frequency of about 500 Hz.

Several lineages of snakes have a means of expanding the trachea, which could clearly alter the acoustic nature of the hiss. Three means of expansion are (1) possession of a tracheal lung (see chapter 6), (2) "pleating" of the tracheal membrane, and (3) tracheal diverticula, which are discussed below in relation to growling. The width of the tracheal membrane is taken up by large pleats in the membrane when it is not under tension. Except for the role of diverticula discussed below, the acoustical influence of tracheal expansion has not been well studied or documented.

Bellowing

During defensive hissing in *Pituophis melanoleucus* the epiglottal keel functions merely to divide the flow of air and evidently does not vibrate to contribute a pulsatile quality to the sound. However, during the beginning of a series of hissing sounds produced by *P. melanoleucus* there is a burst of loud (high amplitude), broad-frequency sound that Bruce Young and his collaborators have called a "bellow." The bellow has been distinguished from a hiss in having simple modulation of both amplitude and frequency, evidently due to a brief period of imbalance between the air flow and tension in the laryngeal septum. The brief duration of such bellowing is less than 0.2 of a second. This represents the time lag between dilation of the glottis to emit air flow and an adjustment of tension in the laryngeal septum by means of an associated smooth muscle. The sound of a bellow includes both temporal variation and harmonic elements that result from vibrations of the laryngeal septum.

The bellow is unique to *Pituophis* and has not been described in any other species of snake. The presence of a "vocal cord" (laryngeal septum) and the complex emission of both a bellow and a hiss in these snakes appears to explain the anecdotal reports of the unusual defensive sounds that they emit. I once encountered a Gopher Snake in California that was, in my experience, uniquely bad-tempered. It struck repeatedly, falling forward with violent momentum during each strike. Also, with each strike I remember a very loud raspy hiss, probably with elements of bellowing that I would not have known about at the time. Together, the striking and hissing were most dramatic, and they created as good of a show as the defensive displays of many rattlesnakes or cobras.

Growling

Other sounds emitted from the tracheal airways of snakes have been described by Bruce Young as "growls." The growl of a snake is the noise that is emitted when the exhalant airstream of the trachea passes over openings in the tracheal membrane that lead to adjoining air sacs, or *tracheal diverticula* (see chapter 6). These structures are not found in all snakes, but they potentially enable growling in those species in which they occur. Growling is best known (and evaluated) in the King Cobra (*Ophiophagus hannah*), and has also been recorded from a colubrid snake, the Red-tailed Rat Snake (*Gonyosoma oxycephalum*). In the King Cobra, the growl involves frequencies below 5,000 Hz (and often below 2,500 Hz), with a dominant frequency of approximately 600 Hz. There is evidence for frequency modulation in the growl of the King Cobra, with higher intensity sounds at the beginning and ending of the emitted noise. The defensive growl of the Red-tailed Rat Snake consists of frequencies below 2,000 Hz, and a dominant frequency of about 625 Hz. The growling sounds of both species are distinct from the hisses of snakes.

Modeling of the tracheal diverticula (air sacs; see fig. 6.19) suggests that they act as resonating chambers, which means they essentially dampen or filter out some frequencies while enhancing others. The size and shape of the resonating chambers determine the frequencies that are generated and thus the power spectrum of the produced sound. The larger the diverticula, the lower the dominant frequency of the growl. Both growls and hisses can be intimidating, depending especially on the size and behavior of the snake!

Nasal Hissing

Observers have long had the impression that many snakes, especially vipers, can hiss through the nasal passages. Much of the impression comes from the observation of snakes hissing while the mouth is shut. In a very early experiment, Frank Wall in 1921 observed that the hiss of Russell's Viper (*Daboia russelii*) sounded different after the nares were partially occluded.

It is now believed that, in many snakes, the exhalant airstream passes through the internal nares. A number of species are regarded as obligate nasal hissers, and these include Eastern Hog-nosed Snakes (*Heterodon platyrhinos*), the Puff Adders (*Bitis arietans*), and Russell's Vipers (*Daboia russelii*). The air flow associated with sound production passes through the nasal passageways, which are essentially static and do not actively modulate the sound. During typical defensive behaviors of the rattlesnakes *Crotalus atrox* (Western Diamond-backed Rattlesnake) and *C. adamanteus* (Eastern Diamondback Rattlesnake), air flow occurs only through the nasal passageways. Hissing is produced during inhalation (inspiration), and it is possible that these hisses are acoustically modified during passage through the nasal passageway. In other heavy-bodied viperid snakes, the external nares are variously modified with complex openings (fig. 8.6). These are likely to function with respect to very loud and prominent hissing noises that are made by these snakes during exhalation (expiration) of air.

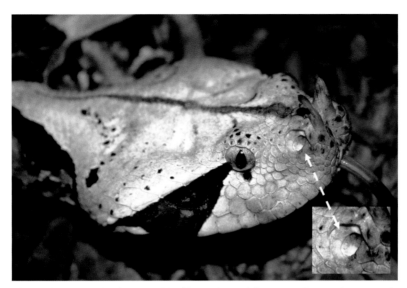

Figure 8.6. Head of a Gaboon Adder (*Bitis gabonica*) illustrating the complex external naris. The **inset** is a higher magnification of the naris, showing there are two levels of circumferential ridges overlying the deep internal opening to the nasal passageway. This snake has the ability to hiss very loudly, and the external opening of the naris possibly acts to produce the loud sound that is heard during hissing. Photograph by the author.

Cloacal Popping

Imagine a snake is making a sound like a popping noise, but the sound is not coming from the head end. There are various anecdotal claims in literature that snakes can produce sounds using the cloaca. Such a phenomenon has been reported in the genera *Ficimia*, *Gyalopion* (hook-nosed snakes), *Micruroides*, and *Micrurus* (coral snakes). Snakes can produce the popping sounds both during, and independent of, cloacal evacuation. The sounds result from a rapid expulsion of air from the cloacal vent, driven primarily by cloacal musculature (principally the *M. Sphincter cloacae*).

The "cloacal pops" recorded from snakes consist of low-amplitude sounds (around 50–70 dB) with a limited frequency range from about 350 to 15,000 Hz, and sometimes harmonics. The sounds are brief (about 0.2 sec) and exhibit a distinct temporal pattern. There is some acoustic variation of cloacal pops both within and between species. The relative size of the cloaca and the associated musculature influence both the amplitude and frequency of the popping sounds that are emitted by an individual snake.

Controlled attempts to elicit cloacal pops from the Eastern Coral Snake (*Micrurus fulvius*) by means of visual and tactile stimulation are generally unsuccessful, unless the head is restrained. However, in the Western Hook-nose Snake (*Gyalopion canum*) cloacal popping can be elicited by light tactile stimulation and is usually associated with thrashing movements. In the Western Coral Snake (*Micruroides euryxanthus*) cloacal popping occurs in conjunction with elevation and curling of the tail. Cloacal popping is characteristic of snakes that have fossorial or

secretive habits, and the phenomenon is sometimes associated with other defensive behaviors. Therefore, Bruce Young and others have concluded that this form of sound production evolved as a defensive behavior. As such, it is likely this mode of sound production occurs in other species that have poorly known natural histories.

Closing Comments

Snakes clearly generate some very interesting sounds, which are used largely in defense. Several considerations are important. First, there are many snake species around the world for which very little is known concerning their natural history, behavior, and ecology. Further studies of a broader range of species might yet reveal other sounds or uses of sound in addition to the ones described here. Second, although the defensive use of sounds seems to be a reasonable conclusion in many contexts that have been widely observed or studied, other uses of sound are possible, including communication with other snakes. With these two thoughts in mind, some additional thoughts arise.

1. A long-considered theory for the evolutionary origin of the rattle of rattlesnakes holds that the structure evolved as a warning device for numerous grazing animals that might not otherwise avoid stepping on a snake. If this were true, why did rattles or similar structures not evolve in other snake lineages that live on the extensive plains of Africa or Australia? Moreover, if the rattle evolved as an acoustic warning device, what was the function of intermediate stages? Gordon Schuett and colleagues have suggested the possibility that an enlarged cap at the tip of the tail could enhance caudal luring (of potential prey) and then subsequently evolved into a rattle. However, other herpetologists dispute this notion and point out there is no evidence to support the idea. The rattle is a complex structure and therefore unlikely to have arisen de novo. So what was the function of an epidermal appendage that led to the eventual complex rattle at the tip of the tail in this clade of snakes? It is of interest to note that Australian death adders, *Acanthophis* spp., have elaborate protrusions of scales at the tip of the tail that suggests to the eye a possible precursor to a rattle (fig. 8.7). What is the function of

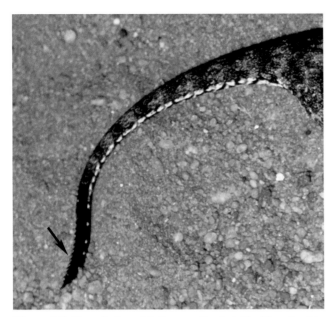

Figure 8.7. The tail of an adult Common Death Adder (*Acanthophis antarcticus*). The tail terminates with an epidermal spine, and there are spinous epidermal appendages arrayed for a short distance along the distal end of the tail (arrow). Photograph by the author.

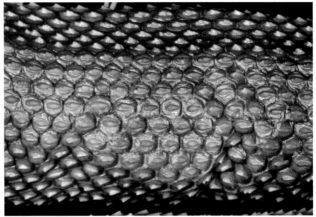

Figure 8.8. Photograph of the skin of a newly discovered sea snake from Australia (*Hydrophis donaldi*). This species was found recently in estuarine habitats in the Gulf of Carpentaria where it might encounter murky or turbid waters. The skin of this new species is strongly spinous, and each scale bears a prominent keel or sharp tubercle that is likely to be sensory. Photograph by Kanishka Ukuwela.

this appendage, and what additional steps involving genetic mutations are required for natural selection to produce a full rattle? Ximena Nelson and colleagues have demonstrated that the motions involved in caudal luring in Common Death Adders (*Acanthophis antarcticus*) mimic the motion characteristics of invertebrates, and the snakes use this deceptive signal to attract agamid lizards. Perhaps the epidermal structures on the tail of death adders also mimic invertebrates (e.g., legs of crickets), reinforcing the possibility that tail structures used in mimicry might precede evolution of the rattle as suggested by Schuett and his colleagues. These and many other intriguing questions relate to the evolution and uses of the wonderful acoustic appendages that decorate the tails of American rattlesnakes.

2. The late Professor Fred White once told me he was convinced that rattlesnakes used their rattle for intraspecific communication. This was said following his return from a visit to a communal den of Prairie Rattlesnakes in the Midwestern United States (located, I believe, in Colorado). At the time, he and a colleague were embarking on a study of the thermal relationships and energetic consequence of mass denning among these snakes during the winter. I do not know Fred's explanation for this particular remark, and he never to my knowledge published on the idea. But I do remember how convinced he appeared when he mentioned this in conjunction with other stories related to the research he was conducting at the den site. One problem with this idea is that the sounds produced by rattlesnake rattles do not overlap the hearing range of the snakes. However, it might be that visual cues are involved with what Fred observed, or that many snakes rattling simultaneously might create vibrational stimuli that could be detected by the sensory systems of the snakes (cutaneous receptors in addition to the inner ear).

3. Fully aquatic snakes such as sea snakes live in aquatic environments where vibrational information is of much value, and their behaviors as well as structure of their skin suggest they are very sensitive to mechanical stimuli (fig. 8.8; see also 7.14). We know almost nothing about the hearing of sea snakes (or other aquatic species) and whether they live in an acoustic world that is much richer and more useful to these animals than most persons might presently suppose.

4. How do sounds, as well as vibrations, affect burrowing species that live subterranean lives, and do some of these species produce sounds that might communicate with other conspecific individuals? Are there sounds that are produced by snakes, either underground or in the sea, which we have not yet noticed or recorded?

As in other areas of snake biology, the production and uses of sounds by these animals are in need of much further study. It is also true that there is a paucity of scientists who have both the interest and training in the relevant areas of physics to properly investigate the open questions. Hopefully, these circumstances will be remedied in the future, and we shall discover many more acoustic secrets that exist in the world of snakes.

Additional Reading

Conley, K. E., and S. L. Lindstedt. 1996. Minimal cost per twitch in rattlesnake shaker muscle. *Nature* (London) 383:71–72.

Cook, P. M., M. P. Rowe, and R. W. Van Devender. 1994. Allometric scaling and interspecific differences in the rattling sounds of rattlesnakes. *Herpetologica* 50:358–368.

Fenton, M. B., and L. E. Licht. 1990. Why rattle snake? *Journal of Herpetology* 24:274–279.

Gans, C., and P. F. A. Maderson. 1973. Sound producing mechanisms in recent reptiles: Review and comment. *American Zoologist* 13:1195–1203.

Kemper, W. F., S. L. Lindstedt, L. K. Hartzler, J. W. Hicks, and K. E. Conley. 2001. Shaking up glycolysis: Sustained, high lactate flux during aerobic rattling. *Proceedings of the National Academy of Sciences* (USA) 98:723–728.

Klauber, L. M. 1997. *Rattlesnakes: Their Habits, Life Histories, and Influence on Mankind.* 2nd edition. 2 vols. Berkeley: University of California Press.

Martin, J. H., and R. M. Bagby. 1973. Properties of rattlesnake shaker muscle. *Journal of Experimental Zoology* 185:293–300.

Moon, B. R. 2001. Muscle physiology and the evolution of the rattling system in rattlesnakes. *Journal of Herpetology* 35:497–500.

Moon, B. R., J. J. Hopp, and K. E. Conley. 2002. Mechanical trade-offs explain how performance increases without increasing cost in rattlesnake tailshaker muscle. *Journal of Experimental Biology* 205:667–675.

Moon, B. R., T. J. LaDuc, R. Dudley, and A. Chang. 2002. A twist to the rattlesnake tail. In P. Alerts, K. D'Aloût, A. Herrel, and R. Van Damme (eds.), *Topics in Functional and Ecological Vertebrate Morphology.* Maastricht, The Netherlands: Shaker Publishing, pp. 63–76.

Moon, B. R., and A. Tullis. 2006. The ontogeny of contractile performance and metabolic capacity in a high-frequency muscle. *Physiological and Biochemical Zoology* 79:20–30.

Nelson, X. J., D. T. Garnett, and C. S. Evans. 2010. Receiver psychology and the design of the deceptive caudal luring signal of the death adder. *Animal Behaviour* 79:555–561.

Rosenberg, H. I. 1973. Functional anatomy of pulmonary ventilation in the garter snake, *Thamnophis elegans. Journal of Morphology* 140:171–184.

Schaeffer, P. J., K. E. Conley, and S. Lindstedt. 1996. Structural correlates of speed and endurance in skeletal muscle: The rattlesnake tailshaker muscle. *Journal of Experimental Biology* 199:351–358.

Schuett, G. W., D. L. Clark, and F. Kraus. 1984. Feeding mimicry in the rattlesnake, *Sistrurus catenatus,* with comments on the evolution of the rattle. *Animal Behaviour* 32:625–626.

Young, B. A. 1991. Morphological basis of "growling" in the King Cobra, *Ophiophagus hannah. Journal of Experimental Zoology* 260:275–287.

Young, B. A. 1992. Tracheal diverticula in snakes: Possible functions and evolution. *Journal of Zoology* (London) 227:567–583.

Young, B. A. 2003. Snake bioacoustics: Toward a richer understanding of the behavioral ecology of snakes. *Quarterly Review of Biology* 78:303–325.

Young, B. A., and I. P. Brown. 1993. On the acoustic profile of the rattlesnake rattle. *Amphibia-Reptilia* 14:373–380.

Young, B. A., and I. P. Brown. 1995. The physical basis of the rattling sound in the rattlesnake, *Crotalus viridis oreganus. Journal of Herpetology* 29:80–85.

Young, B., J. Jaggers, N. Nejman, and N. J. Kley. 2001. Buccal expansion during hissing in the Puff Adder, *Bitis arietans. Copeia* 2001:270–273.

Young, B. A., K. Meltzer, and C. Marsit. 1999. Scratching the surface of mimicry: Sound production through scale abrasion in snakes. *Hamadryad* 24:29–38.

Young, B. A., K. Meltzer, C. Marsit, and G. Abishahin. 1999. Cloacal popping in snakes. *Journal of Herpetology* 33:557–566.

Young, B. A., N. Nejman, K. Meltzer, and J. Marvin. 1999. The mechanics of sound production in the puff adder, *Bitis arietans* (Serpentes: Viperidae) and the information content of the snake hiss. *Journal of Experimental Biology* 202:2281–2289.

Young, B. A., S. Sheft, and W. Yost. 1995. Sound production in *Pituophis melanoleucus* (Serpentes: Colubridae) with the first description of a vocal cord in snakes. *Journal of Experimental Zoology* 273:472–481.

COURTSHIP AND REPRODUCTION

9

> Young sea snakes have been found to be extremely numerous at certain seasons, and it is quite possible that the pregnant females resort en masse to protected bays to bear their young.
>
> —*William A. Dunson*, The Biology of Sea Snakes *(1975), p. 22*

At the right time of the year—generally late summer in north temperate regions—various persons may see numerous young snakes that appear very near to one another, and these are the wonderful product of reproduction by a female snake of the same species that is no doubt in the same vicinity. For some it may challenge the imagination how a legless and armless animal crawling around on its belly can be amorous and produce so many young. Fortunately, at least to my thinking, snakes are able to find one another of the opposite sex, court, mate, and reproduce even in the strangest of circumstances. Even so, studies have recently confirmed what many have witnessed: snake populations are in global decline, just like amphibians and many other animals. The disappearance or increasing rarity of snakes adds much emphasis to the importance of understanding how these interesting creatures reproduce.

Snakes reproduce in diverse, complex, and fascinating ways, and there has been much human interest in this subject ranging from folklore to scientific investigations, as well as the economic interests of the herpetoculturists who breed snakes for sale (fig. 5.25). Since ancient times, snakes around the world have been regarded with symbolic and mythical value. The word "serpent" is of Latin origin and means snake, or something that creeps. Hence the serpent is one of the oldest and more widespread symbols in mythology, and reproduction is one of the more important of many varied contexts.

India is a land of many snake worshippers, and there are rich traditions regarding snakes to represent rebirth, death, and mortality (fig. 5.1). There are several temples in Asia devoted to cobras, where it is believed that snakes are symbols of fertility and offer protection (fig. 9.1). Similarly, in West Africa and Haiti a "rainbow-serpent" is a spirit of fertility.

The Rainbow Serpent also is a mythological being for aboriginal people across Australia, where it is part of a creation myth (fig. 9.2). In Fiji there is a serpent god who ruled the underworld and caused fruit trees to bloom. A common symbol in many different religions and customs is a snake that is portrayed eating its own tail in the shape of a circle, and this represents life and rebirth. In ancient Greece it was in serpent form that Zeus was said to have fathered Alexander the Great. And in Christianity it was a serpent who enticed Eve with the promise of forbidden knowledge, and this ultimately led to her mortality and bearing of children with Adam.

The Essentials of Reproduction

Reproduction is, of course, one of the core essential attributes of any living thing, and is part of the definition of life that can be found in elementary biology textbooks. Organisms are the expression of their DNA, the molecular blueprints for their structure and function. Thus, for one living thing to be an offspring or product of another, the DNA must be reproduced and passed from the first generation individual (G_1) to the second generation individual (G_2). If, as in cloning, the G_2 was an exact DNA copy of G_1, both would be exactly alike unless there were accidental spontaneous changes within the DNA (mutations) or the environment changed and affected the expression of DNA in the second individual. Such changes do, in fact, alter individual organisms and contribute to the variation of life that we see. But there is even far greater variation in organisms because of sex: two different individuals of the same species contribute their DNA to a second generation individual, more or less equally, so the traits of the two individuals—one male

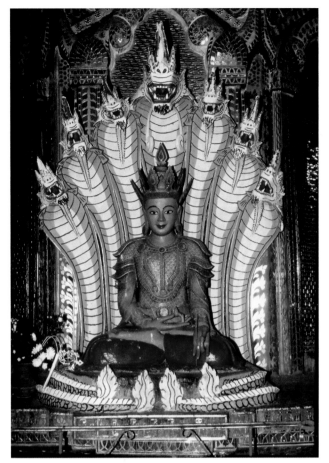

Figure 9.1. A temple to Buddha at Mount Popa, central Myanmar (formerly Burma). The Buddha is under the protective umbrella of a many-headed King Cobra. Photograph by Indraneil Das.

and one female—are combined to produce new variation of traits in the new individual. As this process continues, the thousands of genes, or individual units of inheritance composed of DNA, are recombined in different ways to produce variation among sexually reproducing organisms, including snakes.

Sex

Although individuals of any given species of snake look more or less similar (albeit there is variation in size and color), populations include both male and female individuals. Herpetologists have developed ways of sexing snakes, and these include probing or palping the base of the tale. In younger snakes, these procedures can be difficult and uncertain, but adult snakes of many species exhibit differences in the shape of the tail that can identify the sex of the individual when inspected visually. In comparison with females, the tale of a male tends to be more elongate and is relatively broader near the vent due to internal copulatory organs that are held within a pocket at the base of the tale (fig. 9.3). The copulatory organs can be everted to reveal

them externally (fig. 9.4), or a blunt probe can be inserted into the passageway that allows their eversion during mating. Hence, if one attempts to push a blunt probe gently into the base of the tail (insertion at either side of the midline), it cannot enter the tail of a female but will slide for some distance into the pocket that houses the copulatory organs in a male.

The copulatory organs of male snakes are paired and called *hemipenes*. Yes—the structure we term the penis in humans is paired, and there are two of these in a snake. Each one individually is called a *hemipenis*. In many species, the hemipenes are highly ornamented and may be hooked, bilobed, or bulbous in appearance. The terminal aspects of these structures bear spines or spurs and are rough in surface texture (fig. 9.4). These features secure internal attachment within the cloaca of the female during mating, and their variation among species has been useful as a taxonomic character. Usually only one hemipenis is used during copulation. When erected, internal sinuses become engorged with blood and the structure is turned inside-out while being forced out of the vent. Following copulation the hemipenis is pulled back into the body of the male by a retractor muscle and turns outside-in during the process. When copulating, the erected hemipenis is inserted into the cloaca of the female, and sperm travel down a narrow groove on the hemipenis into the cloaca or vagina (part of the *oviduct*) of the female.

The Gonads

The gonads of snakes are paired organs located in the abdominal cavity, usually in close proximity to the anterior ends of the kidneys and posterior to the gall bladder. The gonads of males are the *testes* (fig. 9.5), and those of the female are *ovaries* (fig. 9.6). In males, the right testis is typically more anterior than the left, and both are generally smooth and elongated, although in blind snakes of the genus *Leptotyphlops* the structures have multiple lobes. The internal location of the testes is different from that in mammals, and the organs develop in close association with the kidneys inside the embryo.

The size of the testes may vary seasonally, with increased size indicative of the production of sperm, called *spermatogenesis*. The sperm are produced from germ cells within *seminiferous tubules*, which are convoluted and comprise the interior of the testis. These tubules are continuous with, and empty into, anterior efferent ducts that are lined with ciliated cells and smooth muscle. The efferent ducts drain to the *epididymis* where sperm will be stored for varying periods until ejaculation. The sperm are ultimately transferred to the hemipenes during copulation.

The female reproductive tract consists of paired *ovaries* and associated pairs of reproductive ducts. Ovaries vary

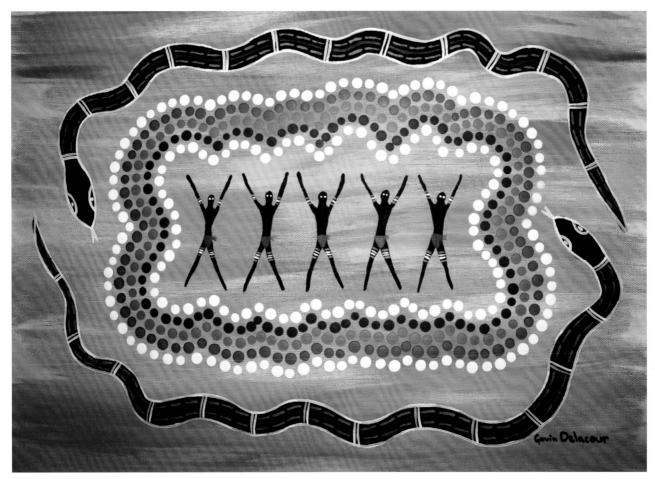

Figure 9.2. The snake is a common motif in the aboriginal art and mythology of Australia. This aboriginal painting depicts people surrounded by snakes, which are associated closely with water, land, fertility, birth, abundance (plants and animals), social relations, and protection. The snake is a creator of human beings, and its life-giving powers send spirits of conception to all the water holes. In essence, the serpent embodies regenerative and reproductive power in nature and in human beings. It is a principal character in major rituals. This painting is by Gavin Delacour, who is an aboriginal painter born at Mt. Isa and presently living in Townsville, Australia.

in their location, but are usually found near the gall-bladder. Each ovary is elongated and contains egg follicles at different stages of development, degeneration, or resorption (fig. 9.6). *Vitellogenesis* refers to the deposition of fat reserves, or accumulation of yolk, in the *ovarian follicles*, and vitellogenic follicles are developing eggs that are being "yolked" within the ovary. The precursors of yolk are synthesized in the liver. Vitellogenic follicles increase in size and become increasingly yellow in color as the process advances (fig. 9.6). Like testes, their status can be influenced by season, and the time that is involved in producing yolk-laden eggs varies among species. Hence, small pre-vitellogenic follicles may characterize quiescent ovaries for much of the year in many species that exhibit seasonal reproduction. The growth of follicles can be quite rapid just before mating in the spring. Ultimately, each individual follicle either releases its egg (termed *ovulation*) or degenerates.

Ovulation releases a mature egg from its follicle, and the egg is now ready to be fertilized. The remaining follicle forms a *corpus luteum*, which becomes an endocrine structure and releases hormones until it regresses following birth of the young or the laying of eggs to hatch outside the body of the female. Ovulated eggs enter the *oviduct*, which is a narrow tube extending from the ovary to the cloaca (see fig. 2.35). It is lined with smooth muscle, both ciliated and nonciliated mucous cells, and various glands. The glands produce various membranes that will surround the developing egg, and their activity varies with the reproductive status of the female. The middle segment of the oviduct where eggs are retained before they are laid contains glands that produce the fibrous and calcium components of the eggshell (see below). This is also the region where embryos are incubated in live-bearing species (see below). The middle part of the oviduct is termed the *uterus* and is homologous to the uterus of mammals.

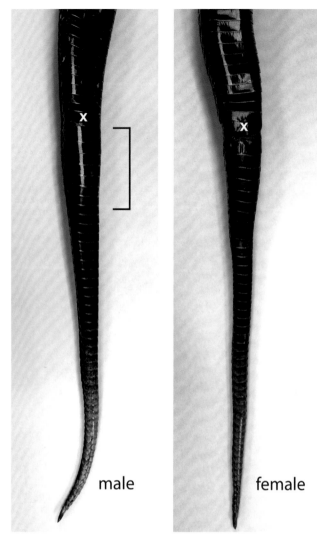

male   female

Figure 9.3. Ventral tail morphologies in Florida Cottonmouths (*Agkistrodon piscivorus conanti*). The male (**left**) shows a somewhat engorged tail near its base, whereas the tail of the female (**right**) is less "turgid" in appearance. The male condition is due to internal presence of hemipenes (bracketed region), which are everted just below the cloaca during mating. The cloacal opening in each photo is immediately below the lowermost ventral scute, which is marked with a white "x" in each photograph. These snakes were lightly anesthetized, and the photographs were taken by the author.

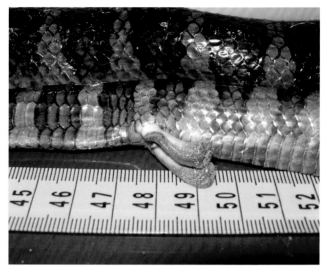

Figure 9.4. Everted hemipenes of a sea krait (*Laticauda semifasciata*) illustrating paired structures, each engorged with blood and showing the sulcus and spiny terminus that assists internal attachment within the cloaca of a female during copulation. A metric rule is shown for scale. Photograph taken in Taiwan by Coleman M. Sheehy III.

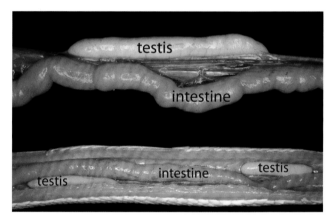

Figure 9.5. Ventral views of the coelomic cavity of a Corn Snake (*Pantherophis guttatus*). The **upper view** features the left testis, which is elongate and lies adjacent to the small intestine. The **lower view** illustrates both testes, the right testis being cranial to the left testis. The cranial direction (toward the head of snake) is to the left in both photos. Photographs by Elliott Jacobson.

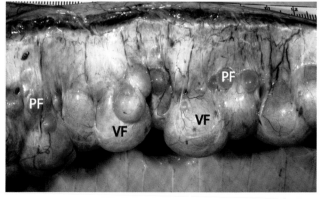

Figure 9.6. Ovary of a Reticulated Python (*Broghammerus reticulatus*) showing multiple previtellogenic follicles (PF) and vitellogenic follicles (VF). Photograph by Elliott Jacobson.

Fertilization

In snakes, and in all reptiles, fertilization occurs internally. Sperm unite with eggs near the upper, or cranial, end of the oviduct following ovulation and prior to the deposition of membranous structures that eventually envelope each egg. Fertilization may occur relatively soon after mating, or following long periods when sperm are stored in the female's reproductive tract. Females of some species can store sperm in *seminal receptacles*, which are pocket-like structures associated with certain segments of the oviduct, primarily in the cranial region. However, sperm aggregations are associated with the lumen or deep furrows of the posterior oviduct in some species (fig. 2.35). One hypothesis related to sperm location is that sperm enter the posterior oviduct following mating, reside for variable periods, and then are attracted to receptacles in the anterior region of the oviduct. Sperm from one or more mating are maintained and nurtured in the storage receptacles. One should also appreciate that viable sperm can be stored in the ducts of the testes and can live within males for long periods.

Female snakes can store sperm for periods of months to years, and thus mating and fertilization do not necessarily coincide closely in time. For example, some species might mate during the late summer or fall, but the young are born the following summer without the female having mated again. Moreover, females are able to produce two or more fertile cohorts of young from a single mating. This capability can be advantageous in circumstances where a population is sparsely distributed and there are relatively few opportunities to mate. There is undoubtedly great variation in the timing of mating, sperm storage, and fertilization in wild populations of snake species that are not yet well studied.

Examples of sperm storage are known largely from accounts of reproduction in captive snakes. Several instances involve females that were kept isolated from males for very long periods and then surprised their owners by giving birth to healthy young snakes. Amazingly, a captive female Arafura File Snake (*Acrochordus arafurae*) was kept in isolation for seven years and following its death was found to contain an apparently viable developing embryo!

Virgin Birth

One of the reasons biology is so fascinating is that almost always there are novel exceptions to the so-called general rules. Hence, there is one species of snake that does not reproduce in a sexual manner as appears to be characteristic of all the other snakes. The Brahminy Blind Snake (*Rhamphotyphlops braminus*) is a small burrowing species, originally from India and Southeast Asia, that has been accidentally introduced in many other parts of the world because of it secretive habits and ability to hide in small containers of soil (fig. 1.11). For this reason it is also called the "Flowerpot Snake." Every individual is a female and, when mature, lays eggs that produce females that are clones of the mother. Each egg develops without the requirement of sperm from another individual and is thus an example of asexual reproduction known as *parthenogenesis*. This condition in *Rhamphotyphlops* is possibly unique among snakes, although it is also known in several species of lizards.

Reproductive Modes

The majority of snake species lay eggs (termed *oviposition*), and this mode of reproduction is called *oviparity* (fig. 9.7). Specialized glands lining segments of the oviduct lay down fibrous structures that envelope the egg, and there may also be superficial layers to which calcium salts are added to impart some rigidity and to provide a likely source of calcium for the developing embryo. These structures are termed the *eggshell* and eggshell membranes, which protect the internal contents of the egg during its development outside the mother's body. Prior to "shelling" of the eggs, the oviparous oviduct exhibits increases in the height of tissue related to growth of the shell glands and thickening of connective tissue and musculature that will envelop the uterus. The oviduct and uterus provide the eggs with water and oxygen prior to oviposition. After the eggs are laid, embryonic development continues outside the female, and the egg yolk provides the energy and nutrients that are required for development of the embryo.

In other species the embryo is retained within the oviduct until development is complete (fig. 9.8). In this condition, the young are born in a developed state in contrast to laying eggs (fig. 9.9). Such reproduction is termed *viviparity*, and snakes that exhibit this mode are *viviparous*. Nutrients and respiratory gases are exchanged across a *placenta*, formed by a close association (apposition) of extraembryonic membranes (the *chorioallantois*) with tissue of the maternal oviduct (uterus), and richly supplied with blood vessels (fig. 9.10). The embryos of viviparous snakes increase in mass due to the uptake of water and nutrients.

There are variable degrees of dependence on a placenta for nutrients. The developing young in some species are nourished by egg yolk, and they hatch or break through the egg membranes immediately before, during, or after the eggs are laid (fig. 9.11).

Whether a species of snake lays eggs or gives birth to developed young depends on the evolutionary history and geography. Viviparity has evolved convergently in 14 principal

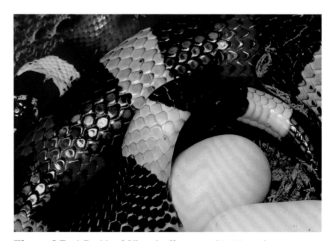

Figure 9.7. A Pueblan Milksnake (*Lampropeltis triangulum campbelli*) with newly oviposited eggs. The white egg near the center of the photograph is just exiting the cloaca where the skin is seen to be stretched. Photograph by David Barker.

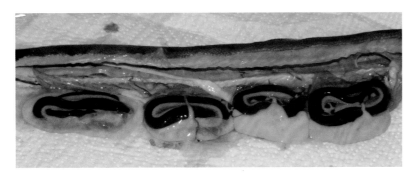

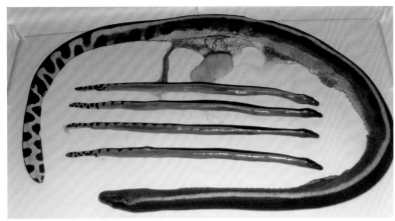

Figure 9.8. In the **upper photo** four embryonic Yellow-bellied Sea Snakes (*Pelamis platurus*) are shown in the condition inside the mother snake immediately before birth. The placental connection to the maternal tissues can be seen in the three embryos to the right. The **lower photo** illustrates the developed condition of these same snakes in relation to the length of the mother. These four neonatal snakes represent the litter size for this particular female. The mother snake died inadvertently for no apparent reason just before these photographs were taken by the author in Costa Rica.

On the other hand, viviparity confers benefits of thermoregulation and permits snakes to exploit environments where suitable sites for nesting are limited or absent. The evolution of viviparity appears to be causally linked to such benefits related to temperature.

The terrestrial live-bearers, or viviparous species, tend to occur at higher altitudes and latitudes, representing locations where temperatures are cooler. Carrying the young snakes inside the mother's body has the advantage that the female can keep the developing embryos warm by basking in warm places (see chapter 4). Such thermoregulation by pregnant females accelerates embryonic development and allows young snakes to be born in time to feed and learn about their environment before cold weather sets in. By comparison, there are fewer sites available where developing eggs could be exposed to warm temperatures that are sufficient to allow development to hatching before the first frosts occur. An important point of this discussion is that carrying developing young inside the mother reduces chances that the vagaries of weather will kill the embryos, because the female snake can respond behaviorally to temperature changes, whereas eggs are dependent totally on the microenvironment in which they are laid. Thus, it is thought that viviparity reduces the mortality of young in colder environments. Species of snakes that inhabit very cold habitats—at the extremes of ranges either by latitude or altitude—are all viviparous.

Similar patterns of reproductive mode and geography occur in lizards. Worldwide, viviparity has evolved independently more than a hundred times in snakes and lizards combined. Thus, it appears that colder climates have stimulated the evolution of live-bearing in many lineages of squamate reptiles. I should mention that the proportion of viviparous species is much higher among snakes than among lizards. For example, Donald Tinkle and Whit Gibbons estimated that among North American reptiles the proportion of viviparous snakes is two to five times greater than that of lizards at comparable latitudes. The reasons for this pattern are not clear. Rick Shine has suggested that the evolution of live-bearing might be favored by defensive capabilities such as large size or venom apparatus, which characterize snakes more so than lizards. Finally, it should be noted that completely aquatic marine snakes are all viviparous, undoubtedly because there are no appropriate places

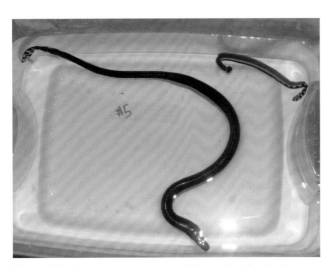

Figure 9.9. A captive newborn baby Yellow-bellied Sea Snake (*Pelamis platurus*) with its mother. Photographed in Costa Rica by the author.

lineages of snakes representing virtually every type of habitat that they utilize. Viviparity can reduce the mobility of female snakes, decrease feeding behavior, and constrain the size of a litter as well as the frequency of reproduction.

for externally oviposited eggs to develop if they were exposed to ocean water.

Placentation evolves together with viviparity in snakes, and the functioning of a placenta requires a thinning of the eggshell as well as changes in its composition. As a consequence, there is an intimate association between the fetal membranes and the lining of the oviduct. Such an important union of tissues gave rise to subsequent specializations for the transfer of oxygen and nutrients from the mother to the embryo (figs. 9.8, 9.10).

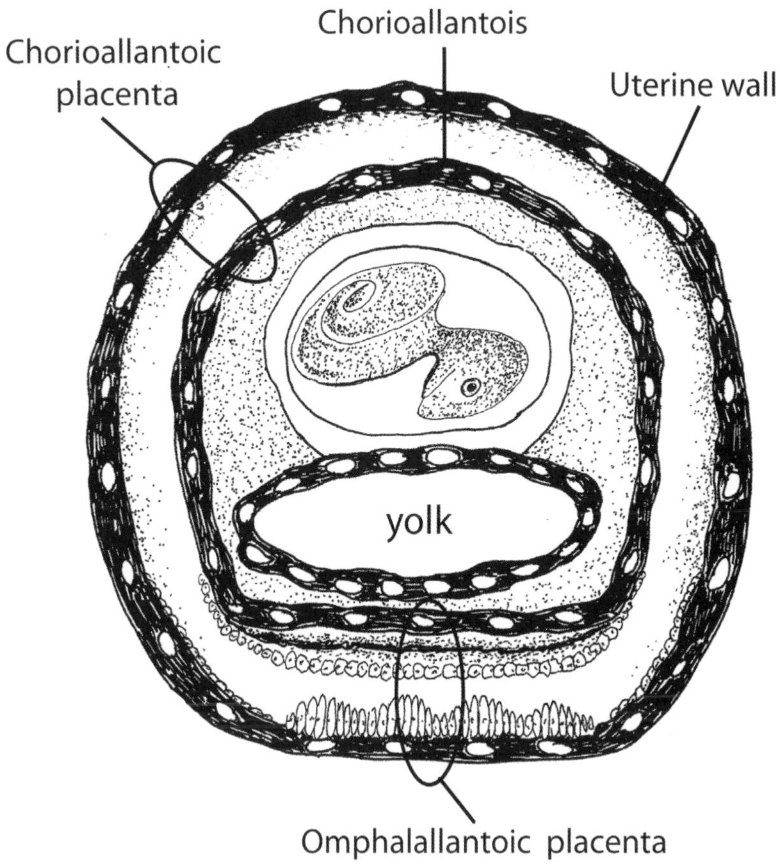

Eggs

The eggs of oviparous snakes vary considerably in size and shape. They are generally ellipsoid, but typically elongate rather than spherical (fig. 9.12). The eggshell is generally leathery and flexible in most oviparous species and consists of two principal layers. The inner layer contains a thin network of proteinaceous and elastic fibers that vary in their size and orientation in different species. These fibers give strength to the shell, but they can also expand as the embryo grows and the egg gains water during its development. Overlain onto this fibrous network is a mineral layer consisting of a sparse covering of calcium carbonate crystals. The mineralized layer is thicker and denser in what are termed "rigid-shelled eggs." These are characteristic of many turtles and crocodilians, and some lizards. However, the mineralized layer of snake eggs is sparser and interspersed with fibers, which renders the eggshell more flexible and variably elastic (fig. 9.13).

The "flexible-shelled eggs" of snakes are very permeable, say compared to avian eggs. They take up water from moist environments during development and tend to expand against the partially mineralized shell. The flexible shell stretches somewhat but also imparts pressure to the internal fluid compartments of the egg. Such eggs may double or triple in mass due to the gain of water (fig. 9.13). On the other hand, these eggs also lose water easily, and the loss can be substantial if the water vapor pressure surrounding an egg is only slightly less than saturated (< 99 percent). The permeability of these eggs has much ecological significance, and eggs can dehydrate lethally if the microenvironment is not appropriate, say because of a drought. In

Figure 9.10. Schematic illustration of the placental membranes investing the embryo of a snake. The chorioallantoic placenta surrounds most of the embryo when its formation is mature, and the omphalallantoic placenta forms the ventral wall of the egg. Each placenta is formed by the union of the fetal membrane with the lining of the uterus. The developing embryo is shown in the center of the illustration. Drawing by Dan Dourson, based on the placental membranes in the natricine snake *Virginia striatula* (Stewart, J.R., and K. R. Brasch, Ultrastructure of the placentae of the natricine snake, *Virginia striatula* (Reptilia: Squamata), *Journal of Morphology* 255:177–201, 2003, and fig. 5.6 in R. D. Aldridge and D. M. Sever (eds.), *Reproductive Biology and Phylogeny of Snakes*, vol. 9 of Reproductive Biology and Phylogeny, B. G. M. Jamieson, series editor (Enfield, NH: Science Publishers, 2011).

contrast with the eggs of snakes, those that are more heavily calcified and rigid can be virtually inflexible and are more resistant to water exchange. Such eggs can be incubated in more open environments than is possible with the less calcified eggs of oviparous snakes.

Inside the egg, the developing embryo is surrounded by other membranes that are internal to the eggshell. These are so-called *extraembryonic membranes*. One of these encloses the yolk to form the yolk sac, while three others surround the embryo in a fluid-filled space and function to transport nutrients, sequester metabolic wastes, and exchange respiratory gases. A network of blood vessels functions to transport nutrients from the yolk to the embryo (fig. 9.11).

Female snakes lay eggs in various places where the temperature and surrounding moisture must meet requirements for

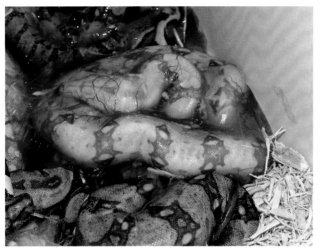

Figure 9.11. Newly born Boa Constrictors (*Boa constrictor*) featuring an albinistic neonate in the center. The young snakes are fully developed at birth and enveloped temporarily within egg membranes, in which blood vessels can be seen. The young break through the membranes very soon after birth. Photograph by Tracy Barker.

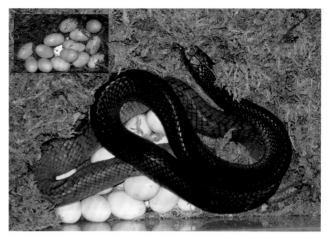

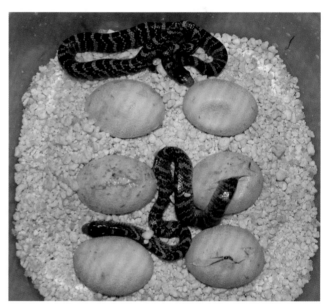

Figure 9.12. A female Yellow-tail Cribo (*Drymarchon corais corais*) from British Guyana, seen here with her clutch of eggs that were oviposited in captivity. The **inset** in the **upper photo** shows the complete clutch of eggs, which number 14. The **lower photo** shows two newborn cribos that have just emerged from their eggshells. Note there are slits in the shell of the lower right-hand egg, made by the egg tooth of the neonate inside the shell. Photographs by Elliott Jacobson.

proper development and hatching. Usually the eggs are buried in moist soil or oviposited in crevices or other places where they are protected from mechanical harm and from drying. Female King Cobras (*Ophiophagus hannah*) actually construct a nest for the eggs, consisting of a mound of leaves and organic debris, which provide a microenvironment that is characterized by moderated and sometimes elevated temperature (fig. 9.14). Also, the eggs are not exposed to the air and are less subject to drying within the leaf mound. Some sea kraits (*Laticauda* spp.) lay their eggs on rock ledges inside moist caves that are adjacent to the sea. These places may be visited by large numbers of snakes, and many females probably return to lay eggs at the same site year after year. There are many species of snakes in which females aggregate communally to gestate and lay eggs in places where the soil conditions are "just right." In some cases, females from a very wide area lay eggs in a communal nesting site, or they aggregate during gestation of the young in areas that are limited in size. Such communal behavior on the part of female snakes likely reflects a scarcity of sites that are suitably moist or warm for eggs or gestation. Unfortunately, there are many species of snakes for which little or nothing is known about reproduction and oviposition.

The proper development and hatching of snake eggs depends on the temperature and moisture of the soil or other medium in which the eggs are laid. These parameters are extremely important during incubation, and they influence the size, shape, growth rate, behavior, and other attributes of hatchling snakes. If temperature or soil moisture conditions are not adequate, the hatching success of eggs can diminish and birth malformations can occur. For example, drier soils can lead to a decreased size of hatchlings, and

smaller hatchling size can decrease the survival rate in some species of snakes. Even when conditions are within a normal range for hatching, subtle changes in these conditions can cause shifts in the trajectories of embryonic development. Such sensitivity suggests there is strong selection pressure for female snakes to recognize and use nesting sites that provide optimal conditions for the eggs to develop and hatch. This probably explains why some sites are used repeatedly for communal nesting year after year.

Just before hatching the baby snake nearly fills the entire space within the confines of the eggshell, and it has to create an opening in the eggshell from which it can emerge at hatching (figs. 9.12, 9.15). There is a deciduous toothlike

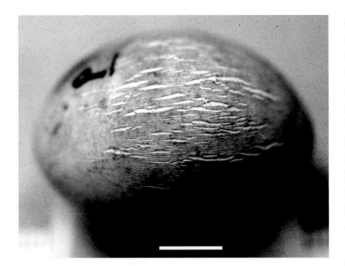

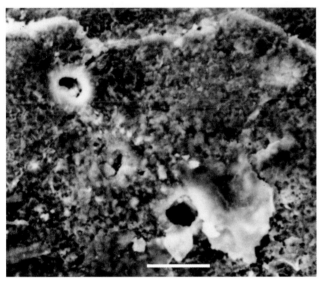

Figure 9.13. The **upper photo** shows the egg of a Black Rat Snake (*Pantherophis obsoletus*) that has completed 80 percent of incubation. The outer shell layers including the calcareous components have fractured because of swelling of the egg from the uptake of water. The **lower photo** is an electronmicrograph featuring the surface of the eggshell and reveals the calcareous layer with pores. The pores presumably enhance the exchange of gases across the eggshell. The bar in the upper photograph equals 1 cm, and that in the lower photograph equals 50 μm. Photographs by the author.

projection from the tip of the premaxillary bone that is termed the "egg tooth." This structure functions to cut or tear an opening in the leathery eggshell, from which the young snake can emerge (figs. 9.12, 9.15). The egg tooth is temporary and is shed away at hatching.

Clutch and Litter Size

There is quite a lot of information that has been published on the number of eggs (*clutch size*) or live young (*litter size*) that characterize reproducing snakes. As a group, snakes

are generally more prolific than lizards and produce clutch or litter sizes that vary from 1 (a few species of boids and colubrids) to more than 100 (some *Thamnophis* species and elapids). Larger clutch sizes are characteristic of some species of boids (e.g., Reticulated Python), and larger litter sizes are characteristic of some species of viperids (e.g., Fer-de-Lance) and natricine snakes (e.g., Northern Water Snake, Plains Gartersnake). Recently an invasive Burmese Python captured in the Florida Everglades was reported to be 17 feet and 7 inches long (a little less than 5 meters) and contained 87 eggs. Most snakes, however, produce young in the range of several to 20 in a single clutch or litter (figs. 9.8, 9.12).

The number of young relative to the length of a female tends to be larger in viviparous than in oviparous species, and in aquatic and semifossorial species compared with arboreal and terrestrial species. Another general finding is that the ratio of the total clutch mass to female mass (called *relative clutch mass*, RCM) is about 20 percent higher in oviparous compared with viviparous species, which implies either a greater brood size or offspring size, or combination of both, in the oviparous species. For a given RCM, the number of eggs produced (clutch size) is related to the energy that is allocated by the female to each individual offspring. Both female size and clutch size vary among snakes, even within a species. In general, marine snakes produce larger young than do terrestrial species. Within marine snakes, larger species produce the larger young, but smaller species also produce relatively large young by reducing the clutch or litter size. If one corrects for female body size, larger clutches generally result in smaller young. Among some oviparous species, larger females tend to lay larger eggs, and for a given size of female, eggs in larger clutches are shorter than those in smaller clutches.

Because the body of a snake is tubular, the volumetric geometry suggests that larger snakes can produce a larger number of similar size offspring and can increase clutch size with less effect on offspring size. All of these factors complicate analysis and generalizations, but suggest there are constraints on the size and number of young—which determine the fitness or reproductive potential of the female. The term *fitness* refers to the ability of an organism to contribute genes to the next generation, and this equates approximately to the number of offspring weighted by the probability that those offspring will survive and reproduce.

When and How Often Do Snakes Reproduce?

This is an important question, and one that is not easily answered because we do not have sufficient knowledge of many species of snakes to generalize with confidence. In places where individuals of a particular species are quite

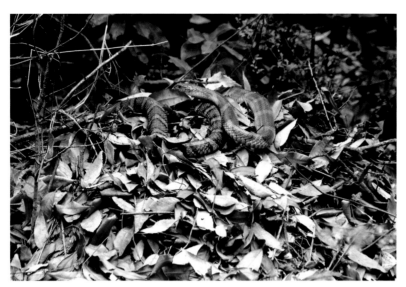

Figure 9.14. A female King Cobra (*Ophiophagus hannah*) photographed while resting on its nest where the eggs are attended in the Western Ghats of India. The female snake constructs the nest by pulling leaves together with coils of its body. Photograph by Gowri Shankar.

common—garter snakes for example—it would seem that at least most females reproduce every year. On the other hand, species that appear to be very rare—sometimes an artifact of human impressions or inability to find specimens—one might assume that reproduction occurs less frequently. The evidence at hand suggests that both situations occur in natural populations of snakes, and that the frequency of reproduction is dependent on the environment and the food resources that are available to a given female.

First, we know much about the captive breeding of snakes through efforts at reproducing species on the part of zoos, private hobbyists, and commercial breeders who have promoted herpetoculture as a significant part of the pet industry (fig. 5.25). Not only are many snakes capable of reproducing every year, but numerous oviparous and several viviparous species are capable of producing more than one clutch or litter during a year. Perhaps the best-known example of an unusually prolific snake is the African house snake (*Lamprophis* spp.), which includes several small- to medium-size species native to sub-Saharan Africa. The species *Lamprophis fulginosus* has become a commonly kept snake because it is easy to maintain in captivity and breeds prolifically. If these snakes are well fed, females will lay clutches of eggs as often as every two months, and the tendency for individuals to mate is not restricted seasonally! Examples of multiple clutches or prolific live-bearing from captive snakes are artificial, however, in the sense that food is available in excess relative to what snakes might actually enjoy as resources in wild populations.

Temperature is an important factor that influences reproductive rates because of its effect in determining activity,

metabolism, and prey availability to females (see chapter 4). Many snakes, especially in temperate climates, reproduce once per year or less frequently depending on both food resources and temperature, which generally equate with the length of the active season. Colder climates generally tend to slow reproduction. For example, European Adders (*Vipera berus*) reproduce approximately yearly in southern Europe, but every two years in northern France and every three years in the Alps.

Environmental Cues Affecting Reproduction

Physical signals from the environment that influence reproduction seem logically to be more important in temperate than in tropical environments. However, we know little about what influences reproductive cycling in the tropics, so this statement is a hypothesis that remains untested. The more logical cues in temperate environments are the amount of day length, or *photoperiod*, and temperature, both of which vary with seasons. Although photoperiod is an important cue for reproductive changes in birds and other animals, temperature is more important for ectothermic reptiles such as snakes. This is especially true in regions where these animals spend much time beneath ground during winter dormancy when changes in the levels and timing of light above ground are not evident below ground.

Increases in temperature—both below and above ground—are thought to play an important role in influencing the spring emergence and subsequent reproductive behavior of many snakes that live in temperate environments. Emergence of hibernating rattlesnakes, for example, is stimulated by increasing temperature, or reversals of temperature gradients, within dens where these snakes spend the winter. However, it seems that increasing temperature is not essential for spring emergence of garter snakes that live in some of the Canadian provinces (fig. 4.7) because they emerge with body temperatures as low as 0.5°C. As in the garter snake, many other species of snake breed seasonally and experience a period of winter dormancy at relatively low temperatures prior to mating in the spring. In cases where reproduction occurs immediately following the emergence from dormancy in the spring, significant changes in reproductive physiology and behavior are likely to occur during the period of winter dormancy.

Because of the difficulties of access, there is, not surprisingly, much "underground" ecology and behavior of snakes that is totally unknown. What are the metabolic status,

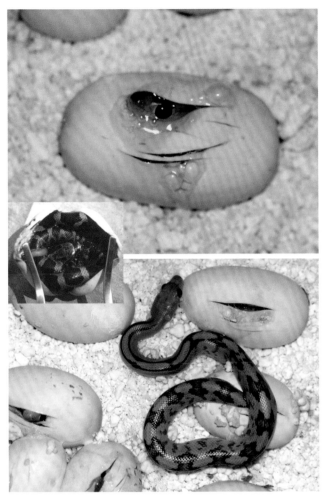

Figure 9.15. A hatchling Trans-Pecos Rat Snake (*Bogertophis subocularis*) as seen (**upper photo**) just as it has pierced the eggshell using the egg tooth (which is now gone) and (**lower photo**) as it appears following emergence from the eggshell. The **inset** illustrates a Black Rat Snake (*Pantherophis obsoletus*) inside its eggshell just prior to hatching. Embryonic fluids can be seen inside the egg and oozing out the openings that were made in the eggs by the respective hatchlings. Photographs by Elliott Jacobson (upper, lower) and the author (inset).

cold, and temperatures could drop to lethal levels for ectotherms within a very short time (less than a day). What happened to the snakes that had been active—which evidently had occupied rather shallow retreat sites and could respond to the brief period of warming? Perhaps they escaped again to underground retreats, or perhaps some had been "caught" by the changes associated with the cold front and were killed in the winter because of their premature emergence. It is interesting to think about this, because there must have been other snakes that were located, and remained, in deeper places where they might not be aware of the brief warming that occurred because of limited ground penetration of the thermal changes.

Warmer temperatures induce courtship and mating behaviors of garter snakes, and they are probably important for activity of the gonads as well. These behaviors are expressed more strongly, and in more individuals, when snakes first experience a lengthy period of low temperature that appears to "reset" an endogenous seasonal clock. Persons who breed snakes subject various captive species to periods of cooling in order to enhance the probability of success when males and females are placed together to encourage mating. More generally, the scientific literature suggests that temperature is the principal environmental cue that regulates reproduction in snakes as well as in other squamate reptiles.

The few snakes that have been studied in tropical locations generally exhibit seasonal reproduction. With respect to populations or species outside of equatorial regions, temperature is a potential environmental cue, although not as extreme in variation as in temperate regions. Seasonality of rainfall can be important, especially in regions that have distinctly seasonal drought. The timing of reproduction might be related to the availability of food resources (which might also be cyclic) to ensure successful vitellogenesis, mating, and embryogenesis in females, and/or to ensure the availability of food for neonates during their early life.

The Neuroendocrine Regulation of Reproduction

Relatively little is known about how nerves and hormones control the reproductive cycles of snakes, relative to the vast literature on this subject that exists for mammals and birds. Moreover, most of the knowledge presently available for snakes is focused on a single species, the Common Garter Snake (*Thamnophis sirtalis*). Generally, signals from the environment related to temperature and light conditions are cues to changes in neural pathways (nervous system), *endocrines* (hormones), and *neuromodulators* that influence reproduction (fig. 9.16). The prefix *neuro-* refers to nerve or neuron. Hence, neuromodulators are chemicals released from nerve endings that "modulate" or change the signaling behavior of neighboring neurons that are part of a common

awareness, and influence of environmental cues for animals that are overwintering very deep beneath the ground and do not immediately experience warming temperatures of spring? Are there endogenous circannual or seasonal cycles that operate to stimulate the timing of emergence? What happens to those animals that happen to occupy sites of refuge that are not very deep? When I was living in eastern Kansas for about 13 years, I noticed that occasionally there were unusual periods of warming that occurred during certain winters. I lived in rural countryside for part of this time, and I observed that certain species of snakes (especially garter snakes) emerged and were active during these warm spells, crossing roads for example. Then what invariably ensued was a cold front would turn the weather bitterly

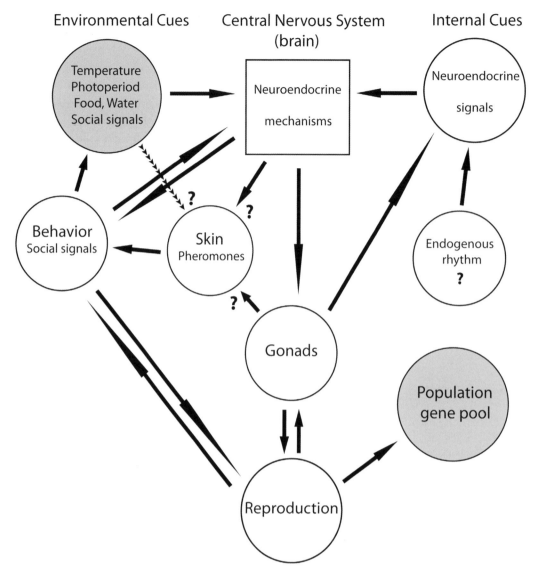

Figure 9.16. Conceptual diagram of the controlling elements in the reproduction of snakes. The gray circles represent factors that reside outside the animal, and the other elements interact within the animal. The scheme of interactions is generalized, and many of the details are not well known in snakes. Drawing by the author.

pathway. Variation in neuroendocrine mechanisms has contributed to evolutionary variation in the patterns of reproduction in these, as well as other, vertebrates.

Environmental temperature plays a key role in regulating reproduction in snakes as well as in other ectothermic vertebrates such as lizards. Temperature influences important centers of the brain, especially specific parts of the *hypothalamus* and the *pineal gland*, a small organ that is formed near the roof of the forebrain. The pineal gland secretes *melatonin*, which is synthesized and released rhythmically in response to environmental cues of temperature and photoperiod. Levels of melatonin (which circulate in blood) are higher during night, or darkness, and therefore exhibit a *circadian* (daily) *rhythm* that is related to daily cycles of light and dark. Melatonin is also produced at other places in the body (e.g., retina, brain, and intestine), but the principal source is the pineal gland. Melatonin influences both physiology and behavior, and it is therefore an important communicator between environmental cues of light and temperature and the internal functions that affect reproduction.

In the absence of light, temperature alone can modulate the level of melatonin in garter snakes that are in winter dormancy. Studies by Deborah Lutterschmidt and Robert Mason showed that melatonin levels are lower in garter snakes exposed to low temperature, but the amplitude of cyclic melatonin release is increased following a prolonged period at low temperature. Other studies indicate that surgical removal of the pineal gland can change the courtship behaviors of snakes. While the precise actions of melatonin are not understood, these and other investigations appear to establish that pineal secretions of melatonin both modulate and synchronize reproduction with environmental cues. Additionally, melatonin also plays a role in synchronizing daily patterns of activity with reproductive behaviors.

A specific region of the brain—including the anterior part of the hypothalamus and the nearby pituitary gland—is an important center for integrating external and internal cues related to reproduction. This site in the central nervous system also is important for responses to temperature and the orchestration of behaviors related to temperature regulation. With respect to reproduction, *gonadotropic hormones* that stimulate the gonads (follicle stimulating hormone, leutinizing hormone) are synthesized in this region—largely in the pituitary—and released into the blood circulation by the external signals that synchronize reproduction. Yet other factors called *gonadotropin-releasing hormones* act in between to stimulate the release of the gonadotropic hormones (also called *gonadotropins*) when activated by signals related to the external cues. This describes the generally characteristic hierarchical control of gonadal function in tetrapod vertebrates, including many reptiles, but we have very sketchy information about the mechanisms that govern this system specifically in snakes. For purposes of this discussion, we will assume that episodic secretion of gonadotropin-releasing hormones and, secondarily, the release of gonadotropins from the hypothalamus, are required for normal reproduction in snakes.

At the level of the gonads—testes in males and ovaries in females—steroids are secreted and stimulate gonadal tissues as well as other distant target organs via circulation in the blood. The principal gonadal steroids in tetrapod vertebrates are *progesterone*, *estrogens*, and *testosterone*. Progesterone is essential for the development of eggs and embryos. Estrogens have many effects including the development and maturation of egg follicles, vitellogenesis, and growth of the oviduct, in addition to secondary sexual characteristics (changes in body coloration, for example) and reproductive behaviors. Testosterone is synthesized in the testes and regulates the secondary sexual characteristics of males. Testosterone belongs to a class of sex steroid hormones called *androgens*. In both male and female reptiles, androgens can be converted to estrogens in the central nervous system and elsewhere (see below). These conversions in the brain affect the reproductive behaviors of both male and female animals, but very little is known about these effects in snakes.

Various other peptide molecules and neuromodulators potentially influence reproduction and the reproductive behaviors of snakes. As with the other factors mentioned above, very little is known about these chemicals and their probable actions in modulating the reproductive system in snakes. Therefore, further discussion of these is not warranted.

Reproductive Cycles

The periodicity of reproduction in snakes is variable among species, with underlying mechanisms or even changes being not well understood except for a few species. Robert Aldridge and his colleagues (in addition to others) have described several types of cyclic reproduction in snakes, with various terminologies being applied to them. Here I shall attempt to simplify the description into basic patterns.

Reproductive processes cycle when the gonads or accessory organs become quiescent for a period of the year. This seems to be widespread in both temperate and tropical species. Spermatogenesis does not need to coincide with mating, and sperm that are produced at another time can be stored in the ducts that are used for transporting sperm in males, or in the oviducts of females (e.g., if mating occurs during the fall). Another pattern occurs when the gonads or accessory organs exhibit a reduction of activity during part of the year but do not become completely quiescent. Such a phenomenon has been inferred to exist in snakes, but the details are not completely verified. Finally, the gonads might remain more or less constantly active without any pronounced cycling in the level of activity. Again, this pattern has been inferred to exist, but the evidence is not conclusive.

Whatever the pattern, variation occurs among species with respect to the phase relationships between reproductive behaviors and the cycling of activity of the gonads. There can also be considerable variation among individuals within a species, although generally speaking, reproduction is highly synchronous among individuals of a population. The majority of snake species that have been studied exhibit seasonal reproduction, and the synchrony of reproduction becomes stronger as the latitude increases away from the tropics. Fewer species have nonseasonal reproduction, and all of these occur in tropical or equatorial areas.

Investigations of reproductive patterns are challenging, and it is sometimes difficult to adequately judge the reproductive condition of the gonads, especially testes. For example, Selma Maria Almeida-Santos and colleagues demonstrated that male Brazilian Rattlesnakes (*Crotalus durissus terrificus*) retain sperm in reproductive ducts throughout the year. Although the volume of semen appears not to vary, the highest counts of sperm are observed just prior to the mating season.

The Common Garter Snake exhibits what is called a "dissociated reproductive cycle." This term refers to mating when the circulating levels of sex steroid hormones are low

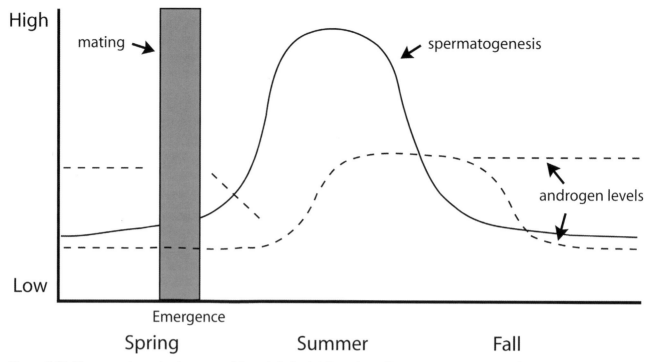

Figure 9.17. The seasonal reproductive pattern of the male Red-sided Garter Snake (*Thamnophis sirtalis parietalis*). The variation of androgen levels (high or low during spring emergence) is hypothesized to be related to annual variation in the severity of winter temperatures. Redrawn by the author after fig. 8.2, p. 293 in R. D. Aldridge and D. M. Sever (eds.), *Reproductive Biology and Phylogeny of Snakes*, vol. 9 of Reproductive Biology and Phylogeny, B. G. M. Jamieson, series editor (Enfield, NH: Science Publishers, 2011).

because of quiescent condition of the gonads (fig. 9.17), which contrasts with most vertebrates, in which mating occurs during periods when gonads are maximally active and circulating levels of sex steroids are elevated. In the garter snake, levels of androgens vary during spring emergence when mating occurs, evidently attributable to metabolic clearance of the hormones depending on the temperatures affecting snakes during winter dormancy following high gonadal activity in the summer and fall (fig. 9.17). Thus, the perception of the extent of "dissociation" of the reproductive cycle in this species is temporal and might be attributable to the variation of temperature during any particular winter dormancy. The pattern of reproduction in this garter snake is unusual when compared to many other species of reptiles, likely due to the evolutionary influence of the extreme winter conditions to which these snakes are subjected in the populations that have been studied. Research with snakes that experience "extreme" conditions in their environment can be very useful in elucidating the regulatory mechanisms that underlie reproduction generally.

cues that trigger specific behavioral interactions between male and female snakes. Males also interact with other males to compete more successfully for access to females. Courtship, mating, and aggressive behaviors are complex and can vary among species. The expression of such activity in snakes can be quite spectacular, but due to the cryptic nature of many species, courtship and mating are rarely observed. Detailed knowledge of reproductive behaviors is known for relatively few species of snakes, and is particularly lacking in secretive, primitive, fossorial, and tropical species.

James Gillingham has categorized the reproductive behavior of snakes into three distinct phases: precourtship, courtship, and postmating. There is a wealth of natural history observations related to the courtship behaviors of snakes, but these are often not consistent in details, terminology, or interpretation. Robust investigations involving both field observations and laboratory experimentation have advanced our understanding of courtship behaviors considerably—especially in recent years—but are lacking for many taxa of snakes.

Courtship and Reproductive Behaviors

Like other vertebrates, snakes engage in ritualized courtship behavior prior to mating and the insemination of females. Courtship depends on visual, tactile, and chemical

Precourtship Behaviors

Many snakes are not particularly social during much of the year, and we could imagine that encounters between individuals of the same species might be somewhat rare (similarly to the rarity of encounters with humans). However, the persistence of a species or population depends on male and female individuals finding one another, and in the snakes' world, awareness of one's neighbors is probably much greater than we imagine. If you are a snake, knowing or finding your neighbors depends largely on communication with chemical cues, as far as we know. Chemicals on the skin of snakes adhere to the substrate over which they move, and other individuals have the capability to detect these chemicals and to derive important information from such "signals." These provide chemical trails, and are a means by which one individual can locate another. The ability of one individual to follow and locate another has been termed *trailing behavior*.

How do snakes detect a chemical trail, and what is the basis of perception that is used to follow it? Watch a snake that is moving through its environment in an exploratory manner, undisturbed by any human observer, and you will notice it is frequently flicking its tongue to sample the chemical cues associated with its surroundings. The tongue collects the chemical cues and transfers them to the vomeronasal organ in the roof of the mouth, where the chemicals are sensed and the information is transmitted to the brain (see chapter 7). These chemical "cues" communicate between individuals and therefore function as *pheromones* (see chapter 5). Thus, pheromones are used in the trailing behavior of snakes, and certain ones also elicit sexual behaviors in snakes.

The vomeronasal system primarily influences courtship behavior, and olfaction plays a lesser or negligible role. Male garter snakes will not court female garter snakes if the vomeronasal nerves are cut, whereas eliminating input from the olfactory nerves does not eliminate courtship.

The vomeronasal system is most responsive to nonvolatile chemicals, which are also most persistent in the environment. The reproductive pheromones produced by snakes reside in the skin. Discharge from the cloacal glands plays either no role whatsoever or perhaps a secondary role that remains to be documented. The "sexual attractiveness pheromone" of garter snakes is well studied and is the only pheromone that is adequately documented in reptiles. It is a mixture of lipids consisting of long-chain methyl ketones. How such compounds are produced and sequestered in the skin for communication with other snakes is not well understood.

Skin-based pheromones are the basis of trailing behavior in which male snakes follow females to initiate courtship. Trailing by males is complex and can involve multiple males trailing a single female, for example in some colubrid species with seasonal occurrence of mating (garter snakes, racers). If the pheromone trail is disrupted, either by configuration of the environmental substrate or by the movement of multiple males, a trailing male relies on visual cues as well as chemical ones to locate or relocate the female. Pheromone-based trailing behavior is presumably widespread among snakes, being known for representatives of caenophidian, boid, and pythonid species. Much evidence suggests that nonvolatile cutaneous lipids may communicate information about the species, sex, reproductive state, size, condition, and other properties of the individual snake that is the source of such pheromones. In some species, the ability of male snakes to trail females is seasonal and occurs only during the mating season.

Lipids that are dispersed from the skin are presumably less effective for intraspecific communication in aquatic environments than in terrestrial ones. Richard Shine has shown that pheromones appear to play no role in trailing behavior of the entirely marine Turtle-headed Sea Snake (*Emydocephalus annulatus*), which depends on visual cues to locate potential mates.

So what about chemical cues that go airborne? One study by Robert Aldridge and colleagues suggests that airborne chemicals can, in fact, be used to locate mates in the Northern Water Snake (*Nerodia sipedon*). Male individuals of this species orient preferentially to aerial cages that contained conspecific females. The use of volatile chemical cues might be more important than previously supposed, particularly in arboreal environments where chemical trailways can be interrupted by gaps in the vegetation.

Courtship Behavior

Courtship behaviors are elicited by pheromones that render a snake sexually attractive as well as eliciting trailing behavior. Once a male has located a female, whether by trailing or by closer association (e.g., simultaneous emergence from overwintering dens), the lipid products in the skin of the female elicit a characteristic sequence of behaviors that are well studied in garter snakes and are also known with little variation in some other species. There is an important connection here between the production of cutaneous pheromones and the act of skin shedding. Courtship is sometimes linked with the timing of ecdysis, and freshly shed females are particularly attractive to males (fig. 9.18). The components of cutaneous pheromones are also found in the older epidermis that is shed from female snakes.

During periods of courtship male snakes that are competing for females engage in ritualized behavior referred to as *combat dance*. This is a behavior in which one male challenges another, usually of the same species, by elevating the anterior body and pushing the opponent in an attempt to knock the individual to the ground. In some species, the two males engaged in "combat" both assume a nearly vertical posture and wave the fore-body, which may intertwine (with each other) when contact is made between the two snakes (fig. 9.19). Biting is not part of the ritual, but rather pushing the opponent to the ground and maintaining a higher position. Characteristically, the loser of the "combat" crawls away when it is defeated.

Typically, larger males are dominant and win out in contests that involve ritualized combat. In some species of snakes, larger males are more successful in mating with females than are smaller males. Characteristically, male snakes tend to grow larger than females of the same species if intermale combat is part of the species' reproductive behavior. Also, the tail of a male snake is typically somewhat longer than is that of a female (fig. 9.3), which could be advantageous for successful mating when courtship involves "tail-wrestling" for cloacal alignment (see below).

Once a male snake has access to a female, courtship begins with the male orienting toward the female and flicking the tongue intensely. The tongue samples the chemical cues from the skin, while both touch and vision are used during these behaviors. Once the male has contacted the female, it rubs its chin along the back of the female while continuing to flick the tongue rapidly and maintaining contact. Biting the body of the female is sometimes involved during this stage of interaction, or even before. I have seen a male cottonmouth trailing a female and, when in close range, crawl quickly forward and gently nip the female on the posterior body near the tail. Usually, however, biting is observed on the dorsal surface of the female, closer to the neck. Such biting seldom damages tissue, but it stimulates the female to assume a more tractable position prior to coitus. Biting during courtship seems to occur principally in colubrid snakes.

At the next stage, the male attempts to align his body with that of the female, and he orients his head in the same direction as hers. The male next engages in *caudocephalic waves*, which are horizontally undulating waves of the body that gently contact the female while lying upon or beside her. These waves move from the posterior part of the body toward the head and are thought to stimulate mating. Sometimes the wave movements are in the opposite direction, from head toward the tail. The last stage of courtship involves movements in which the male attempts to align his cloaca with that of the female and then engage in copulation (fig. 9.20). In boas, courting male snakes use pelvic spurs to stimulate

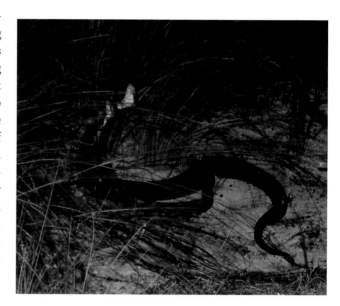

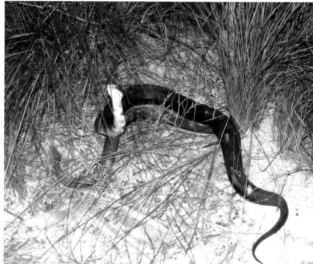

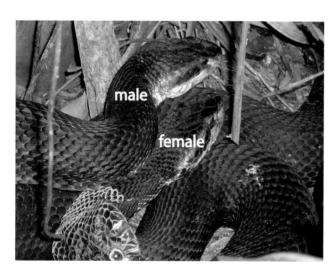

Figure 9.18. A pair of Florida Cottonmouth Snakes (*Agkistrodon piscivorus conanti*) resting together during a spring mating season. The female snake is beginning to shed its skin (visible in the lower part of photo), which imparts maximum attractiveness of the sexual pheromones in the skin. Photographed by the author at Seahorse Key, Levy County, Florida.

Figure 9.19. Ritualized combat behavior between two male Florida Cottonmouth Snakes (*Agkistrodon piscivorus conanti*) at Seahorse Key, Levy County, Florida. The **upper photo** shows the two males with heads elevated in combat. The **lower photo** shows the same two males with the dominant male elevated over the snake that lost the contest and eventually crawled away. Photographs by the author.

cloacal opening of the female just before insertion of the hemipenis (fig. 9.21). Courting snakes may vibrate or jerk the tail in rapid movements during the period just before coitus.

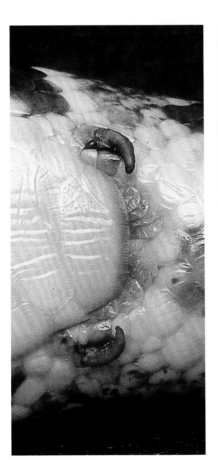

Figure 9.20. A pair of copulating Northern Copperheads (*Agkistrodon contortrix mokasen*) with the tails entwined (arrow) just prior to coitus. Photographed in Kentucky by Dan Dourson.

The use of chemical cues during courtship is documented only in certain snakes, including viperids, natricine colubrids, and elapids. Other snakes such as boas and pythons appear to rely principally on touch and body contact once a potential mate has been identified. Although sea snakes do not use pheromones for trailing, chemical cues are probably important when mating pairs are engaged at close range.

Some intriguing research by Michael LeMaster, Robert Mason, Richard Shine, and colleagues have shown that male garter snakes can assess the body condition of a female based solely on the information that resides in the chemical cues from the cutaneous lipids of a female. The cue evidently depends on the amazing fact that the mix of lipids in the pheromone of a female becomes increasingly dominated by longer-chain molecules as the length and body condition of the female increases. The male snakes prefer to mate with females that are longer and in better body condition.

During copulation the male engages the cloaca of the female by inserting a single hemipenis into the cloaca or into one of her vaginas (see figs. 9.4 and 2.35). The spiny distal surfaces of the hemipenis help to maintain the physical union between the two snakes. I once observed a dramatic example

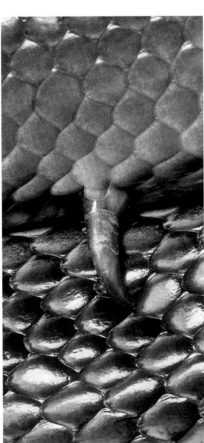

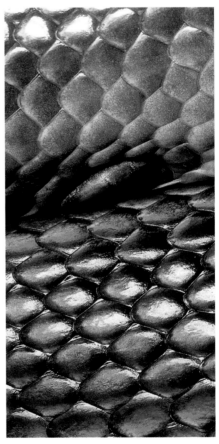

Figure 9.21. Photographs of cloacal spurs in pythons. The photo at the **left** shows the paired spurs of a Ball Python (*Python regius*). The photos in the **center** and at the **right** illustrate a single spur of a Water Python (*Liasis fuscus*), in use during mating and inactive respectively. Photographs by David Barker.

of just how strong this union can be when I watched a male Eastern Yellow-bellied Racer (*Coluber constrictor flaviventris*) pull and drag a female nearly straight up into a pine tree that was being climbed while the two snakes were in copulation. For part of the distance the female climbed upward and parallel with the male in what appeared to be a cooperative effort to ascend together. However, there were moments during this ascent when the female was facing head-down in a direction opposite to that of the male, and she was being pulled upward solely by the means of physical contact at the cloaca. Thus, the full weight of the female was suspended by the hemipenis of the male! Once these two snakes had ascended quite high into the tree, they came to rest in a horizontal position upon some branches that were bearing pine needles, where presumably copulation continued. In snakes generally, the duration of coitus varies from several minutes to many hours.

Following the successful mating of garter snakes, the male deposits a *seminal plug* (sometimes termed *copulatory plug*) in the cloaca of the female. Dried seminal secretions serve as a physical barrier to prevent the female from immediately mating again by blocking her vaginal opening. The plug may also serve to prevent leakage of sperm from the cloaca of the female. There is furthermore some evidence that copulatory fluids from an actively mating male garter snake contain an inhibitory pheromone that renders the female partner sexually unattractive for some while.

One very interesting behavior of snakes is the aggregation of large numbers of individuals during courtship to form what is termed a *mating ball*. This is especially common in garter snakes. There are anecdotal reports of the phenomenon in other species, including sea snakes, but some of the accounts are questionable. In garter snakes, males typically outnumber females in breeding aggregations when 10–100 males simultaneously court a single receptive female. In northern populations, numerous garter snakes emerge near-simultaneously from overwinter dens where they engage in courtship and mating before dispersing for the active season (see fig. 4.7). I have witnessed this phenomenon in eastern Kansas, where I once found hundreds of garter snakes (*Thamnophis sirtalis*) in a so-called mating ball at the base of a dead tree near the edge of a lake. I was most amazed to see how intense the males tongue-flicked and moved with jerky motions in attempt to court a female. There is intense competition among males for a female, and each male works to push other competing males out of the way. To be successful at mating, a male must physically push aside and outmaneuver other males to engage the cloaca of a female in coitus. I picked up several individuals and held them in my hand. Each of these snakes seemed completely oblivious to being handled and steadfastly persisted in rapid tongue-flicking while the body and head continued to jerk rhythmically. I could not be sure about the ratio of males to females in this circumstance.

Another interesting aspect of the mating aggregations of garter snakes is the presence of "she-males," which are male snakes that are courted as females because they produce female pheromones. The pheromones produced by she-males are close enough to that of true females to confound discrimination. Generally, however, larger females receive more intense courtship than do she-males. Current work by Robert Mason and others suggests that androgens are converted to estrogens locally in the skin of male garter snakes. Most, or nearly all, males emerge from winter dormancy with some degree of "feminized" skin, but the amount and quality of the female pheromones diminish with time. Several hypotheses regarding the supposed benefits for having a presence of she-males have been put forward, but the phenomenon is presently poorly understood.

Postmating Behavior

Following mating there is probably little or no social behavior that continues between male and female snakes in most species. However, aggregations of gravid females have been described in several species of viperid, colubrid, and elapid snakes. Reports of female snakes attending eggs following oviposition are numerous, especially involving colubrid and elapid snakes, pythons and pit vipers. Probably all pythons attend or brood their eggs as described in chapter 4, but there is little evidence for parental care of young snakes following their birth or hatching.

Some interesting observations of pit viper behaviors should be mentioned here. Newborn pit vipers of several species remain with the mother snake for short periods following birth, usually a matter of just a few days to two weeks until the very first shedding of skin by the neonates. Thereafter the young snakes disperse. There is little evidence for the adult female actively caring for the young during this period, but the newborn are tolerated and typically coil en masse with their bodies in close contact with the mother. One function of such behavior could be protection from rapid evaporative water loss through the skin, which builds a more protective barrier to water loss during the first ecdysis in some species. The South American Rattlesnake (*Crotalus durissus*), having a tropical lowland distribution, is the only species of rattlesnake that is known *not* to engage in the parental attendance of neonates.

The newborn young of Florida Cottonmouths (*Agkistrodon piscivorus conanti*) remain in close association with their mother until their first ecdysis, as is known in several species of rattlesnakes. I have observed this on several occasions at the Gulf coast island of Seahorse Key. On one occasion, I found the newborn young of a cottonmouth in attendance by both a male and female adult snake. Among the larger adults on the island, male and female pairs are found in close association during all months of the year, and this possibly reflects some degree of pair-bonding in this species. It seems highly likely that the pair of snakes that I found in association with the newborn snakes was a mated pair. These social behaviors of cottonmouths are presently the subject of more intensive investigation.

Growth and Sexual Maturation of Snakes

The rates of growth and sexual maturation of snakes are important features of life history that determine the evolutionary success of a species and its persistence in nature. The investment of females in their offspring is reflected not only in the number of young that are born, but also in the size of the neonate and the amount of embryonic yolk that remains to help fuel its metabolism. Newborn snakes that contain some residual embryonic yolk can grow in length without feeding for variable periods of time, depending on the amount of yolk that is present at birth. It is the presence of residual embryonic yolk that permits some snakes that are born in the late summer to make it through their first winter without feeding if they happen to have bad luck in finding food during their very early life.

Eventually young snakes begin feeding, and the rates of growth that are achieved depend on the genetic constitution of the individual, the availability of heat and water in its environment, and the success of the snake in capturing and digesting prey. There is considerable variation in rates of growth and sexual maturation among snakes, and the differences are not always based in the "hard-wiring" of genetic limitations. Rates of growth in captive snakes can exceed those of the same species in nature because of the constant availability of food and water. However, there are situations in which growth rates that are achieved in the wild are similar to those of captive snakes. The rate of growth in snakes is indeed flexible, being determined partly by genes and partly by the environment in which the nutrition of an individual is based. Within a species, the growth of individuals can vary depending on the quality of habitat, the availability of resources, variation in weather patterns, sex, and other attributes of morphology and physiology that can vary among individual animals.

The growth and maturation of snakes also depend on the size of the individual at birth, and generally larger species of snakes produce larger offspring. However, in many species of snakes in which the adult size is small, offspring are proportionately larger (relative to the size of adults) than are those of larger species. This also is true among some other animals such as certain lizards, birds, and mammals. Thomas Madsen, Richard Shine, and others have also found that young snakes growing with relative rapidity during the first year of life because of a favorable abundance of prey continue to grow more rapidly than average during their subsequent years of life. Thus, the eventual maximum size of a snake can depend, in part, on this "silver spoon" effect.

How rapidly can snakes grow? First, we need to distinguish numerous anecdotes concerning rapid growth rates and the large sizes of snakes that are raised in captivity. Captive pythons generally increase their length nearly fourfold during the first year of life. David Barker has informed me that Burmese and African Rock Pythons in his care have increased in length as much as sixfold during the first year. It is also important to note that many captive individuals can be obese and very large in mass (weight) due to the "overfeeding" of such snakes by their owners. Nonetheless, growth of snakes can also be very rapid in nature. Species of snakes living in warmer climates more than double in length during the first year of life and may achieve sexual maturity within one to two years. In some elapid species of snakes that were studied by Richard Shine, females first mated at one year of age. Relatively early sexual maturation appears to be common among the Elapidae as well as some colubrid snakes, and many species will mate within the first one to three years after birth. In contrast, species of snakes that live in colder climates (either at higher latitudes or higher altitudes) grow and reach sexual maturation more slowly. For example, growth rates in colubrid and viperid species living in colder climates are roughly half the rate of species living in warmer, tropical environments. Sexual maturation in the former species may require four to nine years. Viperid snakes as a group tend to exhibit "delayed" sexual maturity, as do freshwater file snakes (*Acrochordus arafurae*). In the latter species, males mature at five years and females mature at seven years. Regardless of the environment, male and female snakes characteristically achieve sexual maturity at different times; females are generally later than males by several months to a full year or more.

Growth of snakes is more rapid during the early years of life and is generally most rapid during the first one to two years. This fact has great significance because smaller snakes are generally more vulnerable to predation and to death from other causes (such as dehydration). Also, growth is required for snakes to reach sexual maturity. Research of wild snake populations has documented repeatedly that growth is faster, and survivorship lower, in younger snakes compared with older individuals. In some sea snakes, only 10–20 percent of neonates survive their first year, and only 6 percent of the females live to reproduce.

Snakes continue to grow as adults, unlike many species of mammals. However, the rates of growth slow considerably as a snake ages, and larger snakes that are near their maximum size grow very slowly, or negligibly. Typically, growth rates decline markedly when snakes reach sexual maturity, likely as a result of increasing energy investment to structures and behaviors that are related to reproduction (rather than growth). The energy demands for reproduction can be quite different between the sexes. For the multiple reasons discussed here, length is not a reliable indicator of age, and it is difficult to compare the growth rates among species if one uses a single metric for comparison. As a very rough generalization, most snakes are likely to achieve nearly half of their maximum body length during the first three to four years of growth, including larger species such as pythons that grow to lengths of several meters or longer (see chapter 1).

The longevity of snakes tends to fall in between that of lizards and turtles. Snakes in captivity tend to live from 10 to 20 years, with some aging up to 30+ years. A Ball Python in the Philadelphia Zoo lived to be a little older than 47 years. Demographic studies of snakes have shown that life spans in the wild may be similar to that in captivity, with maxima ranging typically between 15 and 30 years. Olive Sea Snakes on the Great Barrier Reef live to about 15 years.

Snakes on Islands

Studies of reproduction in snakes that live on islands are interesting because of the nature of resources, which can be limited, ephemeral, or literally "boom or bust." Clutch size and/or the mass of a young snake are significantly greater during years when prey resources are more abundant and when females have a better condition of energy storage for the production of young. In snakes generally, however, the relations between variation of resources and reproduction are complex, and measures of reproductive output can bear little relationship to the costs of reproduction in a given system. Assuming that resources are adequate or "normal," other factors can intervene to reduce the reproductive output of a female. In many species of snakes reproduction is associated with a decrease in the feeding rates of females, and gravid females may even exhibit anorexia! Such anorexic females may not easily survive after parturition owing either to starvation and depletion of energy reserves, or to being susceptible to predation.

Various interpretations of this phenomenon have identified several advantages of females not feeding. These include easier and more careful thermoregulation by females, which can also move more easily without prey in the digestive tract. Locomotion can already be physically constrained due to the bodily distension from oviductal eggs. François Brischoux and several coworkers have investigated the reproduction of sea kraits (*Laticauda* spp.) on some islets at New Caledonia. They report that female snakes cease feeding as their eggs develop, seemingly because the distension of the body tends to impede locomotion. Therefore, these females would be less effective in movements and more vulnerable to aquatic predators if they continued to feed. The feeding rate decreases progressively with increasing follicle size, suggesting there is a lack of a "threshold" effect on the behavior. Rather, increasing degrees of burdening due to egg development render foraging less productive and increasingly risky in relation to predators.

Snakes and the Future

It seems fitting in this chapter to add a concluding comment about the future of snakes. Indeed, this topic is tied closely to the future of the world as it relates to impacts of human population, technology, and climatic changes. Like many other vertebrates, snakes are documented to be in decline, and the phenomenon appears to be global. What is further alarming is the impression in some parts of the world that the numbers of snakes are decreasing not only where human presence offers obvious causes, but also in relatively pristine regions where there appears to be little, or no, direct human impact. The reasons might relate in various places to the indirect influence of invasive (introduced) wildlife, effects of atmospheric pollutants or radiation, climatic changes, or the subtle collapse of trophic systems. Of course, there could be unknown single or multiple effects of which we are totally unaware.

As long as appropriate habitat remains, I think that some species of snakes will survive even amid broad-scale reductions in other forms of wildlife. Smaller burrowing species, for example, might remain prevalent in suburban areas or even cities, and aquatic species might persist in bodies of water across varied landscapes. Some species might even thrive in agricultural landscapes, whereon a food base of rodents tends to thrive. And there is an important question regarding human impact that begs for more research. Do certain snake species become increasingly rare because of reduced numbers in the population, or is the rarity due (perhaps in part) to a "switching" of behavior to more secretive habits when encounters with humans increases?

What does appear certain is that larger, more spectacular species will disappear from landscapes where human impact is a dominant force. Loss of habitat, direct killing upon highways and roads, predatory losses to dogs and cats that accompany human inhabitants in increasing numbers, use of chemical pesticides, reduction in food base (frogs, for example), and of course direct killing by humans all act with multiplicity to reduce the numbers of snakes that are present in a given area. Despite many years of education regarding the place and value of snakes, far too many people still have misconceptions about snakes, fear them irrationally, and will kill one at each opportunity. This may be especially true in rural areas, where people tend to kill snakes or, at best, want them removed from their property. I contrast this with a personal impression I have that many Australians are well educated and tolerant of snakes, even though numerous species they encounter are venomous. It seems to me that Australians have learned to live with snakes being present in their surroundings, at least in comparison with some other cultures. I emphasize this is a strong impression that is based in my personal experiences, and not a statistically tested statement.

As one example, I knew an Australian couple who had two children and lived in a rural setting. They not only tolerated, but in fact quite enjoyed, the presence of a Red-bellied Black Snake (*Pseudechis porphyriacus*), which on some mornings sunned itself on an open porch that was attached to the house. This snake had been given a name, as was a goanna that also appeared on somewhat regular occasion. The snake was part of the natural environment that was both noticed and appreciated by the family. On the other hand, I cannot imagine many folks in Florida who would tolerate such presence of an Eastern Diamondback Rattlesnake (*Crotalus adamanteus*). The first response would likely be to kill the animal and remove it from the property. There are exceptions to this statement, of course.

So I appeal to the readers of this book to please share some of your excitement about the biology of snakes—what they do and how they live—with others, especially children. I believe that most people are fundamentally curious about snakes, especially if they have not been taught to fear them. This reminds me also to entreat filmmakers to show people the many fascinating behaviors of snakes and to avoid the all-too-common tendency to feature snakes predominantly in defensive postures or attitudes, which gives viewers the wrong impression that a snake is always ready to attack and to harm you. If people change their behaviors and cease to kill snakes, we will come a long way toward preserving and appreciating environments in which rich and varied wildlife entertain the senses and evoke imagination. Remember there is nothing more practical and edifying than to learn about the world around you. For many, one or more species of snakes will be an important part of that world. Together we will celebrate each time a snake is born.

Additional Reading

Aldridge, R., A. Bufalino, and A. Reeves. 2005. Pheromone communication in the watersnake, *Nerodia sipedon*: A mechanistic difference between semi-aquatic and terrestrial species. *American Midland Naturalist* 154:412–422.

Aldridge, R. D., and D. M. Sever (eds.). 2011. *Reproductive Biology and Phylogeny of Snakes*. Vol. 9 of Reproductive Biology and Phylogeny, B. G. M. Jamieson, series editor. Enfield, NH: Science Publishers.

Almeida-Santos, S. M., F. M. F. Abdalla, P. F. Silveira, N. Yamanouye, M. C. Breno, and M. G. Salomão. 2004. Reproductive cycle of the neotropical *Crotalus durissus terrificus*: I. Seasonal levels and interplay between steroid hormones and vasotocinase. *General and Comparative Endocrinology* 139:143–150.

Andren, C., and G. Nilson. 1983. Reproductive tactics in an island population of adders, *Vipera berus* (L.), with a fluctuating food resource. *Amphibia-Reptilia* 4:63–79.

Blackburn, D. G. 1998. Structure, function, and evolution of the oviducts of squamate reptiles, with special reference to viviparity and placentation. *Journal of Experimental Zoology* 282:560–617.

Blackburn, D. G. 2006. Squamate reptiles as model organisms for the evolution of viviparity. *Herpetological Monographs* 20:131–146.

Blackburn, D. G., K. E. Anderson, A. R. Johnson, S. R. Knight, and G. S. Gavelis. 2009. Histology and ultrastructure of the placental membranes of the viviparous Brown snake, *Storeria dekayi* (Colubridae: Natricinae). *Journal of Morphology* 270:1137–1154.

Brischoux, F., X. Bonnet, and R. Shine. 2010. Conflicts between feeding and reproduction in amphibious snakes (sea kraits, *Laticauda spp.*). *Australian Ecology* 36: 46–52.

Burns, G., and H. Heatwole. 2000. Growth, sexual dimorphism, and population biology of the olive sea snake, *Aipysurus laevis*, on the Great Barrier Reef of Australia. *Amphibia-Reptilia* 21:289–300.

Crews, D., and W. Garstka. 1982. The ecological physiology of reproduction in the Canadian red-sided garter snake. *Scientific American* 247:159–168.

Ford, N. 1986. The role of pheromone trails in the sociobiology of snakes. In D. Duvall, D. Mueller-Schwarze, and R. Silverstein (eds.), *Chemical Signals in Vertebrates 4*. New York: Plenum Press, pp. 261–278.

Gillingham, J. 1987. Social behavior. In R. Seigel, J. Collins, and S. Novak (eds.), *Snakes: Ecology and Evolutionary Biology*. New York: McGraw-Hill, pp. 211–217.

Greene, M., and R. Mason. 2000. Courtship, mating, and male combat of the brown tree snake, *Boiga irregularis*. *Herpetologica* 56:166–175.

Kubie, J., A. Vagvolgyi, and M. Halpern. 1978. Roles of the vomeronasal and olfactory systems in courtship behavior of male garter snakes. *Journal of Comparative Physiology and Psychology* 92:627–641.

LeMaster, M., and R. Mason. 2002. Variation in a female sexual attractiveness pheromone controls male mate choice in garter snakes. *Journal of Chemical Ecology* 28:1269–1285.

Lillywhite, H. B. 1985. Trailing movements and sexual behavior in *Coluber constrictor*. *Journal of Herpetology* 19:306–308.

Luboschek, V., M. Beger, D. Ceccarelli, Z. Richards, and M. Pratchett. 2013. Enigmatic declines of Australia's sea snakes from a biodiversity hotspot. *Biological Conservation* 166:191–202.

Lutterschmidt, D. I., and R. Mason. 2009. Endocrine mechanisms mediating temperature-induced reproductive behavior in red-sided garter snakes (*Thamnophis sirtalis parietalis*). *Journal of Experimental Biology* 212:3108–3118.

Madsen, T., and R. Shine. 1993. Costs of reproduction in a population of European adders. *Oecologia* 94:488–495.

Mason, R. T., and M. R. Parker. 2010. Social behavior and pheromonal communication in reptiles. *Journal of Comparative Physiology* A196:729–749.

Mason, R., H. Fales, T. Jones, L. Pannell, J. Chinn, and D. Crews. 1989. Sex pheromones in snakes. *Science* 245:290–293.

Mason, R., T. Jones, H. Fales, L. Pannell, and D. Crews. 1990. Characterization, synthesis, and behavioral responses to sex attractiveness pheromones of red-sided garter snakes (*Thamnophis sirtalis parietalis*). *Journal of Chemical Ecology* 16:2353–2369.

Mullin, S. J., and R. A. Seigel (eds.) 2009. *Snakes: Ecology and Conservation*. Ithaca, NY: Cornell University Press.

Parker, M., and R. Mason. 2009. Low temperature dormancy affects the quantity and quality of the female sexual attractiveness pheromone in red-sided garter snakes. *Journal of Chemical Ecology* 35:1234–1241.

Parker, W. S., and M. V. Plummer. 1987. Population ecology. In R. A. Seigel, J. R. Collins, and S. S. Novak (eds.), *Snakes, Ecology and Evolutionary Biology*. New York: Macmillan, pp. 253–301.

Reading, C. J., L. M. Luiselli, G. C. Akani, X. Bonnet, G. Amori, J. M. Ballouard, E. Filippi, G. Naulleau, D. Pearson, and L. Rugiero. 2010. Are snake populations in widespread decline? *Biology Letters* 6:777–780.

Rigley, L. 1971. "Combat dance" of the black rat snake, *Elaphe o. obsoleta*. *Journal of Herpetology* 5:65–66.

Ross, P., and D. Crews. 1977. Influence of the seminal plug on mating behaviour in the garter snake. *Nature* 267:344–345.

Schuett, G. W., S. Carlisle, A. Holycross, J. O'Leile, D. Hardy, E. Van Kirk, and W. Murdoch. 2002. Mating system of male Mojave rattlesnakes (*Crotalus scutulatus*): Seasonal timing of mating, agonistic behavior, spermatogenesis, sexual segment of the kidney, and plasma sex steroids. In G. W. Schuett, M. Hoggren, M. Douglas, and H. Greene (eds.), *Biology of the Vipers*. Eagle Mountain, UT: Eagle Mountain Publishing, pp. 515–532.

Shine, R. 1985. The evolution of viviparity in reptiles: An ecological analysis. In C. Gans and F. Billett (eds.), *Biology of the Reptilia*, vol. 15. New York: John Wiley, pp. 606–694.

Shine, R. 1988. Constraints on reproductive investment: A comparison between aquatic and terrestrial snakes. *Evolution* 42:17–27.

Shine, R. 1992. Relative clutch mass and body shape in lizards and snakes: Is reproductive investment constrained or optimized? *Evolution* 46:828–833.

Shine, R. 1994. Sexual size dimorphism in snakes revisited. *Copeia* 1994:326–346.

Shine, R. 2003. Reproductive strategies in snakes. *Proceedings Royal Society London* B 270:995–1004.

Shine, R. 2005. All at sea: Aquatic life modifies mate-recognition modalities in sea snakes (*Emydocephalus annulatus*, Hydrophiidae). *Behavioral Ecology and Sociobiology* 57:591–598.

Shine, R., and X. Bonnet. 2009. Reproductive biology, population viability, and options for field management. In S. J. Mullin and R. A. Seigel (eds.), *Snakes, Ecology and Conservation*. Ithaca, NY: Cornell University Press, pp. 172–200.

Shine, R., B. Phillips, H. Wayne, M. LeMaster, and R. Mason. 2003. Chemosensory cues allow courting male garter snakes to assess body length and body condition of potential mates. *Behavioral Ecology and Sociobiology* 54:162–166.

Shine, R., J. Webb, A. Lane, and R. Mason. 2005. Mate location tactics in garter snakes: Effects of rival males, interrupted trails and non-pheromonal cues. *Ecology* 19:1017–1024.

Slip, D. J., and R. Shine. 1988. The reproductive biology and mating system of diamond pythons, *Morelia spilota* (Serpentes: Boidae). *Herpetologica* 4:396–404.

Stewart, J. R., and K. R. Brasch. 2003. Ultrastructure of the placentae of the natricine snake, *Virginia striatula* (Reptilia: Squamata). *Journal of Morphology* 255:177–201.

Sun, L.-X., R. Shine, D. Zhao, and T. Zhengren. 2002. Low costs, high output: Reproduction in an insular pit-viper (*Gloydius shedaoensis*, Viperidae) from north-eastern China. *Journal of Zoology* 256:511–521.

Tinkle, D. W., and J. W. Gibbons. 1977. The distribution and evolution of viviparity in reptiles. *Miscellaneous Publications of the Museum of Natural History, University of Michigan* 154:1–55.

GLOSSARY OF TERMS

abduction (*v.* abduct). Movement of a part away from the medial axis or plane of the body, or movement of two parts away from each other. Cf. *adduction*.

acclimation. A reversible change in morphology, behavior, or physiology that occurs in response to a prolonged change in the condition of a laboratory environment (e.g., temperature). Cf. *acclimatization*.

acclimatization. A reversible change in morphology, behavior, or physiology that occurs in response to a prolonged change in the condition of the natural environment (e.g., temperature). Cf. *acclimation*.

accommodation. The eye's action or ability to bring an object into focus.

acetylcholine. An important neurotransmitter in many different types of neurons, having actions on the heart, smooth muscle of blood vessels, and the activation of muscle at neuromuscular junctions.

action potential. A nerve "impulse" or propagated bioelectric change in a nerve membrane. This is the unit of signaling in the nervous system.

active forager. An animal that moves through its environment actively searching for potential prey.

adduction (*v.* adduct). Movement of a part toward the medial axis or plane of the body, or movement of two parts together. Cf. *abduction*.

aglyph (*adj*. -ous). A snake in which teeth lack a groove or canal, therefore unable to transport venom effectively.

air sac. See *tracheal air sac*.

alimentary canal. See *gastrointestinal tract*.

allantois. See *extraembryonic membranes*.

allele. Shorthand form of allelomorph, representing one of a number of possible alternate heritable forms of a given gene.

allometry. Changes in the relative proportion of a body part in relation to the rate of growth of the whole body, or another body part, as total body size increases. Such changes can be either positive or negative.

alpha (α) keratin. See *keratin*.

ambush forager. Reference to an animal that remains sedentary for periods, usually in strategic locations, and waits for prey to come within capture distance.

amelanistic partial albinism. A condition where skin color lacks melanin, but other pigments are present to impart some, or partial, color.

amnion. See *extraembryonic membranes*.

androgen. A class of sex steroid *hormones* that stimulate male characteristics and promote protein synthesis. In female reptiles, androgens can be converted in the central nervous system to *estrogens* or other steroids. This also occurs in males.

ankylosis. A rigid union between two parts, usually with reference to attachment between teeth and bone by hard mineralized tissue.

aorta. See *dorsal aorta*.

aortic arches. Two (right and left) outflow vessels of the ventricle, which convey systemic blood and join to form the *dorsal aorta*.

apical pit. A sense organ recessed in a small depression usually on the posterior tip of the dorsal scales of certain reptiles, particularly snakes. Little is known about the function of these structures.

apnea. Breath-hold; cessation of breathing.

aposematism (adj. aposematic). Reference to characters, especially coloration, that advertises an organism as dangerous or unpleasant to potential predators.

arteriole. A smaller artery that immediately precedes capillaries.

artery. A blood vessel that conveys generally well-oxygenated blood from the heart to tissues. Pulmonary arteries convey relatively deoxygenated blood to the lung. Cf. *vein*.

ATP. Adenosine triphosphate, an energy-rich nucleotide used as a common energy currency in all living cells.

atrioventricular valves. Valves separating and regulating the flow of blood from the atria to ventricle of the heart.

atrium (*pl.* atria). One of the receiving chambers of the heart, filling with blood returning from veins and emptying to the *ventricle*.

baroreceptor. A sensory receptor that is stimulated by changes in pressure. Typically, this term refers to receptors in the walls of central blood vessels where they detect stretch or distension of the vessel wall due to increased blood pressure.

basal. Reference to the earliest lineage, or early lineages, in a *phylogeny*. The internal nodes of a phylogeny in contrast with terminal branches.

basilar membrane. The delicate strand of elastic tissue bearing the auditory *hair cells* in the *inner ear*.

behavioral thermoregulation. Regulation of body temperature attributable to behaviors of an animal that control its interactions with environmental heat sources. See *thermoregulation*.

beta (β) keratin. See *keratin*.

binocular vision. Overlapping visual fields involving two eyes, such that images are focused on both of two retinas simultaneously and thereby enhance the perception of depth and distance.

body wall. The part of the animal body that encloses the internal body cavity.

boundary layer. A layer of fluid (air or water) adjacent to a physical boundary or surface, in which motion of the fluid is affected by the boundary and exhibits a mean velocity that is less than the free stream velocity away from the boundary. This region is responsible for frictional *drag* of moving objects.

brille. See *spectacle*.

buoyancy. The tendency to float or sink in a fluid environment, water or air.

button. The first permanent and distal segment on the rattle of a rattlesnake, the *prebutton* being lost at the first *ecdysis*.

cantilever. A projecting beam or body that is supported at only one end.

capillary (*pl.*-ies). The smallest (microscopic) blood vessels that are lined by a highly permeable endothelium and exchange gases and chemical substances with tissues through which they pass.

cardiac. Reference to the heart.

cardiac output. The volume rate of blood outflow from the heart, expressed as volume of blood leaving the *ventricle* per time. In snakes with a single ventricle, it is best to specify the cardiac outflow as systemic, pulmonary, or total.

cardiovascular system. See *circulation*.

catecholamines. A group of molecules that act as *neurotransmitters* and *hormones*, including *epinephrine* and *norepinephrine*. These play important roles in accelerating the heart and constricting blood vessels in the cardiovascular system.

caudocephalic wave. A horizontal undulating wave of the body that results in gentle body contacts between a female snake and a courting male that produces the movement while lying beside or upon her. The undulation characteristically moves from posterior to anterior and is thought to stimulate mating.

cavum arteriosum. One of three cavities in the single ventricle of noncrocodilian reptiles, which receives oxygenated blood from the left atrium but has no direct connection to an outflow tract.

cavum pulmonale. One of three cavities in the single ventricle of noncrocodilian reptiles, which lies on the left side of the *vertical septum* and conveys blood into the pulmonary outflow tract.

cavum venosum. One of three cavities in the single ventricle of noncrocodilian reptiles, which lies to the right side of the *vertical septum* and conveys blood to the systemic *aortic arches*.

centrifugal. Acting in a direction outward from a center of rotation.

character, or character state. Reference to an observable phenotypic property or trait of an organism. It represents the particular condition or expression of a feature that might have variable expressions in different organisms.

chorioallantois, chorioallantoic membrane. An extraembryonic membrane formed by union of the chorion and allantois (see *extraembryonic membranes*).

chorion. See *extraembryonic membranes*.

chromatophore. A generalized term for a cell that contains pigment and imparts color to skin.

chyme. Partially digested food (also called *digesta*) in the form of a liquefied mass after it enters the intestine.

circadian rhythm. A cycle of behavior or physiological process that is repeated daily on a 23–25 h interval (roughly one day), attributable to an "internal clock" but synchronized to time-related factors in the environment.

circulation (also blood circulation, cardiovascular system, transport system) The heart and blood vessels, which in aggregate move blood throughout the body. The *pulmonary circulation* transports blood to and from the lungs (where it becomes oxygenated), and the *systemic circulation* transports blood to and from all the other body tissues.

clade. A *monophyletic* lineage of organisms. A single species and its descendants, representing a distinct branch on a *phylogenetic tree*.

clear layer. A term given to the innermost living cells of an *outer epidermal generation* during skin shedding of squamates.

cloaca. The common chamber and passageway where reproductive, urinary, and digestive ducts or canals release their contents. This chamber receives feces from the large intestine and voids its contents to the exterior through the *vent* or cloacal opening.

cloacal pop, popping. Rapid extrusion and retraction of the cloaca, which results in the rapid expulsion of air from the vent in certain North American snakes. The action produces a clearly audible popping sound while the tail is held aloft as a defensive action.

clutch size. The collective number of eggs that are ovulated and laid by a single female at one time. Cf. *litter size*.

coefficient of friction. A dimensionless value that describes the ratio of the force of friction between two bodies and the force pressing them together. This value is an empirical measurement that is determined experimentally.

color polymorphism. See *polymorphism*.

columella. The auditory ossicle (bone or cartilaginous element) that crosses the middle ear cavity and transmits sound or vibrational stimuli from the surrounding tissues of the head (in snakes) to the *oval window* and fluid of the *inner ear*.

combat dance. A challenge behavior between two male snakes, usually of the same species, involving vertical postures, intertwining of bodies, and pushing of the opponent in attempt to force the individual to the ground. Such behavior occurs typically during the mating season of the species involved.

concertina locomotion. A mode of locomotion in snakes, characterized by sequential extension and contraction of the body from one anchored or stationary site to the next as the animal moves with accordion-like appearance in one direction.

cone. A photoreceptor in the *retina*, functioning in bright light and differentially sensitive to light of different wavelengths (thus imparting color vision). Cf. *rod*.

contact zone. See *resistance site*.

conus arteriosus. A thickened part of the amphibian heart between the ventricle and distributing vessels of the systemic and pulmonary circulations. This structure is not present in reptiles.

convection. The mass transfer of heat or matter due to bulk transport in a moving fluid (gas or liquid).

convergence, convergent character. Reference to *homoplasy* or the independent evolution of similar character states in unrelated lineages, usually attributable to similar selection pressures associated with similarity of one or more common features of the environment.

copulatory plug. See *seminal plug*.

cornea. The transparent surface covering the iris and pupil, through which light passes as it enters the eye.

corneous, cornified. Descriptive of keratinized epithelium, as the *stratum corneum* of the epidermis.

corpus luteum (*pl*. corpora lutea). The remnants of a ruptured egg follicle following ovulation, which secrete relatively large volumes of progesterone until late pregnancy in viviparous reptiles.

costocutaneous muscles. The muscles that run between the ribs and overlying skin of snakes.

cranial kinesis. Movements between parts of the skull, usually in contexts related to feeding of snakes.

critical thermal maximum (*pl*. -a) (CTMax). The temperature at which a species, when heated gradually, becomes incapacitated such that long-term survival is not possible at this or higher temperatures.

critical thermal minimum (*pl*. -a) (CTMin). The temperature at which a species, when cooled gradually, becomes incapacitated such that long-term survival is not possible at this or lower temperatures.

crypsis, cryptic. A condition of being camouflaged; concealed.

defensive strike. A strike made by a snake as a defensive movement to thwart a potential predator. Cf. *predatory strike*.

derived, or derived character. Reference to a more recent character or feature that departs from the ancestral condition in a lineage. Opposite to *primitive*.

dermis. The inner layer of skin beneath the epidermis, containing fibrous connective tissue, blood vessels, nerves, and chromatophores.

diagnostic character. A specific character state that distinguishes unambiguously one species or clade of organisms from another.

diapsid. Reference to a reptilian skull in which there are two temporal, or postorbital, openings.

diastole. Relaxation of muscles of the ventricle while filling with blood from the atria, prior to contraction. Cf. *systole*.

dietary water. Preformed water that is present in the food that an animal consumes.

diffusion. Movement of atoms, molecules, or ions as a result of random thermal motion from a region of higher to lower concentration.

digesta. See *chyme*.

digestive tract. See *gastrointestinal tract*.

diverticulum (*pl*. -a). A circumscribed pouch or sac.

dorsal aorta. The principal systemic blood vessel that conveys blood to the body tissues posterior to the heart, formed by the union of the right and left *aortic arches*.

down-regulation. Control of a physiological activity by a decrease in receptor density in a target cell membrane. Cf. *up-regulation*.

drag. The resistance to movement of an object through a fluid, which increases with the viscosity and density of the medium and varies with the shape and surface area and properties of an object. A drag force acts parallel to the relative movement of fluid and opposite to the direction of movement.

ecdysis. The shedding or sloughing of the *stratum corneum* of the *epidermis*, which periodically renews the outer covering of the skin.

ectothermy (*adj*. ectothermic). Reference to an animal that depends on external heat sources to regulate body temperature. Cf. *endothermy*.

eggshell. The shell or outer covering of an egg, consisting of fibers and variable amounts of calcium carbonate crystals.

electromyography. The recording (and study) of electrical activity of muscles.

endocrine (*adj*. or *n*.) Secreting (chemical messengers) into the blood circulation. See *hormone*.

endothermy (*adj*. endothermic). Reference to organisms (e.g., birds, mammals) wherein regulated body temperature is attributable largely to internal heat production arising from relatively high rates of energy metabolism. Cf. *ectothermy*.

endurance. The ability of an organism to exert itself and to move or remain active for a long period of time.

epaxial muscles. Muscles of the trunk that lie, or originate, dorsal to the vertebral column or body axis.

epidermal generation. A unit of lepidosaurian *epidermis* that is periodically formed and shed in *ecdysis*. A complete, mature generation of epidermis when superficial in position just before it is shed to the environment is called an *outer epidermal generation*. During renewal of the epidermis during the shedding cycle, the newly forming unit, lying beneath the outer generation that is about to be shed, is called the *inner epidermal generation*.

epidermis. The outer layer of skin of a vertebrate, overlying the *dermis*. The epidermis contains the *stratum corneum* and living cells having the capacity to form keratin.

epididymis. The largely convoluted tubule that drains the efferent ducts of the testis into the urethra. This structure lies at the surface of the testis and functions to store sperm until they are released to the exterior.

epinephrine. See *catecholamines*.

esophagus. The region of the gut located between the mouth and stomach, functioning to transport ingested food to the region of digestion.

estrogens. A family of sex steroids synthesized primarily in the *ovary*, but some are produced in the adrenal cortex, brain, and testis. These hormones play a central role in stimulating the female system during reproductive cycles and the development of *secondary sexual characteristics*. They also function to prepare the reproductive system for fertilization, and are essential for *vitellogenesis* and egg development.

evaporative cooling. Removal of body heat attributable to evaporation of water, whether passive or actively enhanced by *panting*.

exhalation. See *expiration*.

expiration. Active or passive movement of air out of the lung (to the external environment). *Exhalation*. Cf. *Inspiration*.

external respiration. See *ventilation*.

extraembryonic membranes. Structures formed around the embryo that eliminate wastes (*allantois*), provide food (yolk sac) and oxygen, and protect the embryo (*amnion* and *chorion*).

eyecap. See *spectacle*.

facial pit. See *pit organ*.

facultative endothermy. Endothermic heat production by an animal that is not obligatory, but may or may not occur depending on circumstances.

fang. A grooved or tubular tooth that is used to inject venom.

fascia. A band of connective tissue that forms a sheath, as around a muscle or blood vessel.

faveolus (*pl.*-i). A functional unit of reptilian lung *parenchyma*, consisting of an individual membranous compartment bounded by neighboring units in the form of a honeycomb.

fenestra (*pl.*-ae). A large opening, usually within or between bones.

fitness. The ability of an organism to contribute its genes to the next generation; roughly expressed as the number of offspring contributed to the next generation weighted by the probability of surviving to reproduce.

flow. Movement of fluid, or the quantity of fluid moving, usually expressed as volume per time.

footplate. The expanded base of the *columella* providing contact with the *oval window* of the *inner ear*.

foramen. A hole or opening that allows passage through a tissue wall.

friction. Mechanical resistance to relative motion between two solid surfaces that are in contact. *Static friction* is the force that has to be overcome in order to induce forward motion of an object along a surface that it contacts.

Sliding friction is the force that has to be overcome in order to keep one of two contacting objects moving at a constant velocity.

frontal. Of, or pertaining to, the front of the head or skull of an animal, especially the large and prominent dermal bone on the dorsal roof of the skull, lying between the eye orbits.

fusiform. Spindle-shaped, with tapering toward each end.

gas exchange. In context of physiology, the exchange of respiratory gases (O_2 and CO_2) between an organism and its environment.

gas exchanger. Any permeable organ that exchanges respiratory gases with the environment: lung, gills, or skin.

gastric glands. Glands in the wall of the stomach that secrete mucus, acid, and proteolytic enzymes.

gastrointestinal tract. A hollow, tubular cavity extending through an animal and open at both ends. This structure functions in ingestion, digestion, and absorption of food materials. Also called *alimentary canal*, *digestive tract*, or simply *gut*.

genetic drift. Evolutionary change due to random fluctuations of gene frequencies, independent of selection and most evident in small populations.

genotype. The genetic makeup of an individual, which along with other factors such as the environment determines the organism's *phenotype*. Cf. *phenotype*.

gliding. A form of aerial locomotion involving largely passive but controlled movement through air. In snakes, a flattened body is used as an airfoil to reduce the angle of descent after launching from an elevated site.

glottis. The opening from the pharynx (throat) to the *trachea* or *larynx*.

glycolysis (*adj.* glycolytic). Pertaining to the enzymatic conversion of glucose to the simpler compound of *lactate* (or pyruvate), resulting in production of energy as ATP without a requirement for oxygen. This constitutes the principal route of carbohydrate breakdown and oxidation and is an important aspect of activity metabolism in snakes (and other reptiles) that utilize glycolysis for ATP production in muscle during short but intense bursts of activity.

gonad. A reproductive organ in which either eggs (*ovary*) or sperm (*testis*) are produced. The *ovary* or *testis* is a primary sexual character.

gonadotropin, gonadotropic hormone. Hormones that influence the activity of the *gonads*, particularly those secreted by the anterior pituitary-follicle stimulating hormone and luteinizing hormone.

gonadotropin-releasing hormone. A hormone secreted from the *hypothalamus* and which stimulates the release of *gonadotropins* from the *pituitary*.

gravitational pressure. The component of pressure in a fluid that is attributable to gravity. Also called *hydrostatic pressure*.

gut. See *gastrointestinal tract*.

hair cells. Mechanosensory epithelial cells bearing minute hairlike structures that are bent by sound or vibrational stimuli, which alters the membrane properties and creates bioelectric "signals" that are transmitted to the auditory nerve. These cells are arrayed along the *basilar membrane* of the *inner ear*.

harmonic. In bioacoustics, an overtone whose frequency is an integral multiple of a fundamental frequency.

head pits. Structures similar to *apical pits* and having variable appearances and distribution on the head scales of snakes. Also called *parietal pits*.

heart. The central muscular pump of the cardiovascular system, consisting of two atria and a single ventricle in snakes.

heart rate. The frequency of heart contractions that provide the force to move blood through the circulation. Heart rate is typically measured as the number of heartbeats (or contraction cycles) per time.

hematocrit. The percentage of total blood volume occupied by red blood cells, typically measured in a sample of whole blood.

heme. The ringlike molecular component of hemoglobin containing iron that is responsible for binding oxygen within a structural surrounding of carrier protein.

hemipenis (*pl.*-es). Either of paired copulatory organs lying in a cavity at the base of the tail in squamate reptiles.

hemoglobin. The pigment inside red blood cells responsible for the reversible binding and transport of oxygen.

hemotoxic. A property of snake venoms that impairs blood vessels and lymphatic vessels.

hertz (Hz). Cycles per second (a derived unit of frequency).

hinge. The softer, pliable region of skin between overlapping scales of reptiles, especially squamates.

homology. Similarity of characters due to common ancestry.

homoplasy, homoplastic. Reference to similarity of *character states*, or function, attributable to *convergent* or parallel evolution and not due directly to inheritance from common ancestry.

horizontal undulatory progression. See *lateral undulation*.

hormone. A chemical messenger that is secreted into the blood circulation or intercellular space and affects target tissues. Cf. *endocrine*.

hydrophobic. Repelling water; nonwettable.

hydrostatic indifferent point. That point in a contained horizontal fluid where the pressure does not change when the contained volume (say a tube) is tilted upright.

hydrostatic pressure. See *gravitational pressure*.

hypothalamus. That part of the brain that forms the floor of the median (third) ventricle.

inertia. The tendency of an object to remain at rest or in uniform motion in a straight line unless acted upon by external forces.

inhalation. See *inspiration*.

inner ear. The internal part of the ear, comprising a sensory organ responsible for balance and equilibrium sense in addition to the sense of hearing.

inner epidermal generation. See *epidermal generation*.

inspiration. Active movement of air into the lung. *Inhalation*. Cf. *expiration*.

integument. A covering. The skin and its derivatives.

interaortic foramen. A small opening between the left and right *aortic arches*, located at their base near the *ventricle*.

interstitial fluid. Liquid within the spaces surrounding (outside of) cells, generally similar to blood plasma but with lower content of protein.

interventricular canal. A space within the ventricle of non-crocodilian reptiles that allows communication (flow of blood) between the *cavum arteriosum* and *cavum venosum*.

intracardiac shunt. See *shunt*.

iridescent color. Bright and changing color attributable to reflection due to structural properties of a surface (and not due to pigments).

iris. A muscular disc with a contractile hole situated in front of the eye lens that acts as an adjustable aperture.

Jacobson's organ. See *vomeronasal organ*.

keeled scale. A scale that bears a prominent central keel or protruding midline, detectable by touch or by eye. Cf. *smooth scale*.

keratin. A hard or tough, fibrous, nonsoluble protein produced by the epidermis and forming the outermost *stratum corneum. Alpha (α) keratin* consists of helical, hairlike molecules, whereas *beta (β) keratin* is a pleated sheet and feather-like. The latter is more rigid and generally tougher than is alpha keratin.

keratinocyte. An epidermal cell that has capacity to synthesize keratins.

kinematics. The study of animal motion, its course and patterns.

kinesis. Generally, reference to physical movement. This word is descriptive of movements between parts of the skull (*cranial kinesis*), usually in contexts related to feeding of snakes.

labial pit. See *pit organ*.

lactate, lactic acid. A product of the incomplete oxidation of carbohydrate via the pathway of *glycolysis* in the absence of oxygen. Lactate is a salt of lactic acid, typically produced in muscle during very intense activity.

lacunar cells. A cell type present in the epidermis of squamates during the shedding cycle, located between *α-keratin* above and the *clear layer* below, and characterized by misshapen nuclei that appear to lie in a vacuole.

lamellar granules. Discreet lipid-enriched secretory organelles that are present in the epidermis and from which lipids are released to the extracellular spaces where they become part of the epidermal *permeability barrier*.

large intestine. The posterior segment of the intestine, usually a comparatively straight tube of large diameter passing to the *cloaca*.

larynx. A complex of cartilaginous elements, fibers, and muscles at the pharyngeal opening of the *trachea* that functions to protect the opening and, in some species of reptiles, permits vocalization.

lateral undulation (or horizontal undulatory progression). The most commonly used mode of terrestrial locomotion in snakes, involving horizontal waves that travel down alternate sides of the body axis and generate a reaction force at fixed points in the animal's physical environment—usually surface irregularities in the substrate.

left aortic arch. See *aortic arches*.

left-to-right (L-R) shunt. See *shunt*.

lepidosaur. Any member of a clade of reptiles (Lepidosauria) inclusive of snakes, lizards, amphisbaenians, and tuatara.

lens. The principal light-focusing structure in the eye.

litter size. The collective number of animals that are born at one time in a viviparous species. Cf. *clutch size*.

loreal pit. See *pit organ*.

lymph, lymphatic fluid. Clear plasma-like fluid that is carried in lymphatic vessels.

mandibular raking. An unusual feeding mechanism in which the tooth-bearing elements of the lower jaw rotate synchronously in and out of the mouth, thereby dragging prey into the esophagus. This has been described in small, burrowing thread snakes.

mating ball. A mating phenomenon seen in some snake species, especially garter snakes, in which males outnumber females in breeding aggregations; from 10 to 100 or more males surround and simultaneously court a single receptive female.

mean selected temperature. See *preferred body temperature*.

melanin. A dark pigment derived from oxidation products of tyrosine and dihydroxyphenol compounds, present in skin and internal *peritoneum*.

melanism. Excessive pigmentation or blackening of the skin or other tissues, usually of genetic origin.

melanophore. A chromatophore that contains *melanin*, which is generally dark brown to black in color.

melanophore stimulating hormone (MSH). A hormone formed in, and secreted from, the pituitary gland and which acts on melanocytes to stimulate the dispersion of melanin granules within these cells and thereby cause darkening of the skin.

melatonin. A predominant hormone associated with the pineal gland, but also found in the brain and eyes of ectothermic vertebrates. Synthesis of melatonin is largely under light control, and levels fluctuate rhythmically with light cycles. Melatonin is an important communicator between environmental cues of light and temperature and affects both physiology and behavior, including reproduction in snakes.

mesos layer. A stratum of differentiated cells within the *stratum corneum*, consisting of α-keratinized cells that are alternately sandwiched between lamellar lipids in many species. This layer comprises the *permeability barrier* to flux of water across the skin.

metabolic water. Water that is formed during oxidative cellular metabolism.

microarchitecture. See *microsculpture*.

microdermatoglyphics. See *microsculpture*.

microornamentation. See *microsculpture*.

microsculpture, microsculpturing. Reference to microscopic features of surface morphology that are present on scales of squamate reptiles. Also called *microarchitecture*, *microdermatoglyphics*, and *microornamentation*.

microstructure. In context of scale morphology, see *microsculpture*.

microvasculature. The small peripheral blood vessels that distribute blood within tissues, including arterioles, capillaries, and venules.

microvillus (*pl.*-i). A minute, cylindrical projection of a cell membrane that increases the surface area of absorptive epithelia, as in the intestine.

mimicry. The phenomenon where organisms resemble one another in context of gaining an advantage in avoiding predators.

modality. The state or quality of a stimulus or sensation (light, sound, etc.).

molecular clock. Reference to a constant rate of nucleotide substitutions in DNA when averaged across the entire genome of a species. A *phylogenetic tree* that is constructed on the assumption of a molecular clock has all the terminal taxa equidistant from the root.

monophyletic, monophyletic lineage. Reference to a condition in which a group of species have all been derived from a single common ancestor.

morphological color change. Color changes that occur over days, weeks, or longer due to developmental, ontogenetic, or seasonal changes in chromatophore patterns. Cf. *physiological color change*.

MSH. See *melanophore stimulating hormone*.

muscular ridge. A muscular septum in the ventricle of noncrocodilian reptiles that partially divides the ventricle by separating the *cavum pulmonale* from the *cavum arteriosum* and *cavum venosum*.

nanoscale. Reference to a scale of measurement on the order of a billionth (10^{-9}) of a meter.

naris (*pl.*-es). The nostril or nasal opening, usually paired.

neck sacs. See *tracheal air sac*.

nerve. A bundle of neurons, or processes of neurons that are enveloped by connective tissue. Cf. *neuron*.

net cost of transport. The amount of energy that is used to transport a given mass of an animal a given distance.

neuro-. A prefix meaning nerve or *neuron*.

neuromodulator. A chemical messenger that alters the function or actions of neurons.

neuron. An individual nerve cell and fundamental unit of the nervous system. Cf. *nerve*.

neurotoxic. A property of snake venoms that is destructive to the nervous system, including neuromuscular junctions.

neurotransmitter. A "chemical messenger" that is released from nerve terminals to affect other nerves or cells on which the nerve terminals act.

node. A branching point in a *phylogenetic tree*.

norepinephrine. See *catecholamines*.

oberhautchen. The outermost layer of β-keratin that forms the external *microsculpturing* overlying the *epidermis* of lepidosaurs. The original spelling of this term is Öberhautchen. However, Ernest Williams pointed out in 1988 that the term was now appearing in the English literature so frequently that capitalization with an umlaut was unnecessary.

ontogeny (*adj.*ontogenetic). Reference to complete development of an organism, from fertilized egg to adult.

opisthoglyph (*adj.*-ous). A condition in venomous snakes where the posterior pair of teeth on each maxilla are enlarged or grooved to function as fangs.

outer epidermal generation. See *epidermal generation*.

oval window. The membranous area on the lateral or ventral wall of the *inner ear*, adjoining the *footplate* of the *columella*.

ovarian follicle. The structure of the *ovary* that contains the developing egg.

ovary (*pl.*-ies). The female reproductive organ (*gonad*) that produces ova or eggs.

oviduct. The tube that conveys eggs from the *ovary* to the *uterus* or to the exterior via the *cloaca*.

oviparity (*adj.* oviparous). A mode of reproduction in which underdeveloped eggs are laid by the female. Developing embryos are encased within membranes overlain by a shell, and these are deposited in the environment outside the body before hatching. Cf. *viviparity, viparous*.

oviposition, oviposit. The act of laying or depositing eggs in the environment. Cf. *ovulation*.

ovulation. The release of an ovum or egg from the *ovary*. Cf. *oviposition*.

pant, panting. Increased breathing frequency that increases the rate of ventilated air movement and hence evaporation of water and removal of heat from membranes associated with the upper respiratory airways, throat, and mouth.

parenchyma. The essential and distinctive functional tissue of an organ.

parietal. Either of a pair of dermal bones forming a principal part of the braincase at the roof of the skull (located between the frontals and occipitals). Generally, this term is used in reference to the dorsal part of the head.

parietal pits. See *head pits*.

parthenogenesis (*adj.* parthenogenetic). Reproduction in which an egg develops into an embryo without fertilization by a sperm.

passage time. With reference to the gut, the time elapsed from ingestion to defecation

PBT. See *preferred body temperature*.

performance. The relative measure of key tasks or functions such as feeding, digesting, moving, growing, etc., that are important for survival and reproduction.

performance breadth. Reference to some measure of the thermal range over which *performance* has some subjective value to the organism.

peripheral resistance. The resistance to blood flow attributable to the smaller peripheral blood vessels.

peristalsis. A traveling wave of constriction (followed by relaxation) in tubular tissue such as the gut, produced by constriction of circular muscle. In the gut, these movements serve to move objects through the lumen.

peritoneum. A membrane that lines the body cavity and invests internal organs therein.

perivascular lymphatic. A lymphatic vessel that surrounds and is concentric with a blood vessel. These structures are common in snakes.

permeability barrier. In this book, reference to the specialized layer of lipids that is located in the stratum corneum of the epidermis, limiting the flux of water across the skin.

phenotype. The physical characteristics of an organism, related to its genetic expression and sometimes modified by environment. Cf. *genotype*.

phenotypic plasticity. Variation of phenotype attributable to environmental influence on the phenotype, caused by environment interaction with genetic expression related to the particular phenotype in question. See also *reaction norm*.

pheromone. A chemical substance produced by an individual and released into the environment for the purpose of signaling a social response between (among) individuals of the same species.

photoperiod. The period of light in 24 h.

phylogeny, or phylogenetic tree. A diagram that depicts the relationships of groups of organisms according to their evolutionary history. The diagrammatic tree represents hypothesized genealogical ties and sequence of historical, ancestor-dependent relationships that link taxa.

physiological color change. Color changes that occur quickly due to nervous, hormonal, or local control mechanisms. Cf. *morphological color change*.

pigment. In biological usage, a molecular substance in cells or tissues that imparts color.

pineal gland. An organ formed from the roof of the forebrain that acts to measure light, produces *melatonin*, and regulates the hormonal output of other *endocrine* structures.

pit organ. Specialized infrared receptors having evolved independently several times within the Boidae and once within Colubroidea (Crotalinae). Boid pit organs are located in upper and lower labial scales (and/or rostral scales) and called *labial pits*, whereas crotaline pit organs are present as single structures between the eye and nostril on either side of the head and called *facial pits* or sometimes *loreal pits*. Pit organs consist of a thin, innervated membrane stretched across an open cavity in pit vipers, permitting rapid and sensitive detection of changes in infrared radiation. The labial pits of boids are similar except the membrane lines the inner recess of a labial pocket.

placenta. A vascular, nutritive connection between fetal and maternal tissues, through which the developing embryo exchanges nutrients, respiratory gases, and metabolic waste products. The wall of the *uterus* is typically the maternal connection in placental reptiles.

pleurodont. Reference to an anchoring condition of teeth in which rootless teeth are attached to the inner side of the jawbone, set in a shelf-like inner, lingual wall. This is a common mode of *ankylosis* in lizards and snakes.

polymorphism. The sustained occurrence of two or more distinct and genetically determined forms (e.g., color pattern) in a single species. This usually represents two or more genetically distinct classes in the same interbreeding population.

postprandial calorigenic response, metabolic response, or thermogenesis. See *specific dynamic action*.

power. The rate of doing work, equal to work per time.

prebutton. The small, first segment on the tip of the tail of rattlesnakes, present at birth and lost at the first ecdysis. Cf. *button*.

predatory strike. A strike by a snake that is made with intention of capturing prey. Cf. *defensive strike*.

preferred body temperature (PBT). The mean selected temperature that is maintained by an ectothermic animal in a gradient or mosaic of thermal environments.

pressure. Force per unit area.

pressure shunting. See *shunt*.

prey transport. Reference to swallowing a prey item, including manipulation by various active elements of the jaws and mouth.

prezygapophyses. See *zygapophysis*.

primitive, or primitive character. Reference to a character or feature that is basal or of ancient evolutionary origin. Opposite to *derived*.

progesterone. A steroid *hormone* secreted from the *ovary* and *corpus luteum*, essential for egg retention and pregnancy in *viviparous* species. It has many effects that support egg and embryo development.

prokinesis. A condition of cranial kinesis in which the line of movement is located between the nasal and frontal elements, anterior to the orbit.

proprioceptors. Sensory receptors located primarily in muscles, tendons, or joints that sense tension and provide information about the position and relative motion of body parts.

propulsive force. A force exerted against the environment that results in a *reaction force* that is equal and opposite in direction. The reaction force is equal to *thrust* and enables forward movement of the object or animal exerting the propulsive force.

proteroglyph (*adj.-ous*). A snake or condition in which a relatively long maxilla bears a single, hollow, venom-conducting fang on its anterior end. The fang is fixed and followed posteriorly by non-venom-conducting teeth (characteristic of elapids).

pulmonary. Reference to the lung.

pulmonary circulation. See *circulation*.

punctuated equilibrium or evolution. Reference to relatively brief episodes of speciation, followed by long periods of stability of species.

pupil. The aperture in the center of the iris through which light enters the eye.

push point. See *resistance site*.

pyloris. The distal aperture of the stomach, opening into the small intestine.

radio telemetry. Study of the location, movements, behavior, or physiology of animals using remote detection and transmission equipment involving radio signals.

RCM. See *relative clutch mass*.

reaction force. See *thrust* and *propulsive force*.

reaction norm. The variability of *phenotypic* traits exhibited by a given *genotype* under a range of natural conditions common to the habitat of the species, or under standard experimental conditions. See also *phenotypic plasticity*.

reaction zone. See *resistance site*.

receptor. A nerve or modified sensory cell that receives and *transduces* a *stimulus*.

rectilinear locomotion. A mode of snake locomotion in which the animal moves forward in a straight line, with no lateral movement. Muscles act bilaterally to pull the skin forward relative to the ribs, following which the ventral scales anchor the body to the substrate. Other muscles then pull the ribs and vertebral column forward relative to the stationary ventral skin.

refraction. The bending of light rays when they pass between two media of differing density (e.g., air to water).

relative clutch mass (RCM). The ratio of the total mass of a clutch to the body mass of the associated female, expressed as a decimal fraction or a percentage. Cf. *clutch size*.

resistance. Generally, a property or aggregate properties that impede the movement or flow of something in a circuit or flow system. In context of locomotion, the forces that resist forward movement.

resistance site (site of resistance). In context of snake locomotion, any physical point in the environment against which the body can apply force either to "anchor" a position, or to enable forward movement. Also called *contact zone, reaction zone, push point*.

resonance (resonate, resonating). A physical process whereby an oscillating phenomenon is amplified.

respiration. Strictly, the intracellular oxidation of organic substrates by molecular oxygen, resulting in the generation of ATP energy and the by-products of CO_2 and H_2O.

retina. The innermost, light-sensitive, multimembrane layer of the eye, containing the sensory cells that *transduce* light into vision.

rhinokinesis. A condition of *cranial kinesis* in which mobility of the nasal elements (four snout bones) enables unusual rotations of the snout tip during swallowing movements made by natricine snakes.

right aortic arch. See *aortic arches*.

right-to-left (R-L) shunt. See *shunt*.

rod. A photoreceptor cell of the *retina* that is sensitive to light because of cellular properties responding to low light intensities. Cf. *cone*.

ruga (*pl.*-ae). A ridge or fold.

saccular lung. The segment of lung that consists of thin, membranous tissue with only nutritive blood supply and nonfunctional in gas exchange. Typically, this segment terminates at the blind posterior end of the lung. Cf. *vascular lung*.

sacculus. The smaller and more ventral of two saclike divisions of the fluid system of the *inner ear*, and part of the *vestibular apparatus*.

salt glands. Extrarenal glands that secrete highly concentrated solutions of salt. In snakes, these are located in sublingual or premaxillary locations in marine species.

sand swimming. Reference to rapid burial and burrowing movements of sand-dwelling snakes.

scansorial. Proclivity, or adaptation, for climbing.

sclera. The tough, fibrous outer coat of the eye.

scutes. The ventral scales of a snake.

SDA. See *specific dynamic action*.

secondary sexual characteristics. Reference to phenotypic differences between sexes other than the reproductive organs.

semicircular canals. One of the equilibrium organs in the *inner ear*, which functions to sense acceleration of the head with respect to the gravitational field. See *vestibular system*.

seminal plug (also copulatory plug). Dried semen that obstructs the female's reproductive tract or genitalia.

seminal receptacle. In general, a cavity or structure for storage of sperm. In snakes this is a branched glandular sac in the lumen of the oviduct.

seminiferous tubules. Long, convoluted structures within the testis that support developing sperm.

septum (*pl.*-a). A dividing wall or partition.

shaker muscle. Specialized muscle in the tail of rattlesnakes, used to shake the rattle. This muscle is characterized by having numerous mitochondria, a rich supply of blood vessels, and biochemical properties that confer rapid twitch cycles.

shedding, skin shedding. See *ecdysis*.

shunt. An alternate pathway. With respect to *intracardiac shunts* (within the heart), a *right-to-left shunt (R-L shunt)* results in partial or complete pulmonary bypass (blood normally intended for the pulmonary artery enters the systemic vessels), and a *left-to-right shunt (L-R shunt)* results in partial or complete systemic bypass (blood normally intended for the systemic vessels instead enters the pulmonary artery). Increases in pressure within either of these circuits (whether active or passive) can create shunting, and these mechanisms are called *pressure shunting*. Alternatively, a passive mechanism that also creates shunting occurs when blood that is located in a space of the ventricle common to both pulmonary and systemic circulations at different phases of the heart cycle is subsequently "washed" into the "wrong" circulation by inflowing or outflowing blood moving in the "correct" direction. This mechanism is called *washout shunting*.

shuttling. A thermoregulatory behavior, which involves active movement between contrasting warm and cooler parts of the environment.

sidewinding locomotion. A mode of locomotion in snakes while moving over low-friction or shifting substrates such as desert sands. The movement is characterized by alternate lifting of sections of the body, which are moved forward and then placed down to "roll out" on the substrate, producing a series of separate, parallel tracks, each oriented at an angle to the direction of travel. During these movements the snake is in static contact with the ground at two points.

sinus venosus. The first heart chamber to receive blood from systemic veins and convey it to the *atrium*.

sister taxon. Reference to two taxa having the same immediate common ancestor. These appear on a phylogenetic tree as lineages or branches that arise from a single divergence node.

site of resistance. See *resistance site*.

slide-pushing. See *slipping undulation*.

sliding friction. See *friction*.

slipping undulation (also slide pushing). A mode of snake locomotion employed on low-friction substrates, whereon backward moving body waves (undulations) are propagated rapidly and generate a sliding friction sufficient to produce a reaction force that propels the snake forward. Alternating waves of body motion are similar to those in lateral undulation, but the forward reaction forces are generated without the use of fixed points on the substrate.

small intestine. The anterior segment of intestine and the principal site of digestion, extending between the stomach and large intestine.

smooth scale. Reference to a scale of squamate reptiles that lacks prominent keels or central ridges, detectable by touch or by eye. Cf. *keeled scale.*

snakebot. A robot modeled or fashioned after a snake.

solenoglyph (*adj.-ous*). A snake, or condition, in which each fang is erected by rotation of a reduced maxilla on the prefrontal bone, characteristic of viperid and atractaspidid snakes.

specific dynamic action (SDA). Increase of metabolic rate that follows ingestion of a meal.

spectacle. The fixed and transparent eye covering of a snake, consisting of epidermis that is fused with the *sclera* of the eye. Also called *brille* or *eyecap.*

spermatogenesis. The development of mature spermatozoa in the male *testis.*

spur. A corneous spine projecting from either side of the cloacal opening in certain species of snakes representing basal lineages.

static friction. See *friction.*

stimulus. A quality of the environment that stimulates a *receptor.*

stratum corneum. The keratinized, outermost layers of the *epidermis.*

stratum germinativum. The basal or innermost layer of living cells of the *epidermis,* which by means of cell division gives rise to the cell layers of the epidermis above it.

streptostyly. A condition of *cranial kinesis* in which the quadrate forms a mobile joint with the squamosal element, resulting from the evolutionary loss of the lower temporal arch.

structural color. A color seen on the surface of an animal, attributable to physical or structural attributes that differentially reflect light in various ways, not due to the presence of pigment.

supercooling. Reference to cooling below the physical freezing (= melting) point of body fluids without formation of ice crystals.

supranasal sac. A recess formed by invaginated skin beneath the supranasal scale, having an inconspicuous slit-like opening between the supranasal and nasal scales. This structure is present in many snake species of the subfamily Viperinae and the related Causinae. These structures are innervated and possibly function as heat detectors, similarly to the *facial pits* of pit vipers.

systemic circulation. See *circulation.*

systole. Contraction of the ventricle to eject blood into the arterial system. Cf. *diastole.*

temporal arches. Reference to the upper or lower arches or bars formed by skull bones as a consequence of fenestration.

tendon. A band or cord of fibrous connective tissue that is continuous with muscle fibers and attaches muscle to bone or cartilage.

testis (*pl.-es*). The male *gonad* in which sperm are produced.

testosterone. A steroid *androgen* synthesized in the *testes* and responsible for the appearance and maintenance of male *secondary characteristics.*

thermal intertia. A tendency to slow the gain or loss of heat due to the contribution of an animal's mass to its capacity for heat. Larger objects (or animals) heat and cool more slowly than do smaller objects (or animals), and they are said to exhibit greater thermal inertia.

thermal preferendum. See *preferred body temperature.*

thermoreceptor. A sensory nerve ending specifically responsive to temperature changes.

thermoregulation. Regulation of temperature. See *behavioral thermoregulation.*

thrust. A forward-acting force that produces forward motion. Cf. *propulsive force.*

topology. The branching order of a *phylogenetic tree.*

trachea. A membranous and cartilaginous tube that conducts air between the throat and lung. See also *tracheal lung, tracheal air sac.*

tracheal air sac. Membranous diverticula that are accessory outgrowths of the tracheal airway and function in defensive displays or sound production in various Asian species of snakes.

tracheal chambers or diverticula. See *tracheal air sac.*

tracheal lung. Vascular, functional lung that arises along an expanded tracheal membrane, anterior to the heart in certain species of snakes. See *vascular lung.*

trailing behavior. Reference to one individual following another (usually conspecific) individual, largely by means of a chemical trail that results from adherence of skin *pheromones* to the substrate over which a snake moves.

transducer. A device that changes the form of energy that impinges on it or is an input signal.

truncus arteriosus. Literally arterial trunk, with reference to the three outflow tracts (*right* and *left aortic arches*, and *pulmonary* artery) where they are joined by common elements of fibrous *fascia* near their origins at the *ventricle* of the heart.

undulation. Reference to movement in waves, or sinusoidal movement from side to side.

up-regulation. Control of a physiological activity by an increase in receptor density in a target cell membrane. Cf. *down-regulation*.

urates, uric acid. The crystalline waste product of nitrogen metabolism. Urates are salts of uric acid, which is poorly soluble in water and can be excreted in a precipitated form with minimal loss of water.

uterus. A glandular part of the oviduct (middle region in snakes) responsible for the production of fibrous and calcium components of the *eggshell* in reptiles.

utriculus. The larger of two saclike divisions of the fluid system of the *inner ear*, associated with the sense of equilibrium. See *vestibular system*.

vascular lung. The functional segment of the lung, characterized by a spongy appearance and rich blood supply. Cf. *saccular lung*.

vasoconstriction. Constriction of smooth muscle in blood vessels, usually smaller arteries.

vasodilation. Relaxation of smooth muscle in blood vessels, usually smaller arteries, which results in dilation of the vessel(s) in question.

vein. A blood vessel that returns blood from tissue capillary beds toward the heart. Cf. *artery*.

venom. A toxic or potentially toxic substance normally secreted by an animal and injected by a stinger, fang, or bite.

venom delivery system. With reference to snakes, this term refers to venom, associated glands for production and storage, and the muscles and specialized teeth that are used for delivery.

vent. The cloacal opening from cloaca to exterior.

ventilation. In respiration physiology, the process of moving air or water between the gas exchanger (lung or gill) and the ambient medium (= breathing and sometimes called *external respiration*).

ventricle. The muscular chamber of the heart that receives blood from the two *atria* and pumps it via outflow tracts to tissues of the body.

venule. A smaller blood vessel that connects a capillary bed with a vein.

vertebral column. The spinal skeleton consisting of a series of articulating vertebrae extending from the skull to the tip of the tail.

vertical septum. An incomplete septum in the ventricle of noncrocodilian reptiles that partially separates the *cavum arteriosum* from the *cavum venosum*.

vestibular system. The collective organs of equilibrium in the *inner ear*.

villus (*pl.*-i). One of numerous small, fingerlike projections of tissue that function as absorptive structures in the intestine.

viscosity. A physical property of a fluid that impedes the tendency for adjacent layers of the fluid to move past each other. The internal friction of a fluid causing resistance to flow.

vitellogenesis. The production of yolk, or "yolking" of an egg in the ovary.

viviparity (*adj.* viviparous). The retention of embryos within the oviduct until development is complete, thus giving birth to developed young instead of laying eggs. Cf. *oviparity, oviparous*.

vomeronasal organ. A specialized chemosensory chamber that forms a major sense organ above the roof of the mouth in snakes (and other reptiles). It is lined with sensory epithelium that detects odorant particles that are brought into the mouth on the tongue. Also called *Jacobson's organ*.

washout shunt. See *shunt*.

zygapophysis (*pl.*-es). Each of four processes on the border of the neural arch, which articulates with its opposite member on adjacent vertebrae, providing additional strength to the articulation and preventing undue torsion. Anterior zygapophyses (called *prezygapophyses*) are directed upward and somewhat inward, whereas posterior zygapophyses (called *postzygapophyses*) are directed downward and slightly outward.

INDEX

birth (and hatching), 126, 198, **fig.** 9.15
Bitia hydroides, 33
biting, bite force, *See* behavior
Bitis, 21, 22
    Bitis arietans, 21, 176, 186–187
    Bitis caudalis, 95
    Bitis gabonica, 21, 69, 170, **figs.** 1.6, 1.28, 2.25, 8.6
    Bitis nasicornis, 21, **figs.** 1.28, 2.25
Black-headed Python, **fig.** 7.8
Black-headed Sea Snake, **fig.** 3.6
Black Mamba, **fig.** 2.6
Black Milk Snake, **fig.** 5.19
black peritoneum, 135
Black Racer, **fig.** 5.8
Black Rat Snake, **figs.** 1.48, 2.37, 9.13, 9.15
Blacktail Cribo, 45, **fig.** 1.48
Black-tailed Rattlesnake, **fig.** 1.29
Black Threadsnake, **fig.** 1.12
Black Tiger Snake, **fig.** 4.15
blind snakes, 4, 13, 90, 127, 192
    Braminy Blind Snake, **fig.** 1.11
    dawn blind snakes, 11
"Blocked-flight aggression," *See* behavior
blood, 59, 70, 127, 142–144, 147–148, 155–157, 160, 202, **figs.** 2.26, 6.1, 6.6, 6.15
    blood circulation, 63, 65–66, 97, 113, 141–153, 156, 203, **figs.** 6.1, 6.9
        pulmonary circulation, 143
        systemic circulation, 143
    blood flow, 46, 113, 147, 149, 151, 159, 175, 184
    blood oxygen capacity, *See* oxygen capacity
    blood plasma, 70, 113, 142, 147, 151, 156–157
    "blood pooling," *See* pooling
    blood pressure (arterial), 58, 145, 147–153
        diastolic pressure, 149
        systolic pressure, 149
        venous pressures, 149
    blood supply, *See* vasculature
    blood vessel, 58, 143, 145–149, 151–152, 197–198, **fig.** 6.5
    blood volume, 147–148, 157
Blotched Palm Viper, *See* palm viper
Blue-banded Sea Krait, **fig.** 1.43
Bluestriped Garter Snake, **fig.** 1.46
Blunt-headed vine snake, 32
    Blunt-headed Tree Snake, **fig.** 1.51
boa, 5, 12, 15–16, 34, 50, 55, 67, 78, 91, 97, 107, 120, 173–174, 176
Boa Constrictor, *Boa constrictor*, 16, 53, 96, 107, 136, **figs.** 1.21, 2.31, 9.11
body, body wall, 19–20, 26, 37, 48, 77–78, 81, 83, 85, 87–95, 97, 99, 103, 106–109, 112, 123, 152, 155–156, 158, 168, 174, 181, 185–186, 193, 196, 199, 206, 210, **figs.** 1.20, 1.22, 1.30, 1.31, 1.36, 1.42, 2.32, 3.1, 3.6, 3.11–3.13, 4.10, 5.15

body cavity, 78, 147, 156, 159, **figs.** 6.12, 9.5, *See also* abdominal cavity
body fluids, 71, **fig.** 6.8
body size, length or mass, 78, 88, 91, 92–93, 98, 163, 186, 192, 196, 199, 205, 209
body temperature, *See* temperature
    flattening, compression, *See* behavior
    trunk, 86, 88, 92–93, 95, **fig.** 3.3
Bogertophis subocularis, **fig.** 9.15
boid (Boidae), 16, 68, 123, 136, 155, 175, 177, 199, 205
Boiga, 30, 57
    Boiga irregularis, 30, 60, 96
Bolyeria multocarinata, 16
bolyeriid (Bolyeriidae), 15, 136
bone, 54, **fig.** 2.23
Booidea, 12
Boomslang, 58
Bothriechis, 22
    Bothriechis supraciliaris, **fig.** 1.34
Bothriopsis, 22
Bothrochilus boa, **fig.** 4.12
Bothrops, 22
    Bothrops asper, **fig.** 5.11
    Bothrops jararaca, 62
Boulengerina, 26
boundary layer, 84–85, 123, **fig.** 3.7
Brahminy Blind Snake, 195, **fig.** 1.11
branch (of phylogenetic tree), 9, 12, 34, **fig.** 1.9
brain, braincase, 38, 40–41, 46, 50, 51, 57, 78, 112, 117, 149, 151–152, 163–164, 169–170, 172, 175, 178, 202, 205, **fig.** 2.6
Brazilian Coral Snake, **fig.** 5.19
Brazilian Hawkmoth caterpillar, **fig.** 5.21
Brazilian Rattlesnake, 203
breathing, *See* ventilation
brille, *See* spectacle
Broghammerus reticulatus, 14, 16, **figs.** 1.17, 2.23, 9.6
bronchus, bronchial airway, 153, **figs.** 6.4, 6.11
brooding, *See* behavior
brown snake, 26, 89
Brown Tree Snake, 30, 96
Brown Vine Snake, **figs.** 1.48, 2.18, 5.18
buffer, buffering, 157
Bull Snake, 47, 111, 182, 186
Bungarus, 26
    Bungarus multicinctus, **fig.** 1.40
buoyancy, 84, 86, 155, 159, **fig.** 6.14
Burmese Python, 16, 67, 69, 111, 175, 199, **figs.** 2.36, 4.10, 6.4
burrow, burrowing, *See* behavior
Burton's Snake Lizard, **fig.** 1.4
bushmaster, 22, 47
    South American Bushmaster, **fig.** 1.33
bush vipers, 21
button (of rattle), 182, **fig.** 8.3

caduceus, **fig.** 5.1
caecilian, 3, 19
caenophidian (Caenophidia), 12–13, 15, 17, 146, 205
Caisson disease, *See* decompression illness
calcium, 193, 195
    calcium carbonate, 197
California King Snake, 111, 126, 138, **figs.** 2.7, 5.26
Calliophis, 26
    Calliophis sauteri, **fig.** 1.41
Calloselasma rhodostoma, 22, 62
camouflage, *See* crypsis
cannibalization, *See* behavior
cantilever, *See* behavior
capillary, 141–143, 145–148, 155–157, 183, **figs.** 5.3, 6.4, 6.12, 6.15
capitulum, **fig.** 3.2
captive breeding, 200–201, **fig.** 5.25
carbohydrates, 66
carbon dioxide, *See* respiratory gases
Carboniferous period, 5, **figs.** 1.7–1.8
cardiac muscle, *See* muscle
cardiac output , 149, 151
Caretta caretta, **fig.** 2.14
carotene, *See* pigment
carotid artery, 146, 151, **fig.** 6.5
Carphophiinae, 32
Carphophis, 32
carrion, *See* prey
cartilage, **fig.** 6.11
Casarea dussumieri, 15
catecholamines, 149
Cat-eyed Snake, **figs.** 2.17, 3.3
cat snake, 30
caudal luring, *See* behavior
caudocephalic waves, *See* behavior
causine (Causinae), 176
Causus, 21, 155
    Causus maculatus, **fig.** 1.26
caval vein, 147, **fig.** 6.5
cavum arteriosum, 144, **figs.** 6.2–6.3
cavum pulmonale, 144, **figs.** 6.2–6.3
cavum venosum, 144, **figs.** 6.2–6.3
Central American Coral Snake, **fig.** 5.19
Central American Indigo Snake, **fig.** 1.48
Central American Jumping Pit Viper, *See* jumping pit viper
Central American Rattlesnake, **fig.** 2.39
Central American Speckled Racer, **fig.** 1.48
central nervous system, *See* nervous system
centrifugal acceleration, 84
Cerastes cerastes, 169
Cerberus rhynchops, 34, 167
chameleon, 117
character, character state, 9–11
character evolution, 9–10
Charina, 16
    Charina bottae, 110

chemical cues or signals, *See* chemoreception

chemoreception, 49, 118, 169–173, 205

chemosensory receptors, *See* receptor

Chinese Cobra, **fig.** 2.26

Chinese Green Tree Viper, 115, **figs.** 1.31, 5.6

Chinese Moccasin, 22, **figs.** 7.11–7.12

Chinese Sea Krait, **figs.** 1.43, 6.14, 6.16

Chionactis occipitalis, 94

chorioallantoic placenta, *See* placenta

chorioallantois, *See* extraembryonic membranes

chromatophore, **See** pigments

Chrysopelea, 30, 98

    Chrysopelea paradisi, 98, **fig.** 3.19

chyme, 64–65, 67

ciliary muscle, *See* muscle

circadian rhythm, 110, 202

circannual cycle, 201

circulatory system, 142–153, 160

clade, 10, 27

cladogram, *See* phylogenetic tree

classification (taxonomic), 4–5, 10, 27

clear layer (of skin), 126, **fig.** 5.4

climatic change, 210

climbing, *See* behavior

cloaca, *See* gastrointestinal tract

cloacal gland, *See* gland

cloacal popping, *See* behavior

clock (season or rhythm), 201

Cloudy Snail Sucker, **fig.** 2.8

clutch, clutch and litter size, 199–200, 210, **figs.** 9.8, 9.12

CO₂, *See* respiratory gases
(CO$_2$, *See* respiratory gases)

Coachwhip, 67

coagulation, 58

cobra, 19, 24–26, 46, 56, 59, 61, 96, 108, 187, 191, **figs.** 1.39, 2.26

    King Cobra, 26, 159–160, 187, 198, **figs.** 1.39, 2.11, 4.5, 9.1, 9.14

cochlear duct, 168, **fig.** 7.7

coefficient of friction, *See* friction

coelomic cavity, *See* body

coil, coiling, *See* behavior

coitus, *See* behavior: reproductive behavior

collagen, 118–119, 155

Collared Lizard, **fig.** 4.2

color, coloration, 3, 5, 10, 12, 16, 19, 22, 26, 61, 117, 127–140, 167, 192, **figs.** 1.22, 1.31, 1.34, 5.24–5.25, 6.18, *See also* pigments

    background color match, **fig.** 6.18

    color change, 135–136

        morphological color change, 136

        ontogenetic color change, 136, 138

        physiological color change, 136

    color polymorphism, 138, **figs.** 5.26–5.27

color vision, 166

    genetics, 136–139

    structural color, 123, 127–128, **fig.** 5.12

Coluber, 30

    Coluber constrictor, 99, 135, **fig.** 5.8

    Coluber constrictor constrictor, 137

    Coluber constrictor flaviventris, 208

colubrid (Colubridae), 10, 12, 17, 19, 26, 29, 32, 34, 42, 47, 54–55, 57, 61, 67, 85, 98, 113, 120, 131, 136, 151, 159, 166–167, 173, 199, 205–206, 208–209, **fig.** 31

Colubrinae, 29, 32, **fig.** 1.48

colubroid, (Colubroidea), 12–13, 17, 29, 34, 56–58, 60

columella, 168–169, 181, **fig.** 7.7

combat behavior or dance, *See* behavior

Common Death Adder, 48, 189, **figs.** 1.42, 8.7

Common Garter Snake, 201, 203

communal nesting, *See* behavior

compound bone, 51

compression (body or tail), *See* behavior

compressor glandulae, *See* muscle

compressor muscle, *See* muscle

concertina locomotion, *See* behavior: locomotion

cones (of eye), *See* receptor: visual receptors

connective tissue, 54, 78, 118, 155, 173

constriction, *See* behavior

constrictor laryngis, *See* muscle

contact zone, *See* resistance site

Contia, 32

conus arteriosus, 143

convection, 141–142, 158, **fig.** 6.1

convergence

    convergent evolution, 10, 26, 33, 48, 132, 195, **figs.** 1.22, 1.53, 1.42, 3.8

    convergence in neural circuits, 173

copperhead, 22, 49

    Northern Copperhead, **fig.** 1.32

copulation, *See* behavior: reproductive behavior

copulatory organ, *See* hemipenes

copulatory plug, *See* seminal plug

coral snake, 24–26, 46, 131–132, 188, **fig.** 5.19

Corallus

    Corallus caninus, 17, **figs.** 1.22, 7.4

    Corallus grenadensis, **figs.** 2.20, 3.17

    Corallus hortulanus, **fig.** 2.16

"corkscrew," (of portal vein), 147, **fig.** 6.6

cornea, *See* eye

corneous, cornified, 119

Corn Snake, 96, **fig.** 9.5

coronary arteries, **fig.** 6.2

corpus luteum, 193

"costal pump," 186

costocutaneous muscle, *See* muscle

Cottonmouth, 21–22, 48, 50–51, 53, 95, 135–136, 182, **fig.** 3.2

    Florida Cottonmouth, 46, 53, 66, 137, 208–209, **figs.** 1.3, 1.5, 1.32, 2.2, 2.13, 2.33, 2.35, 2.38, 5.24, 6.2, 6.13, 7.11, 7.13, 9.3, 9.18–9.19

cotylosaur, 5, **fig.** 1.8

countercurrent heat exchanger, 110

courtship, *See* behavior: reproductive behavior

cranial kinesis, *See* streptostyly

cratering, *See* behavior

Crayfish Snake, 29, **fig.** 2.22

Cretaceous period, 6, 12

cricoid cartilage, 186

critical thermal maximum (CTMax), 113

critical thermal minimum (CTMin), 113

crocodile, crocodilian, 5, 10, 80, 118, 143, 145, 197

Cross-barred Tree Snake, **fig.** 5.12

crotaline (Crotalinae), 20, 22, 24, 50, 173–176

Crotalus, 22, 49, 173, 182–185

    Crotalus adamanteus, 22, 80, 187, 211, **figs.** 1.29, 2.5, 5.9, 5.17, 8.3

    Crotalus atrox, 22, 66, 176, 182–183, 187, **figs.** 6.17, 8.3–8.4

    Crotalus catalinensis, 22

    Crotalus cerastes, 67, 92, 99, **figs.** 3.13–3.14, 3.16, 7.10

    Crotalus cerberus, 134, **fig.** 5.22

    Crotalus durissus, 111, 208, **figs.** 4.1, 4.13, 7.12

        Crotalus durissus unicolor, **fig.** 1.29

        Crotalus durissus terrificus, 203

    Crotalus horridus, 50, 66, **figs.** 1.29, 2.32, 7.2

    Crotalus lepidus, **fig.** 1.29

    Crotalus mitchellii, 136

        Crotalus mitchellii pyrrhus, 134, **fig.** 5.23

    Crotalus molossus, **fig.** 1.29

    Crotalus oreganus, 173

        Crotalus oreganus helleri, 134, **figs.** 2.25, 4.6

    Crotalus ruber, 80, 185

        Crotalus ruber lorenzoensis, 22

    Crotalus simus, **fig.** 2.39

    Crotalus viridis nuntius, **fig.** 1.29

Crotaphytus collaris, **fig.** 4.2

crypsis, cryptic, 22, 26, 129–132, 134–136, 167, 204, **figs.** 1.25, 1.28, 1.31, 1.36, 3.16, 5.17, 5.22–5.23, *See also* background color match

CTMax, *See* critical thermal maximum

CTMin, *See* critical thermal minimum

cutaneous evaporative water loss, *See* evaporation

cutaneous gas exchange, *See* gas exchange

cutaneous receptor, *See* receptor

Cylindrophiidae, 13

mating "ball," *See* behavior: reproductive behavior

maxilla, maxillary bone, 16, 19, 40–42, 50, 51, 54–57, 61, **figs.** 2.5–2.6, 2.24

mean selected temperature, *See* preferred body temperature

measurement of temperature, **fig.** 4.4

mechanical cues or signals, *See* mechanoreception

mechanical work, 183–184

mechanoreception, 49, 123, 177–178, 189, 206

mechanoreceptor, *See* receptor

melanin, *See* pigment

melanism, 132, 134–135, 138

melanocyte, *See* pigment

melanophore, *See* pigment

melanophore stimulating hormone (MSH), 136

melatonin, 136, 202–203

membrane, 22, 65, 70, 163, 168, 173, 175, 185, 193–195, **fig.** 7.11

eggshell membrane, 195, **fig.** 9.11

mesos layer (of skin), 119, 125, **figs.** 5.3–5.5

metabolic water, *See* water

metabolism, 70, 209

rate of (metabolic rate), 46, 66–67, 69, 103, 106, 114–115, 135, 157, 200, **fig.** 2.36

metabolic heat production, 105–107, 111–112, **fig.** 4.1, 4.13

metabolic wastes, 197

methyl ketone, 118, 205

Mexican Burrowing Python, 13, **figs.** 1.16, 3.15

Mexican Vine Snake, *See* Brown Vine Snake

microarchitecture, *See* microsculpturing

microbe, 117

microdermatoglyphics, *See* microsculpturing

"microfacets," 172

microfibril, *See* microsculpturing

microgravity, 169

"micro-hairs," *See* microsculpturing

microornamentation, *See* microsculpturing

micropit, 174–175

micropore, 124

microsculpturing (of scales), 121–125, 127, 136, 177, **figs.** 5.10, 5.13

microfibril, 123

"micro-hairs," 123

nanoscale structure, 123

microstructure, *See* microsculpturing

microvasculature, 148

microvilli, 172

Micruroides, 131, 188

Micruroides euryxanthus, 188

Micrurus, 131, 188

Micrurus decoratus, **fig.** 5.19

Micrurus fulvius, 188, **fig.** 5.19

Micrurus nigrocinctus, **fig.** 5.19

midbrain, 169

milk snake, 30

mimicry, 132, 189, **figs.** 5.19, 5.21

mineralized shell, *See* egg: eggshell: "rigid-shelled egg"

mitochondria, 141, 156, 182

mobility of jaw or joints, 78, *See* also behavior, kinesis, streptostyly

modality (of stimulus), 163

"mode," of locomotion, *See* behavior

"mode," reproductive, *See* reproduction

moisture, 198

molecular data, methods, properties, or studies, 4, 9, 13, 24, 34, 62, 166, **fig.** 1.9

mole vipers, 19–20, **fig.** 1.24

momentum, 95, **fig.** 3.12

monitor lizard, *See* lizard: varanid

monophyletic lineage, 7, 10, 11, 17, 32, 34

monotypic, 27, **fig.** 1.14

Morelia

Morelia amethystine, 17

Morelia spilota, 111, **fig.** 6.12

Morelia viridis, 17, **figs.** 1.22, 7.1

morphology, 34

morphological color change, *See* color: color change

mortality, 196

mosasaur, 7, **fig.** 1.8

motor sensory system, 175

mouth, 11, 20, 37, 49, 51, 56, 61–62, 72, 172–173, **figs.** 2.16, 2.19, 2.25, 5.18, 8.5

MSH, *See* melanophore stimulating hormone

mucosa, mucosal cells, 60, 65, 67, 72, **fig.** 2.34

mucus, 56, 64, 176

mucous cells, glands or secretions, 62, 172, 193

Mud Snake, 32, **fig.** 1.50

muscle, musculature, 13, 22, 40, 51, 57–58, 60–62, 72, 77–78, 80, 85, 87–91, 96, 111, 113–114, 118, 143, 146, 156, 158, 160, 165, 169, 182, 183, 185–186, 188, 195, **figs.** 3.5, 6.16, 7.10

axial muscle, 78–79, 87, 92, **figs.** 3.3, 3.9

cardiac muscle, 143–144, 148–149

ciliary muscle, 165

costocutaneous muscle, 91, **fig.** 3.12

compressor glandulae, 60

compressor muscle, 60

constrictor laryngis, 186

epaxial muscle, 78, 88, 97

M. iliocostalis, 78, 183, **fig.** 3.3

M. longissimus dorsi, 78, 183, **fig.** 3.3

M. sphincter cloacae, 188

M. spinalis-semispinalis, 78, 183, **fig.** 3.3

M. supracostalis lateralis, 183

smooth muscle, 65–66, 145, 149, 158, 175, 187, 192–193, **figs.** 2.34, 6.11

tension, 111

twitch, 183–184

muscular ridge, **fig.** 6.3

musk, 182

musk gland, *See* gland

mutation (genetic), 9, 62, 138, 189, 191

Myrichthys colubrinus, **fig.** 1.4

mythology, 117, 124, 191, **figs.** 5.1, 5.14, 9.1–9.2

Naja

Naja atra, **figs.** 1.39, 2.26

Naja shrionegrina, 6

nanopit, 174

nanoscale, *See* microsculpture

narial or nasal valve, *See* valve

naris, nares, *See* nostril

nasal bone, 40

nasal cavity or passages, 169–170, 187, **fig.** 7.9

nasal hissing, *See* behavior

"nasal pore," 176

nasal receptors, *See* receptor

natricine (Natricinae), 29, 40, 42, 46–47, 122, 199, **fig.** 9.10

Natrix, 29

natural history, 204

natural selection, 10, 59, 62–63, 130, 136, 152, 189

neck, 62, 87, 92–93, **figs.** 3.5–3.6

neck sac, *See* tracheal air sac

necrosis, 58

neonate or hatchling, 126, 198, 201, 208–209, **figs.** 9.9, 9.11–9.12, 9.15

Neotropical Bird Snake, *See* Puffing Snake

Neotropical racer, **fig.** 1.48

Nerodia, 29, 40, **figs.** 1.3, 1.47

Nerodia clarkii, 44

Nerodia fasciata, 85

Nerodia fasciata pictiventris, **fig.** 1.47

Nerodia floridana, **figs.** 1.47, 4.8, 5.8

Nerodia sipedon, 48, 205

nerve or neuron, 66, 111, 113, 117, 127, 163, 168, 172, 175–177, 201

free nerve ending, 173, 177

nerve growth factor, 58

nerve signal, *See* action potential

nervous control, 145, 201, **fig.** 6.9

nervous system, 149, 177, 201

central nervous system, 78, 110, 149, 163, 173, 177, 181, 203

nest, 198, **fig.** 9.14

net cost of transport, 99

neural arch, **fig.** 3.2

neuroendocrine regulation, 201–202, **fig.** 9.16

neuromodulator, 201, 203

pit viper, 20, 22, 24, 47–48, 56, 120, 126, 158, 173, 175–176, 208, **figs.** 1.33, 7.11

placenta, placentation , 195, 197, **figs.** 9.8, 9.10

    chorioallantoic placenta, **fig.** 9.10

    omphalallantoic placenta, **fig.** 9.10

    placental membranes, **fig.** 9.10

Plains Gartersnake, 199

plants, 68

plasma, *See* blood plasma

plasticity (developmental, ontogenetic, physiological, phenotypic), 53, 86, 114, **fig.** 4.14

pleurodont, 54, **fig.** 2.21

"Plumed Serpent," **fig.** 5.14

Pogona vitticeps, **fig.** 2.5

point of force application, *See* resistance site

poison, 57–58

polymorphism, 132, *See* also color

polypeptide, 58

polyphyletic, 34

pooling (of blood), 151–152, **figs.** 6.7–6.8

pore, 172, 174, 176, **figs.** 5.13, 9.13

portal vein, *See* hepatic portal vein

Porthidium, 22

    Porthidium nasutum, **fig.** 1.35

postcloacal musk gland, *See* gland

postmating behavior, *See* behavior: reproductive behavior

postprandial calorigenic response, *See* specific dynamic action

postprandial metabolic response, *See* specific dynamic action

postprandial thermogenesis, *See* specific dynamic action

posture, *See* behavior

power, 80, 85

power spectrum, 187

Prairie Rattlesnake, **fig.** 1.29

Prairie Ringneck Snake, **fig.** 1.50

prebutton (of rattle), 182

precourtship behavior, *See* behavior: reproductive behavior

predator, predation, *See* behavior

preferred body temperature (PBT), 109–110, 113, 148

preferred range, *See* preferred body temperature

prefrontal bone, 40, 50, 56

prehensile tail, *See* behavior

premaxilla, premaxillary bone, 55, 71, 198

pressure

    blood pressure, *See* blood

    in fluids, 150, 169, **fig.** 6.7

    in lung, 156, 186

    oxygen, *See* partial pressure

    transmural pressure, **fig.** 6.7

    water vapor, *See* water

pressure shunting, *See* shunt: intracardiac shunt

prey, 3, 20, 22, 25, 33, 37–38, 40–41, 46, 48–51, 53–54, 56, 59, 61–63, 66–68, 95–96, 115, 120, 152, 167, 173, 175, 188, 200, 209–210, **fig.** 1.24

    amphibians, 33, 48

        anurans (frogs, toads), 21, 32, 38, 45–46, 48, 50, 53, 62, 66–67

    birds, 16, 20, 38, 45–46, 48, 50, 53, 67–68, 97, **fig.** 2.37

    caecilians, 19

    carrion, 21, 45

    eggs, 37, 45, 47, 97, **figs.** 2.1, 2.14, 2.19, 2.30, 3.15

    fish or fish eggs, 13, 19, 26–27, 33, 38, 45–48, 50–51, 54, 56, 64, 67, 84, 178, **figs.** 1.44, 2.10, 2.13, 7.14

        eel, 13, 27, 46, 50

    invertebrates, 33, 38, 45, 189

        crabs, 33, 38

        centipedes, 19–20

        crustaceans, 19, 33, 67, **fig.** 2.22

        earthworms, 13, 20, 32, 38

        gastropods (slugs, snails), 32–33, 42, 56, **fig.** 2.8

        insects, 12, 21, 37–38, 45, 67, 167

            larvae or pupae, 41

    mammals, 13, 16, 20, 38, 46, 48, 50, 67–68, **fig.** 2.32

        deer, **fig.** 2.1

        rodents, 20, 49–50, 176, **figs.** 2.36, 3.16

            mice, 13, 38, 45, 50, 53, 63, 169, **figs.** 2.7, 2.16, 4.13

        shrews, 20

    reptiles, 13, 20–21, 25

        lizards, 13, 32, 45–46, 48, 62, 167, 189, **fig.** 3.16

        geckos, 16

        skinks, 16, 19, 54

        snakes, 13, 19, **fig.** 2.11

        turtles, 47, **figs** 2.12, 2.14

    vertebrates, 20

prey handling time, 59

prey transport, 38–42, 45, 66–70, **figs.** 2.11. 2.13–2.14, 2.19, 2.37–2.38

primitive trait or lineage, *See* basal

progesterone, *See* hormone: sex steroids

prokinesis, 40

proprioceptors, 169

propulsive force, *See* force

protease, 58, 65

protein, 4, 62, 65–67, 69–70, 113, 166, 182

proteolytic enzymes, 58, 64

proteroglyph, 57, 61

Protobothrops

    Protobothrops flavoviridis, 22, **fig.** 1.30

    Protobothrops jerdoni, **fig.** 1.30

protraction , 41

Psammophis, 20

    Psammophis subtaeniatus, **figs.** 5.10, 5.13

Pseudechis porphyriacus, 25, 27, 108, 211, **fig.** 4.9

Pseudonaja

    Pseudonaja nuchalis, 26–27

    Pseudonaja textilis, 27

Pseustes poecilonotus, **figs.** 1.48, 2.18

pteridine, *See* pigment

pterygoid bone, 41, 42, 50, 55, **fig.** 2.5

Pueblan Milksnake, **fig.** 9.7

Puff Adder, 21–22, 176, 186–187

Puff-faced Water Snake, **fig.** 1.54

Puffing Snake, **figs.** 1.48, 2.18, 8.5

pulmonary artery or trunk, 143–147, **figs.** 6.3, 6.5, 6.16

pulmonary circulation, 147

pulmonary vein, 147, **fig.** 6.5

pupil, *See* eye

purine, 128

push point, *See* resistance site

pygmy rattlesnake, 22

pylorus, 64

    pyloric valve, 64

python, 5, 8, 12–16, 34, 50, 55, 67, 69, 91, 108–111, 120, 172–174, 176, 208–210

    Python brongersmai, **fig.** 5.25

    Python curtis, 69

    Python molurus, 16, 67, 69, 111, 175, **figs.** 2.36, 4.10, 6.4

    Python regius, 16, 166, 168

    Python reticulatus, 14, 16, **fig.** 1.17

    Python sebae, 16

pythonid (Pythonidae), 16, 205

quadrate bone, 6, 39–40, 51, 168–169, **figs.** 2.5–2.6

quadratojugal bone, 6

quadrupedal, 77

Queen Snake, 29

racer, 26, 30, 45–46, 77, 89, 96, 99, 135, 181, 205

radiation (electromagnetic)

    infrared, 22, 173–176

    solar, 107, 117, 158, **fig.** 4.11

    ultraviolet, 135, 174–175

    visible, 163–165, 174–175, 201

radiation (evolutionary), *See* evolution

radiotelemetry, radio transmitter, 47, 105, 109, **figs.** 4.4–4.5, 4.9

Rainbow Boa, **fig.** 5.12

"Rainbow Serpent" (of mythology), 191

Ramphotyphlops braminus, **fig.** 1.11

rat snake, 30, 46–47, 78, 96–97, 111, 151, 169, **figs.** 2.26, 3.3, 6.5, 6.9, 6.19

rattle (of rattlesnake), 182–185, 188–189, **figs.** 5.14, 8.2–8.4

rattling, *See* behavior

rattlesnake, 22, 47–49, 51, 56, 63, 66, 80, 112, 136, 173, 175–176, 182–185, 187–189, 200, 208, **figs.** 1.29, 5.14, 6.9, 8.2

RCM, *See* relative clutch mass

reabsorption, 54

reaction force, *See* force

reaction norm, 114

reaction site, *See* resistance site

rear-fanged, 50

receptor, 58, 127, 149, 163, 168, 172–175, 177, **fig.** 1.5

 baroreceptor, 149

 chemosensory receptors, 173

 cutaneous receptors, 177, 189

 hair cell receptors, 168–169, 177, **fig.** 7.7

 infrared receptors, 173–175, **fig.** 1.5, *See* also facial pits

 mechanoreceptor, 45, 176–178, **fig.** 2.10

 nasal receptors, 170

 olfactory receptors, 170

 photoreceptor, 166, 177–178, **fig.** 7.3

 stretch receptor, 149, *See* also baroreceptor

 thermoreceptors, 173–177

 visual receptors, 127, 164

  cones, 164, 166–167

  rods, 164, 166

 vomeronasal receptors, 172–173

rectilinear locomotion, See behavior: locomotion

Red-bellied Black Snake, 25, 27, 108, 211, **fig.** 4.9

red blood cell, 142, 148, 156–157

Red Blood Python, **fig.** 5.25

Red Coffee Snake, **fig.** 5.20

Red Diamond Rattlesnake, 80, 185

Red-sided Garter Snake, **figs.** 4.2, 4.7, 9.17

Red-spotted Pit Viper, **fig.** 1.30

Red-tailed Rat Snake, 132, 159–160, 187, **figs.** 5.18, 6.19

reflectance (of light), 128

refraction, 165

Regina, 29

 Regina rigida, **fig.** 2.22

relative clutch mass (RCM), 199

renal vein, 147

renewal stage (of shedding cycle), *See* ecdysis

replacement (teeth), 55, **fig.** 2.23

reproduction, 66, 115, 135, 191–212, **fig.** 9.16

 reproductive cycles, 201, 203–204, **fig.** 9.17

 reproductive mode, 195–197

 reproductive tract, 65

reptile (Reptilia), 5, 10, 39–40, 71, 80, 114, 145, 156, 173, 194, 196, 200, 203–204, **figs.** 1.8, 1.10

 non-avian reptile, 10

resistance

 forces, 87

 to blood flow, 143–145

  peripheral resistance, 148–149

 to evaporative water loss, 124, 126

 to thrust in locomotion, 84–85, 87

  drag, 84–85

friction, 87, 93, 99

 gravitational vertical force, 84

 inertial, 84–85, 89

 viscosity, 84

resistance site, 80, 87–88, 93–94, 96, **figs.** 3.4, 3.9, 3.12

resources, 200–201

respiration , 114, 141, 143, 156, 158

respiratory gases 117, 145, 148, 153, 155–157, 185, 195, 197

 exchange, *See* gas exchange

 carbon dioxide, 117, 141, 146, 153, 156–158, 185, **fig.** 6.1

 oxygen, 46, 113, 117, 141–142, 145–146, 148, 153, 156–158, 160, 185, 195, 197, **figs.** 6.1, 6.15

respiratory gas transport, **fig.** 6.1

resting stage (of shedding cycle), *See* ecdysis

Reticulated Python, 14, 16, 199, **figs.** 1.17, 2.23, 9.6

retina, *See* eye

retraction, retractor muscle, 192

Rhamphotyphlops braminus, 12, 195, **fig.** 1.11

Rhineura floridana, **fig.** 1.4

Rhinoceros Viper, 21, **figs.** 1.28, 2.25

rhinokinesis, 40

rib, 3, 6, 78–79, 85, 88, 91, 97–98, 156, 159, 186, **fig.** 3.12

ribbon snake, 29

Rice Paddy Snake, **fig.** 7.6

right-to-left shunt (R-L shunt), *See* shunt

rigid-shelled egg, *See* egg: eggshell

Ringed Python, **fig.** 4.12

ringneck snake, 26, 32

robotics, 99–100, **fig.** 3.20

Rock Rattlesnake, **fig.** 1.29

rod (of eye), *See* receptor: visual receptors

rodent, 94, 103, 210

rostral scale, 11, 94, **figs.** 1.11, 1.20

Rosy Boa, 16

Rough-scaled Bush Viper, **figs.** 1.27, 5.8

Round Island Boa, 16

rubber boa, 16

rugae, 64

Russell's Viper, 176, 187, **fig.** 5.10

sacculus, 168–169, **fig.** 7.7

salamander, 77, 99

salivary gland, 59

salivary secretions, 62

salt, 71

 salt gland, 71

sand boa, 16

 Kenya Sand Boa, **fig.** 1.20

San Diego Gopher Snake, 104

sand snake, 20

sand swimming, *See* behavior

San Lorenzo Island Rattlesnake, 22

Santa Catalina Island Rattlesnake, 22

Saw-scaled Viper, 182, **fig.** 8.1

scale, 3, 10–11, 13, 51, 54, 89, 93, 117, 119–124, 126–127, 175, 177, 188, **figs.** 1.6, 1.23, 5.6, 5.8–5.12, 7.11

 granular, 18–19, 120

 head plates or scales, 11, 21–22, 51, 120, 177, **fig.** 1.15

 hinge, 120

 keeled, 19–20, 44, 120, 182, **figs.** 5.9–5.10, 8.1, 8.8

 labial, 16

 scute or ventral, 11, 18, 78, 87, 89–91, 120, **figs.** 3.1, 3.12, 5.6–5.7, 5.9, 5.12, 9.3

 smooth, 11, 13, 19, 21–22 120, **figs.** 1.11, 5.8

 spine or spinous, 18, 121, 177, **fig.** 5.8–5.9, 8.8

 tuberculate, 18, **fig.** 5.9

scanning electron microscopy (SEM), 121, 174, **fig.** 5.10

scansorial, *See* behavior: locomotion: climbing

scattering (of light), 128

Schultheis thermometer, 105, **fig.** 4.4

sclera, *See* eye

scolecophidian (Scolecophidia), 11, 12, 34, 41, 55, 173

Scrub Python, 17

scute, *See* scale

SDA, *See* specific dynamic action

sea krait, 27, 50, 71, 85, 198, 210, **figs.** 3.8, 5.11, 6.8, 9.4

sea snake, 24–25, 27, 29, 46, 48, 56, 78, 81, 83–85, 124, 126, 132, 145, 152–153, 157–159, 169–170, 173, 177, 189, 208–209, **figs.** 1.4, 2.15, 6.9–6.10, 8.8

season, seasonality, 114, 193, 201, **figs.** 4.15, 9.17

sea turtle, 47

secondary sexual characteristics, 203

secretion, 11, 57, 66, 71

segment (of rattle), **fig.** 8.2

selection pressure, *See* natural selection

SEM, *See* scanning electron microscopy

semiaquatic, *See* habitat, habits

semicircular canals, 168–169, **fig.** 7.7

seminal or copulatory plug, 208

seminal receptacles, 194

Seminatrix pygaea, 29

seminiferous tubules, 192

serous cells or gland, 60

"serpent," 191

Serpentes, *See* Ophidia

sex, 62, 110, 191–192, 205

sex steroids, *See* hormone

"sexual attractiveness pheromone," *See* pheromone

sexual maturation, 209–210

shaker muscle (of rattlesnake), 182–185, **fig.** 8.4

D1250744

Quality Improvement
for Nurse Managers
Engage Staff and Improve Patient Outcomes

Cynthia Barnard, MBA, MSJS, CPHQ • Barbara J. Hannon, RN, MSN, CPHQ

HCPro

Cynthia Barnard, Author
Barbara J. Hannon, Author
Tami Swartz, Editor
Michael Briddon, Executive Editor
Emily Sheahan, Group Publisher
Janell Lukac, Graphic Artist

Audrey Doyle, Copyeditor
Amy Cohen, Proofreader
Matt Sharpe, Production Supervisor
Susan Darbyshire, Art Director
Jean St. Pierre, Director of Operations

Contents

Figure List

All figures are also available on the included CD.

About the Authors

Cynthia Barnard

Cynthia Barnard, MBA, MSJS, CPHQ, is the director of Quality Strategies at Northwestern Memorial Hospital, the primary teaching hospital of Northwestern University's Feinberg School of Medicine in Chicago, and is research assistant professor in the Institute for Healthcare Studies at the medical school.

At Northwestern Memorial, she is responsible for patient safety, accreditation and regulatory compliance, infection control, and medical ethics. In the Institute for Healthcare Studies, she is codirector of the advanced course in quality improvement (QI) in the Master's Program in Healthcare Quality and Patient Safety.

Barnard is the author of several books, including *Benchmarking Basics: A Resource Guide for Healthcare Managers* and *Performance Improvement Basics: A Resource Guide for Healthcare Managers* (currently in its second edition), and coauthor of *Performance Improvement: Winning Strategies for Quality and Joint Commission Compliance*, currently in its fourth edition and winner of the 2002 David L. Stumph Award for Excellence in Publication from the National Association for Healthcare Quality.

Barbara J. Hannon

Barbara J. Hannon, RN, MSN, CPHQ, is the coordinator of the ANCC Magnet Recognition Program® (MRP) for the University of Iowa Hospitals & Clinics. She chairs the Professional Nursing Practice Committee and Nursing Retention Committee and is involved in QI activities for the department. In 2007, she was selected as one of Iowa's "100 Best Nurses" and in 2009 was profiled in "20 People Who Make Healthcare Better" by *HealthLeaders* magazine.

As the MRP coordinator for the University of Iowa Hospitals & Clinics, she successfully guided the hospital to MRP designation as the 101st MRP hospital in January 2004 and to redesignation in 2008.

Hannon has been a contributing author for *The Image of Nursing: Perspectives on Shaping, Empowering, and Elevating the Nursing Profession* and reviewer of *A Practical Guide to Managing the Multigenerational Workforce*. She is also a frequent contributor to *HCPro's Advisor to the ANCC Magnet Recognition Program®*.

Introduction

Healthcare reform is dominating the national political and legislative agenda. Although healthcare delivery models will undergo major changes in the coming years, one thing that will not change is the public and government demand for quality patient outcomes and safe, affordable care. Key to improving patient quality outcomes and safety are professional nurses. More than 90% of all direct patient care is done by nurses; therefore, to improve patient outcomes, nurses must be actively involved in all aspects of QI. This requires nurse leaders to be knowledgeable about basic QI concepts to facilitate collaboration with other departments in carrying out interdisciplinary improvement processes, as well as developing and implementing their own QI projects for improving and controlling nursing-sensitive indicators (NSI).

This handbook is designed to engage nurses in QI at the organizational level and to help them develop and implement QI measures to improve NSIs at the unit level. It is responsive to important developments and influences from:

- External agencies, such as the Centers for Medicare & Medicaid Services, The Joint Commission, and consumer and payer groups such as The Leapfrog Group

- Industry research and leaders of improvement, such as the Institute for Healthcare Improvement, the National Quality Forum, the Institute of Medicine, and the Agency for Healthcare Research and Quality

- The National Database of Nursing-Sensitive Indicators®

- The ANCC Magnet Recognition Program® and the American Nurses Association

- Your own patients, community, and internal customers, who demand and deserve excellence, and your own professional integrity and commitment to improvement

It is designed with these assumptions:

- You are a nurse manager or director of a nursing division, department, or unit. Whether you serve patients directly or support those who do, you are committed to continual improvement and excellence and you understand your department's operations.

- You want a more solid understanding of QI techniques, accreditation requirements, or statistics and data analysis.

- You want practical, convenient, and useful tools to focus your quality program on delivering effective results rapidly—but you're busy.

This book is a working tool with concepts you can apply to your own program. Throughout the book, you will find examples of how these concepts might apply to your program.

Chapter 1

Quality Improvement
as a Management Tool

LEARNING OBJECTIVES

- Identify potential benefits quality improvement can bring to a unit
- Identify common quality improvement errors

Why Quality Improvement Matters

Your role as a manager is to deliver a defined level of service and technical quality at an appropriate cost, while advancing the organization's goals through leadership. In other words, your success depends on the quality of your department or unit. Quality improvement (QI) is a science and a discipline that can help you get there.

Your customers evaluate your services every day. As a manager, you need to know what those customers experience and determine whether that experience is the one you want them to have—or, if not, how it can be improved.

If you try to improve your department's operations without a deep understanding of its quality, you are

likely to make the situation worse and introduce error and failure. You'll be tinkering with a process you don't fully comprehend.

And if you merely study your department's quality without a focus on continuous improvement, you are likely to find that your customers and even your staff will become frustrated. Quality and productivity may actually decline, and your professional development and excitement may wane (a condition known as *analysis paralysis*).

The answer is to look for new ideas from outside the walls of your department, to bring improvement and stimulation to your team, and to ensure that your customers receive the service they deserve. Your customers may not know whether they are receiving the best possible care and service. This is common in healthcare because a patient rarely can evaluate the technical aspects of care or know what to expect or demand. So it is our ethical obligation to evaluate the quality of our care and service for all of our customers, hold ourselves to a high standard, and continuously improve on their behalf.

QI is a science that brings disciplined measurement, innovation, and focus to the delivery of any product or service. It can apply to almost any process or product

and can be an effective vehicle to build teamwork, professional satisfaction, and improved patient care and customer service.

The History of QI in Healthcare Delivery

The history of QI in healthcare is remarkably brief. The nature of medical care has always been one of constant improvement through learning from each patient's response to care and systematic learning for generalized knowledge through clinical research. But applying these principles to the delivery of healthcare became widely established only in the 1980s and 1990s, spurred by the evolution of the quality assurance standards of The Joint Commission, the creation of the National Committee for Quality Assurance, and revised Medicare payment systems (i.e., diagnosis-related groups) and *Conditions of Participation*.

The past three decades have seen an explosion of inquiry into how quality actually works in the delivery of care, from back-office functions to bedside care of complex, acutely ill patients. Systematic attention has been paid to process design, measurement, and strategies to improve processes and outcomes.[1]

Particularly in the past decade, attention has focused on the perspective of the patient and family. What does it mean to meet the needs of the patient? How does patient satisfaction contribute to better health outcomes, fewer lawsuits, more satisfied staff members, and lower costs? How do we produce patient satisfaction, anyway?[2]

The History of QI in Nursing

Nursing as a profession is coming late to the QI arena. Historically, although many healthcare institutions have had QI departments, these existed as a separate entity, and they were usually led by physicians more concerned with tracking outcomes of medical care than nursing care; nursing as a profession was minimally involved. But as healthcare organizations transition from separate silos into flattened structures with interdisciplinary team collaboration, nurses are finding themselves participants in improving processes that transcend individual disciplines.

A new body of quality metrics, classified as "nursing-sensitive indicators" (NSI) and endorsed by the National Quality Forum (NQF), requires hospitals to now take a look at patient outcomes that can be improved by attention to nursing practices and nurse staffing. Improving and ensuring consistent performance on these NSIs is squarely in the scope of the nursing practice and should be performed by nurses with a quality background.

Additionally, in recent years, the American Nurses Association and the ANCC Magnet Recognition Program® (MRP) have influenced further development of a body of QI measures based on NSIs. The new requirements for MRP hospital designation and redesignation in the *2008 edition of the ANCC Magnet Recognition Program® Manual* require that hospitals outperform the mean of multiple NSIs. This requirement has resulted in nurses developing QI projects to improve nursing care and patient outcomes in relation to these NSIs, has increased evidence-based literature and research on NSI outcomes, and has led to the creation of specific nursing

quality national databases. Nurses now have data they can use to define, implement, and control nursing practices in their own organizations to improve patient care.

Public Disclosure of Quality Data

Perhaps one of the most pressing developments in quality in recent years has been the public disclosure of quality and outcomes, which customers can use to select a provider. The most significant new developments include:

- The Medicare Web site, which details processes and outcomes data from hospitals, home health agencies, and nursing homes[3]

- Attempts by The Leapfrog Group,[4] a consortium of payers and employers, to require providers to disclose their compliance with an array of processes believed to be related to higher quality and safety (for publication on its Web site)

- The measures on The Joint Commission's Web site, which are similar to Medicare's measures for hospitals, as well as scores of providers' compliance with The Joint Commission's National Patient Safety Goals

Several private companies also publish self-described quality evaluations of hospitals and other providers based on proprietary analysis of publicly available databases. At a minimum, you should be familiar with any data reflecting your organization's quality on major Web sites, such as those of Medicare, Leapfrog, and The Joint Commission.

What Is Quality?

Your organization may have a definition of quality. A commonly used definition is the one published by the Institute of Medicine (IOM): "The degree to which health services for individuals and populations increase the likelihood of desired health outcomes and are consistent with current professional knowledge."

A definition of quality applies beyond direct healthcare service; you may simply have a different customer base. For example, if you work in materials management, your customers include the nurse whose customer is the patient. Draw a clear line from your work to those who provide direct care and services, and understand how your work can increase the likelihood of a successful outcome for your customers.

Quality Is a Property of a System

The IOM series on the current status of the healthcare delivery system[5] is an important quality resource. At a minimum, healthcare leaders should be familiar with the executive summaries of two major reports published by the IOM in 1999 and 2001, *To Err Is Human* and *Crossing the Quality Chasm*, respectively.

The latter report described six characteristics of a quality healthcare system (consider the mnemonic STEEEP):

1. Safe

2. Timely

3. Effective

4. Efficient

5. Equitable

6. Patient-centered

The report also made the fundamental argument—still not fully embraced by healthcare professionals—that quality comes from having appropriate systems in place. As a leader, it is your job to participate in building those systems and making sure they focus on consistent delivery of high-quality care and service.

Your staff members and colleagues may still perceive quality as the product of individual effort and competence (or lack thereof). Current thinking in quality acknowledges the importance of individual quality and competence, but it also emphasizes that individual competence is insufficient to produce consistently high quality. Most medical errors and quality failures occur in the course of work performed by capable people. The breakdowns stem from lack of information, poor communication, inadequate technology, and normal human fallibility in the context of poor work design. Therefore, it is the system that must be evaluated and improved. Better designs can avert quality failures and errors; a vast national effort is under way to discover strategies to develop these designs and disseminate them.[6]

Finally, one of the most exciting developments of the past decade has been the creative application of insights from other industries to the improvement of healthcare. Notably, this has included aviation and nuclear power—high-reliability organizations that operate in high-risk contexts that are similar to healthcare. Evidence of this approach has been building since the late 1980s with the use of quality theory from the great pioneers in manufacturing and process quality (e.g., Deming, Juran, and Ishikawa) to apply to healthcare.[7] A science of high-reliability organizations is developing to help translate this work to practical application.[8]

Quality Improvement and Patient Safety

Your goal is to develop a quality plan that ensures that you deliver the right services, and that you deliver them without errors. The IOM's definition of safe care is avoiding injuries to patients when providing care that is intended to help them.

The patient wants health services that, in the IOM's words, "increase the likelihood of desired health outcomes and are consistent with current professional knowledge." From the patient's perspective, anything that is not safe, or is error-prone, does not meet this definition.

Both quality and safety are properties of a system. In the end, the work you do to measure and improve your systems should contribute to safer and higher-quality care. In Chapter 4, we look at the kinds of measures you can define and implement to accomplish these objectives.

What Do Leaders Do to Improve Quality?

Figures 1.1 and 1.2 summarize The Joint Commission's basic expectations of you as a leader. Regardless of whether you are part of an accredited organization, the lists are an excellent place to start, and they establish a credible foundation for a leader's essential role in QI.

Common Pitfalls

Vigorous managers have the ability to drive process improvement to a successful outcome. Key to this is an in-depth knowledge of the system being improved and thoughtful application of improvement science to the specific organization and team. Common pitfalls in management of improvement initiatives occur when managers lead teams to try to improve a process or pro-

cesses they do not really understand, or when they try to impose solutions that are outside the competence or culture of the teams.

Improvement science in healthcare depends on comprehensive technical knowledge of the performance of human beings in systems. As a leader, you have an obligation to master the improvement methodology and to implement improvement through effective teamwork and organizational savvy.

Weick and Sutcliffe remind us that a high-reliability organization is characterized by deference to expertise and mindfulness of potential failure (see the bibliography). As a leader, you are in a position to influence the improvement team to focus on objective data, process mapping, and the insights of frontline staff members. The chapters that follow will assist you in taking a methodical and thorough approach to increase the likelihood of effective and sustained improvement.

	FIGURE 1.1 ▶ THE ROLE OF LEADERS

2009 JOINT COMMISSION LEADERSHIP AND PERFORMANCE IMPROVEMENT STANDARDS SUMMARY

Standard	Content
Developing Your Performance Improvement Plan	
LD.01.03.01	The governing body is accountable for the safety and quality of care
LD.01.05.01	The organized medical staff oversees the quality of care, treatment, and services provided by those who have clinical privileges
LD.03.03.01	Leaders use organizationwide planning to establish structures and processes that focus on safety and quality
LD.04.04.01	Leaders set priorities for performance improvement
Designing Your Performance Improvement Approach	
LD.04.04.03	Any processes that are new or modified are well designed
LD.04.04.07	The organization considers clinical practice guidelines during design or process improvement
Collecting and Measuring Data	
PI.01.01.01	The organization collects data to monitor its performance
Evaluating Data	
LD.03.02.01	The organization uses data to guide decisions and understand variation in the performance of processes that support safety and quality
PI.02.01.01	The organization analyzes and compiles data
Making Improvements	
LD.03.05.01	Leaders implement changes in existing processes to improve the performance of the organization
LD.03.06.01	Those who work in the organization are focused on improving quality and safety
PI.03.01.01	The organization improves its performance
PI.04.01.01	The organization uses data from clinical/service screening indicators and HR screening indicators for assessing and continuously improving staffing effectiveness
Proactive Prevention and Reduction of Adverse Events	
LD.03.01.01	A culture of safety and quality is created and maintained by leaders throughout the organization
LD.03.04.01	The organization communicates information about quality and safety to those who need it, including staff members, licensed independent practitioners, patients, families, and interested external parties
LD.04.04.05	The organization has a facilitywide integrated patient safety program

Source: The Joint Commission, *www.jointcommission.org*

FIGURE 1.2 ▶ LEADERS' RESPONSIBILITIES TO IMPROVE PERFORMANCE	

Line operations managers should regularly assess their compliance with these common Performance Improvement requirements:

❑ Yes ❑ No	The manager can describe the hospital's PI goals for the year and how his or her department can help achieve those goals.
❑ Yes ❑ No	The manager can describe how he or she has allocated resources, such as staff time and information support, to accomplish the hospital's PI goals.
❑ Yes ❑ No	The manager can describe specific improvements that have been made in his or her department.
❑ Yes ❑ No	The manager can describe collaborative improvement projects undertaken with other departments and/or disciplines.
❑ Yes ❑ No	The manager can describe specific measurements that he or she monitors regularly to ensure that processes and outcomes are under control in the department, with specific focus on statistical and benchmarking tools to ensure meaningful assessment.
❑ Yes ❑ No	The manager can describe hospital/organization initiatives to reduce medical errors (as appropriate to department) and his or her role in these initiatives.
❑ Yes ❑ No	The manager can describe PI goals he or she would like to pursue and why they are meaningful to the patient or customer population served by his or her department.

SELF-ASSESSMENT CHECKLIST

▶ You have reviewed the executive summaries of the IOM studies *To Err Is Human* and *Crossing the Quality Chasm*

▶ You are familiar with the IOM's definitions of quality and safety

▶ You are familiar with The Joint Commission's expectations for management of quality and safety

▶ You have reviewed the NQF's endorsed nursing-sensitive indicators

▶ You've looked at your organization's quality results as reflected on the Joint Commission and Medicare Web sites (if applicable)

▶ You are familiar with The Joint Commission's list of responsibilities of effective leaders

▶ You can discuss the importance of a just culture in improving quality and patient safety

▶ You have reviewed the bibliography in this book to become familiar with some of the principal Web sites and resources on quality

Endnotes

1. See, for example, the work of Berwick and the Institute for Healthcare Improvement (see the bibliography).

2. See, for example, the groundbreaking book *Through the Patient's Eyes: Understanding and Promoting Patient-Centered Care*, by Margaret Gerteis, Susan Edgman-Levitan, Jennifer Daley, et al. (eds.); see the bibliography.

3. See *www.cms.gov.*

4. See *www.leapfroggroup.org.*

5. Reports in the IOM's Health Care Quality Initiative that should be familiar to healthcare leaders include *To Err Is Human, Crossing the Quality Chasm,* and *Envisioning the National Health Care Quality Report* (see the bibliography).

6. See, for example, the work of the Institute for Healthcare Improvement and the National Quality Forum. An excellent, brief, and inexpensive videotape that makes this point compelling is *Beyond Blame,* developed by Bridge Medical and distributed by the Institute for Safe Medication Practice *(www.ismp.org).*

7. See the bibliography for more reading about these developments.

8. See the excellent work of Karl E. Weick and Kathleen M. Sutcliffe (2007), *Managing the Unexpected: Resilient Performance in an Age of Uncertainty* (San Francisco: Jossey-Bass).

The Role of Nursing in QI

Nurses at Every Level

The role of professional nurses in quality improvement (QI) is twofold: to carry out interdisciplinary processes to meet organizational QI goals and to measure, improve, and control nursing-sensitive indicators (NSI) affecting patient outcomes specific to nursing practices. All levels of nurses, from the direct care bedside nurse to the chief nursing officer (CNO), play a part in promoting QI within the healthcare provider organization.

The CNO

The CNO sets the tone for the nursing department's participation in QI. As a member of administrative leadership, the CNO must integrate nursing practices into the organizational goals for excellence in patient outcomes through communication of strategic goals to all levels of staff. The CNO must advocate for and allocate resources to meet nursing QI needs. For example, this may include budgeting for more full-time equivalents for QI-trained nurses or wound and skin nurses, or enough secretarial staffing to handle input of large quantities of data. The CNO also must advocate for and allocate resources to enable directors and nurse managers (NM) to plan and improve NSIs unique to their patient populations at the unit level. In addition, the CNO must support a culture of education for directors and NMs in the principles and methods of QI. Although many NMs are educated in management principles, QI concepts may be new to them. The CNO must support a culture of education and learning to help NMs integrate QI on their units or divisions and provide them with the skills and resources to collect data and improve and control processes unique to their patient populations.

For a CNO to create a culture that encourages excellence, he or she must communicate key information and obtain necessary resources. The following is an example of how a CNO might accomplish this:

A healthcare organization's administrators are concerned about budget losses due to reduced reimbursement from the Centers for Medicare & Medicaid Services for several patients who developed advanced stage pressure ulcers

while inpatients. The administrators ask the CNO to determine what can be done to reduce the number of hospital-acquired skin ulcers. The CNO in turn communicates this to the directors and NMs; then the CNO provides the resources needed to fund a departmentwide nursing skin assessment team, supplies additional secretarial support to handle the data collected, and funds nurse researchers to develop evidence-based strategies to improve skin integrity outcomes directly related to nursing practices.

The NM or nursing director

The NM or nursing director is responsible for communicating and operationalizing the organization's QI goals and processes to the bedside nurse, identifying specific NSIs that need improvement according to his or her particular patient population, and coordinating QI processes to improve these at the unit level.

The NM is in a key position to operationalize the culture of safety and quality from organization and department QI activities down to the bedside nurse. Although the NM is frequently overloaded with jobs and responsibilities, accountability for patient outcomes on his or her unit should be of utmost importance, as it is the key product of the patient care delivered by the nurses under his or her supervision. NMs must implement the organizational QI processes and ensure that their staff members follow those interventions defined for nursing. In addition, NMs must look at specific nursing-sensitive indicators that are unique to the patient population being cared for on their units, and focus on those that can be improved by evidence-based nursing processes. NMs contribute creativity and en-

ergy to interdisciplinary improvement efforts as well as specifically nursing-sensitive care outcomes by providing education and support enabling direct care nurses to deliver appropriate care. NMs must then hold their nurses accountable to deliver competent, professional practice.

An example of how an NM could successfully work with the organizational QI team follows:

The NM of an ICU is part of an interdisciplinary team charged with reducing the incidence of ventilator-associated pneumonia (VAP) in the hospital's ICU population. The team develops a VAP bundle that has specific interventions for nurses, physicians, and respiratory therapists. The NM communicates to his nurses the pieces of the new VAP bundle that are nurses' responsibility, as well as those that are implemented through teamwork. For example, the nurse is responsible to maintain the head of the patient's bed at 30 degrees and to perform oral hygiene for the patient at designated intervals. The nurse is also responsible to work with the medical team to assure a daily "sedation holiday" and to assess the patient's readiness to wean from the ventilator at least once daily. After implementing the bundle, the NM holds his nurses accountable for following the bundle elements in daily walk-rounds, periodic reports of compliance, and ultimately performance reviews.

Here is another example; this time of how an NM can successfully address a unit-based NSI:

The NM on an acute neurosurgical unit with a patient population of acute neck/spinal injuries is asked by the CNO to identify an NSI unique to her patient population and to develop an improvement process. Though falls are not an issue on her unit, the NM notes that many of her patients are in cervical neck collars for the long term and is concerned about the incidence of pressure ulcers under the collar. The NM then utilizes departmental evidence-based practice researchers to find best practices in collar usage and participated in the development of an evidence-based standard of care protocol for patients in cervical collars. The NM then educates her nurses on the new protocol, ensures that the right supplies, skin products, and equipment were available to protect patients' skin and monitors the results, while holding her nurses accountable to follow the protocol.

The direct care nurse

The direct care bedside nurse is the key to quality patient outcomes, carrying out the protocols and standards of care shown by evidence to improve patient care. Without bedside nurses committed to following these QI processes, quality outcomes will not be achieved. No QI program designed to improve patient care succeeds from the top down; it must begin with those closest to the patient, the bedside nurse.. Being a QI expert at the bedside may seem like a new role for the bedside nurse, but actually it's what nursing practice has always been about. Each day, bedside nurses must approach their role of providing care by thinking: "How do I prevent my patient from getting a pressure ulcer today?" or "How can I prevent my patient from

getting a VAP or central line infection, or from falling out of bed today?"

QI is really not a new role for bedside nurses. QI has much in common with many time-honored nursing practices such as the daily nurse care plan, defining nursing diagnoses, or planning interventions for the day—an activity which nurses have been performing for years. QI requires that bedside nurses gear nursing care around NSIs unique to the population they are caring for, and utilize the standards and protocols designed by departmental, unit, or organizational teams from the best evidence available. When the bedside nurse follows the bundles, protocols, and standards of care established through best evidence, these bedside nurses are rewarded with improved patient outcomes.

An example of staff nurse engagement in a QI process to reduce heel ulcers follows:

The NM of an ICU is alerted by the departmental skin team of an increase in heel ulcers in her unit after the quarterly prevalence survey. During a staff meeting the NM communicates a new protocol from the departmental skin assessment team to her nurses. The protocol is for nurses to assess their patients' heels every two hours and utilize a new process for elevating heels off the bed. Staff nurses agree to follow the protocol and closely monitor patients' heels, communicating assessments shift to shift to other staff nurses and ensuring consistency in heel ulcer prevention. At the next quarterly prevalence survey, a decrease in heel ulcers is found and the NM recognizes the contributions of the bedside nurses that have im-

proved patient outcomes. The manager and staff agree to continue the effort.

Barriers to Nurse Participation

'I'm too busy to learn something new'

One of the most common complaints staff nurses use to justify a lack of participation in QI activities at the bedside is that they are "too busy" to learn a new nursing activity. Nurse leaders can deal with this common misconception by educating staff members on what QI is and showing them how it is not a new nursing activity. Explaining and demonstrating that QI is part of what they are already doing, but under another name, is helpful.

Nurses have been doing QI (i.e., they have been monitoring and implementing patient interventions and evaluating patient outcomes from those interventions) for as long as nursing has been a profession. Although nursing has not called this process "QI" or "QM," nurses have nonetheless performed QI because QI is really just part of the nursing process. The nursing process is a patient-centered, goal-oriented method of caring that provides a framework for nursing care, involving assessment, nursing diagnosis, planning, implementation/intervention, and evaluation. First, the nurse assesses to determine the situation. Then the nurse diagnoses, or determines the problem. Next, the nurse plans how to fix the problem. Then the nurse puts the plan into action. And finally, the nurse evaluates whether the plan was successful. If NMs have bedside nurses look at QI compared to the nursing process, it is clearly evident that QI and the nursing process involve the same steps. While bedside care focuses on one patient at a time, QI integrates data from many patients to draw a portrait of nursing care and its effects.

Nurses have also been involved in QI through the use of the nursing classification systems, Nurse Interventions Classification (NIC) and Nurse Outcomes Classification (NOC), to plan nursing care for approximately three decades. The NIC describes the treatments that nurses perform. It consists of 433 different interventions that can be measured. The NOC system describes patient outcomes sensitive to nursing intervention and evaluates the effects of NIC interventions as a part of healthcare. The NOC contains 330 outcomes, each with a label, a definition, and a set of indicators and measures to determine achievement of the nursing outcome. Furthermore, the Nursing Minimum Data Set is a classification system that allows for the standardized collection of essential nursing data and the analysis and comparison of nursing data across populations, settings, geographic areas, and time. All of these nursing processes, diagnoses, and interventions use the same fundamental concepts which are used in QI and quality management.

Contemporary thinking about professional nursing certainly emphasizes the role of frontline nurses in collaborating on interdisciplinary quality improvement and leading improvement of nurse-sensitive indicator outcomes. There is an opportunity to link QI to professionalism and to emphasize that the opportunity to participate in QI is an excellent asset in any organization's effort to recruit and retain the best nurses. Understanding that this activity has always been an essential piece of nursing practice sets the stage for nurse participation in QI.

'Quality improvement takes too much time'

Another barrier to direct care nurse engagement in QI is a perception that following a new QI protocol or participating in a new QI process requires more time than performing a practice the old way. A nurse leader can engage nurses struggling with this perception by sharing examples of past QI processes that have actually reduced nursing time to show how QI can help nurses over the long term. An example of a QI project that ended up saving ICU nurses time follows:

Incontinence-associated dermatitis (IAD) is a painful condition suffered by ICU patients with chronic urinary incontinence. The moisture from the incontinence can cause perineal skin breakdown, redness, and a painful rash. An NM in an ICU notes the large amount of time her nurses spend trying to prevent and treat IAD noting there was a lack of standardized product selection and a lack of evidence-based information available to the ICU nurses. For example, she notices her nurses might spend an hour applying a product such as zinc oxide only to have a nurse on the following shift spend an hour removing it and applying something else. In addition, the unit is experiencing an increasing rate of pressure ulcer incidence from the IAD, again increasing bedside nurses' time in treating the ulcers with various modalities, and potentially contributing to longer patient lengths of stay, morbidity, cost, and infection.

The NM helps to decide that a protocol for preventing and treating IAD will help reduce the time her staff nurses spend dealing with this patient care issue. With the help of the departmental researchers, an evidence-based protocol is developed as the standard of care for the unit. The resulting protocol eventually reduces the time her nurse spend trying to figure out what to do for the patients with IAD, resulting in better patient outcomes and increased staff satisfaction.

'QI is not in the scope of nursing practice'

Another barrier to staff nurse participation is a misconception that QI is not in the scope of professional nursing practice, and therefore staff nurses should not be held accountable for it.

As we described earlier, QI really is a part of the nursing process, and therefore is definitely in the scope of nursing practice. In addition, most state boards of nursing require nurses to utilize the nursing process.

For example, the Iowa Board of Nursing states in the Iowa Administrative Code (655—6.1[152]), under the minimum standards of nursing practice for registered nurses, that:

The registered nurse shall utilize the nursing process in the practice of nursing, consistent with accepted and prevailing practice. The nursing process is ongoing and includes:

a. Nursing assessments about the health status of an individual or group.

b. Formulation of a nursing diagnosis based on analysis of the data from the nursing assessment.

c. Planning of nursing care which includes determining goals and priorities for actions which are based on the nursing diagnosis.

d. Nursing interventions implementing the plan of care.

e. Evaluation of the individual's or group's status in relation to established goals and the plan of care.

Holding direct care nurses accountable for nursing-sensitive patient outcomes can be a challenge. The barrier is a perception that if QI participation is not in a bedside nurse's job description, he or she cannot be held accountable for lack of participation in QI on his or her unit. Certainly, engagement in QI should be reflected in any professional nurse role description, annual goals, department quality plan, and feedback reports. Also, to enable NMs to have some influence in getting direct care nurses to participate in QI, QI participation should be placed in the yearly performance appraisal tool as an expectation of bedside nursing practice. Staff nurses have to be held accountable for the care they provide, and the annual performance appraisal is an excellent way to put some teeth in direct care nurse participation in QI.

Common Pitfalls

A common pitfall is failing to use your organization's QI experts for assistance in the development of nursing-sensitive indicator improvement projects.

Nurses have a history of trying to do it all themselves. QI is a science that takes education, preparation, and practice. Though departmental nurse clinical experts and nurse researchers are invaluable to creating a successful nursing QI program, nurse leaders should also maximize their resources and utilize the expertise of organizational QI experts if available. Using all the resources when designing and conducting QI projects leads to improvement in patient outcomes. Not doing so could run the risk of wasting precious time.

SELF-ASSESSMENT CHECKLIST

Before you move on, you may want to ensure that:

▶ You have reviewed the roles of the CNO, the NM, and the staff nurse in regards to QI.

▶ You have a plan to actively engage nurses in QI and to hold them accountable.

▶ Annual performance appraisals include involvement of QI

▶ You are familiar with common misconceptions nurses often have about QI, and have planned strategies to avoid them.

Quality Improvement Planning

LEARNING OBJECTIVES

- Identify the steps involved when planning a quality improvement program

- Explain common errors in quality improvement planning

The first step in developing any quality improvement (QI) plan is to define the mission, leadership, and customers of a work unit or team in the context of the organization's mission and strategic plan.

By the end of this chapter, you will be able to:

- Sketch the framework for your quality plan

- Assure yourself that it fits effectively into the organization's overall plans

- Begin thinking about selecting specific quality measures

As you work through this chapter, fill in the sections of Figure 3.1. Also, consider the questions posed throughout the chapter and use them to make your planning more effective.

Mission, Strategy, Leaders, and Customers

Quality always occurs in a context.

> *Example:* A small rural hospital does not seek to become a national leader in neurosurgery but is committed to developing excellent triage and transfer capabilities. A major urban academic center decides primary care is best left to local providers and concentrates its resources on secondary and tertiary levels of care.

No program can be all things to all people, and the following examples demonstrate that the mission and identity of an organization drive choices:

- What is the mission of your organization, and how can you draw a clear line from that mission to your own department?

- What is the strategic plan of your organization, and how can you draw a clear line from that plan to your own department?

FIGURE 3.1 ▶ SUMMARY OF THE STRATEGIC AND QI PLANNING PROCESS

The strategic plan drives quality definition and priorities. Add your own organization's information at each stage of the chart.

Strategic plan *(Write your organization's strategic goal(s) here.)*

↓

Definition of community, patients/customers, and priorities *(Who are your organization's customers?)*

↓

Annual organizational goals *(List the organization's major goals this year. Select at least those that drive compensation and those that directly affect your department.)*

↓

Managers' annual and long-term goal setting *(List your own departmental and personal goals for the year or longer.)*

↓

Priorities for monitoring and improving quality. And, for each priority, budgets and resource allocation decisions and a link to employees' individual performance goals *(List the areas of quality you plan to improve that are consistent with the management, organizational, and strategic goals previously listed. Review this list as you prepare your budget so that necessary resources are requested. See how you can build these quality goals into the personal goals of each employee in your department. If other departments are collaborating with you to deliver these improvements, ensure that those managers have done the same.)*

Before you can measure and improve quality, you need to know who you are serving and with what goal. The organization's mission and strategy should give you an overall framework and within that, you need to define the mission of your own department.

> **Example:** *A community hospital values its relationship with a local nursing school and places a high priority on providing an excellent experience for the nursing students who are assigned there for clinical training. For a given nursing unit, then, this high priority of the organization translates into a specific goal for the unit: meet targets for supervision and mentoring of students. Success of this goal will translate into more satisfactory care for patients and a higher rate of successful recruitment of students when they complete their education.*

Describe the specific scope of care or service in your department and its mission.

What is the link between your department's mission and that of the organization? If you have not written a formal mission statement, make that a goal for the next quarter. Involve staff members, your boss, and any medical staff leaders with significant influence and involvement in the department. Follow your organization's process, if there is one, to develop and document the mission statement.

Define the scope of your services and who is served by your department or program. If you deliver patient care, the scope of care and services should include the ages and cultural mix of your clientele. This helps you to meet relevant Joint Commission and Medicare requirements to ensure that you have prepared staff

members appropriately to take care of these patients. Customers all have different needs. For a nursing unit, customers include not only patients but families and physicians, and each has a unique set of needs. A pathology department serves not only patients but the attending physician as well. Nontraditional customers (physicians) have needs that go beyond those of traditional customers (patients). They want the same timely and accurate results, but they may also want access to the results online or by fax, certain values to be phoned to them as critical test results, the ability to add on tests without a patient redraw, and other aspects of service that you need to provide.

Who are your customers, what do they want, and how do you know it?

If you are unsure of what your customers want—for example, what an acceptable turnaround time is or how long you may ask a patient to wait past an appointment time—do some research. Research can range from surveying a few dozen customers to studying best practice benchmarks locally or nationally or conducting a comprehensive formal market research study. Compare results within an organization; for example, multiple nursing units can compare results on pain management or timely medication administration and select the best practices as a target for other units.

Think about what customers want by using a comprehensive framework (see Figure 3.2). With your knowledge of your scope of service and your customer base, identify which of these dimensions matter in your area. They won't all apply to all programs; for example, if you run a housekeeping department, timeliness might be quite important, but accessibility doesn't really apply.

FIGURE 3.2 ▶ DIMENSIONS OF QUALITY PERFORMANCE

Tip: Consider the mnemonic **STEEEP** to remember the dimensions of quality.

Safety

- Environmental safety

- Protect patients from harm resulting from the care process (e.g., medical error)

Timeliness

- Accessibility

- Same level of care 24/7 if needed clinically

Effectiveness

- Appropriateness

- Continuity across the episode of illness/treatment

Efficiency

- Cost, rework, time, materials

Equity

- Regardless of factors unrelated to clinical need

Patient-/Customer-Centered

- Includes family, visitors

Adapted from Institute of Medicine's characteristics of quality care (www.iom.edu).

Select two or three of these dimensions and see whether you can evaluate your customers' needs quantitatively. For example:

- **Patient (customer) perspective.** At least 90% of patients rate our nurses as "very good"

- **Accessibility.** Patients can obtain an appointment within 24 hours

- **Continuity.** Every patient leaves with a list of discharge medications and instructions

- **Efficiency.** Costs are at or below the median for the community

- **Timeliness.** Call lights are answered within five minutes

Are your patients'/customers' needs documented in your quality plan?

Talk to your organization's QI department, and find out whether there is a standard method in use for describing patient/customer needs in a QI plan.

Management Goals

With a clear line from the organization's mission and strategy to your department mission and an understanding of what your customers want, consider one more piece of the context for quality: What are your goals for the department? Perhaps you are expanding, adding services, reducing costs, or trying to improve

outcomes or patient satisfaction. Many of these goals either drive a quality goal directly or help you select a relevant quality goal.

For example, if you are reducing costs, measure an important outcome to ensure that it's not compromised. If you are expanding, you might be concerned about unintentionally compromising wait times. If you are trying to improve a particular outcome, then, of course, it needs to be measured. In Chapter 4, you'll determine where you need to develop specific quality goals. Goals typically are prepared annually, but a mature organization has flexibility in revising goals and setting new targets whenever needed. For now, keep track of your management goals for the year so that the quality plan is well integrated.

What are your management goals for the year?

> **Example:** A large group practice has determined that expansion of services to those who speak Japanese and Polish is important. The HR department recognizes that its role in this strategy is the successful recruitment of qualified bilingual employees and physicians.

Establishing meaningful clinical or service goals depends on knowledge of your customers. This will allow you to decide what your priorities are for goal planning. For example, a wait time of 10 minutes may be acceptable or, perhaps, a fantastic experience in one area (e.g., the emergency department). But it creates an unacceptably frustrating experience in another area (e.g., being on hold on the telephone to ask a billing question). This is not the time to select specific measures.

What are the elements of quality your department delivers to patients/customers?

Be able to describe the elements of your care and service that matter to your customers. These might include family information, patient education, specific clinical tests and procedures, billing, delivering a product to a unit, or meeting psychosocial needs.

Budgeting and Resource Allocation

Quality monitoring and improvement activities often identify opportunities to use resources more efficiently and effectively to achieve priority objectives. Use the findings to recommend resource allocation to deliver improved quality at reduced cost.

As noted previously in discussing management goals, quality monitoring has a special role to play when cost reduction or cost management is a priority (as it usually is). Whenever significant operational change is under way (e.g., reducing or reorganizing staff, changing processes or implementing new computer systems), it is critical to continue to measure the basic processes and outcomes of your department to ensure that they are not unintentionally compromised.

Next steps

The last step in this planning phase is to document all the information you have collected and distilled. Your organization's quality department probably has a format that you should use to document your quality plan. Include, at a minimum, the following elements:

- Leadership of the department (you and medical leaders)

- Customers and what they need/want

- Scope of care and service provided by the department (including ages of clients served, if a patient-care area; also consider cultural mix)

- Elements of quality process and outcomes, evaluated to identify those that are high risk, high volume, and problem prone

- Specific quality levels that the department aspires to meet

If you don't have a standard format, the model in Figure 3.3 may be helpful.

Common Pitfalls

Haste is the most common problem in developing a quality plan. It's easy to quickly define indicators and measures of quality without giving enough thought to which measures are truly the most important.

What makes a measure important is simply this: If you improve this measure, your customers receive better care and service that is of value to them. Also, your organization's significant goals are measurably advanced.

Chapter 4 addresses considerations in well-developed measures. But for now, ensure that you work through the quality planning process to develop significant aspects of your department's quality—not excellent measures of trivia!

FIGURE 3.3 ▶ QUALITY PLAN MODEL

SAMPLE LEADERSHIP/SCOPE/SERVICE INVENTORY

Department name: _____

Leader(s) (administrative/medical leader, if any):

_____

_____

Organizational mission and current goals (those that are linked to compensation or otherwise established as key goals for everyone in the organization):

_____

_____

Departmental mission and current goals (of manager and department):

_____

_____

Internal customers (within the organization; e.g., physicians, nurses, pharmacists, employees, board of directors, etc.):

_____

External customers (e.g., patients, families, payers, regulators, vendors, etc.):

_____

Scope of care/service:

- List the processes, procedures, and services you provide: _____

  _____

- List the days/times/sites for which you provide them: _____

  _____

- Describe the staffing model (ratio, mix of staff): _____

  _____

Waste is the second most common problem at this stage. Develop a vigorous, creative, thoughtful quality plan that can become your department's blueprint for the year.

If you actually use this plan as a management tool, you can make truly impressive changes, in collaboration with your staff members and other departments (see Chapter 1 for quality theory and Appendix A for more on the practical aspects of communication about quality). Now is the time to be visionary and to stretch your imagination a little to see what your department can become.

Related concepts

There are a few additional terms you should be familiar with as you think about quality in your department. (See Figure 3.4.) They are often misunderstood and misused, and a good, clear recognition of their place in the quality system will make your program more effective.

FIGURE 3.4 ▶ QUALITY IN YOUR DEPARTMENT—ADDITIONAL TERMS

TERM	HOW DOES IT FIT WITH QI?
Sentinel Event	
If your organization is accredited by The Joint Commission, then you must have a definition of sentinel event as it is used in your organization. The standard Joint Commission definition is "an unexpected occurrence involving death or serious physical or psychological injury, or the risk thereof. Serious injury specifically includes loss of limb or function. The phrase 'or the risk thereof' includes any process variation for which a recurrence would carry a significant chance of a serious adverse outcome."	Why is it important to define "sentinel event"? If you are in an accredited organization, then there are specific investigation and resolution procedures that must be followed on a short timeline when a sentinel event is identified. Even if you are not in an accredited organization, the concept is useful because such an event could signal a potential opportunity for improvement in the processes of care. Sentinel events, however, are not counted as a measure of quality nor are they reduced as part of a quality plan. The only goal for the number of sentinel events in any organization is zero. If a sentinel event occurs, get assistance immediately from the QI or risk management departments in your organization. Once the investigation is complete, those departments can help you determine what improvements to incorporate into your quality plan to ensure that root causes of the event are systematically addressed. Sentinel events are not useful as a quality measure. Because they are rare, you would never use a rate of sentinel events as a quality metric with a threshold. Manage them as a separate signal with a special form of response.
Root-Cause Analysis	
A root-cause analysis (RCA) is simply what the name implies: a search for the deepest underlying cause of a problem, event, or pattern. In the case of a sentinel event, you'll want to determine whether there is a system or process that effectively could have avoided the undesirable outcome.	An RCA can be performed to understand any system, process, or event. It is not applicable only to sentinel events, although it is required in those situations. An RCA may be viewed as one approach to the first step in any quality model—the "plan" or "definition" stage in which you ensure that you thoroughly understand the problem before you begin to design improvements.

FIGURE 3.4 ▶ QUALITY IN YOUR DEPARTMENT—ADDITIONAL TERMS (CONT.)

TERM	HOW DOES IT FIT WITH QI?
Never Events	
The term "never events" is applied to a list of "Serious Reportable Events in Healthcare" developed by the National Quality Forum (see Bibliography). These events (the list currently includes 28) are believed to be preventable much of the time, although not always, if healthcare systems work optimally. The term "never events" is used, for example, by the Leapfrog Group (see Bibliography) in asking hospitals to adopt a four-point transparency policy when such events occur: apologize to the patient; refrain from billing for hospital costs associated with the event; conduct an RCA of the event; and report the event to any appropriate agency dedicated to improvement (a state-reporting database, The Joint Commission, a Patient Safety Organization, etc.).	Many never events are also sentinel events, and the same principles apply. In the majority of cases, these events are not measured or trended, and their rates improved because the only appropriate goal is zero. However, at least two of the items on the never event list may be suitable for QI measures in a given organization because they continue to occur with some frequency and require close organizational attention to improve the systems dedicated to their prevention. Typically, these include patient falls and pressure ulcers (bedsores).
Peer Review	
Although peer review means that professional peers conduct a review of care provided (typically by a physician or nurse), the actual implementation of this process varies. The purpose of peer review is to ensure that any practice that appears to stray from the standard of care can be thoroughly evaluated by those who understand it best. Most states have statutes affording some degree of protection from subpoena for the work of such peer panels, if they are convened properly, to encourage open and candid discussion and recommendations that improve the quality of care. The Joint Commission has recently revised its standards to require that each organization better define when a review by physician peers is needed and how it is to be performed. According to Joint Commission standards, peers can come from the same organization or outside it, but the process of physician peer review must be governed by the organized medical staff, and peer review of nurses is controlled by the chief nurse executive.	Ongoing professional practice evaluation (The Joint Commission's term) provides regular periodic data and feedback for physicians or others. If there is evidence of potential poor quality from these data or any individual event, then focused evaluation of a physician's quality is implemented. Truly effective peer review should pay vigorous attention to system breakdowns and opportunities for improvement in all aspects of patient care. A focus on the specific quality of a particular physician or provider is useful but not sufficient. Results of such an analysis of system problems should be shared with those who are in a position to improve those systems. Medical staff quality committees determine when physician peer review is indicated and oversee the process. They keep track of the findings of peer review panels and monitor to ensure that the process is fair, consistent, and yields useful information.

FIGURE 3.4 ▶ QUALITY IN YOUR DEPARTMENT—ADDITIONAL TERMS (CONT.)	
TERM	**HOW DOES IT FIT WITH QI?**
Peer Review (Cont.)	
	If you are not a physician, it is unlikely that you will participate in physician peer review. However, it is certainly possible that a peer review panel might identify opportunities for improvement in a system that you manage.

The nursing profession is increasing its interest in peer review as a potentially useful process to engage and improve professionalism among nurses. Check with professional society resources for evolving approaches. |

SELF-ASSESSMENT CHECKLIST

▶ What is the mission and strategy of your organization, and how can you draw a clear line from that mission to your own department?

▶ Describe the specific scope of care or service in your department and its mission. What is the link between your department's mission and that of the organization?

▶ Have you obtained a copy of your organization's standard format for documenting a quality plan, if applicable?

▶ Who are your customers, what do they want, and how do you know it? Have you documented your patients'/customers' needs in your quality plan?

▶ What are your management goals for the year?

▶ What are the elements of quality that your department delivers to patients/customers? Have you documented them in the plan?

▶ What QI model is in use in your organization? Do you understand the vocabulary and approach?

Quality Measurement, Monitoring, and Analysis

Developing the right metrics—valid, reliable, feasible, meaningful, and action-oriented—is critical to the success of a quality improvement (QI) program. Measurement can seem costly in time and energy, but it should be an investment that yields significant benefits for patients/customers and process improvement. Measurement is most expensive when it is performed poorly, because it leads to waste and missed opportunities.

As discussed in Chapter 1, your organization probably has a definition of quality, and by the time you read this chapter, you have located and reviewed it. A commonly used definition is that shared by The Joint Commission (TJC) and the Institute of Medicine (IOM): "The degree to which health services for individuals and populations increase the likelihood of desired health outcomes and are consistent with current professional knowledge."

In a world in which measurement, proof, and evidence are ever more valued—even demanded by more payers as a condition of contracting—it is both practically and ethically incumbent on healthcare professionals to develop measures that evaluate their performance in increasing the likelihood of desired health outcomes.

By now you have developed a departmental quality plan (see Chapter 3) and you have defined your role in providing needed services to your customers according to both their own assessment of needs and what you know about relevant professional research and standards.

Introduction to Measurement

Performance and quality simply do not exist in the absence of measurement. These concepts are rooted in the idea of evaluation or assessment, whether in the form of a patient's subjective rating of the courtesy of staff members or an intricately constructed, statistically dense, risk-adjusted mortality rate model.

Measurement will give you the tools to focus the energy of your work teams on achieving productive and effective improvement. You will be investing time, money, and other resources in improving care and service ac-

cording to these measures. In so doing, you will also make the implicit decision not to invest in other QI opportunities, so select meaningful, well-constructed measures.

What should be measured?

In the quality plan for your department, you identified your customers, the scope of your patient care or service, and the most important aspects of care and service for your customers. This was an inventory of the big picture of what your department does.

Now you are ready to move to the next level of detail: the specific metrics that you'll use to evaluate your department's performance.

When you developed your plan, you also considered which aspects of care and service are high volume, high risk, or problem prone. These are all qualitative, not quantitative, characterizations.

In a small department, a service performed three or four times a day may be "high volume." And the "risk" of a high-risk process may be a clinical, financial, safety, or publicity risk. "Problem prone" may mean that the process fails once a week or once an hour.

You should assess the priority for measurement and improvement, and there are well-accepted characterizations (codified in the Joint Commission standards for many years) that can help you do that.

Pull out the quality plan you have drafted, and keep it handy as you work through this chapter.

Types of measurements

Divide metrics into the following (see Figure 4.1 for definitions of the terms):

1. **Foundation** measures and basics, which typically are not monitored

2. **Baseline** measures, which are monitored monthly or less often

3. **Process improvement** metrics, which are used to assess progress while an entire process is redesigned and significantly improved

Baseline monitoring measures of performance

Baseline measures are typically found in the quality plan with monthly, quarterly, or sometimes less frequent monitoring.

These are areas of performance that you believe to be instrumental in producing improved health outcomes or important results to your customers. Keep your attention focused on these measures to ensure that performance is solid and acceptable. They should be performing adequately or near an acceptable level. You may be working on modest improvement efforts but have not yet decided that it is time to launch a formal process improvement team. Hence, you can think of these as a baseline from which you'll decide whether performance is satisfactory or needs a significant improvement initiative.

FIGURE 4.1 ▶ SUMMARY OF DEFINITIONS USED IN MEASUREMENTS

Baseline quality monitoring is the measurement of performance in areas that we know to be fundamental to the provision of high-quality service to patients/customers and according to accepted methodologies and procedures. (We know what to do, we know how to do it, we know it is important; now let's measure to ensure that we are in fact doing it!) A baseline indicator is one we want to measure routinely to evaluate performance. We may or may not be performing as well as we would like on this indicator.

Process improvement is an initiative undertaken after thoughtful review reveals that a careful investment of time and energy is needed to reevaluate and possibly redesign a process that is important to patients and other customers. (We know this process is important; we have reason to believe that the process itself is not optimally designed to produce the results our patients/customers want; let's use our quality improvement methodology to analyze the process and its outcomes and redesign it as needed.)

Indicator is a word commonly used in quality measurement and improvement to describe a discrete measurement of a structure, process, or outcome.

- **Structure** indicators are elements that facilitate care/service, such as resources, equipment, or numbers and qualifications of staff. Example: *All equipment is maintained according to the manufacturer's standard; staff hours per patient day meet plan.*

- **Process** indicators are those functions carried out by practitioners/staff, such as assessment, treatment planning, medication administration, and treatment or other procedures, which ultimately affect outcomes for the patient or customer. Example: *Admissions meet criteria for appropriateness; lab turnaround time meets goal; documentation is timely and complete per policy.*

- **Outcome** indicators include satisfactory recovery of function, specific functional results of care, observable products of a process, complications, adverse events, and other short- and long-term results of treatment/management and processes. Example: *Infection rate is within department standard; mortality rate is below risk-adjusted benchmark; patient satisfaction meets or exceeds department goals.*

Indicators may be revised in the plan during a year, particularly if data indicate that the measure is stable, priorities change to suggest that another indicator is more important to the customer population, etc.

Criteria need to be the indicator when the indicator is not measurable by itself but requires further definition. For instance, "preoperative evaluation is complete" requires further explanation about what constitutes "complete." The criteria may be contained in a policy, procedure, standard of care, standard of practice, clinical path, etc.

Threshold defines a minimum desired level of performance for an indicator. As long as performance reaches this level, we believe that we are performing acceptably. If we fail to reach this level in a consistent fashion, we believe there is a substantive need for improvement. Thresholds are evidence-based whenever possible and derived from professional literature, clinical data, customer satisfaction/expectation data, historical experience, etc.

Goals define the optimal desired level of performance for an indicator. Efforts are directed to improve performance until it reaches or exceeds this level. We may provide fundamentally safe and effective care but still not reach the goal, which may reflect a "stretch" or challenge. Examples might include patient satisfaction ratings in the top quartile when we believe we can further improve; an infection rate that is within the standard of care for a particular patient population but that we believe we can improve with some new approaches to preoperative antibiotic administration. Goals are derived from the same sources as threshold but with a different view: not "what's the minimal acceptable performance level?" but "what's the best performance possible in our setting?"

A WORD ABOUT SENTINEL OR NEVER EVENTS IN YOUR QI PLAN

As described in Chapter 3, sentinel events and never events are classifications by The Joint Commission and the Leapfrog Group/National Quality Forum of adverse events that should be preventable most of the time if healthcare systems work effectively. By definition, these would not seem to be suitable QI metrics, as the only appropriate incidence of these events is zero and they should be individually addressed through root-cause analysis.

However, there are two reasons that you may address these events in your QI plan.

First, it is important to optimize systems for prevention. As an example, use of the Joint Commission's Universal Protocol™ can aid in prevention of wrong-patient, wrong-site, or wrong-procedure surgery (these are sentinel and never events). A thorough process improvement effort can be coupled with a root-cause analysis, if any of these events occur, to optimize safe care and protect patients.

Second, two of the never events in particular reflect rather common problems in healthcare: patient falls and pressure ulcers. Although serious outcomes such as disability or death are uncommon, most healthcare organizations have determined that prevention of falls and pressure ulcers (with or without serious adverse outcomes) does belong in the QI plan.

Baseline monitoring answers the question, "Because we know how to perform this process correctly, are we in fact doing so?" If you decide that the process needs redesign, go into a process improvement phase and set up appropriate measurements. (Read on for the "improvement" category. See Figure 4.2 to determine which category is the right one for a given measure, and see Chapter 7 for more about process improvement.)

If a measure of performance in your department is being reported publicly—for instance, on a state, Medicare, or Joint Commission Web site—then it definitely belongs on your own quality plan. Even if performance is strong, you should monitor it at some frequency. Monitor at the same frequency with which you report data, typically quarterly, so that you and your staff are always aware of these measures, before they are released to the public and used to judge your organization.

Every quality plan should include baseline measures. There is no absolute number of measures; the important considerations are as follows:

- **How many are "mandatory"?** This refers to those required by your organization because they are strategically targeted, submitted to external agencies, posted for public access, etc.

- **How many are substantially in control and at or near desired performance levels?** If you are monitoring several measures, but most of them are performing well, this is manageable. (Read on for a discussion of measures which are "in control" or "out of statistical control.")

FIGURE 4.2 ▶ IS THIS BASELINE OR PROCESS IMPROVEMENT?		
Questions to Consider	**Baseline**	**Process Improvement**
Do we believe we know how to perform this process correctly, efficiently, and appropriately? If yes ...	×	
Do we believe that this process needs a complete analysis and possible overhaul of how it is done? If yes ...		×
Do we feel the process is probably in need of an overhaul but aren't sure exactly how it is performing currently? If yes ... usually baseline while we establish measures, then, if it appears that the process is not performing as desired, it may be a candidate for a focused improvement effort.	× for a period of time	
Is this measurement or indicator dictated by a regulatory agency or made available publicly as part of state, federal, or accreditation programs? If yes ...	× (usually)	
We are meeting our target, goal, or threshold.	×	
We are not meeting our target, goal, or threshold. It could be either baseline or process improvement depending on the degree and scope of improvement needed.	×	×

- **How many have problematic performance levels?** This is the critical group. You cannot expect to focus on more than a few areas for improvement at once. You might be able to reasonably work on two or three baseline measures for improvement—that is, measures that are largely in control and near targeted levels of performance but which need a steady focus—and no more than one to three major process improvement efforts (see Chapter 7).

In summary, you may need to include many baseline measures because you need to monitor them steadily. Not all will be on your schedule for monthly review; some may be quarterly or less often. You may not need

to raise them for discussion at your monthly meetings but might post the results for the staff to see and might include a brief summary statement at the meeting, such as "All the measures we are tracking for The Joint Commission and Medicare continue to be in control and meeting or achieving targeted levels this quarter; see the Quality Management bulletin board for details." And you are more likely to achieve successful and sustainable performance improvements (PI) if you target no more than two or three areas at once for improvement for a given work team (see "Process improvement teams and associated measures" later in this chapter).

Synchronize measures among different departments' plans as relevant. For most effectiveness, the baseline measures you select should be synchronous with

those of other departments that can help you to advance performance.

> **Example:** *A nursing unit has established a length-of-stay goal and performance metric. This will be most effective if medical staff, pharmacy, and radiology share the same goal because they all have a role to play in timely decision-making and in services to facilitate discharge.*

Reflect organizational goals in your quality plan. Consider the organizationwide goals for the year or quarter. If the entire organization has set a goal for shorter wait times, then it will be most effective if every appropriate department shares that goal and has a specific metric in place. Ideally, the measurement will be developed collaboratively so that there are consistent definitions in all areas.

> **Example:** *A large multi-site group practice has set a goal of "wait times shorter than 10 minutes after scheduled appointment time." Every location in the practice measures in the same way, using a sampling methodology and computerized patient arrival and scheduling logs. The goal is shared by schedulers, physicians, reception staff, and clinical ancillary personnel, so that priorities are well aligned. Leadership decides to reward the entire organization based on overall average groupwide results, with additional recognition/reward to individual offices that beat the target.*

> **Example:** *A hospital establishes goals to reduce restraint use. The goal is developed and supported by medical staff members, who re-view and revise the order form for restraints to emphasize alternatives to be attempted before restraints are ordered. The group redesigning the order form includes nurses, who contribute ideas for restraint alternatives, design a cost-effective sitter program, and set up documentation so that patients who are restrained are monitored properly and can be released from restraints as early as is safely possible. Other departments involved with patient care (e.g., security, social work, and pharmacy) offer strategies to assist. And the quality department involves information systems staff so that data collection to monitor all aspects of the program is automated as much as possible.*

Process improvement teams and associated measures

From time to time, you will come across an element of your department's performance that is important but not something you think you can tweak into an acceptable range.

Maybe you have been trying to improve it for some time without success and you are frustrated. Maybe it's become clear that you can't improve by simply reminding staff each month to pay attention to this process; there is something fundamentally wrong in the system design that needs focus. See Chapter 7 for much more about this topic.

Preliminary list of measures or indicators

The term "indicator" is intimidating. An indicator is simply a measurement that is supposed to gauge whether the underlying process is performing as you would like. As QI and the science of measurement, statistical process control, and evidence-based care has matured, the

term "measure" or "metric" is preferred to "indicator." This book will use the latter terms, but you may have colleagues who still use the term "indicator."

Your next step

Refer to your quality plan and look at the important aspects of care and service for your customers as you defined them and determine what you might measure for each. Perform brainstorming and inventory exercises during a staff meeting or special session with medical and staff leaders. Don't worry about the specific metrics or details at this point—just capture ideas for what might be quantified.

Here are some hints on how to proceed:

- View the process as if you were a patient, family member, or other customer

- Consider the compliments and complaints you have received in the past

- Review the relevant professional literature on exceptional performance

- For examples and to complete your own worksheet, see Figure 4.3

Turning Ideas into Measures

Now it is time to prune the list of ideas to a short list of:

- Mandatory measures (public, regulatory, and strategic).

- Important monitoring measures that you believe are in control and performing adequately or better. These may not need frequent monitoring, but you will want to maintain some level of oversight.

- Important monitoring measures that you believe need improvement (ideally, no more than two or three in this category). Note: As you monitor these over time, you may identify one or two areas in which you need to entirely overhaul and redesign a process. That effort is addressed in Chapter 7.

Pruning your list involves the following two steps to select a small number of measures and refine them into practical, useful, and reliable metrics:

Step 1: Select a small number of measures.

Using your brainstormed list and the additional insights gained by reviewing the list according to the IOM and other dimensions, classify each measure on your list using the tool in Figure 4.4.

If you are Joint Commission–accredited, note that the process of selecting measures is part of the leadership standards (see Chapter 1, Figure 1.1, and Figure 1.2). Briefly documenting your rationale in making these selections will help demonstrate compliance. A simple "memo to the file" or an e-mail or memo to the members of the group who helped select the measures will suffice. Figure 4.4 gives an example of selected measures.

FIGURE 4.3 ▶ INITIAL BRAINSTORMING: EXAMPLES OF POTENTIAL MEASURES

Important Aspects of Care and Service	Examples of Potential Measures
Safe and effective nursing care	• Correct patient identification • Timely vital signs and assessments • Accurate verbal orders • Correct medication administration • Quick response to call light • Adequate staffing
Effective clinical care	• Timeliness to PTCA for patients presenting to ED with AMI • Anticoagulation timeliness • Correct antibiotic selection for community-acquired pneumonia • Optimal practices for prevention of surgical-site infection
Compassionate care	• Patient satisfaction with courtesy, response to special needs • Timely response to referrals to chaplain • Effective pain management
Continuity of care	• Complete, timely discharge instructions • Patient satisfaction with information about medications and care at home • No avoidable readmissions • Patient follows up with next visit as agreed to in care plan • Handoffs at each transfer point are documented, medications are reconciled, and care plan is fully implemented

Your Brainstorming:

Important aspects of care and service

_____
_____
_____
_____

Potential measures

_____
_____
_____
_____

FIGURE 4.4 ▶ SELECTING MEASURES

Examples:

This department has identified three categories of measures that are "mandatory," three that seem to be performing adequately but should be monitored (two monthly, one quarterly), and two areas that need improvement as part of an organizationwide improvement effort.

Important Aspects of Care and Service	Potential Measures	Mandatory (e.g., public, regulatory)	Monitor, in Control	Needs Improvement	Proposed Frequency of Monitoring
Safe and effective nursing care	Correct patient identification	• The Joint Commission (TJC)	Focus on insulin		Quarterly
	Timely vital signs and assessments				Defer for now
	Accurate verbal orders				Quarterly
	Correct medication administration	• TJC			Monthly (high risk)
	Quick response to call light				Defer for now
	Adequate staffing	• State mandate			Quarterly
Compassionate care	Patient satisfaction with courtesy, response to special needs	• HCAHPS on The Centers for Medicare & Medicaid Services (CMS) Web site	Monitor	Organization goal	Monthly
	Timely response to referrals to chaplain				Defer for now
	Effective pain management				Monthly
Continuity of care	Complete, timely discharge instructions	• CMS Heart Failure and HCAHPS measures	Monitor	Organization goal	Defer for now
	Patient satisfaction with information about medications and home care				Monthly
	No avoidable readmissions	• TJC			Quarterly
	Patient follows up with next visit as agreed in care plan				Defer
	Handoffs at each transfer point are documented, medications are reconciled, and care plan is fully implemented				Defer

Your Classification of Your Measures:

Important Aspects of Care and Service	Potential Measures	Mandatory (e.g., public, regulatory)	Monitor, in Control	Needs Improvement	Proposed Frequency of Monitoring

Step 2: Turn your ideas into practical, useful, reliable metrics.

Baseline metrics should be designed to measure a component of the process that generally tells how well things are working—something that indicates whether the process is performing acceptably. Not every component of a process needs to be measured for you to determine whether the process is performing acceptably. For example, if you turn on your television and see a picture, this indicates that the underlying electronics are functioning adequately.

Remember, too, that the metrics will disclose only the performance of a portion of the process. So if you are monitoring an outpatient diagnostic test process, you may have terrific wait time data, indicating that the logistics of the patient experience are performing very well. At the same time, the technical performance of the procedure itself may be suffering from high staff turnover, poor training, and unreliable equipment. If you have selected a solid measurement and collected and analyzed it reliably and if the measurement shows good results, it can be assumed the process is performing acceptably. If the measure indicates poor results, it can be assumed the process is not performing acceptably.

Step 3: Establish scope of measurement.

Establishing the scope of measurement is one of your key functions. The most critical question to repeatedly ask yourself is: "What do I want the final data to look like?" The key to choosing data for collection is anticipating what you will need to learn from the data, including investigation of deeper causes of performance problems.

Read the section about data analysis and sketch out the type of report or graph you want to see.

Tips for Designing Effective Measurements

Important characteristics of your measures include validity, reliability, and feasibility. To be valid, the measure must reflect the underlying process or characteristic that you want to investigate.

Example: A measure is developed to count incidents of reported adverse drug reactions to penicillin. It is valid in that it correctly counts those reactions that are recognized and reported.

It would not be a valid measure of prevalence of adverse drug reactions, however, because it depends on spontaneous and voluntary reporting. Reliability is inherent in a measure that will produce the same findings if it is repeated.

Example: A rate of patient complications that is computed based on medical records coding is reliable, because every time the records are counted, the same results will be produced.

However, it will be important to investigate the reliability of the underlying medical records coding process as well. If three coders examine the record, will they produce the same conclusions and codes? If not, you lack inter-rater reliability, which is essential to use these data for reliable metrics. As both of these examples demonstrate, you need to be aware of the sources of the data you are using in QI measurement, and you need to assess the validity and reliability of those sources first.

You may certainly decide to use data that are not perfectly valid or reliable. Sometimes this is the best and

most efficient way to perform initial screening for later deeper investigation.

For example, many QI metrics rely on medical records coding (the International Classification of Diseases [ICD] or current procedural terminology [CPT] codes). It is well established that there are two possible sources of variability, or lack of reliability, in this coding: The medical record documentation may be limited so that the coder cannot discern that the patient experienced a complication, or the coders may vary in their ability to read and interpret the record. Nonetheless, these data are efficient, readily available, and widely used to screen patient records for possible quality problems. As long as the limitations of the data are acknowledged and the next phase of the review involves more intensive analysis of specific records, this can be an appropriate way to consider screening for quality measures. Measure consistently. For example, explicitly define when a procedure starts and stops before measuring the turnaround time for the procedure.

> *Example: Staff members are asked to keep a log of patient wait times, with no other instructions. During one shift, a receptionist keeps a list of patients and the number of minutes they sit in the waiting area before they are called. During another shift, another receptionist keeps a list of patients and the number of minutes after their scheduled appointment time before they are called. Both measures are valid, but they are certainly not the same and should not be combined or averaged together.*

Later, you will write a specific definition of every metric you plan to use in your quality program. You will itemize numerators, denominators, and specific ICD or CPT or other codes and characteristics that will identify quality performance. Consistent definitions mean that you will ensure reliability, so that:

- All staff members performing the measurement have a common understanding of how the measurement is taken

- If you engage in benchmarking with other departments or other organizations, you can use a clear definition of the measurement

Measures also need to be practical and feasible. If the definition of the measure is too subjective or complex, or data abstraction takes hours from other important work, you may find that the benefit of measurement is outweighed by an unsupportable cost. You need to find the right balance through testing and refinement of the measure.

Simplicity is bliss. Measure only what is important and in a way that gives you only the information you need. For example, if you only need to know compliance with a turnaround time standard, tracking "yes" (within standard) and "no" (not within standard) may be a lot simpler than tracking and analyzing the exact turnaround time.

Similarly, if you know a process is not performing acceptably, does knowing how unacceptably it is performing provide you with important information? If final reports are not consistently filed within 72 hours, is it imperative to know whether the average time to file is 110 or 125 hours? Taking a baseline measure of the percent within standard and monitoring after improvement efforts may be as effective but less difficult.

Although there are certainly valid reasons for measuring a process in detail, aim for simplicity, especially for baseline measurement or for processes that are "in control" or not highly variable. (See "Data analysis" later in the chapter for more on processes that are "in control.")

- Wherever possible, use measurements that are already a part of the work flow and data elements that are a byproduct of work tasks. Examples might include patient satisfaction data on existing surveys; data produced by an existing computer system; or, as a last resort, manual logs and data sheets that serve a useful purpose in daily work.

- Where data collection is not a byproduct of work or of automated systems, measure on a sample basis. Often seemingly small sample sizes give surprisingly precise estimates.

- Measure on an ongoing basis to permit management intervention in a timelier manner than periodic gathering of historical data.

- Measure as infrequently as possible. Spend little time performing measurement for its own sake, but ensure that the data are complete and accurate enough to support conclusions and that the sample is statistically valid.

It may also be valuable to track related data that will help in analysis.

Example: Patients have complained about wait time in an area. Your analysis of overall average wait time shows that it is quite short. However, you expand your data collection to include details about patient appointment time, day of week, and appointment type; this richer data set is more helpful in isolating the root cause of the problem and guiding solutions. You discover that certain types of appointments, days of the week, or times of day appear to be problematic, but this was not apparent in the overall average.

Type of metric

This process of designing output will help you decide how to define the actual metric. Again ask, "What do I want to know?" What kind of number will answer the question, "How is this process performing?" This will help you choose the right statistic. It may be a rate, a percentage, an average, a gross number, a "time between events," or a distribution of numbers.

Sketching the output chart before you have any data will challenge you to focus on what matters in evaluating your process, and you will increase the likelihood of collecting meaningful and useful data the first time around.

DESIGNING OUTPUT

Example: Patient falls with injury (*See also discussion of sentinel and never events earlier in this chapter.*)

Time between = during this time interval (e.g., this month), the greatest number of days between falls with injury

Percentage = number of falls with injury divided by the number of patient days this month

Sample size

How much data do you need to analyze? How precise does the analysis need to be? Sampling may be appropriate, especially for in-control baseline indicators. (The concept of measures that are in control is discussed later in this chapter.)

For most healthcare operations processes, standard rules of thumb for sample size are as follows:

- If data are collected as a byproduct of a process and are automated, use all the data you have.

- If you are performing manual data collection, aim for a minimum of 30 observations in a given time period.

- If the process is high volume, 30 observations may not be enough to reflect the diversity of events. Increase the sample size up to as much as 5% of the total number of events.

A word about benchmarks and goals

The word "benchmark" is used in several ways. It can be a simple comparison, a target or goal, a best practice, or a minimum threshold.

Benchmarks or comparisons in QI are often problematic. Because the concept of quality in healthcare largely lacks standardized definitions, it can be difficult to compare performance of two organizations. Even when there are standard definitions, for example, based on diagnosis or procedures coded under ICD-9-CM, there can be significant variation among organizations in how they apply the codes.

However, progress over the past few years has been significant. The Centers for Medicare & Medicaid Services (CMS) has been particularly assertive in creating and enforcing systems to collect and publish reasonably comparable data in home health, nursing homes, and hospitals. In recent years, this has expanded in both clinical measures and evaluation of patient satisfaction with services (in hospitals, the HCAHPS measures). The National Committee for Quality Assurance's Healthcare Effectiveness Data and Information Set measures have had comparison data for several years. Many state hospital associations are assisting their members by providing databases and comparisons. Leading nursing and QI organizations have published standard definitions and, in some cases, benchmarks for important quality indicators. The Agency for Healthcare Research and Quality has developed and published what it calls "empiric" rates for quality and patient safety metrics computed from national databases of millions of hospital discharges, and sponsors the National Guideline Clearinghouse (see Bibliography).

Within a single organization, consortium, or other group, you can compare or benchmark performance among units, departments, and areas. Clinics can compare wait times. Units can compare documentation practices or patient satisfaction. Across a region, hospitals can compare clinical outcomes. See Chapter 5 for more specific information on benchmarking in nursing and how to use nursing-sensitive quality indicators in your quality measurement.

It is definitely necessary to establish a goal, target, or threshold for all quality metrics. In many cases, a benchmark's availability can help you to decide what is realistic as a goal. Examples of goals might include the following:

- Improve patient satisfaction to the 90th percentile compared with peer organizations

- Reduce healthcare-acquired infection rate to below the Centers for Disease Control and Prevention's published rates for a comparable patient population

- Reduce patient falls with injuries to below the benchmark and work toward zero falls (see discussion of sentinel and never events in Chapter 3 and earlier in this chapter)

- Improve all elements of acute myocardial infarction care, per CMS definitions, to exceed statewide benchmarks and approach 100% compliance with optimal practice

- Improve wait time to <15 minutes for 90% of patients and 30 minutes for all

Draft your metrics

You are ready to define your quality and performance metrics. They'll be refined later, but you have almost all the elements at this time. For each of your tentative measures, sketch a possible outcome chart that you want to see. Document your planned metrics with:

- The basic measure (e.g., wait time, satisfaction, or complications) and your performance goal

- The unit of time (e.g., week, month, or quarter) you'll measure

- Additional stratification or levels of detail

you plan to collect (e.g., age groups, day of week, shift, or clinical problem)

- Sample size

- A brief description of how you will obtain the data (e.g., via existing computer systems, a manual log or data maintained as part of care or service, or a special log just for QI data)

- Notes and comments on possible issues with reliability, effort, cost, and complexity associated with this measure

See Figure 4.5 for an example of how to define metrics.

Finalize your metrics

There are two steps remaining before you finalize your specific measures:

- Write down the specific definitions of all relevant data elements

- Develop a data collection tool and test it

Specific definitions

A clear and consistent data definition is critical for successful and meaningful performance evaluation. Every element of data needs a clear definition. (See the following "Example Data Definitions.")

In the examples that follow, various definitions are used. These definitions may not necessarily be the right ones for your situation, but they do demonstrate the importance of being specific once you select a metric.

FIGURE 4.5 ▶ DEFINING METRICS

Examples

Measure	When	Stratification	Sample	Data Source and Methodology	Notes and Comments
Pain management: Percentage of patients with moderate or severe pain who received timely and effective intervention. Goal: 100%.		Just medicine units for now	10 patients per week, 40 per month	Medical record audit of patients with pain scores of 4–10. • Timely: Determine what % received a timely intervention (within 30 minutes per policy) and reassessment within one hour. Goal: 100%. • Effective: Determine what % resulted in reduction of pain to level of 0–3. Goal: 100%.	10 pain events per week may not be enough, but this can be a time-consuming audit. Pilot for a month or two in the medicine units and then reevaluate. There is no benchmark for this, but our organizational goal is 100%.

Specific Definitions:

(a1) Timely intervention

- Numerator: Number of patients who received a documented pain intervention within 30 minutes of a recorded score of 4+

- Denominator: Number with a documented pain score of 4+

(a2) Timely reassessment

- Numerator: Number of patients with a documented reassessment within one hour after intervention

- Denominator: Number with a documented pain intervention

(b) Effective pain relief

- Numerator: Number of patients with a pain score of 0–3, following a documented pain intervention for a score of 4+

- Denominator: Number of patients with a pain score of 4+ and a documented intervention

FIGURE 4.5 ▶ DEFINING METRICS (CONT.)

Examples

Measure	When	Stratification	Sample	Data Source and Methodology	Notes and Comments
Pain management: Percentage of patients with moderate or severe pain who received timely and effective intervention. Goal: 100%.		Just medicine units for now	10 patients per week, 40 per month	Weekly, enter data into a spreadsheet with day/time arrived and time seen. Use every 10th patient on the logs (10% sample, estimate 30–40 per week based on average volume).	Spreadsheet is time-consuming; see whether we can automate it.

Specific Definitions:

Select every 10th patient from the registration log

Record day, time arrived, and time seen

Calculate total: time waited = time seen − time arrived

Do not record patient identifiers

(a) Average wait time
    Numerator: Sum of the minutes all patients waited

  – Denominator: Number of patients

(b) Range of wait times

  – Histogram showing the number of patients who waited under 15 minutes, 15–30, and 30+

(c) Day of week and a.m./p.m.

  – Be able to produce the histogram for any day of the week separately and for day/morning or day/afternoon

EXAMPLE DATA DEFINITIONS

Patient satisfaction: Percent of patients rating nursing care "excellent"
- *Numerator:* Number of patients giving nursing care a top score
- *Denominator:* Number of surveys received with any answer to this question

Overall average satisfaction: On a 0–100 scale
- *Calculation:* Compute the average score on each survey (sum of all questions' scores divided by the number of questions answered); compute the average score across all patients (sum of all average scores, divided by the number of patients)

Mortality rate (usually for a specific population): Percent of patients who expire during hospitalization
- *Numerator:* Number of patients who expire in hospital (e.g., in a specific clinical group, defined by diagnosis-related group, ICD-9-CM, or other characteristics)
- *Denominator:* Number of patients admitted during the time period in that clinical group
- *Exclusions:* This measure might exclude patients enrolled in hospice, neonates under 500 grams, or other groups, depending on the situation

Pain management: Timely intervention for pain
- *Numerator:* Patients with a pain intervention within 30 minutes of a recorded pain score of 4 or greater
- *Denominator:* Patients with a pain score of 4 or greater

Skin integrity in ICU: Avoid skin breakdown in hospital
- *Numerator:* Patients with grade 1 (or greater) pressure ulcers developing more than 72 hours after admission
- *Denominator:* All ICU adult admissions of 72 hours or longer

Image quality in a technical area: Measure for each technologist (sample of 30 images or more per technologist per modality, perhaps quarterly)
- *Numerator:* Number of images that are of acceptable quality, according to your clinicians' criteria (preferably rated objectively/without knowledge of the technologist's identity)
- *Denominator:* Number of images processed by this technologist

Note: With these data, you will also be able to aggregate the data for a quality metric for the entire department for each modality.

Testing your metrics

The final step in developing a metric is to ensure that it's really feasible, practical, clearly defined, and useful.

If you are collecting data from an automated or computerized system, this will be relatively easy to test. If you need to conduct manual data collection, now is the time to develop your data collection tool and test it with a few patients/events.

See Figure 4.6 for a model of a data collection tool.

FIGURE 4.6 ▶ SAMPLE DATA COLLECTION TOOL

Wait Times

Goal: No patient waits longer than 30 minutes. Average is less than 15 minutes.

Department X			
Wait time sample. Select every 10th patient from registration logs			
A	B	C	D (compute C-B)
Day	Time arrived	Time seen	Wait

Analysis:

Using the spreadsheet program, produce these reports:

(a) Average wait time

- Numerator: Sum of the minutes all patients waited (column D)

- Denominator: Number of patients (sum of the rows)

(b) Range of wait times

- Histogram showing the number of patients who waited less than 15 minutes, 15–30, and 30+

(c) Day of week and a.m./p.m.

- Be able to produce the histogram for any day of the week separately and for day/morning or day/afternoon

Data Analysis—An Overview

Good data collection is designed with a thoughtful anticipation of how you will analyze the data. And in-depth analysis leads to improved data collection for future cycles. The two processes are appropriately cyclical, and over time you will become more adept at planning effective measurement.

You have already taken important steps in anticipating data analysis. You designed your planned measurement output, report, or graph before you finalized it. You reviewed your process, the literature, and your experience in order to establish a reasonable sampling plan and to try to be sure you were collecting all necessary supporting data, such as day of week or patient gender/comorbidities. You were careful not to collect too much data or to make the process too complex for reliable use.

The most important additional concept is whether a process is in control. Would you prefer that your department deliver performance with an average of two errors per 10 events or one error per 10 events? It's a trick question, and you need to know how stable the process is before you answer.

Much QI theory focuses on the importance of making processes stable or predictable. The idea is that it is preferable to have a stable, predictable result of, for example, two errors for every 10 events than to have a highly variable result that may average, for example, one error for every 10 events but will sometimes be zero errors per 10 events or eight errors per 10 events or somewhere in between. Why? Consider the sports analogy. Would you rather have a baseball player on your team who is a reliable .300 hitter or one who can go several games without

out a hit and once in a while hit a terrific homer? The idea is that you can work with the .300 hitter to identify strengths and weaknesses and coach him into still-stable but better performance. With the unpredictable hitter, it's hard to know where to begin because performance is so inconsistent.

Once a process is in control (i.e., predictable and stable), examine points in the process that can be modified to produce a better result. As long as the process is producing highly unpredictable results, you have no way of knowing which points should be modified and, in fact, you are likely to do more harm than good if you "tinker" with the process.

Thus, a legitimate goal for process improvement can sometimes be simply to make a result more predictable rather than to show improvement in an overall average or other performance metric. Ultimately, of course, we intend to see processes that are both highly predictable and producing optimal results.

Is this process in control?

The definition of control is a statistical one. You can vary the parameters to call for tighter control or less rigor, depending on how important it is to deliver highly reliable performance.

A process that is in control operates steadily within control limits. A control limit is a statistic that predicts the normal variability in the process. Typically, there will be an upper and lower control limit. These statistics provide a range of predictability. The statistics are usually calculated based on a run of data that you've collected over a period of time, ideally at least 20 samples. A simplified form of control charts is fine for most applications in healthcare operations QI. The upper and

lower control limits are set at three standard deviations from the mean value of the performance statistic (see examples that follow). This means that, as long as the process continues to perform consistently, 99% of the observations will be expected to fall within these limits.

Thus, if you observe that performance is outside the control limits, you know that something unusual has occurred in this process. It may be a single unusual event, or it may be that the process itself has changed and is performing differently.

There are half dozen types of control charts you may wish to compute, each with slightly different statistical considerations and methods. Let's look at the general principle for control chart use.

The control chart
Percentage effective care

You are analyzing the percent of patients for whom documentation demonstrates timely and effective pain management. You can graph the data over a year using a run chart. You notice what looks like a definite improvement trend. See Figure 4.7 for an example of a control chart.

Rules of thumb for a run chart

- A run of 6 or 7 points on either side of the average requires investigation

- A run of 6 or 7 points steadily up or steadily down requires investigation

These trends may indicate that the process you are measuring is undergoing some type of systematic change.

In the example in Figure 4.7, notice that the second of these criteria is not quite met—there are two runs of 5 points of improving percentages. But there certainly seems to be a trend, and the first criterion is met: There are 7 points above the average, beginning in June.

Is this a meaningful change in the pain management process? Based on a couple years of prior data, you will compute the control limits for this process. This will help you to decide whether the process has changed statistically.

(If you don't have data from prior years, compute the control limits using all or part of this same data set for the current year. The problem is that you already suspect that the process is improving, and it would be best if you could define the control limits based on past performance to see most clearly whether it has changed. This is not always feasible given the available data.)

Simple computation of control limits

The upper control limit is equal to the average, plus three standard deviations. The lower control limit is equal to the average, minus three standard deviations. This is easy to compute in any spreadsheet program. If a data point falls outside the control limits, it requires investigation. It suggests that the process may no longer be in control. Or you may be seeing a one-time event—a special cause variation that should be explained but does not mean that the process itself has changed.

Example: Patient satisfaction has been stable for many months, but due to a local community catastrophe on a single day, many staff members had to respond to an influx of patients. Your department was unable to keep up with the

FIGURE 4.7 ► CONTROL CHART FOR A PERCENTAGE MEASURE

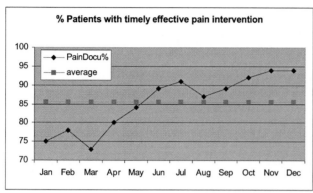

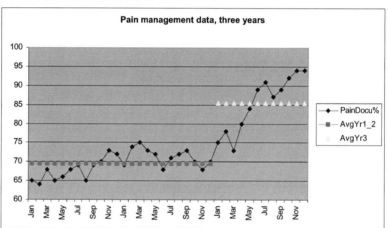

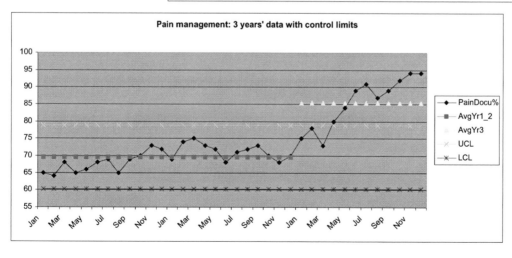

FIGURE 4.7 ▶ CONTROL CHART FOR A PERCENTAGE MEASURE (CONT.)

Supporting Data (SD) Sheet

Month	Pain Documentation%	Avg Yr 1–2	Avg Yr 3	UCL	LCL
Jan	65	69.5		78.9	60.2
Feb	64	69.5		78.9	60.2
Mar	68	69.5		78.9	60.2
Apr	65	69.5		78.9	60.2
May	66	69.5		78.9	60.2
Jun	68	69.5		78.9	60.2
Jul	69	69.5		78.9	60.2
Aug	65	69.5		78.9	60.2
Sep	69	69.5		78.9	60.2
Oct	70	69.5		78.9	60.2
Nov	73	69.5		78.9	60.2
Dec	72	69.5		78.9	60.2
Jan	69	69.5		78.9	60.2
Feb	74	69.5		78.9	60.2
Mar	75	69.5		78.9	60.2
Apr	73	69.5		78.9	60.2
May	72	69.5		78.9	60.2
Jun	68	69.5		78.9	60.2
Jul	71	69.5		78.9	60.2
Aug	72	69.5		78.9	60.2
Sep	73	69.5		78.9	60.2
Oct	70	69.5		78.9	60.2
Nov	68		85.5	78.9	60.2
Dec	70		85.5	78.9	60.2
Jan	75		85.5	78.9	60.2
Feb	78		85.5	78.9	60.2
Mar	73		85.5	78.9	60.2
Apr	80		85.5	78.9	60.2
May	84		85.5	78.9	60.2
Jun	89		85.5	78.9	60.2
Jul	91		85.5	78.9	60.2
Aug	87		85.5	78.9	60.2
Sep	89		85.5	78.9	60.2
Oct	92		85.5	78.9	60.2
Nov	94		85.5	78.9	60.2
Dec	94		85.5	78.9	60.2

Average years 1 and 2: 69.5
SD years 1 and 2: 3.1
Average year 3: 85.5

UCL = average during the baseline period (years 1 and 2) plus three standard deviations
LCL = average during the baseline period (years 1 and 2) minus three standard deviations

Upper control limit (UCL) and lower control limit (LCL): The process should perform within these two limits unless it has changed significantly. The limits identify underlying process change. See text for more discussion about common cause and special cause variation.

usual daily volume with so few staff remaining, and wait times soared. On that one day, satisfaction was very poor, and this caused the weekly statistics to dip below the lower control limit. This is a special cause variation and, once explained, does not need further intervention to improve the process because the routine process was not performing poorly. In fact, if you tried to improve patient satisfaction based on that one day's unusual events, you'd likely waste time and possibly interfere with otherwise very satisfactory operations.

It is certainly legitimate to respond to special cause variation with a properly targeted improvement effort in case the special cause recurs—in this example, you might want to design emergency communication procedures as part of your disaster plan. But you would not want to try to redesign the department's normal work flows because of an unusual or special cause event.

If several data points fall outside the control limits or if an extended series of points falls within the control limits but above or below the mean, your process has probably changed. Recall the rules for reviewing a run chart for possible common cause variation:

- A run of 6 or 7 points on either side of the average requires investigation

- A run of 6 or 7 points steadily up or steadily down requires investigation

The definitions of common cause and special cause variation used by The Joint Commission, which require attention to statistical process control as one element of a comprehensive PI system, are:

- **Special cause.** A factor that intermittently and unpredictably induces variation over and above what is inherent in the system. It often appears as an extreme point (such as a point beyond the control limits on a control chart) or some specific, identifiable pattern in data.

- **Common cause.** A factor that results from variation inherent in the process or system. The risk of a common cause can be reduced by redesigning the process or system.[1]

In our example, the process has improved, as we can see in both the run of improving points and the points that are above the upper control limit. In Figure 4.7, in the third chart, we can see the whole story: the prior two years' data and the resulting control limits.

> *Example: In our example, a hospitalwide effort to improve pain management involved many departments and improved physician and nurse awareness and patient education, bolstered electronic reminder and documentation systems, and strengthened pharmacy support. As a result, performance is significantly different than it was in the past, and the control chart demonstrates this.*

What observations can you make from this chart? It contains a great deal of information, such as:

- The process was in control during year one and year two. It performed consistently within the expected control limits.

- In May of year three, something changed in

this process. Not just one or two but all future data points exceeded the upper control limit.

We could enrich the chart further with a line showing a benchmark (best practice) for patient satisfaction if we have that information and/or a line showing our goal for the year. With this information, you should then:

- Confirm that the process has changed. Can you identify policy, procedure, training, process flow, environmental, or other changes?

- Recompute the control limits to reflect the new process. You will do this by using just the new process data (e.g., since May of year three). Be-cause you don't have the recommended 20 or more data points, these control limits may be a little less stable—and a little wider—than de-sired, but they will help you make sense of future performance.

- Observe performance until you are confident that the new process is in control in its new limits. (As you accumulate more months of data, keep recomputing the control limits beginning with May of year three, until you have at least 20 months of data.)

Other types of control charts

There are other types and tools to refine the statistical approach beyond the simplified one presented here. Our example displayed data that reflected the percentage of correct events (pain documentation). Types of data that can be plotted on control charts (in parentheses) and the technical names of the charts include:

- Percentage of events that meet or don't meet criteria (e.g., percentage of patients with timely and effective pain management [called the "p chart"])

- Number of errors found when you examine an equal number of events in each time period (e.g., examine 10 medical records coded each week and count the number that are inaccurate [called the "np chart"])

- Average performance over time (e.g., patient satisfaction ratings on a 0–100 scale; the number of patients who respond may vary each month [called the "8 chart"])

In your organization, you may have a set of standards or rules that help to determine what kinds of charts should be used for which data and how to compute control limits. If not, see Appendix C for a few references to assist you in computing and interpreting these charts.

How to look at data

In the last section, we looked at run charts and control charts. These are useful for examining trends over time.

Other important data formats to consider include the following (see Figure 4.8 for samples):

- **Histogram.** A chart that displays frequency of events in different categories. It is used to see differences among groups and often leads to more analysis. To make sense of this chart, you might compute the average satisfaction for the entire organization and then determine whether each group's

FIGURE 4.8 ▶ EXAMPLES OF DATA ANALYSIS TOOLS

A. Histogram

A chart that displays frequency of events in different categories. Used to see differences among groups; often leads to more analysis.

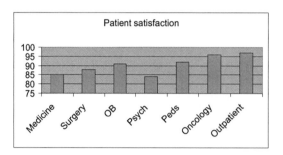

B. Run chart

Displayed using bars, showing a single group's quality metric over time. Used to see change over time.

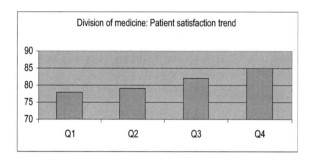

C. Pareto diagram

A histogram organized from most frequent event to least frequent event. Used to identify the most important factors or groups in a level of performance; often leads to more analysis.

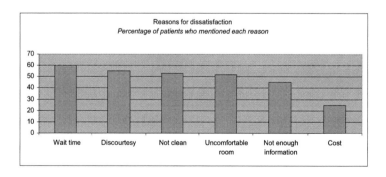

FIGURE 4.8 ▶ EXAMPLES OF DATA ANALYSIS TOOLS (CONT.)

D. Scatter diagram

Used to show the relationship between two continuous numeric variables; the method for displaying a possible "correlation" between the variables.

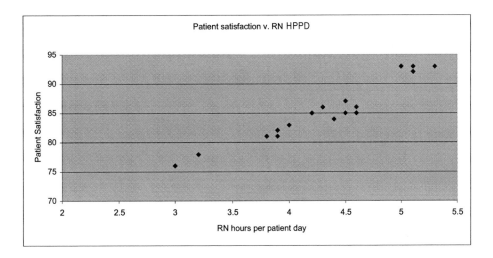

Note: Your spreadsheet program can probably compute an equation and display a trend line for the relationship. For example:

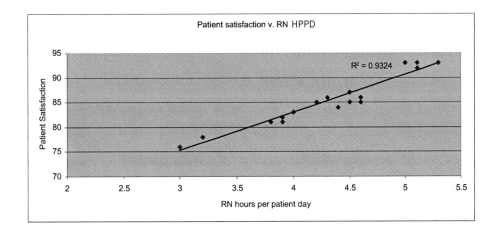

QUALITY IMPROVEMENT FOR NURSE MANAGERS

FIGURE 4.8 ▶ EXAMPLES OF DATA ANALYSIS TOOLS (CONT.)

E. Radar ("spider web") Diagram

This chart is somewhat complex but can be a powerful tool as a snapshot of performance. Choose several metrics (usually about five) that portray a composite picture of performance in a department or program.

In this case, the metrics offer a balanced portrait. Note that they are all set up so that higher scores represent *better* performance:

- Patient satisfaction

- Staff turnover (percent retained each year)

- Timely results (reports within 24 hours)

- Rapid patient access to care (less than 10 minutes)

- Efficient service (percentile performance according to an external benchmark, where 100th percentile would be most efficient/lowest cost)

The results quickly highlight a decline in performance from last year to this year and suggest that possibly the increase in "efficiency" (lower cost) may have been achieved at the expense of timely service and patient satisfaction. Results show:

- Lower patient satisfaction

- Higher turnover

- Slower access to care

- Fewer results posted within 24 hours

- More efficient/lower cost of service

Perhaps the team neglected to implement the cost reductions with accompanying process redesign to ensure the same level of service.

The radar diagram provides a quick comparison on several metrics at once, and the "webs" can reflect two points in time for a single department (as in this example), or you may wish to show your department performance as one web and an external set of benchmarks as the other web.

FIGURE 4.8 ▶ EXAMPLES OF DATA ANALYSIS TOOLS (CONT.)

Data Sheet	This Year	Last Year
Satisfaction (% top box)	85	90
Timely (%<10 minutes)	80	87
Cost/service (benchmark percentile)	85	75
Effective (% reports within 24 hours)	65	86
Staff turnover (% retention/year)	75	92

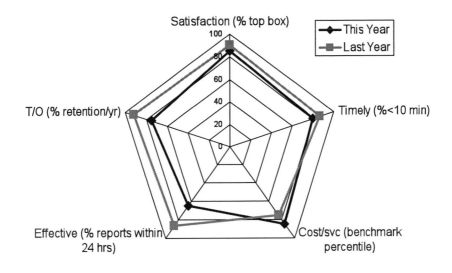

score was statistically significantly different from the overall mean. You may also want to study each group's score independently over time using a bar chart. (See chart A in Figure 4.8.)

- **Run chart.** A graphic display of data in sequence chronologically, with the x-axis displaying time or successive samples/ events. It is used to discern patterns over time. See chart B in Figure 4.8 for an example of a run chart. See Figure 4.7 and the earlier discussion of control charts for a step-by-step approach to make sense of a run chart using statistical process control methods.

- **Pareto diagram.** A histogram organized from most frequent event to least frequent event. It is used to identify the most important factors or groups in a level of performance and often leads to more analysis. If you discover that three factors or subgroups contain 80% of the problems or defects in your measure, you certainly will use that information to focus on those groups. This can be a powerful tool to determine where the core process problem may be. (See chart C in Figure 4.8.)

- **Scatter diagram.** Shows the relationship between two continuous numeric variables; displays a possible "correlation" between the variables. It may be useful to compute a correlation coefficient (your spreadsheet program should do this) between two variables.

For example, you may suspect that patient satisfaction is related to the percentage of agency staff hours on any given day. If you gather data for 15 or more time periods, with both percentage agency staffing and satisfaction score or percentage, you can use the correlation to determine whether these are statistically related. You could then study the survey data to look at the specific questions and how they may be answered differently by a sample of patients who encountered agency staff and another sample who encountered employee staff. (See chart D in Figure 4.8.)

TO DO

Revisit your metrics and the plan you constructed for analysis. Did you select the right data displays to make sense of the data?

If your data are continuous measures over time, and if you have historical data, develop a control chart and determine whether the process is in control.

Common Pitfalls in Defining and Selecting Measures

- Over measuring: Sampling too many records; using chart review and complex audit tools rather than readily available data from other, possibly less familiar sources; computing precise rates with labor-intensive manual data collection rather than tracking and trending simple incidence with recourse to more sophisticated tools, if indicated

- Measuring and focusing on a symptom of a process failure rather than the underlying process that produces a given outcome or result

- Measuring and focusing on random events that are not the product of a definable process or system

- Failing to measure and monitor an important indicator of performance because it is not strictly within the department's control (usually driven by fear of a negative quality report card)

Common Pitfalls in Data Use

The following is a lighthearted summary developed over many years of working with quality data. As you reflect on the plans and measures you have developed, test them against these common errors in data collection, management, and use.

Lies, darn lies, and statistics
Definition: Incorrect, inconsistent, or unclear measurement.

> *Example: Two staff members are measuring wait time. One staff member measures from patient arrival until patient is seen; the other measures from original patient appointment time until patient is seen. They cannot be analyzed as a single data set.*

> *Example: A chart shows the delay time in communicating results from one computer system to another. The chart looks terrific, with zero delays displayed all week. On investigation, it transpires that one of the systems is down completely and the absence of data was charted by a well-meaning staff person as a value of zero.*

Definition: Incorrect analysis.

> *Example: A customer service department finds that afternoons are impossibly busy, and mornings are undemanding. Average time for response to queries in the morning is just a few minutes. Average in the afternoon is a consistent half hour or longer. The manager describes the department's overall average as 15 minutes response time.*

Flinching
Definition: First defined by Donald W. Marquardt,[1] a statistician in 1984, this important concept reflects harmful behaviors of staff members in response to quality metrics that are not well designed. Flinching describes situations in which action is:

- Taken that is harmful to long-term results of an organization, although it causes improvement in short-term reported results

- Motivated by the belief that a good quality report will produce greater rewards or fewer penalties than alternative actions (in other words, it's more important to look good than to be entirely accurate)

Example: Staff members know that their bonus or performance review depends on shortened wait times and higher patient satisfaction. Without directly sabotaging, they carefully choose which patient visits or surveys to sample in compiling the data for the monthly quality data summary.

Example: Maintaining or upgrading equipment will mean a few days of dislocation for staff and patients, causing inconvenience and dissatisfaction. The manager knows that patient satisfaction is the key organizational goal for the year, and so postpones the upgrade repeatedly, risking reliability of the equipment.

The great data dam

Definition: Rejection of data altogether, unwillingness to engage in analysis and improvement.

Example: This can be a significant problem in presenting administrative data to clinicians, who will quickly identify the real limitations in the data. For example, if you don't have risk adjustment in mortality data, it may be utterly rejected by medical staff. On the other hand, you need their engagement and constructive help in order to improve the analysis.

Poetry in motion

Definition: Belief that high levels of visible activity (e.g., data collection, graphs, tables, teams, and meetings) equal actual analysis and improvement.

Example: Unfortunately, this is not uncommon. A symptom can be seen when an executive can proudly tell you there are dozens of quality teams working but can't remember any specific improvements that benefit the customer and that have been actually implemented and measured lately.

Paradise lost

Definition: Obsessive search for perfect measurement and perfect performance, leading to endless refinement and failure to actually improve the process.

Example: If you've worked with a measure for six months or more, and you're still tinkering to get it just right and have neither improved it nor convinced yourself that performance is acceptable, you may suffer from this syndrome. (Or you may have chosen something too difficult to measure with the data and tools you have available.)

Analysis paralysis

Definition: Often found along with "paradise lost." The experience of being afraid of taking a risk or acting in the absence of perfect and complete data.

Example: If your data have shown that there is a consistently higher risk of late medications on second shift when you are the busiest and you're still expanding your sample size, checking a few more variables, and waiting for the local statistician to prove that it's a statistically significant difference, you may be paralyzed.

Slice of life

Definition: By carefully/carelessly selecting a period of reference, a series of data points can take on factitious meaning.

> **Example:** *Consider the two charts in Figure 4.9, and you will quickly see the problem.*

Another definition: Over-analyzing minor variations from threshold, goal, or target that are within the normal range of predictable variability of the process.

> **Example:** *If you don't use control limits, you may erroneously overreact to what looks like a decline in performance over a couple of months; with the use of simple control limits, you may*

be able to show that the trend is to be expected within the normal limits of the process as designed.

Strange bedfellows

Definition: Benchmarking to a group or process that is not comparable instead of comparing "apples to apples."

> **Example:** *An extreme example would be a comparison of wait times between a large urban emergency department and a small rural one. More subtle problems can arise in performing clinical process comparisons without adequate risk adjustment.*

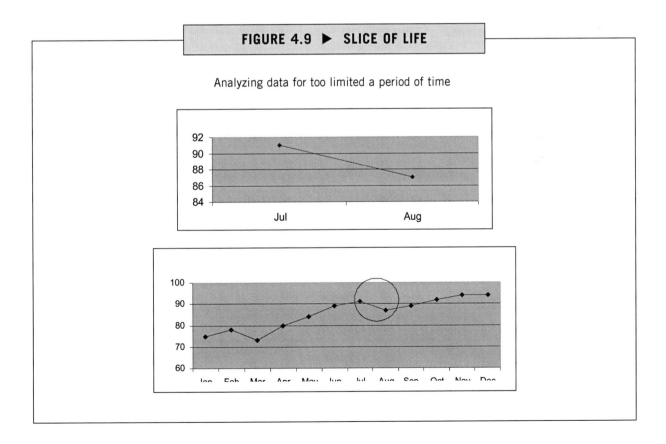

FIGURE 4.9 ▶ SLICE OF LIFE

Analyzing data for too limited a period of time

Trivial pursuit

Definition: Competent and energetic performance measurement and QI efforts applied to processes and outcomes of no particular importance to any patient or customer but possibly convenient and interesting to the principal.

> *Example: Documenting that education was provided to the patient is not, perhaps, trivial, but what really matters is whether the patient understood the education. A better metric might be an objective evaluation of patients' accuracy in a return demonstration of wound care or description of their own discharge instructions or callbacks to patients in a few days to check on compliance.*

Similarly, a materials department may work hard to document that it stocked carts on schedule, but it's more important that items were actually available to clinical staff when they were needed.

The stocking metric may be achieved, but if par levels are wrong or stocking schedules don't match cycles in patient volume, the customer (i.e., clinical staff members who need supplies) will not be well served.

Hawthorne effect

Definition: Often-cited phenomenon of PI consequent solely on an awareness of observation and focus, first described in the late 1920s by Elton Mayo, a Harvard researcher, based on work at the Western Electric Hawthorne Works. The Hawthorne effect poses a problem for QI because observed improvement may be transient and unrelated to actual process changes.

> *Example: Staff members are aware that observers are monitoring hand washing. It's a novelty to have observers on the unit; there's anxiety and amusement, and the entire group finds, without intending it, that hand hygiene is performed more consistently. Humans are social and responsive, and the knowledge that someone is working on a process can stimulate increased interest and focus among the team, no matter what the specific measures or planned improvements may be.*

The blame game

Definition: Attributing variable outcomes or inconsistent performance to individual employee or physician behavior rather than the underlying systems and processes.

> *Example: Three staff members are disciplined for programming an infusion pump incorrectly. Eventually, it is discovered that the pump's software requires an unusual sequence of entries under a rare scenario. The process is guaranteed to produce failures. The real solution is to handle the rare scenario with alerts and forcing functions so that staff members don't have to rely exclusively on vigilance and their memory to use the right sequence of steps.*

SELF-ASSESSMENT CHECKLIST

▶ You used your quality plan to sketch out important aspects of your processes that should be evaluated

▶ You considered external audiences as well as your internal standards for the level of performance you intend to provide

▶ You reviewed the literature and your own experience to be sure that you are collecting the right information about performance

▶ Your metrics meet criteria for validity, reliability, and feasibility

▶ You set performance goals with attention to benchmarks or comparisons when relevant and available

▶ You defined the collection and computation of every metric in detail so that the data can be collected reliably

▶ You tested the metric

▶ You know whether your process is in control or how you will collect enough data to evaluate this

▶ You have confirmed that your data analysis plan is the right one to give you useful data for evaluation and, if necessary, improvement

---

Endnotes

1. Donald W. Marquardt, "Report Card Issues in Quality Management," *Quality Management Journal* (April 1994). Paper first presented at 1984 American Society for Quality Control Fall Technical Conference.

Nursing-Sensitive Indicators

You may think of quality indicators as those which require interdisciplinary or organizationwide collaboration, and those which are nursing-sensitive, or primarily in the scope of nursing control.

Those indicators requiring interdisciplinary collaboration are complex processes and are usually coordinated by an organizational QI department with the ability to involve multiple disciplines. These are organizational indicators. Although nurses participate in many of these organizational QI projects, they are not in the sole domain of nurses to control.

However, within the scope of nursing practice are nursing-sensitive indicators (NSI). These are metrics that improve if there is a greater quantity or quality of nursing care, according to the American Nurses As-

sociation (ANA). In the last few years, an increasing body of knowledge in defining NSIs and their contribution to patient outcomes has been developed for the nursing profession. This has resulted from a number of factors. Research has indicated that patient outcomes improve, complications and mortality are reduced, costs can be reduced, and patient and professional nurse satisfaction can be enhanced with strong performance on nursing-sensitive indicators.

Payment has also become an important factor in spurring additional interest in NSIs. The Centers for Medicare & Medicaid Services (CMS) has implemented a formula which can result in reduced Medicare reimbursement to hospitals if patients experience any of a dozen hospital-acquired conditions. Four of these—pressure ulcers, patient falls, catheter-associated urinary tract infections (CAUTI), central line–associated bloodstream infections (CLABSI)—have been termed "nurse sensitive" by the National Quality Forum (NQF). According to the ANA, they will improve if there is a greater quantity or quality of nursing care.

The ANCC Magnet Recognition Program® (MRP) has also influenced the development of NSIs. The MRP represents achievement of processes and outcomes of nursing care which are among the best in the United

States, according to consensus and evidence-based standards. As of 2008, any hospital applying for MRP designation or redesignation must show clear evidence that patient outcomes in a number of NSIs outperform the mean of a national benchmarking database. In addition, in 1998, the National Database of Nursing Quality Indicators was established by ANA so that nurses would have a national benchmark to which they can compare their outcomes. This has given the profession of nursing a solid core of benchmarkable nursing sensitive indicators that are totally nursing care dependent. In addition, a large body of nursing evidence-based practices (EBP) related to improving these NSI has been developed to help nursing develop standards of care to meet the challenge of improving these NSI outcomes.

Types of Quality Indicators

NSIs are characterized by measures that are in the realm of nurses to improve and control. They are "sensitive" to nursing practices. Organizational indicators are those requiring interdisciplinary collaboration. Development of new indicators occurs when no acceptable existing indicator represents nursing's contributions to patient care.

An example of an NSI follows:

> *Design and implementation of procedures to prevent falling when patients get up to go to the toilet is a process entirely in the control of bedside nurses. Using nursing EBP such as initiation of toileting rounds to prevent falls is en-*

tirely in the realm of nursing practice and does not require physicians or any other disciplines to institute. There is evidence that the quality and quantity of nursing care does influence the rate of patient falls. Thus, this is a nursing sensitive quality indicator.

Two examples of an organizational indicator follow:

- *Reducing average length of stay is a common hospital goal, yet getting patients discharged in a timely manner is a complex process involving many disciplines. The physician must write the discharge instructions, the pharmacy must get the patient's discharge medications packaged, the dietitian must instruct the patient on his or her diet, and the business office must get the discharge papers together. Yet, no matter how much the nurse coordinating all these tasks tries to reduce the time involved, if the physician does not write the discharge prescriptions and the pharmacy fails to get them filled and the dietitian does not get to the bedside, no actions by the nurse are going to make a difference. Nurses cannot control this process alone. It is therefore not solely a nursing-sensitive indicator.*

- *The organization would like to improve its success in decreasing the time it takes to get the initial antibiotic administered to patients with a diagnosis of pneumonia in the ED. No matter how hard a nurse tries, he or she cannot fix this issue alone. A physician must write the order for the antibiotic and the pharmacy must dis-*

pense the drug and get it into the hands of the nurses to administer. Unfortunately, no amount of work by the nurse alone can affect this outcome; the improvement requires an interdisciplinary process that involves getting the MD to write the order, the pharmacy to tag this drug as an emergency and mix it in a timely fashion, then figuring out a quick way to get it into the hands of the nurse.

The Agency for Healthcare Research and Quality has listed a number quality indicators to measure healthcare quality. Some are obviously nursing-sensitive and some physician-sensitive, but many are multidisciplinary and require collaboration to monitor and improve quality. They include:

- Complications of anesthesia (PSI 1)

- Death in low mortality diagnosis-related groups (PSI 2)

- Decubitus ulcer (PSI 3)

- Failure to rescue (PSI 4)

- Foreign body left in during procedure (PSI 5)

- Iatrogenic pneumothorax (PSI 6)

- Selected infections due to medical care (PSI 7)

- Postoperative hip fracture (PSI 8)

- Postoperative hemorrhage or hematoma (PSI 9)

- Postoperative physiologic and metabolic derangements (PSI 10)

- Postoperative respiratory failure (PSI 11)

- Postoperative pulmonary embolism or deep vein thrombosis (PSI 12)

- Postoperative sepsis (PSI 13)

- Postoperative wound dehiscence in abdominopelvic surgical patients (PSI 14)

- Accidental puncture and laceration (PSI 15)

- Transfusion reaction (PSI 16)

- Birth trauma—injury to neonate (PSI 17)

- Obstetric trauma—vaginal delivery with instrument (PSI 18)

- Obstetric trauma—vaginal delivery without instrument (PSI 19)

- Obstetric trauma—cesarean delivery (PSI 20)

Healthcare organizations are required to collect quality measures on a number of medical outcomes. For example, the Centers for Medicare & Medicaid Services

(CMS) require multiple measures, from heart failure parameters to pneumonia care to surgical and obstetrical care to be collected. The Joint Commission suggests hospitals collect data on quality measures from inpatient psychiatric services to deep vein thrombosis prevention to childhood asthma care. Though many of these measures certainly have a nursing participation component, the majority require participation of physicians and a measurement of their performance. Therefore collecting these quality measures remain the responsibility of organizational quality improvement resources. It is out of the scope of nursing practice to monitor and measure physician performance. These measures are not NSIs. Examples of NSIs endorsed by the NQF and required by the MRP to be collected and submitted at the unit level can be viewed in Figure 5.1.

ANCC Magnet Recognition Program® Requirements for NSI Collection

The new MRP model unveiled in 2008 requires MRP hospitals and those aspiring to become MRP designated to showcase exceptional outcomes. Exceptional outcomes defined by the MRP include outperforming the mean in multiple NSIs based on a national benchmark. As shown in Figure 5.1, these include a wide array of indicators. In addition, for those units in which Figure 5.1 indicators do not apply, the applying hospital must

choose other specialty-specific, nationally benchmarked indicators. This MRP requirement has led to an explosion of unit/population specific indicators. MRP listservs and networking platforms have produced a number of indicators as represented in the table below. The list continues to grow as more hospitals become interested in population-specific NSIs.

Examples of specialty-specific indicators for units for which the previous do not apply are shown in Figure 5.2. Additional sources (which include organizational and nursing-sensitive indicator examples) to consult for obtaining quality measures for unique units or settings include:

- Healthy People 2010, *www.healthypeople. gov/LHI/lhiwhat.htm*

- State Healthy People 2010, *www.phf.org/ pmqi/state.htm*

- National Quality Measures Clearinghouse, *www.qualitymeasures.ahrq.gov*

- National specialty organizations, nursing professional societies, and networking with other hospitals, other MRP directors, etc.

- State hospital associations

FIGURE 5.1 ▶ NQF AND ANCC MAGNET RECOGNITION PROGRAM® NSIs

Indicator	NQF–Endorsed	ANCC Magnet Recognition Program®–Required
Nursing hours per patient day	Yes	Yes
Skill mix	Yes	Yes
Nurse vacancy rate	No	Yes
Nurse education and certification rates	No	Yes
Falls	Yes	Yes
Falls with injury	Yes	Yes
Nosocomial pressure ulcers incidence and prevalence	Yes	Yes
Patient satisfaction • Nursing care • Pain management • Education	No	Yes
Nursing satisfaction	Yes	Yes
Central line-associated bloodstream infection	Yes	Yes
Catheter-associated urinary tract infection	Yes	Yes
Ventilator-associated pneumonia	Yes	Yes
Restraint use	Yes	Yes
Pediatric IV infiltrations	No	Yes
Nurse work-related injuries • Needle sticks • Musculoskeletal injuries • Exposures	No	Yes

FIGURE 5.2 ▶ SPECIALTY- AND POPULATION-SPECIFIC MEASURES

Unit/Population Type	Indicator (Nurses may be in control of these process measurements, depending on setting)
Neonatal/pediatric	• Medication error rates/1,000 doses/1,000 days • Respiratory synctial virus rates • Readmission for asthma • Unplanned extubation • Pain management in newborns • Ventilator days for neonates
Mental health	• Elopement • Compliance with suicide risk assessment • Seclusion times • Number of days staff attend training programs per year for assaultive behavior • Years experience among unit RN staff at time of patient restraint • Recidivism rates
Obstetrics	• Satisfaction with pain management • Intent to breast feed • Time from birth to first attempt at breast feeding
Outpatient ambulatory clinics	• No-show rate for second clinic visit • Wait times • Left without being seen • Patient satisfaction with discharge information • Accuracy of diagnostic test transcription (correct lab and x-ray orders) • Follow-up calls regarding abnormal test results • Post-procedure follow-up call rates

FIGURE 5.2 ▶ SPECIALTY- AND POPULATION-SPECIFIC NSI EXAMPLES (CONT.)

Unit/Population Type	Indicator
Emergency department (ED)	• Wait times • Left without being seen • Time from triage to physician exam • ST segment elevation myocardial infarction to cath lab • Diagnostic test transcription accuracy (correct x-ray and lab orders) • Compliance with domestic abuse assessment • Post-ED visit follow-up call rates
Critical care units/EDs	• Blood transfusion errors • Compliance with blood transfusion protocols
ORs/PACUs	• Pain management • Hypothermia rates • Nausea/vomiting prevention protocol compliance • Timeout completion rates • Right site surgery compliance

---

ANCC MAGNET RECOGNITION PROGRAM® REQUIREMENTS

NSIs concerning patient outcomes

During the two-year period before applying for MRP designation or redesignation, organizations must collect NSIs on patient outcome data at the unit level and outperform the mean of a national, external benchmark on the following:

- Patient falls and falls with injury

- Nosocomial pressure ulcer incidence and prevalence

- CLABSI

- CAUTI

- Ventilator-associated pneumonia (VAP)

- Restraint use

- Pediatric IV infiltration

Other specialty-specific nationally benchmarked indicators for those units for which the above indicators may not apply (see Figure 5.2)

NSIs concerning nurse work-related injuries

During the two-year period before applying for MRP designation or redesignation, organizations must collect nurse outcome data on nurse injuries and outperform the mean of a national, external benchmark (if available) on the following:

- Needle sticks

- Musculoskeletal injuries

- Exposure to chemicals, toxins, or external agents

NSIs concerning patient satisfaction with nursing

During a two-year period before applying for MRP designation or redesignation, organizations must collect NSI on patient satisfaction data at the unit level and outperform the mean of a national, external benchmark on four of the following:

- Patient satisfaction with pain management

- Patient satisfaction with education

- Patient satisfaction with nurse response time

- Patient satisfaction with courtesy and respect of nurses

- Patient satisfaction with careful listening by nurses

- Other nurse related survey questions

NSIs concerning nurse job satisfaction

Organizations must collect data on nurse satisfaction and engagement at least every two years and the results must outperform the mean of a national, external benchmark.

Other nurse-sensitive outcomes

Organizations must collect other indicators related to nursing outcomes and outperform the mean of a national, external benchmark in regards to the following:

- Nursing hours per patient day

- Nursing skill mix

- RN turnover and vacancy rate

- Percentage of nurses with certification (both leaders and direct care staff members)

- Educational preparation of nurses (both leaders and direct care staff members)

Source: *2008 ANCC Magnet Recognition Program® Manual.*

How to Choose Your NSIs

Choosing which NSI data to collect and analyze can be difficult. While all of them may be appealing in that they are well grounded in the literature and make a difference in patient outcomes, it is important to be thoughtful in selecting priorities because of the time and resources needed. If you are a MRP hospital or are aspiring to be, the NSIs you need to collect and analyze has been set for you. Even if you are not currently aspiring to MRP status, if application for MRP designation is planned in the future, your department needs to have eight-quarters of data on MRP-designated NSIs to apply. Leaders need to look at the number of NSIs and plan strategically which indicators to begin with and add indicators as resources are increased. Collecting NSI data, participating in a national database, analyzing returned data, and developing QI processes based on evidence and best practices is a very timely and resource-intensive endeavor. For example, doing a quarterly pressure ulcer prevalence survey on every pediatric, neonatal, and adult inpatient in one day is labor-intensive and requires tremendous resources to do properly. It is also important to understand that merely collecting data without a plan to use it in a meaningful way is a waste of time. Start slowly with one or two indicators and increase as resources are available. It is important to choose NSIs at the unit level that will have the most impact for the population on that unit. Careful planning will help the process.

Figure 5.3 is a table of NSIs collected at the unit level. Departments of nursing should create a similar grid to easily track what NSIs are being collected.

Step 1: Collecting data

NSI data needs to be collected at the unit level by experts who understand data collection and are familiar with the definitions and requirements of the database. Improving a process is dependent upon accurate data, so accuracy of the data collected is paramount.

For example, skin integrity data collected during a prevalence survey requires that those nurses doing the survey are experts in identifying the stages of pressure ulcers. The National Database of Nursing Quality Indicators® (NDNQI) national database, for example, requires all nurses collecting the data to pass a tutorial and know the definitions for staging. This provides reliability and supports accuracy of the database. Likewise, participation in a falls database requires those nurses collecting fall data to understand the definitions of falls with injury. All database participants need to be in agreement as to what constitutes minor or moderate injuries or an assisted fall before entering this data. Nosocomial infection data that includes CLABSI, CAUTI, and VAP must be collected by nurses expert not only in obtaining surveillance data, but also knowledgeable about the complex national standard definitions indicating infection. Therefore, departments of nursing must not only train certain nurses to collect data, but also train those entering data so consistent and accurate data and results are obtained.

Many nurses have an interest in infection control surveillance, or safety issues such as falls and skin integrity and are good candidates to send to training courses or conferences to learn accurate techniques of data collection. In many hospitals, NSIs are being collected in large

FIGURE 5.3 ▶ TABLE OF NSIs COLLECTED AT THE UNIT LEVEL

	Hours per patient day	Skill mix	Skin integrity	Falls	Length of stay	Patient satisfaction	Nurse satisfaction	Electronic medical record errors	Blood admin errors	Pain management	RN turnover	Additional
Adult med-surg units	Yes	Yes	Yes	Yes	Yes	Yes	Yes	Yes	Yes	Yes	Yes	• Falls prevention (toileting rounds compliance) • CAUTI
ICU	Yes	Yes	Yes	Yes	Yes	Yes	Yes	Yes	Yes	Yes	Yes	• VAP • Restraints • CAUTI • CLABSI
Pediatric	Yes	Yes	Yes	Yes	Yes	Yes	Yes	Yes	Yes	Yes	Yes	• Pediatric IV infiltration • Nasogastric tube verification • Hand hygiene compliance
Neonatal	Yes	Yes	Yes	No	Yes	Yes	Yes	Yes	Yes	Yes	Yes	• Hand hygiene compliance • STABLE© • Retinopathy of prematurity
Psychiatric	Yes	Yes	No	Yes	Yes	Yes	Yes	Yes	No	Yes	Yes	• Seclusion time • Restraints • Elopement • Suicide Risk Assessment
Labor & delivery	Yes	Yes	No	No	Yes	Yes	Yes	Yes	Yes	Yes	Yes	• Intent to breast feed
OR/PACU	No	No	Yes	In preop areas	No	PACU	Yes	Yes	Yes	Yes	Yes	• Hypothermia rewarming (PACU) • Chlorhexadine preparation
ED	Yes	Yes	No	No	ED LOS	Yes	Yes	Yes	Yes	Yes	Yes	• ST-Segment Elevation Myocardial Infarction (Time to cath lab) • Diagnostic test order errors • Domestic abuse screening compliance • ED wait times
Outpatient and clinic	No	No	No	No	No	Yes	Yes	Yes	No	Yes	Yes	• No show rates • Second visit no show • Incorrect diagnostic test ordering • Telephone follow-up

numbers in order to comply with MRP requirements. It may be helpful to designate a nurse expert with QI expertise to coordinate and supervise data management on NSIs; among MRP organizations, the MRP program director is often the person overseeing data collection. Examples of NSI sources, including who often collects such data, is shown in Figure 5.4.

Step 2: Finding accurate NSI data

To ensure consistent data collection, the nursing director must identify the sources of the NSI data and use the same source consistently. Nurse staffing data including hours per patient day and skill mix can be retrieved from HR data in a consistent method. For example, counting patient days can be achieved by various methods, but must be consistent each time the data is collected. Nurse satisfaction data can be retrieved from nationally recognized surveys and the NDNQI database includes a nursing survey that is free to all member hospitals.

Skin ulcer data needs to come from actual hands-on prevalence surveys conducted by skin nurse experts, and restraint data may be obtained at the same time the skin ulcer prevalence survey is conducted. Falls data usually comes from a hospital incident reporting system. Before attempting to collect falls data, the department must feel satisfied that the incident reporting system is capturing the majority of falls. Blame-free cultures that encourage incident reporting in a nonpunitive environment will produce more accurate data than cultures of fear. A culture that ensures that nurses feel safe reporting incidents is of utmost importance to ensure accuracy of the data you are spending a lot of resources to collect and analyze. For example, collecting data on falls is dependent on nurses admitting

to the falls on incident reports, so nurses must be assured of nonpunitive actions if they report an error.

Also, patient satisfaction with aspects of nursing care is an NSI, which may be essentially free data since your organization may already have a patient satisfaction measurement system in place. Nursing can work with patient satisfaction surveys to ensure that there are specific nursing-related questions as required on the questionnaire.

Creating a blame-free culture

Creating a blame-free culture must be an organizational accomplishment. Historically, nurses have had poor compliance with reporting errors for fear of job loss, punishment, humiliation, embarrassment, or confrontation with a nurse manager or leader. In healthcare organizations with old models that "the nurse is always wrong and physician and patient are always right," it is very difficult to change the mind-set of nurses and convince them to report errors, especially in older nurses.

However, as the healthcare profession moves from a top down authoritarian model to recognition of participatory management, more nurses will lose the fear of administrators and embrace a blame-free culture. In addition, hospitals must develop a process to investigate all errors that resulted in harm or potential harm through a near miss. The organization should provide emotional support for staff members involved in an incident that resulted in patient harm. There also must be systems in place to protect staff from malfunctioning equipment, to provide staff with technology proven to increase patient safety such as electronic medical records and bar code scanning for medication adminis-

FIGURE 5.4 ▶ SOURCES OF NSI DATA

Indicators	Source	Who Collects the Data?
• Skill mix • Hours per patient days	• Human resource (HR) data • Acuity system • Time and attendance systems	• HR personnel • IT • Nurse managers
• Patient satisfaction	• Organizationwide vendor (e.g., Press Ganey, HCAHPS)	• Data specialist • Researchers • Quality personnel • MRP coordinator or designated nurse leader
• Nurse satisfaction	• Vendor (e.g., NDNQI, Morehead, AONE)	• Nurse researchers
• Falls	• Incident reporting system	• Quality and safety personnel • Risk manager • MRP coordinator or designated quality nurse
• Skin ulcer incidence and prevalence	• Actual quarterly survey done at the patient's bedside	• Nurse skin specialists trained in recognition of skin ulcer stages • Nurses certified as wound ostomy care nurses • Nurses who have passed the NDNQI tutorial on skin assessment
• Nursing education/ certification	• HR • Database creation specifically for these elements	• Maintained by nursing administration • MRP coordinator or designated nurse leader
• Restraints	• Patient quarterly survey (can be done when the skin survey is done)	• Nurses doing skin survey (in unites not doing skin survey, a designated nurse or charge nurse)
• Nosocomial infections	• Chart review (labs, device days, physician notes)	• Infection control specialist
• RN injury (needlesticks, etc.)	• Workers' compensation office/ HR/safety department	• Workman's compensation, employee health, HR
• RN vacancy rate	• HR • Nurse managers	• HR personnel, nurse managers

tration. Leadership needs to ensure that there is sufficient staffing, functional equipment, and adequate supplies.

To create a blame-free culture that encourages the report of errors and near misses:

> *An organization proves its commitment to fostering safety by encouraging error reporting in a non punitive environment. This type of environment has been described as a 'just culture.' In a just culture, staff members are not afraid to report a safety issue, even if it involved their own error or that of their colleague. In a just culture, staff members are not disciplined for coming forward to report an error or near miss unless it involved misconduct of some kind. By encouraging the open reporting of errors, it is possible to gather important information regarding which of the organization's safety areas are most vulnerable. Staff members should be encouraged to bring forward near misses, as well as events that affected the patient in some way. Near miss events are rich opportunities to proactively improve systems before any patients are harmed.*
>
> *–Lisa Khanna;* The Patient Safety Officer's Handbook, *May 29, 2008*

Nursing Peer Review

This book focuses on systems to set priorities for improvement, select and implement measures, analyze results, and drive improvement. An important parallel activity emerging in the nursing profession is the development of case-specific nursing peer review. This process can be highly constructive, professional, and complementary to systems improvement.

Nursing peer review councils are composed of staff nurses who review the care provided by nurse peers to discover opportunities to improve practice or nursing processes. These reviews may be based on an identified error, an unexpected outcome, a patient complaint, or other triggers. These nonpunitive councils have helped foster environments of trust for practicing bedside nurses who may otherwise fear reporting an error in anticipation of a punitive response. They are also rich sources of insight into opportunities to improve healthcare delivery systems.

Step 3: Benchmarking your data

Choosing to benchmark your data with other like institutions at the national or state level is a decision that needs to be made at the administrative level. If you are a MRP hospital or an aspiring MRP hospital, you must benchmark your NSI data at the broadest level, which means a national database. Benchmarking has a number of advantages in that it gives you the ability to see how you are performing. However, benchmarking also requires action if your performance is worse than the target.

The Centers for Medicare & Medicaid Services now requires participation in a systematic clinical database registry for nursing-sensitive care.[1]

Step 4: Choosing a database

When choosing a database with which to benchmark, it is very important to ensure that your data is collected absolutely according to the database requirements and their definitions. The key is comparing apples to

apples (i.e., you must make sure that your definition of an assisted fall is the same as the definition of an assisted fall in the participating database). This also holds true in matching units to units. Not all psychiatric units have the same patient populations, nor do all surgical units. Comparing fall rates in a neurosurgical unit to fall rates in an ambulatory GI surgery unit are not the same. Patients with brain tumor resections and aneurysm coils have neuromuscular issues that may increase fall rates, making this population very different from patients who have merely had laparoscopic cholecystectomies. In this case, the patient populations are not "apples to apples" and data will not be accurate. It is therefore extremely important to investigate who is in the database and the acuity of the patients in the units. Examples of databases are shown in Figure 5.5. In addition, other database examples include:

- NDNQI®: Includes skin integrity, falls, skill mix, nurse hours per patient days, nurse satisfaction, nurse education and certification levels, pediatric IV infiltration, pediatric pain cycle, restraints, and assaults

- University Health System Consortium Academic Medical Centers: Includes falls, medication error, transfusion error, equipment failure/error, complication of treatment, behavioral indicators (www.uhc.edu)

- National Association of Neonatal Nurses: Includes neonatal parameters (www.nann.org)

- The National Healthcare Safety Network: Includes VAP, CLABSI, CAUTI, surgical site infections, *Clostridium difficile* infections, and more (www.cdc.gov/nhsn)

- Press Ganey: Includes patient satisfaction data (www.pressganey.com)

- Morehead Associates: Includes nurse satisfaction (www.moreheadassociates.com)

- Vermont Oxford Network: Includes neonatal data (www.vtoxford.org)

Check with your state hospital association, department of public health, or other agencies to determine what data are available at the state level. More and more states are collecting and publishing data on these dimensions of care.

The National Database of Nursing Quality Indicators

Because it is a leading tool for improving nursing performance and nursing-sensitive indicators, NDNQI is profiled in the following paragraphs in more detail.

NDNQI® is the only national nursing database that provides quarterly and annual reporting of structure, process, and outcome indicators for nursing-sensitive quality indicators. NDNQI is coordinated by the National Center for Nursing Quality at the University of Kansas School of Nursing. It collects data from participating hospitals on bedded units that include psychiatric and neonatal and pediatric populations. NDNQI® provides quarterly reports at the unit and aggregate level that can be customized for indicator or hospital type. The reports also provide a mean as well as upper and lower quartiles for each indicator. Units that can report

FIGURE 5.5 ▶ EXAMPLES OF DATABASES FOR NSIs

NSIs	Database Examples	Ranges
• Hours per patient day • Skill mix • Vacancy rates	• The National Database of Nursing Quality Indicators© (NDNQI) (*www.nursingquality.org*) • State hospital associations	• National • State
• Nosocomial pressure ulcer incidence and prevalence	• NDNQI • Novation/KCI	• National • National
• Falls • Falls with injury	• NDNQI • University HealthSystem Consortium (UHC) *(www.uhc.edu)*	• National • Academic medical centers
• Patient satisfaction	• Press Ganey *(www.pressganey.com)*	• National
• Nursing satisfaction	• NDNQI • Morehead Associates *(www.moreheadassociates.com)* • *American Organization of Nurse Executives (www.aone.org)*	• National • National
• Nosocomial infection rates • CLABSI • VAP • CAUTI • *Clostridium difficile*	• NDNQI *(www.nursingquality.org)* • State hospital associations • Centers for Disease Control and Prevention *(www.cdc.gov/)* • The National Healthcare Safety Network *(www.cdc.gov/nhsn)*	• National • State • National • National
• Pediatric and neonatal indicators	• Vermont Oxford Network *(www.vtoxford.org)* • National Association of Neonatal Nurses *(www.nann.org)*	• National
• Medication errors	• UHC	• Academic medical centers
• Restraints	• NDNQI	• National
• Nurse vacancy rates	• NDNQI • State hospital associations	• National • State
• Nurse education and certification rates	• NDNQI • MRP	• National • National

to NDNQI® include: critical care, step-down, medical, surgical, combined med-surg, rehabilitation, and psychiatric. Cohorts for comparison can be selected, such as teaching (academic medical centers) hospitals with MRP status or hospitals with similar bed size. NDNQI® enables participating hospitals to make correlations between nurse staffing levels and patient outcomes through the use of this database. Currently, more than 1,200 facilities in the United States contribute to this growing database, and the benefits include improving RN retention efforts and recruitment, research and education, and satisfying reporting requirements for a regulatory agency.

Step 5: Internal benchmarking

There are times when you may not be able to benchmark your NSIs. This may be due to the lack of a database for the indicator or the inability to match your unit population with another unit in the database. In this case, you can benchmark the data internally in a control chart that enables you to set upper and lower limits and a median target. This allows you to evaluate your performance over time as you implement process improvements. NSIs such as vaccination rates, hand hygiene compliance, screenings compliance, etc. can all be internally benchmarked and trended over time.

Similar benchmarking can be performed for specialized areas such as outpatient units, emergency departments, labor and delivery, or behavioral health units that have unique patient populations or difficult to match NSIs.

Step 6: Strategies to improve and control outcomes based on NSI

Improving outcomes based on NSI data is the goal of the QI process. Choosing the strategy you want to implement to improve your outcomes data should be evidence based and best practice. Nurses are already using EBP to improve and streamline patient care. However, it is important to understand the difference between EBP and QI.

EBP can be defined as the collection, interpretation, and integration of research-derived, best available evidence to improve the quality of practice. EBP work involves a search through current literature to select the best nursing practices available to improve a nursing-sensitive outcome.

QI, on the other hand, is a continuous process of defining, measuring, analyzing, improving, and controlling a process to improve care. Improving and ensuring consistent use of a certain practice utilizes or incorporates best practices found through EBP into the improvement process piece.

At this time, the current literature is full of EBP protocols, standards of care, and other nursing activities directly related to NSIs. There is available literature on falls prevention, pain management, preserving skin integrity, restraint reduction, and nosocomial infection prevention bundles. Networking with other departments of nursing, attendance at EBP conferences, professional society conferences, or utilization of Web sites such as the National Nursing Practice Network are all are invaluable to help nurse leaders utilize EBP in their QI projects instead of unnecessarily reinventing the wheel.

Utilizing best practices culled from the literature to address the most pressing NSI improvement is the best strategy nurse leaders can adopt to improve patient outcomes that are nursing sensitive:

Example: An ICU nurse became concerned about the high incidence of IAD in her patients and admitted confusion to her NM on what products and protocols she should be using to prevent this uncomfortable condition that could lead to skin ulceration and breakdown in her patients. The NM was unsure of what could be done and contacted the departments' EBP experts to help with a comprehensive evidence search. Over the course of one year, the staff nurse searched the literature on prevention of IAD and eventually created an algorithm and protocol on prevention of IAD based on best practice. The protocol involved finding the best product among multiple products, a QI process was developed in which multiple products were tried on the ICU until the exact process was controlled. After the protocol was approved by the Practice Committee and instituted on the ICUs, the incidence of IAD dropped dramatically. In this case, patient outcomes were greatly improved due to the institution of EBP that were incorporated into a QI process at the unit level by direct-care nurses.

Common Pitfalls

- **Choosing too many NSIs to collect at the unit level.** Doing so without adequate resources to collect and manage data should be avoided.

Example: Too often nursing departments get in a rush to collect all of the NSIs required by the MRP and end up overloaded with data they

do not know how to manage within nursing. The risk in moving too quickly and trying to collect too many indicators at once is ending up with inadequate collections and subsequent faulty data, and, therefore, faulty benchmarks. Since it is imperative that nursing leaders act on this data and institute QI plans to improve outcomes, this data must be accurate. Start slowly with one or two indicators in select units and build a system that has adequate resources to collect, manage, and interpret the data.

- **Not choosing the most robust benchmark.** Benchmarking data is only valuable when the database being used is robust. In other words, definitions must match and comparison units must match in an "apples to apples" fashion for the results to be valid and reliable.

Example: Comparing falls across all surgical units is potentially unreliable unless you know what those surgical units are. Not all surgical units are a match! A neurosurgical unit is very different from a general GI surgery unit. Patients who have brain resections are more apt to fall than patients in a general GI surgery unit who have had simple laparoscopic cholecystectomies. Therefore, benchmarking and comparing fall rates in these units would lead to grossly inaccurate benchmarking. You must investigate the cohort of units you will be benchmarked with to make sure they are "like units."

- **Collecting inaccurate data.** QI is dependent upon analyzing and measuring data,

and therefore that data must be valid. Hospitals must ensure that those collecting data are expertly trained to know what it is that they are collecting. A common pitfall involves minimally training collectors instead of spending the time and money necessary to have experts collect data.

Example: *Misidentification of prevalence and stages of pressure ulcers by untrained nurses can lead a department of nursing to falsely believe they do not have a skin integrity issue in their patients. Better to spend the time and money training a valid skin team of nurses.*

SELF-ASSESSMENT CHECKLIST

After you read this chapter, be sure you can:

▶ Describe the difference between organizational QI indicators and NSIs

▶ List NSIs endorsed by the NQF

▶ Describe the role of MRP in defining NSIs

▶ List the basic 10 NSIs required by the MRP to be collected at the unit level by MRP hospitals and those aspiring MRP designation

▶ List some examples of population- and unit-specific NSIs that can be collected for these unique patients

▶ Define what individuals should collect NSI data and what skills they need to ensure valid data is being collected

▶ Explain why it is necessary to create a blame-free culture in your institution

▶ Explain why you should benchmark your data at a national level

▶ List possible national databases with which you might want to benchmark your data

▶ List what indicators you might choose to internally benchmark

▶ Understand what NDNQI is and what indicators are available from their database to help you

▶ Understand the value of using EBP in your QI processes

Endnotes

1. CMS, *www.cms.hhs.gov/HospitalQualityInits/08_HospitalRHQDAPU.asp.*

Chapter 6

Engaging Nurses in QI

LEARNING OBJECTIVES

- Discuss methods to successfully engage staff nurses in quality improvement

- Describe ways to hold staff nurses accountable for quality improvement efforts

Improving nursing-sensitive indicators (NSI) or organizational indicators with a nursing component requires participation of direct-care bedside nurses. QI programs designed by organizational-level experts to improve patient care and driven down from the top will not succeed without buy-in from staff members closest to the patient. It is critical that nurses at the bedside are engaged in QI, carrying out the bundles, protocols, and other processes designed to improve quality and safety. Yet getting direct-care nurses involved in QI is difficult in many hospitals, as bedside nurses complain they are already too busy, they do not have enough staff members to carry out complex QI processes, or they do not

feel QI is in the scope of the nursing practice. Nurse leaders must create a culture of engagement in QI, keeping in mind the following concepts:

- QI must be meaningful to nurses and not seen as just a regulatory requirement

- QI must be linked to professionalism

- The processes used in the protocols must be driven by best practice, and nurses must be able to see a direct link between nursing interventions and patient outcomes

- Nurses must understand (and accept) the data

- Nurses must be involved in the process of improvement and in identifying the interventions, action plans, and monitoring

- Nurses must see their efforts rewarded with improved data

The Rules of Engagement

To engage direct-care nurses, nurse leaders need to follow four basic rules:

1. Be transparent with your staff at all times

2. Make accountability for improvement at the unit and staff nurse levels

3. Give your staff the tools to succeed

4. Continually "reward and recognize" improvement

Be transparent

Information and knowledge are crucial to staff engagement in meeting the strategic goals of the healthcare institution. Staff members will be engaged if they know the facts about their organization. In the past, some staff nurses were disengaged hospital employees, focused on patient care and knowing little about issues such as budget or operating margins or market share. Nurse leaders may even have promoted this attitude, rarely sharing budget-sensitive information with staff nurses. However, emerging insights from healthcare and other industries demonstrate that an engaged and informed workforce is crucial to deliver strong performance and efficiency. Nurses have a special role and opportunity in healthcare organizations as licensed professionals who can make an enormous difference in the success of the overall organization, its culture, teamwork, performance, and safety. In these economic times the need for staff nurses to understand the issues facing their institution.

As valued employees who are integral to the success of their organization, nurses need to see that quality outcomes draw patients to their institution and increase market share. Likewise, they need to understand that poor outcomes may cost their hospital its reputation, as well as financial penalties, loss of managed care contracts, any indirect cost increases associated with inefficiency, rework, readmissions, etc. Continued employment may be at risk for nurses who work in hospitals with decreasing market share or budget difficulties. Therefore, all nurses need to know the facts about their institution (good or bad) and understand that it is their job to promote excellence. Nurse leaders need to share the following:

- Operating and capital budgets, market share, and the role of labor cost in the budget

- Performance on key clinical and business metrics

- Strategic goals of their institution

- Market share

- Labor costs/margins

- Institutional strengths, new programs, and plans

The following is an example of how sharing this information can be helpful:

> ***Example:*** *The chief nursing officer (CNO) of a large hospital was told by the hospital CEO that he had to cut the nursing budget, as the*

hospital had a budget deficit due to a decrease in patient census. The CNO shared this information for the first time with all staff nurses during multiple open forums, indicating that nursing positions might have to be cut unless increased census at the hospital occurred. Staff nurses were shocked at the reality of the budget losses. Each unit, fearing fellow staff nurse cuts, created nursing-driven projects to improve patient satisfaction to ensure a continued census and continued employment. Staff nurses requested weekly updates from the CNO regarding how census and budget numbers were faring, creating a new climate of transparency in the nursing department.

Direct-care nurses and QI data

Nurse leaders also need to share benchmarks with direct-care nurses. Nurses want to know how their institution compares to others, especially hospitals in the same market area, on quality measures, and NSIs. Nurses are interested and will be engaged in questions pertaining to their institution, such as the average length of stay for patients with certain conditions; whether patients experience more falls, more skin ulcers, or more cardiac arrests or deep vein thrombosis than patients at other hospitals; or whether patients are more satisfied with their nursing care than patients at other hospitals. Nurse leaders must share these data, good or bad, with their staff. In addition, it is important that nurse leaders let their staff know the unit targets for improving data and engage staff to participate in establishing and monitoring targets for improving results.

How to share data with direct-care nurses

For the busy bedside nurse who do not have the time to view complex data report sheets, the use of colorful, simple graphs can be used to quickly demonstrate unit performance. For example, if you want to show a unit that it is staying within its targets for falls, you can graph falls on a control chart, showing the trends over time.

Control charts allow for monthly or quarterly data points to be placed, and the resulting frequency line can be viewed quickly by busy unit nurses to check their progress. An example of such a chart can be seen in Figure 6.1.

Another way to show direct-care nurses how they are doing at the unit level is to use a unit scorecard. An example of a unit score card for an orthopedics unit is shown in Figure 6.2.

The following is how a nurse leader can share QI data to improve outcomes:

> **Example:** *The nurse manager (NM) of a medical ICU looked at benchmarked data regarding ventilator-associated pneumonia (VAP) rates in her unit compared to VAP rates in other hospitals in the state through the state hospital association. Analysis revealed that her unit's rate was one of the lowest in the state. She had the QI department make a large, colorful graph showing her unit's low VAP rate against the average rate for all participating hospitals in the state. The graph was colorful and easy to see. Her staff were instantly able to see their performance. She posted the graph and made copies for her staff members for a unit staff meeting in which she praised them for adhering to the VAP bundles. Her staff showed pride in their accomplishment and vowed that the unit's VAP rate would be the 'lowest in the state' by the next quarter.*

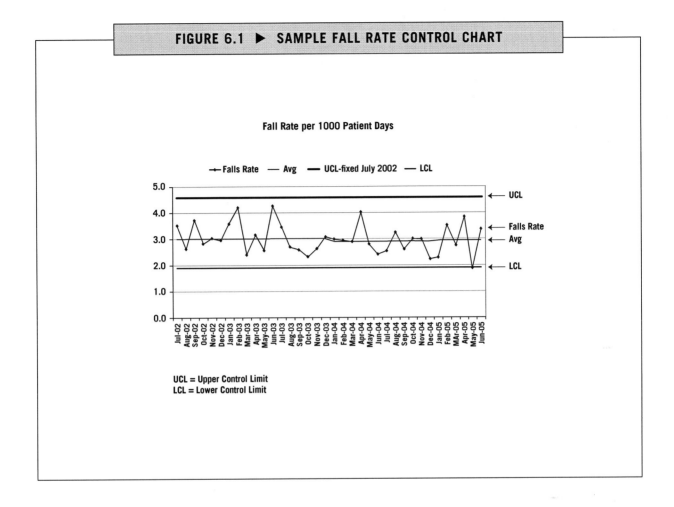

FIGURE 6.1 ▶ SAMPLE FALL RATE CONTROL CHART

FIGURE 6.2 ▶ SAMPLE ORTHOPEDICS UNIT SCORECARD

Orthopedics	FY2006				FY2007		Comments
Quarter	Oct-Dec 05	Jan-Mar 06	Apr-Jun 06	July-Sept 06	Oct-Dec 06	Jan-Mar 07	
Fall prevention project (toileting rounds compliance)	21% 17%	26% 18%	11% 19%	37% 27%	33% 23%	64% 60%	
CAUTI incidence	2.8	1.59	2.06	1.2	0.9*	0.6*	
Skin integrity and pressure ulcer prevalence	0.02	1.23	1.26	2	1.14	0.8	
Patient satisfaction:							
• Overall nursing	82.1%	84.7%	85%	83.5%	81.9%	82.6%	
• Nurse kept patient informed	79.5%	81.5%	81.7%	82.2%	79.4%	81.4%	
• Time nurse spent with patient	78%	79.7%	79.1%	78.3%	77%	78.4%	
RN staff turnover (STN)	3.2%	0%	4.76%	5.4%*	1.00%	1.79%	* 1 STN abandoned job, 1 STN transferred to less acute unit
Unassisted falls /1,000 patient days	0.42	1.59	2.52	2.63	1.25	0.09	
Med error rate/10,000 doses	3.18	3.63	1.3	4.93	4.1	3.37	
Pain assessment compliance	99%	89%	93%	99%	88%	91%	
Hours per patient day (total direct) (target: 7.9)	8.92	8.77	8.44	8.19	8.56	9.3*	* 1;1 patients, higher acuity, increased unit activity (admission/discharge). Budgeted hours per patient day increased from 7.6 to 7.9 on 7/1/06.
Average length of stay (unit # days/percentile)	3.11/16.92%	2.85/6.35%	2.80/7.04%	2.94/15.49%	2.92/11.76 %tile	3.11/8.62%	

Nurse leaders can communicate information about and advertise how their institution is performing in a number of ways:

- Open forums for all nursing staff members

- Newsletters

- Broadcasts/podcasts

- Staff meetings

- Shared governance meetings and quality meetings

- Posted scorecards

- Standardized graphs from benchmarks

- A weekly blog by the CNO

Two examples of how nurse leaders can share this information follow:

- *Every Tuesday, the CNO of a large Midwestern academic medical center writes a personal blog for her staff. The blog is placed on the institution's intranet and is easily accessed from any personal or clinical computer in the hospital. In the blog, the CNO chats about administrative and budget issues in a section called "How are we doing?" The CNO also chooses a couple of quality issues and presents them. For instance, this might be improvement in patient satisfaction data from a unit, or evidence of decreased central line–associated bloodstream*

infection rates in a unit, or comments from a grateful patient.

- *A staff nurse indicated to her NM that she wanted to know how the staff was doing regarding skin ulcer prevention, but she did not have time to read the scorecard posted in the nurses' lounge. In addition, the staff nurse said that all the percentages were confusing to her. The NM asked the organizational quality management department for help in displaying the data in an easier medium and was provided with frequency graphs that showed her unit's data in a bright blue line matched with the benchmark's median in bright red. The next quarter, the same staff nurse said that she noticed their skin ulcer prevalence was below the national median. The NM asked her how she knew this, and she said that she could see their unit's blue line below the red line from across the room while eating her lunch in the lounge.*

Establish accountability at the unit level

The second rule of engagement involves nursing leadership establishing accountability for QI at the unit level. Leaders must establish a culture that reinforces the fact that QI is not some other department's responsibility, but rather is every nurse's job. This makes every unit and every nurse on that unit accountable for improving patient outcomes. Nurse leaders and NMs must communicate this to the staff. During staff meetings, NMs need to share what might be dismal outcomes data and ask the staff, "What are you going to do about it?" They need to share candid information and feedback about progress and areas in which perfor-

mance is poor, even dismal, and challenge the staff to become part of the improvement process.

Strategies may include surveying unit nurses to see what improvement they as a group want to work on first. Or NMs can create unit QI councils with rotating staff members to work on NSIs at the unit level. Goals for improving outcomes should be based on staff consensus; let the staff decide on a target for reducing falls, for example. Staff nurses are more likely to be engaged if they can participate in setting goals, rather than being told by management what goals they must meet, though NMs do need to help staff nurses set appropriate goals. NMs also need to define accountability for quality outcomes in the yearly performance appraisals of their staff members. For instance, the performance appraisal may address goals such as participation in unit quality improvement teams, compliance with safe practices such as hand hygiene or VAP bundle, and mentoring and teaching new staff the fall prevention protocols. All of these can be appropriate professional accountabilities of a bedside staff nurse.

Another example of how nurse leaders can successfully make accountability a priority follows:

> **Example:** The NM of a palliative care unit noted that patient satisfaction with respite care on her unit was far below the national average. Some of the comments on satisfaction surveys included complaints of too much noise, too many interruptions, and lack of comfort for family members staying with them. The NM presented this to her staff and appointed a unit quality council with staff members from all shifts to look at improving patient satisfaction.

> Of the three issues, the unit council with direct-care input decided to tackle the noise issue first. Suggestions were collected from staff members and patients, current literature was reviewed, and a QI plan was created by staff nurses. In two quarters, patient satisfaction increased 25% due to staff nurse efforts. The NM recognized that staff engagement occurred at a high level because this was a program created and driven by staff nurse colleagues, rather than a policy written by nurse leaders that was forced on the staff from the top down.

The design and implementation of improvement occurs most effectively with substantial frontline participation. Many nurse managers create unit QI councils with rotating staff to work on NSIs at the unit level.

Provide the tools needed for better engagement

Bedside staff nurses will not become engaged in QI unless nurse leaders educate them on the basic pieces of QI. This is tricky as the curricula for quality management are abundant, and overwhelming bedside nurses with too much QI information confirms to them that they do not have time to do this, or that QI is not in the scope of nursing. QI and quality management information must be basic, geared toward nursing, and reinforced with practical examples. The following QI questions need to be answered:

- What is QI, why do it, and what is nursing's role?

- What are NSI versus organizational indicators?

- What is benchmarking, why do we need to do this, and what benchmarks do the institution and the unit use to compare outcomes?

- How do I read dashboards, scorecards, frequency graphs, and run or control charts?

- What evidence-based practices (EBP) can be used to improve NSI data?

Bedside nurses can get this information through unit in-services, Web-based programs, or staff meetings where information about data can be shared little by little. An example of what one nursing department did to help increase direct-care nurse knowledge about QI follows:

> **Example:** The department of nursing at an academic medical center requested that the nursing quality department create a four-hour in-service titled 'Nursing QM 101' for bedside staff members. The in-service covered all the basic tools listed previously, with time to practice looking at dashboards and control charts. The in-service was so popular with staff nurses and mid-level managers that it is now offered twice a year.

In addition to educational tools, bedside nurses need time to work on QI projects. NMs need to schedule non-patient care time for staff nurses on QI committees or who are working on unit-based QI projects. Allowing a few hours of nonpatient care or release time to do this will increase engagement and may motivate other

nurses to get involved. An example of how this can be accomplished follows:

> **Example:** The nursing manager of a large medical-surgical floor was concerned about staff nurse satisfaction data that indicated nurses outside her unit disliked floating to this large unit because they did not know how the unit worked or where supplies were. She asked for staff nurse volunteers to create a unit-based QI committee called QIC to look at ways to improve nursing satisfaction through the use of 'pull nurse packets' that gave float nurses what they needed to care for patients on her floor. The three nurses on the committee were given four hours of nonpatient care time a week for four weeks to work on the packets. The packets that resulted from this committee's work increased both float nurses satisfaction rates in regard to floating to the unit and the unit's staff satisfaction with working with floated nurses. In addition, the NM found that many of her direct-care staff wanted to volunteer for other QIC projects.

Reward and recognize nurse involvement in QI

One of the easiest ways to engage staff members in QI is positive reinforcement through reward and recognition of their efforts. Nurses can be recognized at the unit level by their colleagues, or at the divisional, departmental, or institutional level. Examples of ways to recognize and reward nurses include the following:

- Publicize all QI projects on the unit or in the department through newsletters, the

intranet, or other hospital publications. Even utilize local media outlets to publicize nurses and their projects.

- Set aside a day to recognize nurses who have made a difference through QI projects. Utilize poster displays of the projects and post them in the lobby for all to see.

- Publish the QI project and the outcomes in a professional journal.

- Encourage a friendly competition between units to improve NSI with rewards such as food, small gifts, etc.

- Use divisional or departmental rewards for units with the most improved data.

Example: *The department of nursing at an academic medical center has a Nursing Recognition Day every spring in the hospital lobby with high patient, family, and visitor exposure. During this event, nurses set up posters of their QI projects and the outcomes achieved. The posters remain on display in the lobby and on the intranet. In addition, First, Second, and Third Place and Best in Show awards are given to the winning posters, along with a $100 certificate to the winners to put toward an educational event. Each year, the number of posters representing a unit-based staff nurse QI projects increases.*

Example: *The NICU at a large academic hospital recently celebrated 365 days without a*

central line–associated bloodstream infection. Nursing leadership surprised the NICU nurses with a large cake for the unit and a poster placed in the main lobby of the hospital with the NICU nurses' pictures and their accomplishment. A local news reporter who happened to be at the hospital that day requested the opportunity to put a copy of the poster and the achievement in the local newspaper for the entire community to see.

Example: *A friendly competition among units at flu vaccination time occurs in a large Midwestern hospital every year. The goal of the organization and the department of nursing is a 100% healthcare staff vaccination rate. The department of nursing decided to reward the nursing units with the highest vaccination rates with free pizza for every shift. In addition, unit vaccination rates were published on a colorful graph in the main lobby for all patients and visitors to see. This friendly competition has increased staff vaccination rates each year, culminating in multiple units with 100% vaccination compliance rates.*

Engaging nurses in QI can be accomplished with a strategic plan that involves elements of the four rules of engagement as indicated earlier in this chapter. The creation of this culture will not occur overnight, but with continual adherence to an engagement plan, nurses will see the end results. Remember, nurses must see the results of their efforts, have time to do work asked of them (not layered on top of another assignment), be passionate about performing the work, and receive rewards and recognition.

Monitoring and Implementing Different Programs

With the responsibility as a department to improve NSIs, nurse leaders must approach the major NSI at both the departmental and unit levels. We outline some examples in the following sections.

Falls prevention

The following steps can be taken to help reduce falls:

- Create an EBP falls prevention committee at the departmental level.

- Engage patients and families and learn from their concerns and suggestions.

- Develop in-services or continuing education programs for all staff nurses on why patients fall and EBP practices to prevent them.

- Make the department falls committee responsible for falls data obtained through an incident reporting system. The committee should analyze Pareto chart data on the organization's falls and focus on 20% of the units that have 80% of the falls.

- Give the units with the highest falls specific QI projects involving processes gleaned from EBP on falls prevention that involve bedside staff nurse practices such as toileting rounds, low-bed usage, floor mats, foam chairs, family education, bed alarms, and frequent faller protocols.

- Ensure that all units are provided with monthly or quarterly updated control charts and scorecards on falls on their units matched with a national benchmark.

- Reward and recognize at the institutional, departmental, and unit level all successes resulting in fall reductions.

Skin integrity

The nurse leader should take the following steps to reduce ulcer incidence and prevalence:

- Provide trained skin experts such as wound ostomy certified nurses as resources for bedside nurses.

- Create an EBP departmental skin committee with unit-based skin champions.

- Develop in-services or CE programs for all staff nurses on EBP-based skin integrity protocols and practices that protect patients' skin.

- Conduct quarterly incidence and prevalence skin surveys. Skin surveys should be done only by trained skin experts.

- Ensure good tools fare available for skin assessment monitoring documentation, appropriate products are available for skin care and physicians are engaged to address nutrition, skin interventions and other EBP skin treatments.

- Identify areas that need skin integrity improvements and create QI projects that utilize EBP. Unit-based QI projects might include projects to improve heel ulceration in the ICU or reduction of cervical collar ulcers on a neurosurgery unit.

- Recognize at the institutional, departmental, and unit level all successes resulting in skin integrity improvement.

Pain management

The nurse leader should take the following steps to better manage patient pain:

- Create an EBP departmental pain committee.

- Engage patients and families, learning from their concerns and suggestions

- Designate and train certified pain resource nurses who are divisionally based to identify QI opportunities to improve pain management.

- Utilize and analyze pain assessment and intervention audits of the medical record. Examine patient satisfaction surveys and conduct targeted patient interviews to identify areas of opportunity.

- Create a department level continuing education program on pain management techniques and EBP strategies to reduce patient pain.

- Reward and recognize units that have increased patient satisfaction with pain management.

- Create pain improvement QI projects utilizing EBP at the unit level to meet the needs of unique patient populations such as neonates or the elderly.

Vacancy rate

Encourage each unit to create a staff nurse committee to address and improve retention of nurses and reduce vacancy rates. Some unit-based EBP examples include the following:

- Develop a self-scheduling process with a team of staff nurses that addresses scheduling preference, vacation scheduling, and fairness

- Encourage development of social committee programs

- Pair new nurses with older staff members

Examples of departmental-based initiatives include:

- Graduate nurse residency programs

- Shared governance retention committees

- Identify experienced staff nurse mentors at the departmental level willing to provide support to other bedside nurses regardless of unit

Patient satisfaction

The following are examples of nurse-driven QI projects aimed at improving patient satisfaction to a large academic medical center:

- A project to reduce patient and family anxiety and confusion through the use of prepared scripts for a multitude of frequent patient questions.

- Increase patient satisfaction in an outpatient chemotherapy infusion unit by increasing patient throughput.

- Increase patient satisfaction on an orthopedic floor through reduction of average length of stay through redesign of discharge process.

- Increase patient satisfaction through reduction of noise on an oncology unit through the use of EBP on improving patient environments.

- Reduce perineal skin ulceration resulting from incontinence-associated dermatitis through the use of EBP project on a standard skin protocol for ICU patients.

- Increase patient satisfaction in regard to pain management at the unit and departmental levels through the creation of a cohort of trained pain management resource nurses to help bedside nurses manage their patients' pain.

Nurse satisfaction

QI projects to improve nurse satisfaction need to be coordinated at both the departmental and unit levels. Examples of departmental projects include:

- A retention committee to evaluate NM workload

- Older-nurse focus groups

- Increased nursing recognition (via programs such as the DAISY© Award)

- Increased staff nurse membership on departmental retention committee

- Optimal float nurse program design and implementation

- Use of staff nurse council suggestions

- Nurse staffing advisory council

QI projects to address nurse satisfaction at the unit level include:

- Development of unit-based scheduling protocols and self-scheduling

- Development of educational processes on improving collegial relationships at the unit level. This process may include the implementation of social committees, journal clubs, unit projects, intercollegiate task forces to improve interdisciplinary unit staff, including physicians, pharmacists,

social workers, etc., with discussion regarding communication and collaboration.

- Improvement of preceptor programs to provide a preceptor to each new nurse or utilize departmental mentoring program

- Development of methods to ensure release or nonpatient care time for shared governance and preceptor activities

Common Pitfalls

- **Lacking transparency.** Direct-care nurses want to be proud of their care and will become engaged in trying to improve

patient outcomes as long as they know the bare facts. Nurse leaders must share both the good and the bad news with them. Being in the dark only creates confusion ... not action.

- **Not giving direct-care nurses enough recognition.** Nurses are sensitive to lack of recognition for the hard work they do every day. Nurses sometimes feel overlooked, such as when physicians and not bedside nurses are continually praised by an organization in its publications and media. It is important to regularly and systematically recognize and reward bedside staff nurses for their quality improvement work. Celebrate improved data all the time, every time.

SELF-ASSESSMENT CHECKLIST

Before moving on, ensure you can do the following:

- ▶ List the rules of engagement required to ensure that your nurses embrace a quality culture
- ▶ Understand what organization knowledge you should be transparent about with your direct-care nurses
- ▶ Understand the tools you can use to share outcome data with your direct-care staff
- ▶ Describe some activities at the unit level you can use to reward and recognize direct-care staff participation in QI processes
- ▶ List some strategies at the departmental level to improve patient NSI outcomes
- ▶ List some strategies at the unit level to improve patient NSI outcomes

---

Process Improvement Basics

> **LEARNING OBJECTIVES**
>
> - Define process improvement
> - Explain the risks and benefits of process improvement
> - Describe cultural factors that affect process improvement

- Performance fails to meet the target, threshold, or goal consistently

- Performance becomes variable as well as inconsistent

- Patients/customers express dissatisfaction, although performance has been stable (perhaps their needs have changed although your process has not)

- Benchmarks or research suggest that better performance is achievable

- The measure represents an important aspect of care or service for patients/customers so that you are willing to allocate resources and priorities to its improvement

Sometimes performance cannot be improved within the current process. If it is important to improve this particular measure of performance, you may need to step back to review and reengineer the current process, whether administrative or clinical. Process improvement requires a serious investment of time, energy, and staff commitment and, if implemented properly, can result in significant benefits. It also carries significant potential risks.

When Measurement Might Lead to a Process Improvement Effort

Sometimes you'll find that you select a measure and, upon review over a period of time, you discover that your:

If so, this is a process you consider for possible improvement. As we saw in Chapter 4, a process with common cause variation is a good candidate for redesign.

Introduction to Process

A process is a sequence of interrelated activities that convert inputs from suppliers into outputs for customers. A process could be, for example, obtaining a diagnostic test for a patient—composed of a series of separate processes, such as:

- Ordering the test

- Obtaining the specimen

- Labeling the specimen

- Transporting the specimen

- Receiving the specimen

- Selecting the equipment, reagent, or other tools to conduct the test

- Conducting the test

- Recording the results

- Communicating the results

When does a process begin and end? In the example above, it's a comprehensive definition including many steps. The operational definition of a process depends on the purpose of the definition. If all steps in the process appear to be working well except labeling specimens correctly, then you might focus on just that piece of the process.

For a clinical path work group, the process encompasses all activity from scheduling the inpatient stay through discharge or beyond. For a process improvement team within a department, the process may be very limited (e.g., receive, store, and retrieve records efficiently and accurately).

A formal definition of process improvement is to redesign a process to produce a measurably different outcome. This means that the new process is statistically stable (see Chapter 4).

An informal way to describe process improvement is referenced in Figure 4.1 in Chapter 4: "We know this process is important; we have reason to believe that the process is not optimally designed to produce the results our patients/customers want; let's use our quality improvement methodology to analyze the process and its outcomes and redesign it as needed."

Risks and Benefits of Process Improvement

The obvious benefit of process improvement is, of course, improved results for patients or customers. This is fundamental, and if you can't achieve that goal then the undeniably significant effort involved in process improvement won't be worth it. But there are also other benefits and risks.

A secondary important benefit is that process improvement, when implemented competently, builds teamwork, develops a deep understanding of process, continues to produce better and more reliable outcomes over time, and sparks truly creative and innovative ideas for quantum leaps in performance.

Example: A team is formed to work on medication availability. Representatives from pharmacy and nursing work together to understand the process from medication order to delivery of the medication to the inpatient unit. Both groups gain a deeper understanding of their shared process, learn respect for the others' challenges and expertise, and collaboratively design an improved process. Medications are available more quickly to the units, and both departments receive solid data demonstrating the results of their work. Over time, they continue to meet periodically to monitor the data together and are able to flag signs of potential problems and tweak the process to avoid those problems without waiting for them to interfere with the overall outcome before action is taken.

There are both obvious and more subtle risks involved in this teamwork model. The most obvious risk is that you will invest time, energy, money, and other resources and may fail to improve the process. This can unleash additional negative effects such as discouraging staff, impairing management credibility, and creating skepticism for future efforts.

A less obvious risk is that you may improve the performance metric you intended to improve but unintentionally interfere with other elements of the process that work reliably or introduce new sources of variation and potential harm.

Example: A medication availability team is formed in another organization. The group develops good team dynamics and designs a new process that is effective in the short term. However, within a few months, it becomes apparent

that the process does not work well on evening/night and weekend shifts because the team did not thoroughly review all aspects of the process. The team goes back to the drawing board to work on these other shifts.

One change the team makes is to place an increased number of commonly used IV fluids and medications in the floor stock rather than waiting for the pharmacy to deliver them, labeled, for each patient. This definitely speeds up access to the products, and nursing staff are pleased. Within a month, there are one or two medication errors that result from this change because a nurse selects the wrong product from the floor stock. The errors are identified but cause no patient harm and are believed to be due to individual nurse carelessness. Not until a third error causes significant patient harm is it recognized that the process change improved timely availability (on some shifts) but created an unacceptable level of risk in this organization and patient population.

A final risk is one of opportunity cost. By spending a great deal of time on one process improvement, you are implicitly making the decision not to commit the time and energy to other processes and improvement opportunities. If your initial selection was not appropriate, that's not a good use of resources.

Example: A team is formed in the operating room to work on improving turnover time between cases. After several months, the team has succeeded in reducing room turnover time from 30 minutes to 25 minutes, with meaningful although modest cost savings. However, at that point, a Joint Commission survey finds that there is poor compliance with the mandatory Universal Protocol™ to avoid

wrong patient/procedure/site, and the organization is required to implement a very rapid improvement effort and corrective action to come into compliance. A more comprehensive risk assessment should have identified this as a high-risk and problem-prone process that put patients and the organization at risk.

Selecting a process for improvement

The first candidates for process improvement will be those that affect important aspects of care and service for key customer populations. As always, whether a process is high volume, high risk, and problem prone is a key consideration when evaluating it for possible improvement focus. Based on baseline measures, processes that are not in statistical control would also be good candidates.

Most departments don't have the capacity to work on more than one process improvement effort at a time. In addition, if you try to work on two different processes, there is a chance that improvement in one will have an effect on the other. Limit these significant projects to one at a time, and give each one the time and resources it needs to be completed carefully, thoroughly, and accurately before moving on to the next one.

Developing a process improvement opportunity statement

As has been emphasized throughout this book, you won't be able to improve a process or performance measure unless you define it clearly. For a process improvement effort, you will need an opportunity statement or charter (see Figure 7.1). This simple outline answers basic questions, such as:

- What is this process? What are its boundaries?

- How does it affect the performance of important functions?

- Who believes it is important enough to sponsor it and allocate resources?

- Why is it important to our patients/customers at this time?

- Who will work on the improvement?

Answer these questions, and define clear priorities among all who will work on the process improvement before the team is convened.

By now it should be clear to you that process improvement tends to be focused on complex processes. If they were simple and easy to improve, we would have been able to adjust performance levels without a complete redesign. Similarly, processes that need redesign are often those that cross department boundaries (see the previous example of medication availability).

All departments involved in a process redesign need to share the priority and sense of urgency to address the performance problem. Each needs to contribute at least staff time and a commitment to implement the team's recommendations. Only by producing a clear opportunity statement in advance can you ensure that you will have this level of support.

FIGURE 7.1 ▶ SAMPLE PROCESS IMPROVEMENT TEAM CHARTER

Process Improvement Opportunity Statement

Process name/description: Improve surgical timeout	**Team leader:** OR manager
Process begins with what step: Patient enters OR	**Team members:** List all departments involved in this process and representative(s) from each
Process ends with what step or deliverable: Timeout is complete and documented	OR manager OR medical director
Sponsor name: OR medical director and vice president for surgery	OR nurses OR techs
Primary customers: Patients	Surgeons Anesthesiologists
Other customers: All staff in OR	CRNAs

Proposed Measures of Performance
(process and outcome measures as relevant)

Institute of Medicine's dimensions	Applies? Y/N	Current performance	Goal (if known)	Specific metric (if known)
Effective Complete information?	Y	80% complete	100%	All required elements completed.
Safe Always done?	Y	90%	100% (excluding trauma, etc.)	Some surgeons skip this.
Patient-centered Scripted to reassure patient, if awake?	Y	No script in place.	Script in place and used when appropriate.	
Timely Performed immediately before incision?	Y	Don't know.	Document time on the T/O record.	100% documented and immediately before incision.
Efficient Easy to perform, all elements included, documented?	Y	Poor. Staff say that they find it cumbersome.	100% in compliance and staff satisfied.	To be determined.
Equitable	N/A	Not believed to be an issue.		

Link to organization strategic plan:
Our plan calls for safe care according to evidence-based guidelines.

Link to established organization goals:
We have a goal to achieve zero "never" or sentinel events associated with preventable harm, and we know that the timeout is designed to eliminate wrong-patient, wrong-site, wrong-procedure events. We have a goal to achieve accreditation without requirements for improvement.

Specifically, why should this process improvement be a priority at this time?
Our self-assessment indicates that our timeout performance is not reliable. Although we have not had a wrong-patient, wrong-site, or wrong-procedure event, we could place patients at risk and could risk a citation from The Joint Commission. We should invest the time and energy to improve this process.

Establishing a viable process improvement team

Why do you need a team?

Processes can probably be redesigned by management fiat, but in many cases, that will guarantee failure. It is better to convene a team to work on a process because:

- Including frontline staff ensures that you get a real-life and deeper view of the process as it is actually implemented—not as it may be described in policies and procedures.

- Including a variety of people improves the chances that you'll get creative ideas.

- Sharing the effort among departments and management/staff levels builds commitment to the analysis and recommendations.

- In busy hierarchical organizations—characteristics typical of healthcare delivery—there is a tendency for each department to focus exclusively on its own goals and to fail to build a sense of shared process. Teamwork helps to break down these barriers and improves performance much beyond one effort; it contributes to an overall improved culture of quality and improvement throughout the organization.

What is the purpose of a team?

Teams differ from traditional committees and task forces in a couple of core ways. They are convened specifically to research a problem or opportunity with open minds and to contribute unique individual expertise. A team is never convened to build consensus around a predefined outcome—that may be a function of a committee or other group but not a process improvement team.

Teams tend to be more egalitarian than traditional committees and task forces. Each member of the team has been selected for personal knowledge of the process being improved and is expected to contribute advice, ideas, and creative perspectives.

Teams tend to go through interpersonal developmental stages that can be challenging. Relationships are more important in a group conducting a creative, shared investigation than they are in a hierarchically driven committee. See the Bibliography for resources available to assist team leaders in managing effective teams.

Who should participate on a team?

A team should include staff members who are close to the process being analyzed. Often, this will include professional/technical staff, frontline managers, etc.

The team leader may be a manager or a staff member with leadership training and aptitude. Depending on the resources in your organization, the team leader may have a facilitator or process consultant assigned to provide conceptual and technical support as the team conducts its work.

The team must be sponsored by a leader who has the ability to allocate resources and respond to the team's work products constructively. This leader must meet with the team regularly, review its work products, and address the team's recommendations.

Cultural Factors: Systems and Blame

Effective QI demands the involvement of all staff members who participate in the operational process, and it demands their willingness to view themselves as part of a system. If physicians, nurses, management, and others cling to a belief that quality outcomes could be ensured if everyone would just do their jobs more carefully, you won't be able to develop truly high-reliability and high-quality care processes.

Further, as long as staff members believe they will be punished if they reveal personal shortcomings, errors, and potential errors, they will simply not identify those issues that could actually improve the process. The terms "blame-free culture" and "just culture" are beginning to circulate in the healthcare field to denote an environment in which it is openly acknowledged that people make mistakes, care is delivered as part of a system, and improvement of that system is the only way to improve care. Such a culture asserts—and demonstrates—that staff will not be punished for identifying ordinary human error (as opposed to malicious, criminal, or flagrantly reckless conduct). And such a culture proves itself by investing resources in systems improvement that makes the work and care environment safer, more productive, more rewarding, and more deserving of trust.

This kind of culture is not achieved quickly. Not only do physicians maintain a powerful concept of personal accountability, but both physicians and nurses are aware that their licenses can be at risk for certain kinds of errors and quality outcome failures.

Within an individual department, steps you can take toward a just or systems culture include:

- Maintaining an overriding focus on the ultimate goal of your department, such as care or service that measurably meets the needs of the patient/customer

- Paying most of your attention to systems measurement and improvement

- Ensuring that interdisciplinary communication is always respectful and appropriate

- Keeping all discussions of performance focused on the system of care and barriers to the effective use of the system

- Prohibiting group or public discussions that focus on identified individual performance issues

- Building an effective system that screens for individual performance problems and a confidential, effective method to address them

- Adhering to principles of confidentiality, fairness, and equitable treatment of all staff members

Physician Participation on QI Committees and Process Improvement Teams

Sometimes it is just not practical to expect physicians to participate fully on teams. Meetings that last several hours don't accommodate a clinician's schedule. Instead, identify where the physician's contribution is essential. Use the following strategies:

- Include physicians on a team only when they have a substantive role in analyzing past performance and designing new systems, and then include them only at critical points.

- Meet with physicians individually, at their convenience, to rapidly and comprehensively outline the problem, progress, and conclusions to date. Don't allow the physician to veto all that has occurred, but do listen to any concerns raised.

- Focus in particular on physician input on evidence-based guidelines for practice and care decisions and interpretation of the literature.

- Focus on physician input when redesigning the system at points that involve the physician—(e.g., communication, orders, and results) and that affect patients directly.

- Insist on vigorous physician leadership involvement when it is genuinely needed.

Critical Team Success Factors and Important Analytic Tools

There are many resources focused on successful leadership of improvement teams (see Appendix C). Critical success factors for a team include:

- A clear, well-organized opportunity statement or charter that specifies the process and the performance measures

- Strong sponsorship by a leader who can:
  - Allocate resources for data collection and process support
  - Ensure that the team's work has an appropriate priority
  - Give the team marching orders that are realistic in scope

- The collaborative involvement of staff from relevant departments or professions/disciplines, including frontline staff who actually work with the process

- Good support for measurement and analysis, including experts who can consult on statistics and other methodologies (see next section)

- Disciplined leadership and an approach to quality improvement (see Chapter 3) that keep the project on track for accountability and timeliness

- Organizational willingness to act on recommendations

Typical steps in a team process improvement approach will include the well-known Plan, Do, Check/Study, Act (PDCA) or other similar descriptions of methodology (see Chapter 3).

The tools that will be useful to a process improvement team are more extensive and creative than the simple and straightforward measurement strategies outlined in Chapter 4 for baseline monitoring.

As the team moves through each phase of its work, different tools will be relevant. See Figure 7.2 for an outline of typical phases and tools and the Appendixes for additional tools. The following list breaks down the PDCA cycle.

Plan

For an effective improvement effort, the plan phase (including a clear definition of the problem and its root causes) must be comprehensive and accurate. If the diagnosis is incomplete, the therapy won't address it. Do not skimp on this phase. Important tools include the flow chart, Failure Modes and Effects Analysis (FMEA), cause-and-effect diagrams, and a thorough set of data elements to measure the process. Although not a quality improvement tool, the use of thorough literature reviews and benchmarking is appropriate at this phase as well.

Do

The next phase involves setting specific objectives and metrics, designing the improved process, and, usually, pilot testing it. This, too, must be thorough.

In addition, you will be examining the process for any evidence of unintended consequences—other aspects of the process that no longer perform reliably or new sources of error or harm that have been introduced unwittingly into the process. The FMEA tool offers one method to do this prospectively, even before you test the process in actual practice.

If possible, the process should include engineered features such as alerts, reminders, and forcing functions. A good mantra for process design is, "The easiest thing to do should be the effective and safe thing to do." Good process design should also include built-in feedback loops to keep the members of the work group fully informed about progress with the new process.

Check/study

The redesigned process must be tested carefully in theory and then in practice (check phase). You will be looking for improved performance in your primary process measures, of course.

Act

When the team and sponsor are prepared with thorough evidence that the new process works effectively and has not introduced new sources of variation or error, leadership should be ready to implement the process with appropriate resources and continued measurement. At this stage, the tools will be organizational management tools: policies, procedures, accountability for personal and group goals, training, and the features of the process design.

Sustaining the gains achieved by a process improvement team is surprisingly difficult. Change can be challenging, and the redesigned process may take time to settle in and become fully integrated into operations. The feedback loop described in "Do" and other engineered process features will be important to ensure that this occurs.

FIGURE 7.2 ▶ PROCESS IMPROVEMENT PHASES AND TOOLS

PLAN

Actions	Tools
Identify the process, its purpose, and its boundaries	• Data inventories: complaints, performance measures • Brainstorming • Focus groups, interviews
Identify process customers and their expectations, professional literature, and standards	• Brainstorming • Focus groups, interviews, surveys • Literature review
Map the process and identify potential causes of variation and failure	• Flow charts (macro and micro) • Failure Mode and Effects Analysis (FMEA) • Cause-and-effect diagram (fishbone) • Relationship maps • Interviews • Force field analysis • Nominal group technique
Measure and analyze performance and variation	• Data collection from existing and new sources • Basic data analysis graphics: histogram, run chart, control chart, Pareto chart, scattergram, correlation, t-test, analysis of variance • Cost-of-quality analysis • Lean value stream mapping
Identify root causes of actual and potential defects	• Brainstorming • Cause-and-effect diagram • FMEA • "Five whys" • Root-cause analysis framework (The Joint Commission)

DO

Actions	Tools
Create measurable improvement objectives	• Brainstorming • Literature review, benchmarking
Devise strategies to achieve objectives	• Brainstorming • FMEA • Literature, evidence basis, benchmarking • Lean value stream mapping
Develop action plan	• Flow-charting • Action plan format • Organizational framework (policies, procedures)
Implement action, possibly as a pilot test	• Organizational framework (accountability and authority)

FIGURE 7.2 ▶ PROCESS IMPROVEMENT PHASES AND TOOLS (CONT.)

CHECK

Actions	Tools
Collect data on the pilot test or improvement implementation	• Data collection from existing and new sources • Basic data analysis graphics: histogram, run chart, control chart, Pareto chart, scattergram, correlation, t-test, analysis of variance • Cost-of-quality analysis
Analyze the results	• Compare to objectives • Repeat FMEA • Return to Plan and Do to refine the design if needed

ACT

Actions	Tools
Implement the improvement comprehensively	• Organizational framework (accountability, authority, policies, procedures, training, engineered supports such as alerts, reminders, forcing functions, improved equipment, resources, environment, etc.)
Track the improvement to ensure sustained performance for an appropriate period of time	• Quality improvement program

Common Pitfalls

- Undertaking process improvement with a predetermined but not proven idea of the proper improvement or solution

- Underestimating the difficulty of conducting a thorough plan phase

- Skimping on the plan, thoughtful data collection, and investigation

- Underestimating the time commitment and, sometimes, interpersonal challenges in leading a team

- Having difficulty developing creative approaches that improve performance and efficiency (value) simultaneously

- Failing to challenge the team with literature, benchmarks, and best practices from others

- Failing to provide adequate team support for data analysis and use of creative and possibly unfamiliar methodologies, such as FMEA

- Being in too much of a hurry for thoughtful analysis and design

- Being too slow and allowing the team to lose momentum amid other priorities

- Failing to monitor the revised process design for unintended results: introduction of new sources of variation, new failure modes, and risks of defects or harm

- Failing to allocate adequate resources to sustain the improvement over the long term

SELF-ASSESSMENT CHECKLIST

▶ Your team selected a process that was important

▶ The process was demonstrably in need of improvement

▶ The team expectations were realistic

▶ The team had effective sponsorship at a level that was senior enough to allocate resources and priority

▶ The team had technical support in facilitating brainstorming and using methodologies such as FMEA and cause-and-effect diagrams

▶ The team had access to data and tools to analyze the data

▶ The team had enough time but not so much time that it lost momentum

▶ The team had regular opportunities to review its progress with its sponsor and other leaders

▶ The team knew the scope of its work and goal and remained focused and realistic

▶ The recommendations were targeted, well engineered, and in scope

▶ Leaders ensured that the recommendations were thoroughly tested and vetted for effectiveness

▶ The demonstrably useful recommendations were implemented and sustained for an extended monitoring period

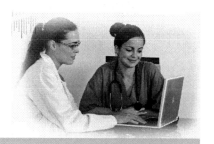

Appendix A

Quality Reporting and Communication

Strong operations management means that you're an effective communicator and leader to your staff. The performance improvement (PI) or quality improvement (QI) plan gives you a tool to organize the work of the department to produce effective results. Steady, consistent information sharing with staff members is critical to ensure their involvement and commitment to mutual improvement goals.

By the end of this appendix, you will have designed a communication flow that ensures that every employee is aware of, and invested in, the quality plan. Each employee will understand how it is possible to take a role in developing and refining the plan, and each employee should be able to describe his or her role in improving the care and service offered by the department.

Further, at the end of this appendix, you will have an effective system in place for documentation of this communication to ensure compliance with relevant Joint Commission and other accreditation/regulatory requirements that pertain to your organization.

The Importance of Communication in QI

Good managers know that quality does not happen by fiat or executive order but is the result of staff members' comprehensive understanding of what is expected of them, why it is appropriate to expect it, how they will be supported to deliver that quality, and how they will be evaluated according to defined criteria. Communication is core to QI in:

- Defining the expectations of the organization for each employee's performance

- Clearly linking those expectations to the mission

- Outlining for employees how their individual and team performances are measured and evaluated, and keeping them informed of the results

- Listening to employees' thoughts and ideas about potential improvement, born of direct experience in delivering care and service

- Sharing with employees the progress and knowledge developed elsewhere in the organization, and outside it, which may help employees improve individual and team performance

Note: The word "employees" is used throughout this appendix, and it applies equally to nonemployed staff members engaged in the work of the unit or department (i.e., volunteers, physicians, agency staff, students, and others, as applicable).

Customer

The core message of QI is that quality is defined and evaluated by the customer. As we have discussed, the customer can be the patient or another external or internal customer, and we have a responsibility to work with all types of customers to identify what level of service is needed and how we can provide it effectively.

As discussed in Chapter 3, the development of a quality plan must be sensitive to the needs of all customers. You may decide not to perform ongoing measurements of all aspects of care and service—in fact, you should not, as it would likely consume more resources to measure than to provide service. In Chapter 4, we address the question of how to select appropriate measurements and how to rotate them over time to ensure that all aspects of care and service are monitored.

> *Example:* In an inpatient nursing unit, the ultimate customer is the patient. The visitor also judges quality on behalf of the patient. In addition, regulatory / accreditation agencies will evaluate quality on behalf of patients. Internal customers include physicians, nurses, and all staff who move in and out of the unit.

> *Example:* In an outpatient surgery program, the ultimate customer is the patient, who will judge quality on the basis of convenience, wait time, compassion, and cleanliness as well as clinical outcomes, perceived safety and information sharing. Physicians will monitor the quality of the nurses' and surgery technologists' work.

Employee Orientation to Quality

Every new employee in your department probably has received some type of organizational orientation. Just as you provide a local orientation, you also need to prepare the employee to take a role in your QI efforts. What does that involve?

For consistent delivery of high-quality care in an atmosphere of teamwork, each employee needs to be able to identify his or her customers for each aspect of the work process. And each employee should know the basic quality goals and measures of the work unit and be able to describe how he or she can contribute to the success of those goals. Employees need to know that their own ideas and contributions to continuous QI are desired and welcomed.

Each new employee should have an opportunity to become acquainted with the key performance measures or indicators that have been selected by the department (see Chapter 4). The orientation should focus on how the employee's responsibilities contribute to the achievement of the department's overall objectives and how the key performance measures have been developed to meet patients'/customers' needs.

Your staff members should realize that they are someone's customers too. As they work to improve quality in your department, they may well identify opportunities for others to do the same. Nurses may recognize inconsistencies in how the pharmacy delivers medications, transporters may suggest a simpler way for nurses to call to schedule patient pickup, or the payroll department may become concerned with chronically late time cards from one department.

These are all QI opportunities as well, and good teamwork reinforces an overall culture of quality and mutual respect in the organization. See the suggested meeting agenda (Figure A.1) for ways to solicit input from staff members that can be forwarded to other departments.

FIGURE A.1 ▶ MODEL QUALITY MEETING AGENDA

[Department name] _____ monthly quality staff meeting

❑ Call to order/attendance/approval of last meeting's minutes

❑ Process improvement team(s) status reports (if any) (see Chapter 7)

- Team name _____
- Team name _____
- Clinical path work group: diagnostic group

❑ Quality monitoring results (baseline) (see Chapter 4)

- List indicators scheduled for monitoring this month, if desired

❑ Patient/customer feedback:

- Trends this month/quarter on patient/customer survey
- Letters, complaints, and anecdotal information this month

❑ Sentinel events:

- Manager reviews pertinent events

❑ Risk and safety and infection control issues, for example:

- Fire drill performance
- Safety committee advisories
- Policy changes

❑ Other QI reports, for example:

- Special employee recognition
- Quality reports from departments who support us

❑ Adjournment

Conducting and Documenting Meetings

You might be expected to give every employee an opportunity to participate in a monthly staff meeting. If logistics preclude an in-person meeting each month, broad-based communication can be achieved for off-shift or casual workers with a meeting minutes notebook that all staff members must review and initial. How-ever, this should not replace all in-person meetings.

A monthly staff meeting is not a regulatory or accreditation requirement. The Joint Commission requirement (see Figure 1.1 in Chapter 1) dictates that the organization "communicates information related to safety and quality to those who need it, including staff... patients, families... Effective communication is vital among individuals and groups within the facility... Poor communication often con-tributes to adverse events and can compromise safety and quality of care, treatment, and services. Effective communication should be timely, accurate, and usable... " As you consider your flow of communication, make sure you can answer the questions you might be asked by a Joint Commission surveyor, state department of health nurse, or other regulator, such as:

- How do you inform your staff of the quality issues and goals for the department?

- If I interview staff members, will they know what you are trying to improve and what the current problem areas are?

- How do you include staff input as you set quality or PI goals?

- Can every employee describe quality control responsibilities?

- Do employees feel empowered to stop a patient care process if they feel it is unsafe or does not meet your criteria for quality? When I interview them, I will ask about these subjects.

- Extensive staff input and involvement is also expected, according to criteria for leading recognition programs such as the Malcolm Baldrige National Quality Award[1] and the ANCC Magnet Recognition Program® of the American Nurses Credentialing Center.[2]

Common Pitfalls in Planning a Meeting

Clearly, there is no dispute over whether involving the frontline work force in quality is the right thing to do. Yet it remains challenging to implement.

Time and logistics are the most common problems. The daily challenges of running a cost-effective operation may easily push a staff meeting to the bottom of the priority list. For example, patient care, and medical staff needs, staffing shortages are high priorities. Make sure you counter such challenges by:

- **Ensuring that the meeting has real value.** Structure substantive agendas so that the meeting is not merely a formality but is actually productive.

- **Conducting the meeting efficiently.** Meetings don't have to last an hour! Much routine information that doesn't need discussion can be assembled and posted in a staff report room or other nonpublic location. Focus the meeting agenda on items that require action, and leave the routine items for staff members to review later.

- **Planning.** It's not always easy, but it is essential to plan ahead to allocate time specifically for staff meetings. Don't try to slip in a meeting without proper notice.

- **Including the right people, and starting and ending on time.** Don't waste anyone's time; begin on time, and ensure that everyone is there who needs to present information. If you want to offer an update on pain management strategies, then the expert on that topic must be present.

- **Providing food.** Budgets don't always permit it, but it can be helpful to offer staff members some edible encouragement and reward for their participation.

Recommendations for Designing Effective Communication

Check with your organization's HR or Quality department to determine whether there are specific requirements in place for your setting. If there are no formal requirements for meeting structure, frequency, and documentation, consider the recommendations that follow. If your organization does have such requirements, the following recommendations can easily be tailored and incorporated into your structure to enrich the content and help you to conduct and document meetings efficiently and effectively:

- Obtain your organization's policy, procedure, or guidelines about how often to conduct staff and quality meetings, mandatory content or agenda structure, and required/recommended formats for meeting documentation.

- Learn who needs copies of your minutes—such as your supervisor or the quality department. Also find out how long you should keep copies of your minutes and the underlying data.

Devote a portion of each monthly staff meeting to quality. This will not always include a review of specific indicators and measurement data; however, the manager should convene the meeting as a quality management or QI review session. The subject material will vary depending on the department.

A word about confidentiality and protection

Quality data are extremely sensitive. There is the potential for embarrassment, litigation, or patient harm if they are released or shared irresponsibly. Key considerations include:

- Privacy of patients

- Privacy of staff members and physicians

- Discoverability

- Risk management

- Corporate/organizational public relations and potential embarrassment

Keep the analysis of these data to a confidential quality committee. What limited protections are available by law recognize the complexity of quality measurement. Even more important, these laws are designed to encourage full and can-did discussion and action by healthcare professionals to improve quality. It is your professional and ethical obligation to ensure that this goal is fulfilled.

The most important legal, regulatory, and accreditation resources on this issue are as follows:

- **Health Insurance Portability and Accountability Act of 1996 (HIPAA):**[3] Identifiable patient information cannot be shared except when there is an appropriate need to know in the context of healthcare treatment, operations, and payment.

- **Patient rights:** Similarly, you are obligated to respect the patient's right to privacy as outlined in the Centers for Medicare & Medicaid Services' Conditions of Participation, Joint Commission standards, state laws and regulations, and other relevant authorities.

- **Discoverability:** There are no national standards for protection of QI information from subpoena and discovery in connection with legal action.[4] Many states, however, uphold specific protections for quality data that are generated and analyzed in a properly constituted quality process, such as a committee that has been authorized by the board or medical staff.

How to protect information appropriately

The following are typical elements of a properly structured quality information flow:

- A quality orientation session for all new quality department staff members or those collecting relevant data

- A confidentiality statement signed by all employees, physicians, volunteers, and students

- A quality committee request for information

- A notation documenting all information collected on behalf of the committee, such as "privileged and confidential data"

- Quality information that is kept physically secure (e.g., locked offices and password protected computers)

  Note: Quality meetings begin with a reminder of the confidentiality provisions and responsibilities.

Query your organization's quality or legal department for any guidelines that de-scribe how to ensure that quality management of information is properly protected.

Holding the Quality Meeting

Remember, the quality meeting must be substantive, efficient, well planned, and well attended. Take the following steps for holding and documenting a quality meeting:

1. Prepare the agenda

2. Prepare data and materials for the meeting:

   - Prepare monitoring/performance data for discussion, such as quality metrics and patient/customer satisfaction.

   - Collect reports from intra-departmental or interdepartmental process improvement teams

   - Identify sentinel, critical, or other special events requiring discussion

   - Collect other information for discussion from sources such as the risk, employee safety, infection control, and support departments' quality updates and other updates.

   - Focus on information that requires action

3. Hold the meeting and document attendance

4. Document the group's conclusions and recommendations and planned follow-up on departmental indicators

5. Document other discussion briefly (e.g., improvement teams' efforts, sentinel events, and safety issues)

6. Route all or part of the minutes to the next level of the management/quality department, as stipulated in your organization's flow and procedures

The Quality Meeting

Discussion, conclusions, recommendations

The most important part of the meeting is that discussion of progress, discussion, conclusions and recommendations. If this part of the quality meeting is well done, it will inform and inspire the team and create momentum for continued improvement.

During the quality meeting with staff, conduct a discussion of each of the projects and measures. The following four basic questions are recommended to organize the discussion:

1. Did our interventions last month/period have the desired effect?

2. Are we meeting our target/goal/threshold?

3. If we are meeting our goal, does this performance appear to be solid, consistent, and reliable? (See Chapter 4 for a discussion of monitoring progress for meaningful improvement using methods such

as trend charts and statistical process control) If we are not meeting our goal based on the data, why not?

4. While reviewing these data, are there other possible improvement opportunities we should consider pursuing later?

Don't skimp on this portion of the discussion. Conduct and document a thorough analysis to ensure that the real underlying factors driving performance are effectively identified and understood. This segment of the meeting should generate vigorous staff discussion and input.

Strategies and Action Plans

With the staff, determine recommended actions that should be undertaken to maintain or further improve performance, based on the conclusions reached. Consider the following:

- Should we revise an action plan we previously developed?

- Who will be responsible, and when, for each action?

The department may undertake some of these actions or recommend them to others. (What will we recommend to whom? Using what rationale? Who will convey the recommendation?)

Follow-up

Finally, the group defines needed follow-up—primarily by identifying groups that should receive status updates or recommendations about this indicator, process, or group of indicators—and when this should be accomplished. Consider these questions:

- How can we share all this information with staff members not present today?

- When are the data shared with the chain of command (e.g., our vice president)?

- When are the data shared with pertinent medical leadership?

- When can we obtain feedback on our recommendations to other areas?

- Do we need consultation regarding matters such as data analysis, HR is-sues and information systems?

- Should we share these data with some of our customer groups?

- Should we share these data with colleagues who provide a similar service and solicit or offer advice?

- When will we review the data again?

Communication with employees, senior management, medical staff, and customers

Communication with employees regarding quality measures should occur at least on orientation and, it is recommended, monthly thereafter.

Communication with senior management can occur when managers' reports are submitted to directors and then to senior management. Not every measure will necessarily be reported to more senior levels; often, selected focus indicators or a "dashboard" of measures will be chosen for attention. Your organization may have a quality council or other occasion during which you present quality reports to other levels of management.

Indicators that are of concern to counterpart medical staff quality committees should be shared regularly. Increasingly, the development of shared indicators between hospital and medical staff departments is encouraged (see Chapter 4).

If your organization or department has matured to the point that you have inter-disciplinary quality committees, then the discussion will include perspectives of all involved staff members (e.g., nurses, technologists, physicians, and aides). In that case, a single report can reflect progress on a shared measure and the conclusions of the interdisciplinary group working on it and can be used for communication to all groups that need to know about progress.

Communicating with physicians who are not actually on the committee is a common problem when working on QI with medical staffs. Physicians in your quality committee meetings may not see it as their role to communicate the conclusions, actions, and reflections of the committee to the remainder of the medical staff. This can be due to time constraints and to the fact that physicians tend to be volunteers on committees and not part of a management hierarchy with defined responsibilities for communication. It can also be due to a lack of simple mechanisms and logistics for such communication.

Query your organization's quality department for guidelines or expectations on how often you should report to your internal customer departments about performance metrics relevant to them. And be sure to ask your customers how often they would like reports.

Recordkeeping

Retain quality meeting minutes for the duration specified by your organization. Three years is typical (the duration of a triennial accreditation survey window), but your organization will have its own guidelines. For indicators dictated by legislation or regulatory or accreditation agencies, guidelines promulgated by the agency may direct

recordkeeping of the detailed data supporting the quality summary data sheets (which are incorporated into meeting minutes). If your department works with the state nuclear safety agency, the U.S. Food and Drug Administration, the AABB, Occupational Safety and Health Administration, Drug Enforcement Agency, the College of American Pathologists, and others, you should check their current requirements.

For process improvement teams, retain the core data used to support the team's work in a binder or file organized by the relevant team leader or sponsor for at least three years or through the next accreditation survey, whichever is longer, in order to support further analysis if performance of the process begins to slip.

Query your organization's quality or legal department for guidelines about record retention, including any work that it has done to inventory the external agencies of interest. You may have an organizational policy that addresses this question.

See Figure A.2 for an example of what should be included in a quality improvement notebook.

FIGURE A.2 ▶ THE DEPARTMENTAL QUALITY IMPROVEMENT NOTEBOOK

Each department should maintain its own QI book or set of resources, including:

Resource materials
Copy of organization's QI plan/goals for the current year

Departmental QI book
Departmental QI plan (current)
Monthly meeting minutes

Correspondence with other quality committees, including:

    ❑ Referral of issues to other departments/committees

    ❑ Receipt of issues referred from other departments

Correspondence with QI department regarding content and development of QI plans

Departmental supplemental records
Detailed records of data, analysis, and other correspondence related to measurement and improvement of specific indicators and processes (these records will be referred to in the monthly meeting minutes)

See text for a discussion of retention periods for documents.

Endnotes

1. See *www.quality.nist.gov/index.html*

2. See *www.nursecredentialing.org/magnet.aspx*

3. See *www.hhs.gov/ocr/hipaa*

4. The Health Care Quality Improvement Act of 1986, amended 1998, Title V of Public Law 99-660, provides a general overarching level of protection insofar as it provides immunity from certain damages, but it does not preclude subpoena. Most (but not all) states have enacted laws that are clearer, more comprehensive, and more fully elaborated through case law.

Appendix B

Data Analysis, Statistical Tools, and Useful PI Methodologies

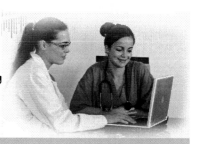

The following pages include introductory overviews of many of the common analytic and statistical tools that are helpful in quality and process improvement.

Defining the problem/process

- Brainstorming

- Data collection tool design and check sheets

- Cause-and-effect (fishbone) diagram

- Failure Modes and Effects Analysis (FMEA)

- Flow charts (macro and micro)

- Root-cause analysis framework and "five whys"

Analyzing the data

- Histogram

- Run charts/control charts

- Pareto diagram

- Scattergram and correlation

- Costs of poor quality and benefit-cost analysis

- Six Sigma

Designing improvement and testing and sustaining it

- Flow-charting

- FMEA

- Action planning

- Balanced scorecard

- Organizational framework

- Quality improvement (QI) program

Defining the Problem/Process

Brainstorming

- **What it is:** Open, nonjudgmental process of generating ideas.

- **How to do it:** Be clear about the question. Are you brainstorming to identify the source of a performance problem? Possible solutions to the problem once you know the source? Or possible failure modes that could occur in a process? These are all different topics. Choose just one at a time for brainstorming. The leader identifies the question and writes it on a board or flip chart. Ask each per-son in the room to offer an answer or idea. Do not comment or permit discussion, just collect ideas until there are no more.

- **When to use it:** In the early stages of diagnosis or problem solving, when you have a team of people who are experienced in the use of the process.

- **When not to use it:** When you don't have people present who actually work in the process but are merely speculating.

- **Common pitfalls:** Being judgmental and stifling potentially good ideas, failing to involve people who know the process and leading the process in a predetermined direction by the way the question is framed.

- **Next steps:** Processes such as affinity diagrams can be used to group the brain-stormed ideas into related categories. If you place each brainstormed idea on an adhesive note, you can move them around until they are grouped in a way the team finds useful. (Then you'll move ahead to analyze the specifics of each category, such as relevance to solving the problem, feasibility, cost, and time frame, etc.)

See the cause-and-effect, or Ishikawa, diagram for a logical next step for using these results in Figure B.1.

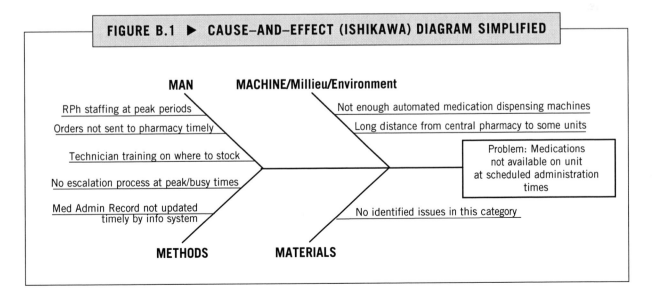

FIGURE B.1 ▶ CAUSE–AND–EFFECT (ISHIKAWA) DIAGRAM SIMPLIFIED

Data collection tool design: Check sheets and logs

- **What it is:** Simple method of collecting clearly defined, useful, and relevant data to answer questions about a process.

- **How to do it:** Set up a data collection tool so that each row of the sheet is a process event (e.g., patient visit or treatment). Each column of the sheet should be a step in the process, such as:
  - Time of arrival
  - Time seen
  - Time dismissed
  - Number of films
  - Quality control score
  - Assessment documented
  - Intervention documented
  - Reassessment documented

On the reverse side of the sheet or clearly marked on the sheet, define specifically what each column means and how to record it. Examples include:
  - Patient name or medical record number
  - Time patient enters the waiting room, in 24-hour clock
  - Quality control score by physician, on a 1–5 scale where 5=best and 1=unacceptable, retake needed
  - Date/time on a 24-hour clock when pain was screened, full assessment was documented, intervention was identified or explicitly declined, and reassessment was performed

Pilot the sheet with staff for a few process events to ensure that it is clearly understood and correctly used. Note that in most cases, you cannot allow the patient to initiate the log by signing in because the patient would then see other patients' names or other identifying information. See Figure B.2 for an example of a sample data collection sheet.

- **When to use it:** Develop new data collection tools only when you know you need the data, you have no alternative method to collect the data from automated systems, and you have a sampling plan to ensure that you have the right amount of data from the right populations (see Chapter 4).

- **When not to use it:** When you have any alternative way of getting adequate data that doesn't require manual effort to collect the information or when you have not fully demonstrated that you truly need it.

- **Common pitfalls:** Poor definitions, so that staff members collect data inconsistently; sloppy use of the tools, especially when staff are busy; illegibility.

FIGURE B.2 ▶ SAMPLE DATA COLLECTION TOOLS

Simple data collection sheet to monitor timeliness of phases of a patient visit. Note that each column is clearly defined.

Clinic Visit Log Sheet

Sequential number and patient initials	Time arrived (hh:mm on 24-hour clock)	Time called to exam room (hh:mm on 24-hour clock)	Time checked out (hh:mm on 24-hour clock)
1. JH	10:03	10:24	11:18
2. LW	13:10	13:25	13:54

Outpatient Department Quality Control Sheet

If you provide a service that is checked for quality and sometimes must be repeated, you may wish to monitor the number of times a retake is needed. This does not necessarily mean that the technologist did a poor job—sometimes it is unavoidable. But you may want to watch for trends.

Technologist initials	Sequential number and patient initials	Modality/type of study	Number of images taken	Number of images repeated for QC issues
JD	1. SW	CXR outpatient	1	0

Outpatient Financial Counseling Volume Monitoring

This simple tick sheet is easy to maintain and can be readily summarized at the end of each work day. It provides data on volume by predetermined time segments.

Date: Monday, June x, 20xx

Hour of day of patient arrival	Medicare	Medicaid	Private payer	Uninsured
0700 until 0800	✓✓✓	✓	✓	✓✓
0800 until 0900	✓✓✓✓✓	✓✓✓✓	✓✓✓✓✓✓	✓✓✓
0900 until 1000	✓✓✓✓✓✓ ✓✓✓✓✓✓	✓✓✓✓✓✓ ✓✓✓✓✓✓	✓✓✓✓✓✓ ✓✓✓✓✓✓	✓✓✓✓✓✓✓
Etc.				
1600 until 1700	✓✓✓✓✓✓ ✓✓✓	✓✓✓✓✓✓ ✓✓✓✓✓✓	✓✓✓✓✓✓	✓✓✓✓
1700 until 1800 (closing)	✓✓✓	✓✓✓✓✓✓ ✓✓✓	✓✓✓✓✓✓ ✓✓✓✓	✓✓✓✓✓✓✓ ✓✓✓

Cause-and-effect (fishbone) diagram

- **What it is:** Published by Kaoru Ishikawa in the 1960s, a valuable approach to classifying sources of a process or performance problem.

- **How to do it:** Draw a "fishbone" (see Figure B.1) with the four "ribs" marked with the following four "M" categories:

    - Man (people, competence, training)

    - Methods (procedures, policies, management)

    - Material (supplies, tools)

    - Machines and milieu/environment (physical space, distance, machine reliability)

Now collect all known or probable failures in each of these categories and draw them as branches off the ribs. If you performed brainstorming and affinity grouping, this will be easy. If time and expertise permit, make sure the final item listed in each category is specific and measurable. You are going to want to see how much each one actually contributes to the performance outcome.

Note: Use additional categories or rename the categories if necessary, although these four categories suit most significant process analyses.

- **When to use it:** To clarify thinking and to confirm that brainstorming was complete and well organized. To challenge the group to see whether something has been overlooked. (e.g., "We are studying medication timeliness and no one mentioned anything about physical space layout.")

- **When not to use it:** It is much easier for most groups to start with brainstorming and use the Ishikawa diagram later to group the results, rather than start with the diagram, which is foreign to most people and may draw a blank stare rather than rich ideas.

- **Common pitfalls:** Most common is failing to define the outcome of interest clearly. "Medication late" is a poorly defined outcome. "Medication not available on nursing unit in proper location at scheduled administration time" is better and still leaves plenty of room for a rich range of contributing factors. Another pitfall is not being specific enough or not pushing the group to come up with measurable and definable causes.

Failure Modes and Effects Analysis

- **What it is:** Developed in the 1970s in aviation and automotive industries, an FMEA tries to predict and mitigate all possible product/process failures. An FMEA is a diagnostic process that includes features of flow-charting, cause-and-effect analysis, and brainstorming. See Figure B.3 for a sample FMEA analysis.

- **How to do it:**

   1. Build a detailed process flow chart. (Note: Quite often, the first attempt won't be detailed enough, and you'll continue to elaborate on it during the remainder of the process as you recognize the complexities in the process.)

   2. For each process step, identify all possible failure modes (i.e., reasons why the process may not work as planned).

   3. For each failure mode, identify F=frequency on a 1–10 scale where 10 is most frequent.

   4. For each failure mode, identify effects that this failure will have on the out-come of the process.

   5. For each effect, identify S=severity on a 1–10 scale where 10 is the most severe (critical) effect on outcome.

   6. For each effect, identify the current process features and controls that are in place to catch the failure before it has an effect (detection/mitigation).

   7. For each, identify D=detectability on a 1–10 scale where 10 is the least likely to be detected in normal operations.

   8. Compute the risk priority number (RPN)=F x S x D (range will be 1–1000).

   9. Arrange the RPNs in descending order.

   10. For any failure mode with severity=10, place an asterisk no matter what the final RPN was.

   11. Examine the process failures with the highest RPNs and all those with a se-verity of 10 (identified with an asterisk) and use to establish priorities for improvement.

- **When to use it:** FMEA is extraordinarily powerful and should always be considered as a valuable tool for any complex and high-risk process. It is labor-intensive but often worth it. For hospitals, The Joint Commission requires use of an FMEA.

FIGURE B.3 ▶ EXAMPLE OF A FAILURE MODE AND EFFECTS ANALYSIS (PARTIAL)

Process Step	Failure Modes	Frequency F	Effects	Severity S	Controls	Detectability D	FxSxD Risk Priority Number
Medication order is sent to pharmacy	Unit secretary is busy	8	Delay	10	No effective controls.	10	800
	Tube system is down	1	Delay	6	Known immediately, backup transport plan in place.	1	6
Pharmacy reviews order	Pharmacy is busy	10	Delay	7	Staff escalation plan, priority orders organized by manager on duty.	6	420
If order requires clarification, pharmacy contacts ordering MD	Cannot locate MD, cannot read pager number, MD does not call back promptly	6	Delay	8	MD pager # should be on order. RPh can escalate to another MD.	8	384
Pharmacy profiles order in pharmacy system	System flags interactions, contraindications	7	Delay	4	RPh contact MD for questions.	2	56
	Out of stock	2	Change in med	4	Always detected.	1	8

- **When not to use it:** For simpler processes, ordinary brainstorming can be sufficient. Don't embark on an FMEA unless you are willing to commit the necessary resources to see it through. Recognize that you will identify many failure modes and will then need to resolve each one—either improve them or determine that they can be tolerated in the current system (e.g., are sufficiently detectable, in-frequent, or have minimal severity).

- **Common pitfalls:** A FMEA is a fundamentally subjective methodology, with all the strengths and weaknesses that implies. It relies on the collective experience, candor, and analytical skills of the group. It is essential to bring together experienced frontline people who use the process, a strong facilitator, and a resource to keep the documentation current and accurate. The atmosphere must be one of trust and a willingness to face—even to welcome—the identification of potential risks. You cannot perform an FMEA in an atmosphere of suspicion and blame because staff members must feel free to acknowledge they have observed process failures or risks of failure.

  If there are data that describe the process failures already, bring them to the table, but remember that your goal is to develop a thorough understanding of process failure modes, including those that have not yet caused detectable problems.

  Don't let the group wrangle over the scoring. Define in advance what you mean by a "severity score of 10" or other points on the scale. In healthcare, it is all too easy to assign a 10 to almost any failure mode. For example, you may theorize that any delay in the medication process could lead to a severe outcome. But if every severity score is 10, then the score is meaningless. The group can establish its own norms to make the scoring meaningful for this particular process.

- **Next steps:** FMEAs create a prioritized set of risks that you have identified. Validate this list by collecting data on how often the various failures actually do occur or how effectively the controls in place really do detect the failures. Once you are satisfied that you have identified the high-priority failure modes with the most critical effects, move to an operational work plan to improve the process. Repeat the FMEA with the new process (either in its design stage or after implementing some or all of the improvements) to determine whether you have reduced the RPNs. The process of the FMEA, prioritization, improvement design, implementation, and evaluation can continue until you are satisfied with the performance of the process and the risks that remain.

Flow charts (macro and micro)

- **What it is:** Graphic display of a process that makes it easier to understand and improve.

- **How to do it:** Brainstorm the process with the group, drawing the step-by-step process as you go. Typical symbols to use include those in Figure B.4.

- **When to use it:** Flow-charting should be the first step in almost any process improvement effort. It can help you decide whether you have defined the process clearly. Do you know when this process begins? When it ends? Who plays roles in it? What the measurable outcome is?

  As with an FMEA, this can be a laborious process but should be well worth the time spent.

- **When not to use it:** If you are not solving a process problem, the flow chart will not be useful. For example, if you have narrowed a performance problem to staff competence in taking vital signs on second shift, then you probably don't have a process problem. However, the vast majority of improvement efforts do involve process review.

- **Common pitfalls**: Failing to involve the right people in the process, thereby sketching an incomplete or inaccurate flow chart; failing to specify each step in detail (e.g., who does it, what they do, and in what sequence); failing to articulate decision points; and making assumptions and oversimplifying.

FIGURE B.4 ▶ FLOWCHARTING

Standard Flow Charting Symbols

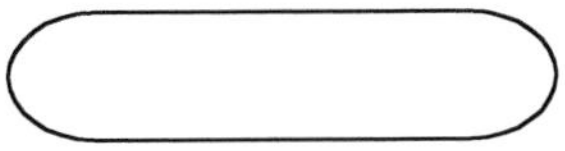

Start or stop a process

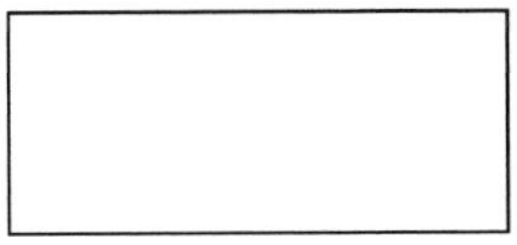

Process step (be sure to specify who performs it)

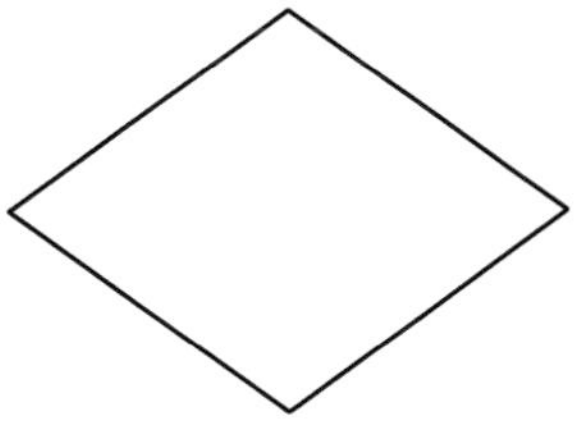

Decision point in the process

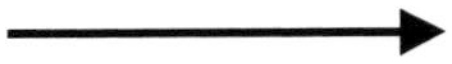

Direction of process flow

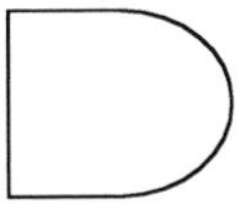

Optional but useful: method of identifying process steps in which a DELAY may occur

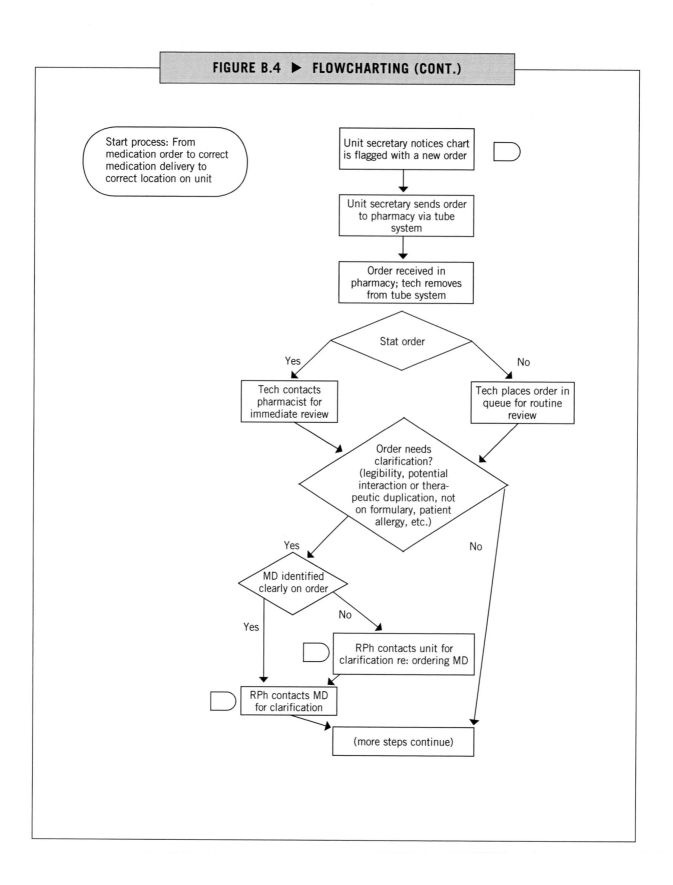

FIGURE B.4 ▶ FLOWCHARTING (CONT.)

Start process: From medication order to correct medication delivery to correct location on unit

Unit secretary notices chart is flagged with a new order

Unit secretary sends order to pharmacy via tube system

Order received in pharmacy; tech removes from tube system

Stat order

Yes — No

Tech contacts pharmacist for immediate review

Tech places order in queue for routine review

Order needs clarification? (legibility, potential interaction or thera-peutic duplication, not on formulary, patient allergy, etc.)

Yes — No

MD identified clearly on order

Yes — No

RPh contacts unit for clarification re: ordering MD

RPh contacts MD for clarification

(more steps continue)

Five whys and root-cause analysis framework (from The Joint Commission)

- **What it is:** The Joint Commission provided the key impetus for the industry's attention to sentinel events and root-cause analysis (RCA). The Joint Commission defines an RCA as:

  A process for identifying the basic or causal factors that underlie variation in performance, including the occurrence or possible occurrence of a sentinel event. An RCA focuses primarily on systems and processes, not the performance of individuals. It progresses from special causes in clinical processes to common causes in organizational processes and identifies potential improvements in processes or systems that could decrease the likelihood of such events in the future, or determines, after analysis, that no such improvement opportunities exist. (The Joint Commission's Comprehensive Accreditation Manual for Hospitals 2009).

- **How to do it:** The Joint Commission has an RCA tool available on its Web site. The tool aims to ensure that you take a thorough and methodical look at all the factors that may contribute to a sentinel event or, indeed, any observed performance problem. The Joint Commission suggests that you address human factors, environmental factors, equipment factors, and external factors. You then drill down to competence, staffing levels, process tolerance for staff variation, orientation and training, access to information, communication among team members, physical environment, emergency response, culture, and prevention.

  The Veterans Administration National Center for Patient Safety (*www.patientsafety.gov*) is another excellent resource. The root-cause framework endorsed there includes detailed attention to:

  - Human factors—communication
  - Human factors—training
  - Human factors—fatigue and scheduling
  - Environment and equipment factors
  - Rules, policies, and procedures
  - Effectiveness of barriers to error and harm

  The term "five whys" is also used in RCAs to emphasize the importance of steadily proceeding to the deepest or true root cause. It does not mean only five whys, however. The point is to keep going until you have found the true organizational systems cause of the error or quality problem. The following is an example:

1. Why did the medication error occur? Because the RN selected the wrong medication from the drawer. (Note: In another step, we'll examine why the RN did not check the medication to the order before administering it.)

2. Why did the RN select the wrong medication? Because the drawer was stocked differently than usual.

3. Why was the drawer stocked differently? Because the technician was new and did not know the usual system.

4. Why did the technician not know the usual system? Because he was hired during a staff crunch, and there was not time to do the usual orientation. (Note: In another step, we'll examine why orientation is the only time we teach staff how to stock this drawer and why there is no immediate in-formation during stocking that would provide cues or directions.)

5. Why was the orientation skipped? Because the manager was juggling a heavy workload with limited staffing.

6. Why was staffing inadequate? Because there is high turnover and increasing census; the manager could not hire during the last quarter due to a budget freeze; and there is no escalation or emergency plan for staffing shortages. (Note: In a future step, we might look at reasons for high turnover and whether the increasing census could have been predicted with an early warning system. We might also look at whether the department needs to staff to projected volumes rather than at a fixed budget.)

7. Why is there no escalation plan for staffing shortages? For this particular set of issues, we may have reached the real systems root cause: The manager did not have organizational support to manage peak volumes with appropriate staffing.

It is obvious that without these root-cause approaches, the immediate response would be simply to discipline the nurse and never uncover the possibility of continuing systems problems in pharmacy staffing. In that case, it would be only a matter of time before the same problem occurred to another staff member.

- **When to use it:** RCA is always employed for sentinel events, under Joint Commission standards, and it is appropriate for use whenever a significant patient safety event or error occurs causing harm or the potential for harm. It will be a management decision whether to apply the full scope of RCA to any given problem short of a sentinel event.

The insights and creative thinking that are taught in RCA can be extremely helpful in all aspects of process improvement. For example, in developing an FMEA or an Ishikawa cause-and-effect diagram, use the RCA categories of analysis to be sure that you have thought about all aspects of the process or problem.

- **When not to use it:** RCA can be laborious and time-consuming and should be applied only when the scope of the problem warrants it.

- **Common pitfalls:** Failure to analyze deep enough into the underlying systems causes of errors. For example, labeling "communication" the root cause of a problem but not exploring why the team did not communicate in a timely or accurate manner.

Analyzing the Data

Histogram

- **What it is:** Display, typically using vertical bars, to show distribution of performance data by category or over time. See Chapter 4 for examples.

- **How to do it:** All spreadsheet programs will generate a histogram from simple columnar data.

- **When to use it:** Histograms are powerful tools to make sense of the relationship among performance metrics.

- **When not to use it:** If you know that the metrics contain disparate subpopulations, it may not be appropriate to use a simple histogram. If you have many, many categories to display, you may want to use a Pareto chart to separate the important from the rest.

  See Figure B.5 for an example of a histogram.

Run charts/control charts

- **What it is:** Graphic display of data over time. See Chapter 4 for examples of run charts. Control charts can be overlaid on the run chart to help discern whether the process being measured is stable and in control or is subject to special cause variation or is changing over time.

- **How to do it:** See Chapter 4 for discussion and examples; also see the Bibliography for more detailed resources.

- **When to use it:** A run chart is appropriate whenever performance is evaluated over time. A control chart is helpful when you have at least 20 time periods of history to use as a basis for the process' upper and lower control limits, and it can be used with caution even when you don't have that much history.

- **When not to use it:** If the process is highly variable, the control limits will be so wide that they will not be useful.

- **Common pitfalls:** Building control limits with inadequate data or choosing the baseline period without adequate rationale.

- **Next steps:** Once the control limits are established, identify special-cause variation and systematic changes in process and explore the source of these developments.

See figure B.5 for an example of a run chart.

Pareto diagram

- **What it is:** A histogram arranged in order from most frequent to least frequent, so that you can focus on the "vital few" events rather than the "trivial many."

- **How to do it:** All spreadsheet programs will do this, if you sort the data in descending order by frequency.

- **When to use it:** Any histogram of event frequency can be clarified by displaying it as a Pareto chart, but particularly those with many groups will benefit from this treatment.

- **When not to use it:** When you have a reason to want to group the data by an-other logical characteristic rather than simply volume.

See Figure B.5 for an example of a Pareto diagram.

FIGURE B.5 ▶ HISTOGRAM, PARETO CHART, RUN CHART, AND CONTROL CHART EXAMPLES

Histogram

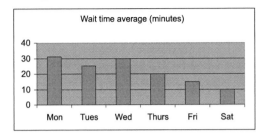

Run Chart: One data series over time

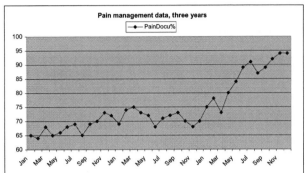

Control Chart

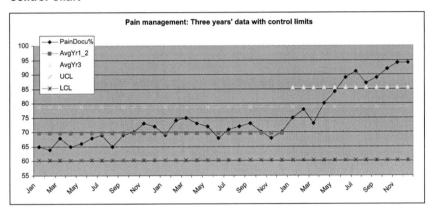

Pareto Chart

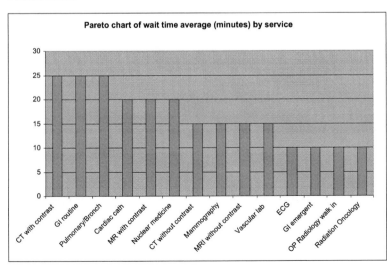

QUALITY IMPROVEMENT FOR NURSE MANAGERS

Scattergram and correlation

- **What it is:** A two-dimensional display of a relationship between two continuous variables. The scattergram is the graph; a correlation is a statistic that can be computed to describe the strength of the relationship.

- **How to do it:** Spreadsheet programs will create a scattergram with ordinary row and column data. They should create the statistic, as well, and some will fit a trend line to the data.

- **When to use it:** When you want to examine the relationship between two variables, particularly if there is a great deal of data. (e.g., nursing hours per patient day on the y-axis or patient falls per 1,000 days measured for each nursing unit each month on the x-axis).

- **When not to use it:** If the data are categorical rather than continuous, this would not be an appropriate approach. Also, if you think that the process has changed during the data collection period (e.g., if you implemented a new fall prevention program in the sixth month of a year-long data collection process on falls and staffing), then you would not want to blend all those data into a single chart. Finally, if the relationship is not linear, this graphic and statistical approach will not work. (Linear means that you expect that as one rises the other will rise as well.)

- **Common pitfalls:** The most common problem is that people do not use this approach often enough. It is not common to have such large databases of potentially related continuous variables, but such questions as staffing in particular can be helpfully illuminated by this method.

- **Next steps:** If you discover that there is a strong relationship between two variables, use more detailed process analysis to understand why the relationship occurs and what you can do to strengthen the benefits demonstrated by the relationship (e.g., if you find that a certain staffing level appears to be related to fewer patient falls).

See Figure B.6 for an example of a scattergram.

FIGURE B.6 ▶ SCATTERGRAM

Unit	Staffing	Patient falls per 1,000 days
	RN HPPD	*Fall Rate*
A	4	2.9
B	3.5	3.2
C	4.7	2.5
D	4.1	2.8
E	4.9	1.9
F	4.3	3
G	4	3.1

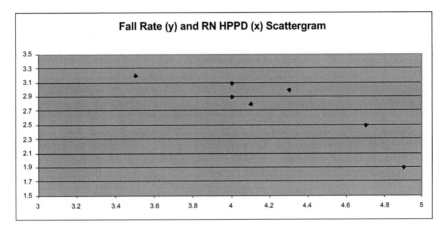

Fall Rate (y) and RN HPPD (x) Scattergram

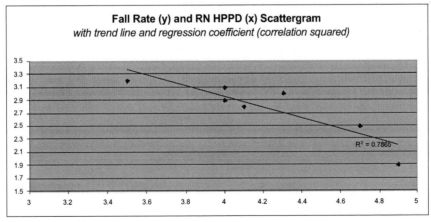

Fall Rate (y) and RN HPPD (x) Scattergram
with trend line and regression coefficient (correlation squared)

Costs of poor quality and benefit-cost analysis

- **What it is:** A systematic and disciplined approach to assessing the costs of delivering less than optimal quality and evaluating the cost and benefit of alternative improvement ideas.

- **How to do it:** There is an extensive science to the measurement of cost and benefit of quality (see Appendix C for a starting point).

As you add up the costs of poor quality, consider these:

- Prevention costs incurred to prevent an error or quality defect (e.g., investing in computer systems to check medication interactions before dispensing or bar coding systems for blood and medications)

- Inspection costs to check quality and problems during the process (e.g., nurses who make daily rounds to ensure that patients are receiving correct therapy according to a care path)

- Internal failure costs incurred before the failure reaches the patient or other customer (e.g., nurses who have to send wrong medications back to pharmacy)

- External failures incurred if the patient or customer experiences the error or quality defect (e.g., patient harm or death, litigation, or damage to reputation of the healthcare organization)

Cost-benefit analysis for a process improvement: Thus far, you have measured the costs of poor quality. Now you have to evaluate the costs of implementing the proposed improvement. To do this comprehensively, include all the costs of implementation, such as staffing, training, computer systems, supplies and equipment, and space renovation. Estimate how much of the costs of poor quality will be mitigated or saved as a result of the improvement.

When to use it: Whenever a process improvement is likely to incur significant costs or eliminate significant costs of poor quality, this is a useful tool. Consult your own organizational financial staff for any guidelines or methodologies that may be in use.

When not to use it: If you feel the costs and benefits are not measurable, clearly this will not be helpful.

Common pitfalls: As noted, cost estimation must be performed in a complete and disciplined manner in order to be credible and useful. In most cases, you need to involve your organization's financial talent.

See Figure B.7 for an example of how to map out the costs of poor quality.

FIGURE B.7 ▶ COSTS OF POOR QUALITY

What does it cost to provide poor quality?

Category of Cost	Example	Cost Today	Cost under Improvement Alternative 1	Cost under Improvement Alternative 2
Prevention costs incurred to prevent an error or quality defect	Computer systems to check medication interactions before			
Inspection costs to check quality and problems during the process	Daily RN rounds to check correct therapy per care path			
Internal failure costs incurred before the failure reaches the patient or other customer	Sending wrong medications back to pharmacy			
External failures incurred if the patient or customer experiences the error or quality defect	Patient harm or death, litigation, damage to			

How will the proposed improvement (or alternatives) change the cost-benefit profile of this process?

Cost-Benefit Analysis of Improvement Alternatives	Improvement Alternative 1	Improvement Alternative 2	Current Process
Start-up costs (computer, software, equipment, renovation, training materials, overtime)			
Annual costs			
Staff			
Training			
Supplies, materials			
Equipment depreciation			
Outside services			
etc.			
Annual benefits			
Incremental revenue (more volume, higher price, better collection% or payer mix)			
Reduced liability, rework, lost output, other "costs of poor quality"			

Six Sigma

- **What it is:** The term "Six Sigma" is a measurement of the reliability of a process or product. Sigma refers to a standard deviation, and a process operating at Six Sigma will experience 3.4 errors per billion events. There is no process in health-care service delivery that approaches this level of reliability. However, Six Sigma has been used to describe an entire science of process improvement that focuses on disciplined measurement and careful use of the kinds of tools outlined in this appendix. Motorola and General Electric are two leading companies that have developed and refined this methodology.

- **How to do it:** Most who claim to be performing Six Sigma process improvement are not, in fact, expecting to reach actual Six Sigma levels of variability. However, their work is characterized by passionate attention to reducing variability to the lowest level possible. Many resources are available to assist in training green belt and black belt Six Sigma experts (the distinction is based on the number and scope of projects they have completed and the commitment of their time). The American Society for Quality provides a starting point (*www.asq.org*).

Designing, Testing, and Sustaining Improvement

Flow-charting

Once you have entered the improvement phase, use the flow chart you have created to pinpoint all the areas you have changed and to update the chart to the new process design. Look for new sources of error, delay, or variability and any unintended consequences of your new process. This is a vital step, particularly when you have made substantial changes.

FMEA

As described earlier, the development of an FMEA results in a prioritized list of high-risk failure modes that must be addressed to reduce frequency of the failure or severity of the effect, or to increase detectability so that the failure can be mitigated before harm occurs. The team will produce alternative designs to accomplish these goals, and then a new FMEA can be produced on one or more of the revised process designs to estimate its probability of failure. The testing process will be to:

- Draw the new flow chart

- Repeat the FMEA on the new process, being careful to challenge all assumptions and identify all failure modes

- Calculate new RPNs

- Focus on:
  - Failure modes from the original FMEA that are still not addressed
  - New failure modes with high RPNs or high severity

- Repeat the process until the team feels that the process has been optimized

- Implement the improvements, in a pilot test mode, if possible

- After a period of settling in (collecting appropriate performance measures and reporting failures if/when they occur), repeat the FMEA with the now experienced team

Action planning

- **What it is:** Action planning is, of course, exactly what it says—a plan for action (see Figure B.8). Many action plans fail to be implemented effectively, and some techniques for action planning can improve your chances of success.

- **How to do it:** The keys in action planning are to:

  – Define the action and a measure of its accomplishment precisely

  – Assign the action to a specific person and ensure that that person accepts the assignment

  – Set a specific time frame for accomplishment and ensure that it is met or adjusted appropriately

- **When to use it:** All action planning should be formally documented and followed up regularly. If possible, link significant action plans to annual performance goals of the department and staff involved.

See Figure B.8 for an example of an action plan.

Balanced scorecard

- **What it is:** First defined by Robert Kaplan and David Norton in the *Harvard Business Review*, the balanced scorecard is a method of selecting a palette of different metrics that ensure that the organization is monitoring all central aspects of its mission.

- **How to do it:** Within your own department, a balanced scorecard (or dashboard, as some call it) might include key:

  – Financial measures

  – Clinical or operational measures of effectiveness

  – Measures of safety (e.g., patient, customer, and employee)

  – Measures of satisfaction (e.g., patient, customer, and employee)

FIGURE B.8 ▶ SAMPLE ACTION PLAN FORMAT

Process: _____

Improvement goal: _____

List the process name here: _____

Select a specific measurable improvement goal

Task	Result	Responsibilities	Target Date
Describe the task specifically	Describe a measurable result	Name of individual	Date

Sample

Process: _____

Improvement goal: _____

Wait time for service in department X: _____

- 90% of patients seen within 10 minutes, 90% of patients "very satisfied"

Task	Result	Responsibilities	Target Date
Purchase headsets for reception staff and technical staff to communicate	All staff have and can use new equipment	CD	Feb 15
Write script for reception staff to greet patients, create correct expectation, alert of any delays	Script available and pilot-tested	XY	Feb 15
Develop escalation procedure if volumes exceed predetermined thresholds	Define thresholds, write procedure	LM	Feb 15
Cross train staff from Department Z who may assist in high-volume volume periods	All staff familiar with expectations and know location of written procedures/refresher	GH	Feb 15
Update computer system so reception staff can enter patient arrival, patient name will appear in technical area as "arrived"	Computer system in place, tested	EF	Feb 15
Train reception staff on new procedure	All reception staff know exactly what to do when a patient arrives	AB	March 1
Train technical staff on what to expect from reception	All technical staff know how they will be contacted by reception staff, how to use new computer system upgrade	JK	March 1
Train technical staff on dealing with patient concerns, complaints about wait time	Role-play and manager evaluation indicates tech staff are competent in this area	PQ	March 1
Implement daily monitoring of wait times for first three months	Daily accurate data in place, time is established for regular staff review and action planning	ST	March 1

- **When to use it:** Consult your organization's quality department to determine whether this approach is in use and what the parameters are for your situation.

Organizational framework

Organizational resources are key to effective implementation of QI. One of the most significant hurdles to continuous QI and performance excellence arises if the management team considers QI a task to be undertaken separately from operational management and leadership.

Virtually all routine organizational structures are relevant to improving performance, such as:

- Management and staff accountability and authority

- Policies, procedures, and training

- Engineered supports such as alerts, reminders, and forcing functions

- Equipment, resources, and environment

QI program

The QI program is, of course, designed to keep a regular focus on performance improvement. If you have followed the tips in Chapters 1, 3, and Appendix A in developing an effective quality plan and communication program with your staff, you are well-positioned to direct your team's energy to effective improvement in important aspects of care and service in your department.

Appendix C

Bibliography and Resources

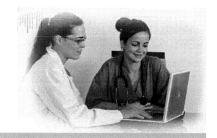

Nursing-Specific Resources

Kozier, Barbara, et al. (2004) *Assessing, Fundamentals of Nursing*: Concepts, Process and Practice, 2nd ed., p. 261

Donahue, M.P.; Brighton, V., "Nursing Outcome Classification: Development and Implementation, " *Journal of Nursing Care Quality*, 1998, 12(5).

Moorhead, S.; Johnson, M.; Maas, M.; el. Al., *Nursing Outcomes Classification*, Elsevier, Fourth Edition, 936 pages, 2007, ISBN 0-323-05408-0

Williams, C. A., "The Nursing Minimum Data Set: a major priority for public health nursing but not a panacea,"*American Journal of Public Health*. 1991 April; 81(4): 413–414.

Quality Improvement/Performance Improvement Philosophies and the Strategic Imperative

Berwick, Donald M., Godfrey, A. Blanton, and Roessner, Jane. *Curing Health Care: New Strategies for Quality Improvement*. Oxford and San Francisco: Jossey-Bass, 1990.

Berwick, Donald M. *Escape Fire: Designs for the Future of Health Care*. San Francisco: Jossey-Bass, 2003.

National Academies Press (*www.nap.edu*) publishes the Institute of Medicine reports. All of them can be read online for free, downloaded, or ordered in hard-copy for a relatively modest cost. IOM reports in its "Health Care Quality Initiative" that should be familiar to healthcare leaders have included:

- Kohn, Linda T., Corrigan, Janet M., and Donaldson, Molla S. *To Err is Human: Building a Safer Health System*, National Academies Press, *www.nap.edu/catalog.php?record_id=9728 (accessed March 10, 2009).*

- Committee on Quality of Health Care in America, Institute of Medicine. *Crossing the Quality Chasm: A New Health System for the 21st Century*, National Academies Press, *www.nap.edu/catalog.php?record_id=10027 (accessed March 10, 2009)*.

- Hurtado, Margarita P., Swift, Elaine K., and Corrigan, Janet M. *Envisioning the National Health Care Quality Report*, National Academies Press, *www.nap.edu/catalog.php?record_id=10073* (accessed March 10, 2009).

Weick, Karl E. and Sutcliffe, Kathleen M. *Managing the Unexpected: Assuring High Performance in an Age of Complexity*. San Francisco: Jossey-Bass, 2001. The second edition is Weick and Sutcliffe. *Managing the Unexpected: Resilient Performance in an Age of Uncertainty*. San Francisco: Jossey-Bass, 2007.

Marx, David. *Patient Safety and the Just Culture: A Primer for Health Care Executives*. Medical Event Reporting System—Transfusion Medicine, *www.mers-tm.org/support/Marx_Primer.pdf* (accessed March 10, 2009).

Rosander, A.C. *Deming's 14 Points Applied to Services*. New York: Marcel Dekker, 1991.

Deming, W.E., *The New Economics: For Industry, Government, Education*. Cambridge, MA: The MIT Press, 1994.

Midwest Business Group on Health in collaboration with Juran Institute, Inc., and The Severyn Group, Inc., *Reducing the Costs of Poor-Quality Health Care Through Responsible Purchasing Leadership*. Chicago: Midwest Business Group on Health, 2002.

Management Tools

Barnard, Cynthia and Eisenberg, Jodi. *Performance Improvement: Winning Strategies for Quality and Joint Commission Compliance*, Fourth Edition. Marble-head, MA: HCPro, Inc., 2009.

Barnard, Cynthia. *Benchmarking Basics: A Resource Guide for Healthcare Managers*. Marblehead, MA: HCPro, Inc., 2006.

Technical Tools

Carey, Raymond G. and Lloyd, Robert C. *Measuring Quality Improvement in Healthcare: A Guide to Statistical Process Control Applications*. Milwaukee, WI: ASQ Press, 1995.

The Joint Commission. *Comprehensive Accreditation Manual for Hospitals*, most recent edition, Root-cause analysis framework, online at *www.jointcommission.org*.

Brassard, Michael and Ritter, Diane. *The Memory Jogger™ II*, Madison, WI: GOAL/QPC/Joiner Associates/Oriel, Inc., 1994.

GOAL/QPC and Oriel, Inc., *The Team Memory Jogger™*, Madison, WI: GOAL/QPC/Joiner Associates/Oriel, Inc., 1995.

Streibel, Barbara J., et al., *The Team Handbook*, Third Edition. Madison, WI: Joiner/Oriel, Inc., 2003.

Musson, David M. and Helmreich, Robert L. "Team Training and Resource Management in Health Care: Current Issues and Future Directions." *Harvard Health Policy Review* Vol. 5, No. 1, (Spring 2004).

American Society for Quality, *www.asq.org*.

National Association for Healthcare Quality, *www.nahq.org*.

Institute for Healthcare Improvement, *www.ihi.org*.

Veterans Health Administration National Center for Patient Safety, *www.patientsafety.gov*.

Evidence-Based Measures

National Guideline Clearinghouse™, *www.guideline.gov*.

National Quality Measures Clearinghouse™, *www.qualitymeasures.ahrq.gov*.

QualityTools™, a clearinghouse for practical, ready-to-use tools for measuring and improving the quality of healthcare, *www.innovations.ahrq.gov/qualitytools*.

U.S. Department of Health and Human Services Agency for Healthcare Re-search and Quality Rockville, MD, National Healthcare Quality Report (December 2003).

American Nurses Association National Database of Nursing Quality Indicators, *www.ana.org/quality*.

ANCC Magnet Recognition Program®, *www.ana.org/ancc*.

Agency for Healthcare Research and Quality, *www.ahrq.gov.* Includes resources such as:

- Monthly Web M&M, excellent case studies in quality and patient safety

- National quality indicators and patient safety indicators literature and soft-ware that you can download and use with your own administrative (billing) data

- Validated survey of "culture of safety" with comparative/benchmark data

- Extensive consumer resources in quality and patient safety

- Listserv for weekly update e-mails

- Bibliographies

Hospital Consumer Assessment of Healthcare Providers and Systems, *www.hcahpsonline.org* and *www.cms.hhs.gov/hospitalqualityinits.*

Centers for Medicare & Medicaid Services, *www.cms.gov.*

The Leapfrog Group, *www.leapfroggroup.org.*

National Quality Forum, *www.qualityforum.org.* Serious Reportable Events fact sheet at *www.qualityforum.org/projects/completed/sre/fact-sheet.asp* (accessed March 10, 2009).

Nursing Education Instructional Guide

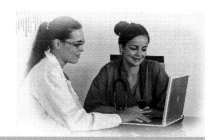

Target audience:

- Nurse managers

- Ancillary managers

- Chief nursing officers

- Directors of nursing

- VPs of nursing

- VPs of patient care services

- Staff development specialists

- Clinical nurse leaders

- Advanced practice nurses

Statement of Need

This 150-page handbook will provide strategies for nurse leaders to improve quality improvement outcomes. It will teach the history of quality improvement in healthcare as well as nursing's role in quality improvement. It will also teach nurse leaders how to plan quality improvement efforts, as well as the basics of quality measurement and analysis and process improvement. This guide also provides information for nursing-sensitive quality indicators and provides strategies for effective communication and successful staff engagement in the quality improvement effort. (This activity is intended for individual use only.)

Educational Objectives

Upon completion of this activity, participants should be able to:

- Identify potential benefits quality improvement can bring to a unit

- Describe common quality improvement errors

- Identify the role of nurses at every level in quality improvement

- Describe barriers to nurse participation in quality improvement

- Identify the steps involved when planning a quality improvement program

- Explain common errors in quality improvement planning

- Explain how to identify measures

- Discuss how to analyze data trends

- Describe common misuses of data

- Define nursing-sensitive indicators

- Describe the necessary steps for choosing nursing-sensitive indicators

- Discuss methods to successfully engage staff nurses in quality improvement

- Describe ways to hold staff nurses accountable for quality improvement efforts

- Define process improvement

- Explain the risks and benefits of process improvement

- Describe cultural factors that affect process improvement

Faculty

Cynthia Barnard, MBA, MSJS, CPHQ, is the director of Quality Strategies at Northwestern Memorial Hospital, the primary teaching hospital of Northwestern University's Feinberg School of Medicine in Chicago, and is research assistant professor in the Institute for Healthcare Studies at the medical school.

At Northwestern Memorial, she is responsible for patient safety, accreditation and regulatory compliance, infection control, and medical ethics. In the Institute for Healthcare Studies, she is co-director of the advanced course in quality improvement (QI) in the Master's Program in Healthcare Quality and Patient Safety.

Barbara J. Hannon, RN, MSN, CPHQ, is the coordinator of the ANCC Magnet Recognition Program® (MRP) for the University of Iowa Hospitals & Clinics. She chairs the Professional Nursing Practice Committee and Nursing Retention Committee and is involved in QI activities for the department. In 2007, she was selected as one of Iowa's "100 Best Nurses" and in 2009 was profiled in "20 People Who Make Healthcare Better" by *HealthLeaders* magazine.

As the MRP coordinator for the University of Iowa Hospitals & Clinics, she successfully guided the hospital to MRP designation as the 101st MRP hospital in January 2004 and to redesignation in 2008.

Continuing Education

Nursing Contact Hours: HCPro is accredited as a provider of continuing nursing education by the American Nurses Credentialing Center Commission on Accreditation.

This educational activity for 3 nursing contact hours is provided by HCPro, Inc.

Faculty Disclosure Statement

HCPro, Inc., has confirmed that none of the faculty or contributors have any relevant financial relationships to disclose related to the content of this educational activity.

Instructions

In order to be eligible to receive your nursing contact hours or physician continuing education credits for this activity, you are required to do the following:

1. Read the book *Quality Improvement for Nurse Managers: Engage Staff and Improve Patient Outcomes*

2. Complete the exam and receive a passing score of 80%

3. Complete the evaluation

4. Provide your contact information on the exam and evaluation

5. Submit exam and evaluation to HCPro, Inc.

Please provide all of the information requested above and mail or fax your completed exam, program evaluation, and contact information to:

HCPro, Inc.

Attn: Continuing Education Manager

P.O. Box 1168

Marblehead, MA 01945

Fax: 781/639-2982

Note: This book and associated exam are intended for individual use only. If you would like to provide this continuing education exam to other members of your nursing or physician staff, please contact our customer service department at 877/727-1728 to place your order. The exam fee schedule is as follows:

Exam Quantity	Fee
1	$0
2 – 25	$15 per person
26 – 50	$12 per person
51 – 100	$8 per person
101+	$5 per person

CONTINUING EDUCATION EXAM

Name: _____

Title: _____

Facility Name: _____

Address: _____

Address: _____

City: _____ State: _____ ZIP: _____

Phone Number: _____ Fax Number: _____

E-mail: _____

Date Completed: _____

1. Which of the following is a potential positive benefit of quality improvement efforts?
   a. Analysis paralysis
   b. Improved patient safety
   c. Busier staff members
   d. Spend more money

2. Which of the following will likely hurt, instead of help, a facility's chances to improve outcomes?
   a. Obtaining a profound knowledge of the system being improved and thoughtful application of improvement science to the specific organization and team
   b. Looking for new ideas from outside the walls of your department
   c. Familiarizing yourself with The Joint Commission's expectations for management of quality and safety
   d. Attempting to impose solutions that are outside the competence or culture of your team

3. Which of the following is the responsibility of the nurse manager or director in regard to quality improvement?
   a. Integrating nursing practices into the organizational goals of the entire facility
   b. Supporting a culture of education for directors and nurse managers/directors in the principles and methods of QI
   c. Carrying out the protocols and standards of care at the bedside
   d. Communicating and operationalizing the organization's QI goals and processes to the bedside nurse

4. For best QI results, nurse leaders should:
   a. Try to tackle all QI efforts themselves
   b. Convince hospital leadership that QI is not a nursing responsibility
   c. Maximize their resources and utilize the expertise of organizational QI experts
   d. Delegate all QI responsibilities to staff nurses

5. Which of the following is a barrier to nurse participation in quality improvement?
   a. A yearly performance appraisal tool that includes QI participation as an expectation of bedside nursing practice
   b. QI projects that make staff nurses' jobs easier and more efficient
   c. The perception that QI and efficient, safe patient care are extremely different concepts
   d. Acknowledgments for staff nurses who adhere to QI protocol and are involved in QI efforts

6. Which of the following answers is NOT a step to creating a quality improvement plan?
   a. Analyzing data and creating control charts for the nursing staff
   b. Creating a mission statement
   c. Defining the scope of your department's services
   d. Identifying goals for your department

7. Which of the following is a common error when planning quality improvement?
   a. Identifying indicators and measures as your first step
   b. Documenting all the information you've collected regarding your department
   c. Using patients' perspective to help develop your plan
   d. Allocating resources and budgeting

8. Which of the following describes part of the process to identify measures?
   a. Creating a mission statement
   b. Teaching staff nurses how to read scattergrams
   c. Identifying your customers
   d. Referring to your quality plan and looking at the important aspects of care and service for your customers as you defined them

9. A benchmark is:
   a. A type of graph
   b. A simple comparison, a target or goal, a best practice, or a minimum threshold
   c. A legal document used to submit data
   d. A concept that reflects harmful behaviors of staff members in response to quality metrics that are not well designed.

10. The most important additional concept is whether a process is in _____.
    a. flux
    b. control
    c. the patient's room
    d. static

11. Which of the following is common misuse of data?
    a. Displaying simple charts where staff nurses can view them easily
    b. Attributing variable outcomes or inconsistent performance to individual employee instead of the underlying systems and processes
    c. Using an "apples to apples" approach
    d. Using control charts

12. Which of the following describes a histogram?
    a. A chart that displays frequency of events in different categories
    b. A chart that shows the relationship between two continuous numeric variables; displays a possible "correlation" between the variables
    c. A survey of patients' histories
    d. A measure that improves if there is a greater quantity or quality of nursing care

13. Those indicators requiring interdisciplinary collaboration are complex processes and usually coordinated by an organizational QI department with the ability to involve multiple disciplines are called _____.
    a. nursing-sensitive indicators
    b. patient indicators
    c. process improvement indicators
    d. organizational indicators

14. What is a nursing-sensitive indicator?
    a. A measurement that only physicians have the power to improve
    b. A cue that a staff nurse is too sensitive to criticism
    c. A measure that improves if there is a greater quantity or quality of nursing care
    d. An indicator that requires interdisciplinary collaboration and is usually coordinated by an organizational QI department with the ability to involve multiple disciplines

15. Which of the following answers consists of steps for choosing nursing-sensitive indicators?
    a. Collect data, benchmark, find strategies to improve data
    b. Create a mission statement, acknowledge staff nurses, create control charts
    c. Allocating resources and budgeting, create a mission statement
    d. Identify organizational indicators, report data

16. Which of the following is a best practice for engaging nursing staff in quality improvement efforts?
    a. Post complex charts about organizational indicators for staff viewing
    b. Be transparent with your staff at all times
    c. Share information only when a staff nurse has requested it
    d. Punish staff who fail to partake in QI efforts

17. Which of the following will help keep staff nurses accountable in regard to QI efforts?
    a. Warning them that if they fail, there might be pay cuts
    b. Controlling every aspect of QI yourself, without input from staff nurses
    c. Empowering staff nurses to decide what to measure and what the unit's goals should be
    d. Reminding staff nurses that the facility requires them to take part in such efforts, and that you do not have power over that decision

18. What is process improvement?
    a. Another term for "benchmarking"
    b. The degree to which health services for individuals and populations increase the likelihood of desired health outcomes and are consistent with current professional knowledge
    c. A concept that patients have the right to confidentiality within the healthcare setting
    d. Redesigning a process to produce a measurably different outcome

19. What is a benefit of process improvement?

    a. It builds teamwork, develops a deep understanding of process, continues to produce better and more reliable outcomes over time, and sparks truly creative and innovative ideas for quantum leaps in performance

    b. It forces you to invest time, energy, money, and other resources, although you might fail to improve the process

    c. It forces unintentional interference with other elements of the process that work reliably or introduce new sources of variation and potential harm

    d. It takes time and resources away from other projects

20. Which of the following is a common cultural barrier to process improvement?

    a. A system that prohibits group or public discussions that focus on identified individual performance issues

    b. A system that adheres to principles of confidentiality, fairness, and equitable treatment of all staff members

    c. All employees cling to a belief that quality outcomes could be ensured if everyone would just do their jobs more carefully

    d. An effective system that screens for individual performance problems and a confidential, effective method to address them

CONTINUING EDUCATION EVALUATION

Name: _____

Title: _____

Facility Name: _____

Address: _____

Address: _____

City: _____ State: _____ ZIP: _____

Phone Number: _____ Fax Number: _____

E-mail: _____

1. This activity met the learning objectives stated:
   ❏ Strongly Agree ❏ Agree ❏ Disagree ❏ Strongly Disagree

2. Objectives were related to the overall purpose/goal of the activity:
   ❏ Strongly Agree ❏ Agree ❏ Disagree ❏ Strongly Disagree

3. This activity was related to my continuing education needs:
   ❏ Strongly Agree ❏ Agree ❏ Disagree ❏ Strongly Disagree

4. The exam for the activity was an accurate test of the knowledge gained:
   ❏ Strongly Agree ❏ Agree ❏ Disagree ❏ Strongly Disagree

5. The activity avoided commercial bias or influence:
   ❏ Strongly Agree ❏ Agree ❏ Disagree ❏ Strongly Disagree

6. This activity met my expectations:
   ❏ Strongly Agree ❏ Agree ❏ Disagree ❏ Strongly Disagree

7. Will this activity enhance your professional practice?
   ❏ Yes ❏ No

8. The format was an appropriate method for delivery of the content for this activity:
   ❏ Strongly Agree ❏ Agree ❏ Disagree ❏ Strongly Disagree

10. If you have any comments on this activity please note them here:

    _____

    _____

11. How much time did it take for you to complete this activity?

    _____

Thank you for completing this evaluation of our continuing education activity!

Return completed form to: **HCPro, Inc. • Attn: Continuing Education Manager • P.O. Box 1168, Marblehead, MA 01945 •Tel 877/727-1728 • Fax 781/639-2982**

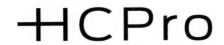